HIV Infection

A Primary Care Manual

HIV Infection

A Primary Care Manual

Third Edition

Howard Libman, M.D.

Assistant Professor of Medicine, Harvard Medical School;
Associate in Medicine, Division of General Medicine and
Primary Care, Beth Israel Hospital, Boston

Robert A. Witzburg, M.D.

Associate Professor of Medicine, Boston University School of
Medicine; Associate Chief of General Internal Medicine, Boston
City Hospital; Medical Director, Neighborhood Health Plan,
Boston

Little, Brown and Company
Boston   New York   Toronto   London

Library of Congress Cataloging-in-Publication Data
HIV infection : a primary care manual / [edited by] Howard Libman, Robert A. Witzburg. — 3rd ed.
     p.   cm.
   Includes bibliographical references and index.
   ISBN 0-316-51160-9 (pbk.)
   1. AIDS (Disease)   2. AIDS (Disease)—Patients—Care.   I. Libman, Howard.   II. Witzburg, Robert A.
   [DNLM: 1. HIV Infections—therapy.   2. HIV Infections—complications.   3. Opportunistic Infections—complications.
4. Opportunistic Infections—therapy.   WC 503.2 H6765 1995]
RC607.A26C58   1995
616.97'92—dc20
DNLM/DLC
for Library of Congress   95-32353
                                                                          CIP

Printed in the United States of America

ICP

Editorial: Nancy E. Chorpenning, Deeth K. Ellis
Production Editor: Marie A. Salter
Copyeditors: Mary Babcock, Libby Dabrowski
Indexer: Dorothy Hoffman
Production Supervisor/Designer: Mike Burggren

The cover image was kindly donated by Dr. Sigfus Nikulasson, Pathology Department, Boston University School of Medicine, Boston.

To the patients and staff
of Boston City and Beth Israel Hospitals

Contents

III. Opportunistic Diseases

IV. Special Topics

Contributing Authors

Nezam H. Afdhal, M.D.
Associate Professor of Medicine, Boston University School of Medicine; Chief, Section of Gastroenterology, Boston City Hospital, Boston

Lawrence M. Barat, M.D., M.P.H.
Assistant Professor of Medicine, Boston University School of Medicine; Medical Director, Immunodeficiency Unit, Boston Specialty and Rehabilitation Hospital, Boston

Thomas W. Barber, M.D.
Assistant Professor of Medicine, Boston University School of Medicine; Associate Director, Housestaff Training, Boston University Medical Center Hospital, Boston

M. Anita Barry, M.D.
Assistant Professor of Medicine and Public Health, Boston University Schools of Medicine and Public Health; Director of Communicable Disease Control, Boston Department of Health and Hospitals, Boston

David L. Battinelli, M.D.
Assistant Professor of Medicine, Boston University School of Medicine; Director, Housestaff Training, Boston University School of Medicine, Residency Program in Medicine, Boston

Alexandra Beckett, M.D.
Assistant Professor of Psychiatry, Harvard Medical School; Director, HIV Psychiatry Service, Beth Israel Hospital, Boston

Kathleen Bennett, M.D.
Assistant Professor of Medicine, Boston University School of Medicine; Attending Physician, Section of General Internal Medicine, Boston City Hospital, Boston

Paul E. Berard, M.D.
Clinical Instructor in Medicine, New York Medical College, Valhalla, New York; Staff, Department of Medicine, Section of Hematology and Oncology, St. Vincent's Medical Center, Bridgeport, Connecticut

Sheilah A. Bernard, M.D.
Assistant Professor of Medicine, Boston University School of Medicine; Director, Clinical Cardiology, Boston City Hospital, Boston

Steven C. Borkan, M.D.
Assistant Professor of Medicine, Boston University School of Medicine; Attending Physician, Renal Section, Boston City Hospital, Boston

Stephen L. Boswell, M.D.
Instructor in Medicine, Harvard Medical School; Medical Director, Fenway Community Health Center, Boston

Mariel Brittis, M.D.
Assistant Professor of Ophthalmology, Cornell University Medical College; Assistant Attending Ophthalmologist, The New York Hospital, New York

Melanie J. Brunt, M.D., M.P.H.
Assistant Professor of Medicine, Boston University School of Medicine; Assistant Director, Diabetes Service, Boston City Hospital, Boston

Robert A. Burke, R.N., M.A., C.I.C.
Nurse Epidemiologist, Department of Hospital Epidemiology, Boston University Medical Center Hospital, Boston

Stuart R. Chipkin, M.D.
Assistant Professor of Medicine, Boston University School of

Medicine; Director, Clinical Endocrinology, Diabetes, and Metabolism, Boston City and Boston University Medical Center Hospitals, Boston

Calvin J. Cohen, M.D., M.Sc.
Clinical Instructor in Medicine, Harvard Medical School, Boston; Research Director, Community Research Initiative of New England, Brookline, Massachusetts

Timothy P. Cooley, M.D.
Assistant Professor of Medicine, Boston University School of Medicine; Attending Physician, Sections of Hematology and Oncology, Boston City Hospital, Boston

Ellen R. Cooper, M.D.
Associate Professor of Pediatric Infectious Diseases, Boston University School of Medicine; Director, Pediatric Infectious Disease Program, Boston City Hospital, Boston

Judith S. Currier, M.D.
Assistant Professor of Clinical Medicine, University of Southern California School of Medicine; Medical Director, Rand Schrader HIV Clinic, Los Angeles County and University of Southern California, Los Angeles

Bret E. Davis, M.D.
Resident in Dermatology, Boston University and Tufts University Medical Centers, Boston

Eileen Dunn, R.D.
Former Staff Dietician, Boston City Hospital, Boston

Harrison W. Farber, M.D.
Professor of Medicine, Boston University School of Medicine; Director, Medical Intensive Care Unit, Boston City Hospital, Boston

Marshall Forstein, M.D.
Instructor in Psychology, Harvard Medical School, Boston; Director, HIV Mental Health Services, The Cambridge Hospital, Cambridge, Massachusetts

Kenneth A. Freedberg, M.D., M.Sc.
Assistant Professor of Medicine and Epidemiology, and
Biostatistics, Boston University School of Medicine; Co-Director,
HIV Diagnostic Evaluation Unit, Boston City Hospital, Boston

Jon D. Fuller, M.D.
Assistant Clinical Professor of Medicine, Boston University
School of Medicine; Assistant Director, Clinical AIDS Program,
Boston City Hospital, Boston

Gail M. Garvin, R.N., M.Ed.
Nurse Epidemiologist, Epidemiology Unit, Boston City
Hospital, Boston

Leonard H. Glantz, J.D.
Professor of Health Law, Boston University Schools of Medicine
and Public Health, Boston

Kevan L. Hartshorn, M.D.
Associate Professor of Medicine, Boston University School of
Medicine; Medical Director, Hematology-Oncology Outpatient
Services, Boston City Hospital, Boston

James J. Heffernan, M.D., M.P.H.
Associate Professor of Medicine, Boston University School of
Medicine; Associate Director, Department of Medicine, Boston
City Hospital, Boston

Lisa R. Hirschhorn, M.D.
Director, HIV Medical Care and Research, Dimock Community
Health Center, Boston

David Ives, M.D.
Instructor in Medicine, Harvard Medical School; Medical
Director, Virology Research Clinic, Beth Israel Hospital, Boston

Helen M. Jacoby, M.D.
Instructor in Medicine, Harvard Medical School; Associate in
Medicine, Division of Infectious Diseases, Beth Israel Hospital,
Boston

Michael S. Karasik, M.D.
Assistant Professor of Medicine, Section of Gastroenterology,
Boston University School of Medicine; GI-AIDS Consultant,
Immunodeficiency Clinic, Boston City Hospital, Boston

Howard K. Koh, M.D., M.P.H.
Professor of Dermatology, Medicine, and Public Health, Boston
University Schools of Medicine and Public Health; Director,
Cancer Prevention and Control, Boston University Medical
Center Hospital, Boston

Howard Libman, M.D.
Assistant Professor of Medicine, Harvard Medical School;
Associate in Medicine, Division of General Medicine and
Primary Care, Beth Israel Hospital, Boston

Harvey J. Makadon, M.D.
Associate Professor of Medicine, Harvard Medical School;
Medical Director, Ambulatory Services, Beth Israel Hospital,
Boston

Colleen Manning Osten, R.D.
Former Director of Nutrition Services, Greenery Rehabilitation
and Skilled Nursing Center, Boston

Stephen I. Pelton, M.D.
Professor of Pediatrics, Boston University School of Medicine;
Coordinator of Pediatric AIDS Program, Boston City Hospital,
Boston

Edward S. Peters, D.M.D., S.M.
Fellow, Department of Oral Health Policy and Epidemiology,
Harvard School of Dental Medicine; Assistant Surgeon,
Department of Oral Medicine and Dentistry, Brigham and
Women's Hospital, Boston

Peter J. Piliero, M.D.
Assistant Professor of Medicine, Albany Medical College;
Attending Physician, Division of HIV Medicine, Albany
Medical Center Hospital, Albany, New York

John A. Rich, M.D., M.P.H.
Assistant Professor of Medicine, Boston University School of
Medicine; Attending Physician, Section of General Internal
Medicine, Boston City Hospital, Boston

Jeffrey H. Samet, M.D., M.P.H., M.A.
Assistant Professor of Medicine, Boston University School of
Medicine; Medical Director, Addiction Services, and Co-
Director, HIV Diagnostic Evaluation Unit, Boston City Hospital,
Boston

Carol A. Saunders, R.N., B.S.N.
Former Director, Clinical Research Associates, Boston

Christopher W. Shanahan, M.D., M.P.H.
Fellow in General Internal Medicine, Harvard Medical School;
Division of General Medicine and Primary Care, Beth Israel
Hospital, Boston

Abby Shevitz, M.D., M.P.H.
Research Fellow in Epidemiology, Harvard School of Public
Health; Staff Physician, Adult Clinic, Martha M. Eliot Health
Center, Boston

Robert W. Simms, M.D.
Associate Professor of Medicine, Boston University School of
Medicine; Director, Arthritis Clinic, Boston City Hospital,
Boston

Judith L. Steinberg, M.D.
Assistant Clinical Professor of Medicine, Boston University
School of Medicine; Program Director, HIV Services, East
Boston Neighborhood Health Plan, Boston

Alan M. Sugar, M.D.
Associate Professor of Medicine, Boston University School of
Medicine; Attending Physician, Section of Infectious Diseases,
Boston University Medical Center Hospital, Boston

Carol A. Sulis, M.D.
Assistant Professor of Medicine, Boston University School of

Medicine; Hospital Epidemiologist, Division of Infectious Diseases, Boston City Hospital, Boston

Thomas L. Treadwell, M.D.
Assistant Professor of Medicine, University of Massachusetts Medical School, Worcester, Massachusetts; Program Director, Department of Medicine, Metrowest Medical Center, Framingham, Massachusetts

Nagagopal Venna, M.D.
Associate Professor of Neurology, Boston University School of Medicine; Director, Clinical Neurology, Boston City Hospital, Boston

Brant L. Viner, M.D.
Assistant Professor of Medicine, University of Massachusetts Medical School; Infectious Diseases Consultant, Medical Center of Central Massachusetts, Worcester, Massachusetts

Randall P. Wagner, M.D.
Former Guest Researcher, Laboratory of Immunology, National Institute of Dental Research, National Institutes of Health, Bethesda, Maryland

Alan A. Wartenberg, M.D.
Assistant Professor of Medicine, Tufts University School of Medicine; Medical Director, Addiction Recovery Program, Faulkner Hospital, Boston

Robert A. Witzburg, M.D.
Associate Professor of Medicine, Boston University School of Medicine; Associate Chief of General Internal Medicine, Boston City Hospital; Medical Director, Neighborhood Health Plan, Boston

Beth Zeeman, M.D.
Assistant Professor of Medicine, Boston University School of Medicine; Attending Physician, Immunodeficiency Clinic, Boston City Hospital, Boston

Preface

As Sicknesse is the greatest misery, so the greatest misery of sicknes is solitude; when the infectiousnes of the disease deterrs them who should assist, from comming . . .

John Donne,
Devotions Upon Emergent Occasions

This manual is intended to support physicians, nurses, and other health professionals in their efforts to provide high-quality primary medical care to adults infected with human immunodeficiency virus (HIV). The text originated in 1988 as a loose-leaf publication for the medical house officers and attending staff of the Department of Medicine at Boston City Hospital. In response to the success of the original effort, a new version entitled *Clinical Manual for Care of the Adult Patient with HIV Infection* was published in 1990 through the New England AIDS Education and Training Center, and a supplement followed in 1991. A second edition, published by Little, Brown and Company, became available in 1993. This third edition represents a substantially revised and expanded work, including updated chapters from the previous edition and new chapters on pathophysiology, endocrinologic manifestations, gastrointestinal parasites, clinical trials, and advanced HIV disease. The text has been further strengthened with contributions by experienced AIDS clinicians from throughout the Boston medical community.

We have attempted to organize the book around clinical management issues, which are accessible from both an organ system and a disease perspective. Part I provides an overview of HIV infection; Part II addresses its clinical manifestations; Part III describes associated opportunistic diseases; and Part IV includes a variety of special topics, such as ambulatory management, risk reduction for health care workers, and HIV infection in specific populations.

The field of HIV-related research is constantly advancing, and standards of clinical practice continue to evolve. There are many unresolved issues concerning the care of patients with HIV infection. We have tried to indicate where uncertainty exists and to present a reasonable approach to management based on current literature and standards of practice. We hope that in areas where optimal therapy is not known, health care providers will make every effort to encourage patients to participate in clinical research trials.

We thank the authors for their informative and timely contributions. We are also indebted to Drs. Harvey Makadon and Timothy Cooley, for their editorial assistance, and to the staff of Little, Brown and Company, for their ongoing support. Finally, we wish to acknowledge the house officers and faculty of Boston City Hospital and Boston University School of Medicine and of Beth Israel Hospital and Harvard Medical School. Their commitment and professionalism continue to inspire us.

H.L.
R.A.W.

Overview of HIV Infection

1

Pathophysiology and Natural History

1

Stephen L. Boswell

Pathophysiology

Significant progress has been made in understanding the viral pathogen that causes acquired immunodeficiency syndrome (AIDS). This lymphotropic virus, human immunodeficiency virus (HIV), was first isolated in 1983 from patients with AIDS-related complex (ARC) and AIDS [1, 2]. It is closely related to two other retroviruses, human T-cell lymphotropic virus, type 1 (HTLV-1) and human T-cell lymphotropic virus, type 2 (HTLV-2). HTLV-1 has been associated with adult T-cell lymphoma/leukemia and with tropical spastic paraparesis. HTLV-2 has been described with hairy cell leukemia and is found in a significant number of American injection drug users [3].

Unlike HTLV-1 and HTLV-2, HIV is a cytopathic virus. It is composed of a central cylindrical core of diploid ribonucleic acid (RNA) surrounded by a spherical lipid envelope. The viral antigen p24 is located in the core and serves as a serologic marker of replication. The binding of the HIV envelope glycoprotein, gp120, to the receptor present on the surface of CD4+ T lymphocytes has been posited to play a direct role in the destruction of these cells [4]. CD4 receptors have a binding site capable of interacting with a viral envelope protein that is noncovalently associated with gp120 (Fig. 1-1). Through this mechanism, HIV is able to fuse with the cell membrane. Once within the cytoplasm of the host cell, the envelope of the virus is shed, and its contents are released. It is then that reverse transcription occurs: Deoxyribonucleic acid (DNA) is made from the viral RNA template. Infected cells remain in a dormant state for a variable period of time. When activation occurs, the

3

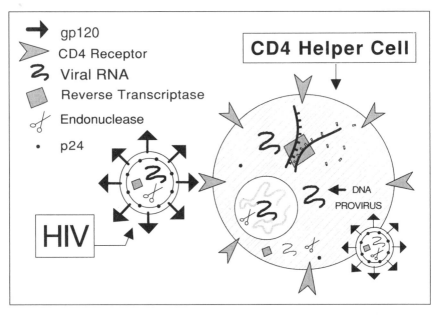

Figure 1-1. HIV/CD4 lymphocyte interaction. (From H Libman. Pathogenesis, natural history, and classification of HIV infection. *Prim Care* 19:1–17, 1992.)

proviral DNA transcribes genomic and messenger RNA. After viral proteins are synthesized, new virions are assembled. On budding from the infected cell, these viruses circulate until they identify new target cells.

The manner in which HIV causes depletion of CD4 cells remains obscure, although several direct and indirect mechanisms have been postulated (Table 1-1). The loss of CD4 lymphocytes plays a central role in the pathogenesis of immune deficiency related to HIV infection. These

Table 1-1 *Proposed mechanisms of HIV cytopathicity*

Direct
    Toxic consequences of viral replication (budding)
    Accumulated nonintegrated viral DNA
    Accumulated viral RNA and aberrant host cell RNA
    Intracellular complexing of HIV envelope and CD4 receptors
Indirect
    Syncytia formation
    Autoantibodies
    Release of soluble toxic substances, e.g., gp120
    Innocent bystander cell killing
    Apoptosis
    HIV infection of stem cells
    Superantigens

lymphocytes interact with large numbers of hematolymphatic cells and help mediate immunologic response to a wide variety of infections and some neoplasms. So important is this loss of CD4 lymphocytes in the pathogenesis of AIDS that the number of these cells in the peripheral blood is a good predictor for disease progression [5, 6]. Other factors, including disruption of the architecture of lymphoid organs, as well as direct and indirect effects on the qualitative function of the CD4 lymphocyte and monocyte-macrophages, may also play a role in the immunopathogenesis of AIDS.

Primary Infection: Selection of Viral Phenotypes

There is increasing evidence that the process of HIV transmission is not random. The heterogeneous viral population found in a person with HIV infection undergoes a highly selective process resulting in the transmission of a relatively narrow group of viruses [7–10]. These are principally nonsyncytium-inducing (NSI) strains characterized by their tropism for macrophages and ability to cause rapid cell death. This selection may be a consequence of a process that limits virus entry, of preferential virus replication after entry of a population of heterogeneous viruses, or both. The predominance of macrophage-tropic virus immediately after transmission has led to speculation that these cells may play an important role in viral entry.

Viremia and Migration to Lymphoid Tissues

Following transmission of HIV, rapid and widespread dissemination of the virus occurs [11, 12]. This process is characterized by a dramatic increase in viral burden during the weeks after transmission. Associated with viremia is a precipitous drop in CD4 lymphocyte count, which may be a consequence of HIV-induced cell killing, the redistribution of circulating CD4 lymphocytes to lymphoid tissues, or both [13, 14]. This increase in viral burden begins to slow with the development of a cellular immune response to the infection, suggesting it may have an important role in controlling viral replication [15, 16]. In addition, humoral immunity may contribute to the clearance of HIV from the plasma and peripheral blood mononuclear cells (PBMCs) [17–19]. As an immune response becomes established, the CD4 lymphocyte count rebounds but generally not to the preinfection level.

The amount of virus found in the peripheral blood falls dramatically after primary infection. Simultaneously, clinical symptoms associated with primary infection resolve, and the HIV-infected person enters a clinically latent phase of the disease. Initially, these observations led to the conclusion that HIV replication is slow during this period of latency and that mechanisms other than HIV-induced cell killing are responsible for the persistent decline in CD4 lymphocytes observed [20]. However, recent studies have demonstrated that lymphoid tissues contain a high viral load throughout the course of the disease, significantly more than are found in the peripheral blood [21, 22]. Newer and more sensitive techniques for quantifying viral load in peripheral blood have demonstrated that large amounts of HIV are produced during clinical latency [23, 24]. There appears to be a vigorous immune response to the virus and a large turnover of CD4 cells in this phase.

The lymph nodes of asymptomatic HIV-infected persons sequester the virus on the surface of follicular dendritic cells, facilitating antigen presentation to immune-competent cells, including CD4 lymphocytes. This may be an important mechanism for ongoing infection of newly recruited and activated cells. Thus, while little HIV can be found in peripheral blood during the clinically latent phase, the amount of virus found in lymphoid tissues increases over time.

Involvement of Nonlymphoid Tissues

CD4 lymphocytes appear to be the primary reservoir of HIV in infected persons. However, several other cells are also susceptible to HIV infection (Table 1-2). Monocyte-macrophages harbor significant amounts of virus in vivo [25]. Unlike CD4 lymphocytes, monocyte-macrophages and follicular dendritic cells may not be destroyed by HIV and may foster viral replication without cell death [25–29]. These cells may be responsible for the movement of the virus to nonlymphoid tissues and play a direct role in the development of HIV-related conditions in several organ systems, including the skin, central nervous system, and gastrointestinal tract [30–32]. HIV infection has been associated with

Table 1-2 *Cells susceptible to HIV infection*

Hematopoietic
    CD4+ T lymphocytes
    Monocyte-macrophages
    Follicular dendritic cells
    B lymphocytes
    Promyelocytes
Nervous system
    Astrocytes
    Oligodendrocytes
    Capillary endothelium
    Macrophages
Skin
    Langerhans' cells
    Fibroblasts
Other
    Bowel epithelium
    Undefined cells in the retina, cervix, and colon
    Tumor cell lines from brain, colon, and liver
    Renal epithelium

adrenal dysfunction, pulmonary disease, cardiac dysfunction, and neuropathy [33–36].

The dynamics of nonlymphoid tissue involvement in HIV disease are currently under study. A comparison of the amount of proviral DNA found in tissues of asymptomatic HIV-infected persons and in those with AIDS demonstrated significant involvement of lymphoid tissues in all patients [37]. However, nonlymphoid tissues, including the brain, lungs, and colon, were not involved in asymptomatic patients but were in several with AIDS. These data suggest that nonlymphoid tissue involvement may be a late-stage phenomenon.

Disease Progression

As the number of CD4 lymphocytes declines, immune dysfunction eventually becomes apparent in the vast majority of HIV-infected persons [38]. The correlation between CD4 cell count and immunodeficiency has become a valuable tool to assess progression of disease. The role of peripheral blood virus quantitation using techniques such as polymerase chain reaction and branched-chain DNA assays is currently under study. The relationship between the degree of immune dysfunction, as reflected in the CD4 lymphocyte count, and specific infections or neoplasms is complex and the subject of considerable ongoing research. Some opportunistic infections are rarely seen until the CD4 lymphocyte count drops below specific thresholds. For example, cytomegalovirus retinitis and disseminated *Mycobacterium avium* complex (MAC) infection are unusual in individuals with absolute CD4 lymphocyte counts greater than 100 cells/mm^3 [39, 40]. This observation suggests that these conditions represent reactivation of latent infections in the context of severe immunodeficiency.

Other HIV-related problems occur throughout the spectrum of CD4 lymphocyte counts. For example, Kaposi's sarcoma (KS) is diagnosed at all stages of HIV disease [41]. This finding suggests a direct role for HIV or for a cofactor such as a coincident viral infection. Recent data suggest that a herpesvirus may play a role in the development of KS [42].

In general, the progression of HIV disease correlates most strongly with the loss of CD4 lymphocytes, the amount of HIV found in the plasma, and the proportion of PBMCs carrying provirus [43–45]. Other clinical and laboratory findings have also been identified as independent predictors of HIV disease progression (Table 1-3).

Changes in Viral Phenotype

Significant changes in viral phenotype occur during the course of HIV disease. Viruses obtained from asymptomatic HIV-infected individuals are characterized by a preponderance of NSI isolates [46–48].

Table 1-3 *Independent predictors of HIV disease progression*

Symptoms
    Constitutional symptoms
Signs
    Hairy leukoplakia
    Oral candidiasis
Laboratory studies
    CD4 cell count
    CD4:CD8 ratio
    Serum β_2-microglobulin
    Serum and urine neopterin
    p24 antigen
    Serum and mononuclear cell HIV titer
    HIV-related anemia
    Erythrocyte sedimentation rate
    Cutaneous anergy

These strains replicate less efficiently, have a monocyte-macrophage tropism, and appear to be less pathogenic than syncytium-inducing (SI) isolates [49]. As HIV disease progresses, SI strains begin to predominate. The question of whether this increasing predominance of SI strains is a cause of or a consequence of progressing immunodeficiency remains unresolved. Clearly, the isolation of SI viruses is not a prerequisite for the development of severe immunodeficiency, since NSI viruses cannot be identified in approximately 50 percent of individuals with AIDS.

Cofactors

Coinfection with additional viral pathogens is common among HIV-infected persons. Several of these viruses may induce the expression of cellular proteins, which facilitate viral gene transcription and upregulate HIV expression. Herpes simplex virus (HSV), type 1; cytomegalovirus (CMV); Epstein-Barr virus (EBV); adenovirus; hepatitis B virus; human herpesvirus, type 6; pseudorabies virus; and HTLV-1 have all been shown to enhance HIV replication [50–52]. HIV and HSV-1 may coinfect cell lines that they are not known to infect separately, and a similar phenomenon has been reported with HIV and CMV [53]. The clinical relevance of these observations has yet to be determined.

Other immunologic components also appear to play a role in HIV disease modulation and progression, including cytokines such as tumor necrosis factor, cell-mediated cytotoxicity, antibody-dependent cellular cytotoxicity, natural killer cells, and cytotoxic T cells.

Natural History

HIV infection in the adolescent and adult is a continuum that can be divided into four phases: (1) primary infection, (2) early HIV infection

(CD4 count > 500 cells/mm³), (3) intermediate HIV infection (CD4 count 200–500/mm³), and (4) late HIV infection, or AIDS (CD4 count < 200/mm³). These categories are theoretical constructs that have evolved as our understanding of HIV disease has advanced. A representation of these disease stages and several corresponding clinical and immunologic parameters is presented in Figure 1-2 [54, 55].

Primary Infection

Primary infection with HIV may be accompanied, in up to 50 percent of patients, by the acute retroviral syndrome [11, 56]. In spite of this fact, only a small portion of those who experience symptomatic primary infection come to medical attention. The syndrome is characterized by an acute mononucleosis-like illness that begins 2 to 4 weeks after viral transmission, is generally mild to moderate in severity, and lasts for 1 to 2 weeks.

The most common features of primary HIV infection are fever, lethargy, lymphadenopathy, pharyngitis, a truncal maculopapular rash, myalgia, and arthralgia [11, 57–59] (Table 1-4). Headaches, photophobia, and diarrhea can also occur. In addition, various neurologic manifestations, including headache, photophobia, meningoencephalitis, myelopathy, peripheral neuropathy, and Guillain-Barré syndrome, have been described [60–70]. The syndrome is most commonly confused with EBV mononucleosis [71] (Table 1-5).

Transient lymphopenia, followed by a lymphocytosis comprised mainly of CD8 lymphocytes, is common in primary HIV infection; one-

Figure 1-2. Natural history of HIV infection. (Courtesy of Dr. Jon Fuller, Boston City Hospital.)

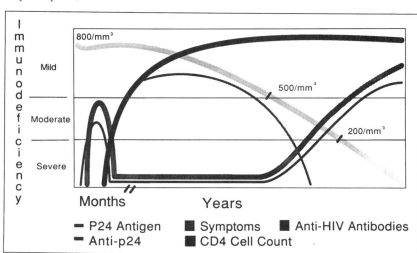

Table 1-4 *Clinical manifestations of primary HIV infection*

General
    Fever
    Lymphadenopathy
    Lethargy
    Myalgia
    Arthralgia
Gastrointestinal
    Pharyngitis
    Diarrhea
    Nausea or vomiting
    Hepatosplenomegaly
    Oral thrush
Neurologic
    Headache
    Meningoencephalitis
    Peripheral neuropathy
Dermatologic
    Truncal maculopapular rash
    Mucocutaneous ulcers
Other
    Thrombocytopenia
    Leukopenia
    Increased liver function tests

third of patients may have atypical lymphocytes on the peripheral blood smear. CD4 lymphocyte counts may drop to levels indicative of advanced HIV disease but typically rebound 2 to 3 weeks later, although generally not to baseline [72]. In some instances, the CD4 lymphocyte count remains suppressed, and this may be a harbinger of a more accelerated course of HIV disease [72]. Mild thrombocytopenia is also common but resolves quickly. Increased serum transaminase levels occur in approximately one-fourth of patients with primary HIV infection and are infrequently associated with clinical hepatitis [71, 73].

Currently no specific treatment is recommended. Clinical investiga-

Table 1-5 *Clinical features distinguishing acute retroviral syndrome from EBV mononucleosis*

Clinical feature	Acute retroviral syndrome	EBV mononucleosis
Onset	Acute	Insidious
Tonsillar hypertrophy	−	+
Enanthem on palate	−	+
Exudative pharyngitis	−	+
Mucocutaneous ulcers	+	−
Rash	+	−
Diarrhea	+	−

+ = present; − = not present.

tions using zidovudine (ZDV) during primary HIV infection have been insufficient to determine whether antiretroviral therapy alters the course of this or subsequent stages of HIV disease [74]. Other agents are currently being evaluated.

Early HIV Infection

Early HIV infection is characterized by CD4 lymphocyte counts in the normal range (≥ 500 cells/mm³). The majority of individuals with this stage of infection have no symptoms of HIV disease. When clinical features are present, they most often include persistent generalized lymphadenopathy and dermatologic conditions, such as seborrheic dermatitis, shingles, and folliculitis. Rarely, oral hairy leukoplakia and recurrent aphthous ulcers occur. In general, manifestations of early HIV infection correlate poorly with the risk of disease progression [38].

Despite the relative paucity of overt clinical symptoms and signs in early HIV infection, the laboratory evaluation often reveals characteristic abnormalities. The complete blood count may show leukopenia or thrombocytopenia, or both, while anemia is seen quite infrequently. Although the leukopenia of early HIV infection is usually mild, thrombocytopenia may, at times, be severe. A polyclonal gammopathy is common and results in an increased total serum globulin level. Transaminase levels may be increased but are usually related to a concomitant disease such as viral hepatitis or medication-related toxicity.

Antiretroviral therapy is not presently recommended for early HIV infection, as data are insufficient to determine its effect on the natural history of the disease at this stage.

Intermediate HIV Infection

Intermediate HIV infection is characterized by CD4 lymphocyte counts between 200 and 500/mm³. The majority of individuals with this stage of infection have few or no symptoms. Clinical features present during early HIV infection may worsen in severity or frequency during the intermediate stage. New problems may also develop, including constitutional symptoms, diarrhea, recurrent HSV infection, and oral or vaginal candidiasis. In addition, conventional bacterial infections involving the sinuses, respiratory tract, and skin become more common during this stage. Laboratory abnormalities are similar to those found in early HIV infection.

The use of ZDV during intermediate HIV infection appears to result in slower rates of disease progression [75]. However, postponing ZDV therapy until the development of symptomatic HIV disease or a fall in the CD4 lymphocyte count below 200 cells/mm³ in patients with asymptomatic HIV infection does not alter the combined endpoint of time to disease progression or death [76]. These observations suggest that ZDV therapy prolongs the intermediate stage of HIV infection.

Acquired Immunodeficiency Syndrome

Acquired immunodeficiency syndrome is defined by a CD4 lymphocyte count of less than $200/mm^3$ or the presence of opportunistic diseases indicative of profound immunodeficiency [77] (see Tables 2-1 and 2-2). Without treatment, this stage of HIV infection is characterized by a 50 to 70 percent risk of developing a new AIDS-related condition or dying within 2 years [78].

One of the most common conditions that characterizes AIDS is *Pneumocystis carinii* pneumonia (PCP). With the advent of PCP prophylaxis and antiretroviral therapy, the risk of PCP has declined significantly [79]. In addition, individuals with a CD4 lymphocyte count less than $200/mm^3$ are at increased risk of developing *Toxoplasma gondii* encephalitis, tuberculosis, cryptosporidiosis, isosporiasis, salmonellosis, and esophageal candidiasis. In addition, many of the problems that characterize earlier stages of HIV infection may worsen when AIDS develops.

Neoplasms such as lymphoma, KS, and invasive cervical cancer are seen more frequently in patients with AIDS. Mononeuritis multiplex, myelitis, cranial nerve palsies, and peripheral neuropathies are but a few examples of the neurologic conditions that may occur. Adrenal insufficiency, testicular atrophy, hypothyroidism, and nephropathy have also been reported [80].

As AIDS progresses and the CD4 cell count declines below $100/mm^3$, new disorders may ensue. Among these are CMV retinitis, disseminated MAC infection, cryptococcal meningitis, progressive multifocal leukoencephalopathy, invasive aspergillosis, disseminated coccidioidomycosis, and disseminated histoplasmosis. HIV-associated dementia may become an important source of morbidity, while wasting syndrome may impede recovery from the many illnesses experienced by those with AIDS.

The use of antiretroviral therapy and prophylaxis against opportunistic infections during this stage of illness has significantly altered the natural history of HIV disease [81, 82]. In one recent study of HIV-infected persons with CD4 lymphocyte counts less than $200/mm^3$, the average life expectancy was 38.1 months, approximately 12 months longer than that found in the early 1980s [79].

Long-term Nonprogressors

A subpopulation of asymptomatic persons with HIV infection and normal CD4 cell counts over 7 to 10 years or more has recently been described [83, 84]. Although they appear to represent an epidemiologically and immunologically heterogeneous group, most have had a vigorous immune response to their infection and have maintained normal lymph node architecture over time. Efforts to isolate infectious virus from their peripheral blood have been unsuccessful or produced a low titer.

References

1. Barre-Sinoussi F, Chermann JC, Rey F, et al. Isolation of a T-lymphotropic retrovirus from a patient at risk for acquired immune deficiency syndrome (AIDS). *Science* 220:868–871, 1983.
2. Gallo S, Popovic M. Frequent detection and isolation of cytopathic retroviruses from patients with AIDS. *Science* 224:500, 1984.
3. Rosenblatt JD, Plaeger-Marshall S, Giorgi JV, et al. A clinical, hematologic, and immunologic analysis of 21 HTLV-II–infected intravenous drug users. (Published erratum appears in *Blood* 76:1901, 1990.) *Blood* 76:409–417, 1990.
4. Fauci AS. HIV: Infectivity and mechanisms of pathogenesis. *Science* 239:617, 1988.
5. Goedert JJ, Kessler CM, Aledort LM, et al. A prospective study of human immunodeficiency virus type 1 infection and the development of AIDS in subjects with hemophilia. *N Engl J Med* 321:1141–1148, 1989.
6. Eyster ME, Ballard JO, Gail MH, et al. Predictive markers for the acquired immunodeficiency syndrome (AIDS) in hemophiliacs: Persistence of p24 antigen and low T4 cell count. *Ann Intern Med* 110:963–969, 1989.
7. Zhu T, Mo H, Wang N, et al. Genotypic and phenotypic characterization of HIV-I patients with primary infection. *Science* 261:1179–1181, 1993.
8. Zhang LQ, MacKenzie P, Cleland A, et al. Selection for specific sequences in the external envelope protein of human immunodeficiency virus type 1 upon primary infection. *J Virol* 67:3345–3356, 1993.
9. Wolfs TF, Zwart G, Bakker M, Goudsmit J. HIV-I genomic RNA diversification following sexual and parenteral virus transmission. *Virology* 189:103–110, 1992.
10. Wolinsky SM, Wike CM, Korber BT, et al. Selective transmission of human immunodeficiency virus type-1 variants from mothers to infants. *Science* 255:1134–1137, 1992.
11. Clark SJ, Saag MS, Decker WD, et al. High titers of cytopathic virus in plasma of patients with symptomatic primary HIV-I infection. *N Engl J Med* 324:954–960, 1991.
12. Dear ES, Moudgil T, Meyer RD, Ho DD. Transient high levels of viremia in patients with primary human immunodeficiency virus type I infection. *N Engl J Med* 324:961–964, 1991.
13. Tindall B, Cooper DA. Primary HIV infection: Host responses and intervention strategies. *AIDS* 5:1–14, 1991.
14. Mackay CR, Marston W, Dudler L. Altered patterns of T cell migration through lymph nodes and skin following antigen challenge. *Eur J Immunol* 22:2205–2210, 1992.
15. Cooper DA, Tindall B, Wilson EJ, et al. Characterization of T lymphocyte responses during primary infection with human immunodeficiency virus. *J Infect Dis* 157:889–896, 1988.
16. Walker CM, Moody DJ, Stites DP, Levy JA. CD8+ lymphocytes can control HIV infection in vitro by suppressing virus replication. *Science* 234:1563–1566, 1986.
17. Boucher CA, de Wolf F, Houweling JT, et al. Antibody response to a syn-

thetic peptide covering a LAV-I/HTLV-M neutralization epitope and disease progression. *AIDS* 3:71–76, 1989.

18. Albert J, Abrahamsson B, Nagy K, et al. Rapid development of isolate-specific neutralizing antibodies after primary HIV-1 infection and consequent emergence of virus variants which resist neutralization by autologous sera. *AIDS* 4:107–112, 1990.

19. Ariyoshi K, Harwood E, Chiengsong-Popov R, Weber J. Is clearance of HIV-I viraemia at seroconversion mediated by neutralizing antibodies? *Lancet* 340:1257–1258, 1992.

20. Brinchmann JE, Albert J, Vandal F. Few infected CD4+ T cells but a high proportion of replication-competent provirus copies in asymptomatic human immunodeficiency virus type I infection. *J. Virol* 65:2019–2023, 1991.

21. Pantaleo G, Graziosi C, Butini L, et al. Lymphoid organs function as major reservoirs for human immunodeficiency virus. *Proc Natl Acad Sci USA* 88:9838–9842, 1991.

22. Pantaleo G, Graziosi C, Demarest JF, et al. HIV infection is active and progressive in lymphoid tissue during the clinically latent stage of disease. *Nature* 362:355–358, 1993.

23. Wei X, et al. Viral dynamics in human immunodeficiency virus type 1 infection. *Nature* 373:117–122, 1995.

24. Ho DD, et al. Rapid turnover of plasma virions and CD4 lymphocytes in HIV-1 infection. *Nature* 373:123–126, 1995.

25. Embretson J, Zupancic M, Ribas JL, et al. Massive covert infection of helper T lymphocyte. *Nature* 362:359–362, 1993.

26. Hammer SM, Gillis JM, Pinkston P, Rose RM. Effect of zidovudine and granulocyte-macrophage colony-stimulating factor on human immunodeficiency virus replication in alveolar macrophages. *Blood* 75:1215–1219, 1990.

27. Ho DD, Rota TR, Hirsch MS. Infection of monocyte/macrophages by human T lymphotropic virus type III. *J Clin Invest* 77:1712–1715, 1986.

28. Pemo CF, Yarchoan R, Cooney DA, et al. Replication of human immunodeficiency virus in monocytes. Granulocyte/macrophage colony-stimulating factor (GM-CSF) potentiates viral production yet enhances the antiviral effect mediated by 3'-azido-2'3'-dideoxythymidine (AZT) and other dideoxynucleoside congeners of thymidine. *J Exp Med* 169:933–951, 1989.

29. Bagasra O, Pomerantz RJ. Human immunodeficiency virus type I provirus is demonstrated in peripheral blood monocytes in vivo: A study utilizing an in situ polymerase chain reaction. *AIDS Res Hum Retroviruses* 9:69–76, 1993.

30. Nelson JA, Wiley CA, Reynolds-Kohler C, et al. Human immunodeficiency virus detected in bowel epithelium from patients with gastrointestinal symptoms. *Lancet* 1:259–262, 1988.

31. Watkins BA, Dom HH, Kelly WB, et al. Specific tropism of HIV-I for microglial cells in primary human brain cultures. *Science* 249:549–553, 1990.

32. Rappersberger K, Gartner S, Schenk P, et al. Langerhans' cells are an actual site of HIV-1 replication. *Intervirology* 29:185–194, 1988.

33. Aronow HA, Brew BJ, Price RW. The management of the neurological

complications of HIV infection and AIDS. *AIDS* 2(suppl 1):S151–S159, 1988.

34. Anderson RM. The role of mathematical models in the study of HIV transmission and the epidemiology of AIDS. *J Acquir Immune Defic Syndr* 1:241–256, 1988.
35. Membreno L, Irony L, Dere W, et al. Adrenocortical function in acquired immunodeficiency syndrome. *J Clin Endocrinol Metab* 65:482–487, 1987.
36. Plata F, Autran B, Martins LP, et al. AIDS virus-specific cytotoxic T lymphocytes in lung disorders. *Nature* 328:348–351, 1987.
37. Donaldson YK, Bell JE, Ironside JW, et al. Redistribution of HIV outside the lymphoid system with onset of AIDS. *Lancet* 343:383–385, 1994.
38. Moss AR, Bacchetti P. Natural history of HIV infection. *AIDS* 3:55–61, 1989.
39. Jacobson MA, Mills J. Serious cytomegalovirus disease in the acquired immunodeficiency syndrome (AIDS). Clinical findings, diagnosis, and treatment. *Ann Intern Med* 108:585–594, 1988.
40. Horsburgh CRJ. *Mycobacterium avium* complex infection in the acquired immunodeficiency syndrome. *N Engl J Med* 324:1332–1338, 1991.
41. Lane HC, Masur H, Gelmann EP, et al. Correlation between immunologic function and clinical subpopulations of patients with the acquired immune deficiency syndrome. *Am J Med* 78:417–422, 1985.
42. Chang Y, Cesarman E, Pessin MS, et al. Identification of herpesvirus-like DNA sequences in AIDS-associated Kaposi's sarcoma. *Science* 266:1865–1869, 1994.
43. Ho DD, Moudgil T, Alam M. Quantification of human immunodeficiency virus type I (HIV-1) in the blood of infected persons. *N Engl J Med* 321:1621–1625, 1989.
44. Coombs R, Collier AC, Allain JP, et al. Plasma viremia in human immunodeficiency virus infection. *N Engl J Med* 321:1626–1631, 1989.
45. Venet A, Lu W, Beldjord K, Andrieu JM. Correlation between CD4 cell counts and cellular and plasma viral load in HIV-I–seropositive individuals. *AIDS* 5:283–288, 1991.
46. Koot M, Vos AH, Keet RP, et al. HIV-I biological phenotype in long-term infected individuals evaluated with an MT-2 cocultivation assay. *AIDS* 6:49–54, 1992.
47. Koot M, Keet RP, Vos AH, et al. Prognostic value of HIV-I syncytium-inducing phenotype for rate of CD4+ cell depletion and progression to AIDS. *Ann Intern Med* 118:681–688, 1993.
48. Connor RI, Mohri H, Cao Y, Ho DD. Increased viral burden and cytopathicity correlate temporally with CD4+ T-lymphocyte decline and clinical progression in human immunodeficiency virus type 1–infected individuals. *J Virol* 67:1772–1777, 1993.
49. Richman DD, Bozzette SA. The impact of the syncytium-inducing phenotype of human immunodeficiency virus on disease progression. *J Infect Dis* 169:968–974, 1994.
50. Rosenberg ZF, Fauci AS. The immunopathogensis of HFV infection. *Adv Immunol* 47:377–431, 1989.
51. Levrero M, Balsano C, Natoli G, et al. Hepatitis B virus X protein transactivates the long terminal repeats of human immunodeficiency virus types 1 and 2. *J Virol* 64:3082–3086, 1990.

52. Bohnlein E, Siekevitz M, Ballard DW, et al. Stimulation of the human immunodeficiency virus type 1 enhanced by the human T-cell leukemia virus type I tax gene product involves the action of inducible cellular proteins. *J Virol* 63:1578–1586, 1989.

53. Heng MC, Heng SY, Allen SG. Co-infection and synergy of human immunodeficiency virus-I and herpes simplex virus-1. *Lancet* 343:255–258, 1994.

54. Piatak M, Jr, Saag MS, Yang LC, et al. High levels of HIV-I in plasma during all stages of infection determined by competitive PCR. *Science* 259:1749–1754, 1993.

55. Weiss RA. How does HIV cause AIDS? *Science* 260:1273–1279, 1993.

56. Cooper DA, Gold J, Maclean P, et al. Acute AIDS retrovirus infection. Definition of a clinical illness associated with seroconversion. *Lancet* 1:537–540, 1985.

57. Ho DD, Samgadharan MG, Resnick L, et al. Primary human T-lymphotropic virus type III infection. *Ann Intern Med* 103 (pt 1):880–883, 1985.

58. Fox R, Eldred LJ, Fuchs EJ. Clinical manifestations of acute infection with human immunodeficiency virus in a cohort of gay men. *AIDS* 1:35–38, 1987.

59. Kessler HA, Blaauw B, Spear J, et al. Diagnosis of human immunodeficiency virus infection in seronegative homosexuals presenting with an acute viral syndrome. *JAMA* 258:1196–1199, 1987.

60. Hardy WD, Dear ES, Sokolov RT, Jr, Ho DD. Acute neurologic deterioration in a young man (clinical conference). *Rev Infect Dis* 13:745–750, 1991.

61. Came CA, Tedder RS, Smith A, et al. Acute encephalopathy coincident with seroconversion for anti-HTLV-111. *Lancet* 2:1206–1208, 1985.

62. Ho DD, Rota TR, Schooley RT, et al. Isolation of HTLV-HI from cerebrospinal fluid and neural tissues of patients with neurologic syndromes related to the acquired immunodeficiency syndrome. *N Engl J Med* 313:1493–1497, 1985.

63. Ho DD, Samgadharan MG, Resnick L, et al. Primary human T-lymphotropic virus type III infection. *Ann Intern Med* 103:880–883, 1985.

64. Calabrese LH, Proffitt MR, Levin KH, et al. Acute infection with the human immunodeficiency virus (HIV) associated with acute brachial neuritis and exanthematous rash. *Ann Intern Med* 107:849–851, 1987.

65. de Ronde A, Reiss P, Dekker J, et al. Seroconversion to HIV-I negative regulation factor (letter). *Lancet* 2:574, 1988.

66. Piette AM, Tusseau F, Vignon D, et al. Acute neuropathy coincident with seroconversion for anti-LAV/HTLV-HI (letter). *Lancet* 1:852, 1986.

67. Wiselka MJ, Nicholson KG, Ward SC, Flower AJ. Acute infection with human immunodeficiency virus associated with facial nerve palsy and neuralgia (letter). *J Infect* 15:189–190, 1987.

68. Paton P, Poly H, Gonnaud PM, et al. Acute meningoradiculitis concomitant with seroconversion to human immunodeficiency virus type 1. *Res Virol* 141:427–433, 1990.

69. Hagberg L, Malmvall BE, Svennerholm L, et al. Guillain-Barré syndrome as an early manifestation of HIV central nervous system infection. *Scand J Infect Dis* 18:591–592, 1986.

70. Rabeneck L, Popovic M, Gartner S, et al. Acute HIV infection presenting

with painful swallowing and esophageal ulcers. *JAMA* 263:2318–2322, 1990.

71. Gaines H, von Sydow M, Pehrson PO, Lundbegh P. Clinical picture of primary HIV infection presenting as a glandular-fever–like illness. *Br Med J* 297:1363–1368, 1988.

72. Stein DS, Korvick JA, Vermund SH. CD4+ lymphocyte cell enumeration for prediction of clinical course of human immunodeficiency virus disease: A review. *J Infect Dis* 165:352–363, 1992.

73. Sinicco A, Fora R, Sciandra M, el al. Risk of developing AIDS after primary acute HIV-1 infection. *J Acquir Immune Defic Syndr* 6:575–581, 1993.

74. Tindall B, Gaines H, Imrie A, et al. Zidovudine in the management of primary HIV-1 infection. *AIDS* 5:477–484, 1991.

75. Hamilton JD, Hartigan PM, Simberkoff MS, et al. A controlled trial of early versus late treatment with zidovudine in symptomatic human immunodeficiency virus infection. Results of the Veterans Affairs Cooperative Study. *N Engl J Med* 326:437–443, 1992.

76. Seligmann M, Warrell DA, Aboulker JP, et al. Concords: MRC/ANRS randomised double-blind controlled trial of immediate and deferred zidovudine in symptom-free HIV infection. *Lancet* 343:871–881, 1994.

77. Centers for Disease Control. 1993 revised classification system for HIV infection and expanded surveillance case definition for AIDS among adolescents and adults. *MMWR* 41(RR-17):1–19, 1992.

78. MacDonell KB, Chmiel JS, Poggensee L, et al. Predicting progression to AIDS: Combined usefulness of CD4 lymphocyte counts and p24 antigenemia. *Am J Med* 89:706–712, 1990.

79. Osmond D, Charlebois E, Lang W, et al. Changes in AIDS survival time in two San Francisco cohorts of homosexual men, 1983 to 1993. *JAMA* 271:1083–1087, 1994.

80. Bourgoignie JJ, Meneses R, Ortiz C, et al. The clinical spectrum of renal disease associated with human immunodeficiency virus. *Am J Kidney Dis* 12:131–137, 1988.

81. Moore RD, Hidalgo J, Sugland BW, Chaisson RE. Zidovudine and the natural history of the acquired immunodeficiency syndrome. *N Engl J Med* 324:1412–1416, 1991.

82. Hoover DR, et al. Clinical manifestations of AIDS in the era of pneumocystis prophylaxis. *N Engl J Med* 329:1922–1926, 1993.

83. Cao Y, Qin L, Zhang L, et al. Virologic and immunologic characterizations of long-term survivors of human imunodeficiency virus type 1 infection. *N Engl J Med* 332:201–208, 1995.

84. Pantaleo G, et al. Studies in subjects with long-term nonprogressive human immunodeficiency virus infection. *N Engl J Med* 332:209–216, 1995.

Classification, Epidemiology, and Transmission

2

M. Anita Barry

Historical Background

The first case reports of AIDS appeared in 1981 with the identification of clusters of *Pneumocystis carinii* pneumonia and Kaposi's sarcoma in previously healthy young homosexual men in California and New York [1–4]. Human immunodeficiency virus was isolated in 1983, and subsequent research studies established the causal relationship between HIV infection and AIDS, although the pathophysiology and role of cofactors in disease progression remain incompletely defined [5–10]. In 1985, four years after the first case reports of AIDS, an enzyme-linked immunosorbent assay (ELISA) to detect antibody to HIV was introduced [11]. The widespread use of HIV antibody testing over the past decade has provided a more complete understanding of the epidemiology and clinical features of the epidemic [12]. During this time, AIDS has become a global pandemic, with an estimated 17 million people infected with HIV worldwide [13].

Classification of HIV Infection

Classification of HIV infection is important to address epidemiologic, clinical, therapeutic, prognostic, and public health issues, and a variety of staging systems have been developed. HIV disease is associated with a broad spectrum of manifestations, ranging from asymptomatic infection to AIDS, a condition characterized by severe immunodeficiency.

AIDS-related complex (ARC) is a term that originally referred to a specific HIV-related syndrome and is still used by some clinicians to identify any important disease manifestations that do not meet diagnostic criteria for AIDS.

The Centers for Disease Control and Prevention (CDC) provides a surveillance definition of AIDS for the purpose of case reporting based on laboratory markers of progression and the presence of opportunistic diseases. The CDC classification system has undergone a series of modifications over the past decade, the most recent being the 1993 revision (Table 2-1). Prior versions included (1) the original surveillance definition, created before the availability of HIV antibody testing and, thus, heavily reliant on the diagnosis of HIV-related opportunistic infections (OIs) and neoplasms; and (2) a 1987 revision, which included additional "indicator diseases" and modified diagnostic criteria [14–17].

The 1993 CDC AIDS criteria are based on several studies that have demonstrated a strong association between HIV-related OIs and the absolute number of circulating CD4 lymphocytes [17–24]. In this classification system, HIV-infected persons with a CD4 cell count less than $200/mm^3$ or with a CD4 percentage less than 14 percent of total T-lymphocyte count meet surveillance criteria for AIDS, regardless of whether HIV-related opportunistic diseases are present. Specific AIDS indicator conditions remain part of the case definition, with pulmonary tuberculosis, recurrent bacterial pneumonia (at least two episodes within a 12-month period), and invasive cervical cancer, added in 1993 (Table 2-2).

Table 2-1 *1993 revised classification system for HIV infection[a] and expanded AIDS surveillance case definition for adolescents and adults[b]*

	Clinical categories		
CD4+ T-cell categories	*(A)* *Asymptomatic, acute (primary) HIV, or PGL*	*(B)* *Symptomatic not (A) or (C) conditions*	*(C)* *AIDS-indicator conditions*
(1) ≥ 500 /mm³	A1	B1	C1
(2) 200–499/mm³	A2	B2	C2
(3) < 200/mm³	A3	B3	C3

PGL = persistent generalized lymphadenopathy.
[a]Criteria for HIV infection for persons aged ≥ 13 years: (a) repeatedly reactive screening test for HIV antibody (e.g., enzyme immunoassay) with specific antibody identified by the use of supplemental tests (e.g., Western blot, immunofluorescence assay); (b) direct identification of virus in host tissues by virus isolation; (c) HIV antigen detection; or (d) a positive result on any other highly specific licensed test for HIV.
[b]Persons with an AIDS-indicator condition (category C) as well as those with CD4+ T-lymphocyte counts < 200/mm³ (categories A3 or B3) are reportable as AIDS cases in the United States and Territories, effective January 1, 1993.
Source: Adapted from Centers for Disease Control. 1993 revised classification system for HIV infection and expanded surveillance case definition for AIDS among adolescents and adults. *MMWR* 41(RR-17):2, 1992.

In addition to the CDC criteria for AIDS, other staging classification systems have been developed, none of which has gained widespread acceptance [25–29]. Justice and associates [29] devised a system that utilizes clinical and laboratory parameters to identify prognostic categories. The World Health Organization has published an HIV classification system, used mainly in developing countries, which is based on clinical criteria [26]. The Walter Reed staging system classifies HIV-infected persons on the basis of CD4 lymphocyte count, response to delayed hypersensitivity testing, and the presence of lymphadenopathy, oral candidiasis, and OIs [25].

AIDS Epidemiology in the United States

Despite the limitations of AIDS case reporting, these data provide the basis for assessment of epidemiologic trends, a crucial step in disease prevention and control. Since national surveillance of AIDS began in

Table 2-2 *Indicator conditions included in the 1993 AIDS surveillance case definition*

Candidiasis of bronchi, trachea, or lungs
Candidiasis, esophageal
Cervical cancer, invasive*
Coccidioidomycosis, disseminated or extrapulmonary
Cryptococcosis, extrapulmonary
Cryptosporidiosis, chronic intestinal (> 1-month duration)
Cytomegalovirus disease (other than liver, spleen, or nodes)
Encephalopathy, HIV-related
Herpes simplex: chronic ulcer(s) (> 1-month duration) or bronchitis, pneumonitis, or esophagitis
Histoplasmosis, disseminated or extrapulmonary
Isosporiasis, chronic intestinal (> 1-month duration)
Kaposi's sarcoma
Lymphoma, Burkitt's (or equivalent term)
Lymphoma, immunoblastic (or equivalent term)
Lymphoma, primary in brain
Mycobacterium avium complex or *Mycobacterium kansasii*, disseminated or extrapulmonary
Mycobacterium tuberculosis, any site (pulmonary* or extrapulmonary)
Pneumocystis carinii pneumonia
Pneumonia, recurrent*
Progressive multifocal leukoencephalopathy
Salmonella septicemia, recurrent
Toxoplasmosis of brain
Wasting syndrome, HIV-related

*Added in the 1993 expansion of the AIDS surveillance case definition.
Source: Adapted from Centers for Disease Control. 1993 revised classification system for HIV infection and expanded surveillance case definition for AIDS among adolescents and adults. *MMWR* 41(RR-17):15, 1992.

the United States, the number of cases reported has increased steadily. However, accurate interpretation of the rate of increase is complicated by the fact that the AIDS surveillance definition has undergone several revisions over time. The most significant changes in the surveillance definition occurred in 1993, when, following the addition of CD4 lymphocyte count as a diagnostic criterion, 105,990 new cases were reported in US adults and adolescents, a marked increase compared to 1992. Information on clinical progression from studies examining the spectrum of HIV disease has been used to permit meaningful comparisons during this period [30]. Adjustments based on this methodology suggest that 63,000 HIV-infected persons would have developed OIs in 1993, an increase of 3 percent compared to the number in 1992.

An estimated 1.0 to 1.5 million persons in the United States are infected with HIV. In 1994, the most recent time period for which data are available, a total of 80,691 AIDS cases were reported, including 79,674 in adults and adolescents 13 years of age or older [31]. While most cases (82%) occurred in men, a pattern noted since surveillance was initiated, the 14,081 cases reported in women reflect a threefold increase compared to 1985 [32]. Based on 1990 data from the National Center for Health Statistics, HIV infection was the leading cause of death among young men in New York, New Jersey, California, Florida, and Massachusetts, and in 64 of 172 cities with a population of 100,000 or more [33, 34] (Fig. 2-1A). It is also now the fourth leading cause of death among young women [33, 34] (Fig. 2-1B).

A disproportionate share of AIDS cases over the years have occurred in racial and ethnic minority populations, a finding likely related to social, economic, and cultural factors. In 1994, 59 percent of reported cases occurred in nonwhites [31]. Evaluation of 1993 AIDS cases by race and ethnicity revealed rates per 100,000 population of 162, 90, and 30 for black non-Hispanics, Hispanics, and white non-Hispanics, respectively [35].

Although homosexual and bisexual men have accounted for a majority of annual AIDS cases since the beginning of the epidemic, the rate of increase in this group has been declining since 1987, particularly in geographic areas where early cases were reported. In contrast, the proportion of AIDS cases resulting from heterosexual transmission has increased continuously over the past decade from 1.9 percent in 1985 to 9 percent in 1993 [36].

Figure 2-2 depicts risk behaviors identified in reported US AIDS patients in 1994. Cases attributable to unprotected homosexual sex accounted for 43.3 percent, injection drug use was responsible for 31.8 percent, unprotected heterosexual sex accounted for 10.3 percent, and receipt of contaminated blood or blood products was responsible for fewer than 2 percent. It is important to note that data for the entire cohort mask variability in risk exposure within specific population groups. For example, of 1,994 women with AIDS, 41 percent reported

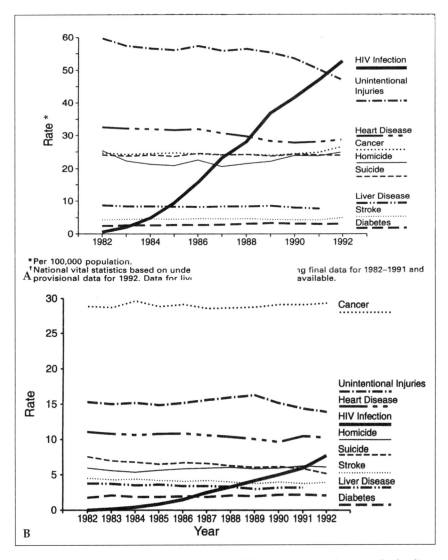

Figure 2-1. A. HIV infection has overtaken all other causes to become the leading cause of death among men aged 25–44 in the United States. **B**. HIV is the fourth leading cause of death among women aged 25–44 in the United States. Rate per 100,000 population. (From Centers for Disease Control. Update: Mortality attributable to HIV infection among persons aged 25–44 years—United States, 1991 and 1992. *MMWR* 42:869–872, 1993.)

injection drug use and 38 percent described heterosexual contact with a partner at risk for, or known to have, HIV infection or AIDS [37]. Similar changes in HIV risk behaviors in women have also been noted in seroprevalence surveys [38].

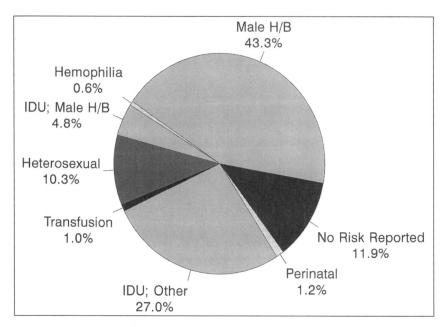

Figure 2-2. Exposure category for 1994 reported AIDS cases in the United States (n = 80,691). IDU = injection drug use; H/B = homosexual/bisexual. (Adapted from Centers for Disease Control. Update: Acquired immunodeficiency syndrome—United States, 1994. *MMWR* 44:65, 1995.)

HIV Seroprevalence Surveys

Using reported AIDS cases alone to estimate the prevalence of HIV infection is problematic. The AIDS case definition is designed primarily to detect severe illness, and the relatively long time period for disease progression suggests that many HIV-infected persons are not identified through the surveillance system. Alternative methods to obtain information on HIV prevalence have included anonymous ("unlinked") serologic surveys in specific populations, including persons attending sexually transmitted disease, drug treatment, or prenatal clinics; applicants for military service and the Job Corps; blood donors; and prisoners [38–42]. Seroprevalence surveys are limited by the fact that they represent selected populations and include only individuals who have undergone phlebotomy as part of clinical care or a screening process. However, these surveys complement data provided through AIDS case surveillance and contribute important information on the geographic variability and temporal trends of the epidemic [39].

Among male patients in sexually transmitted disease clinics, overall HIV seroprevalence has declined in recent years but remains over 15 percent among those who reported sex with men. For injection drug users entering substance abuse treatment programs, HIV seroprevalence in eastern US cities has ranged from 15 to 40 percent, but is less than 7 percent elsewhere in the country. Overall seroprevalence rates have declined among men applying for military service, entering the Job Corps, and donating blood. However, in Job Corps applicants, increased rates were noted in black women. Mean HIV seroprevalence in prisons among men was 1.2 percent compared to 1.8 percent in women [40]. In childbearing women, HIV seroprevalence increased from 0.16 percent in 1989 to 1990 to 0.17 percent in 1991 to 1992, with higher rates noted in the Southeast and declining rates in the northern United States.

Worldwide HIV Epidemiology

Recent estimates are that over six million people, 2.5 percent of the adult population in sub-Saharan Africa, are HIV-infected [43]. In developing countries, particularly parts of Africa and the Caribbean basin, heterosexual contact has played an important role in HIV transmission [44, 45]. An expanding group of HIV-infected women has resulted in substantial numbers of children with perinatally acquired infection in these regions. In Southeast Asia, India, and Malaysia, marked increases in HIV seroprevalence have been associated with injection drug use and prostitution. In other developing countries, transfusion of contaminated blood products and use of unsterile medical equipment continue to play a major role in HIV transmission. Epidemiologic projections using HIV incidence and seroprevalence data, adjusted for reporting efficiency, suggest that further spread will occur in areas that have already experienced high HIV incidence, as well as rapid progression into regions where the incidence has thus far been relatively low [45].

Transmission of HIV

Delineation of HIV risk in an individual is crucial for appropriate clinical intervention as well as to provide education related to modification of future behaviors. Modes of HIV transmission include sexual, blood, and perinatal contact. Within each of these categories, the risk of transmission varies based on factors such as circulating viral concentration and stage of illness in the index case, viral strain, presence of coexisting genital ulcer disease, specific type of contact, and immune status of the person exposed.

Sexual activity, both homosexual and heterosexual, is the major mode of HIV transmission worldwide, with specific trends varying in different geographic areas. Both infectivity of the source and susceptibility of the person exposed affect the sexual transmission of HIV. Factors identified as potentially related to infectivity in the source case include low CD4 lymphocyte count, high CD8 lymphocyte count, presence of antibodies to certain HIV antigens, use of antiretroviral agents, clinical stage of HIV disease, and presence of other sexually transmitted diseases [46]. Recipient-related factors believed to be important in HIV transmission include the presence of genital ulcer disease, other sexually transmitted diseases, and genital or mucosal injury related to mechanical trauma or chemical irritation such as nonoxynol-9 contraceptive sponges [46].

Several studies have evaluated transmission risk and cofactors related to HIV transmission in specific groups. Coates and associates [47] reported that, among gay and bisexual men, sexual contacts of men with AIDS or an HIV-related condition were more likely to be seropositive if they engaged in activities likely to be associated with anorectal mucosal injury. In evaluating heterosexual transmission, Padian and colleagues [48] reported that 23 percent of women with heterosexual contact to HIV-infected male partners were seropositive and that factors associated with infection included the total number of sexual exposures to the index case and the practice of anal intercourse. Seidlin and coworkers [49] evaluated 158 non–injection-drug-using heterosexual partners of HIV-infected persons and found that risk factors for male-to-female transmission included the presence of AIDS or ARC in the index case, history of anal intercourse, and history of bleeding as a result of intercourse. Among heterosexual contacts of persons infected with HIV as a result of transfusion, 18 percent of women and 8 percent of men were infected [50]. In some couples, no transmission occurred despite repeated sexual contact without protection, while in others it was noted after relatively few exposures. These and other data indicate that multiple factors play a role in the sexual transmission of HIV [51, 52].

Risk of parenteral HIV transmission also varies with the nature and type of exposure. In injection drug users, the risk attributable to the use of contaminated paraphernalia is difficult to quantify since HIV infection in this population has been associated with behaviors related specifically to drug use as well as to socioeconomic factors [53]. Schoenbaum and associates [53] evaluated 452 drug users enrolled in a methadone treatment program in New York and concluded that HIV seropositivity was related to the number of injections per month, percentage of injections with used needles, average number of cocaine injections per month, and percentage of injections with needles that were shared with strangers or acquaintances. Heterosexual activity was also found to be an independent risk factor for HIV infection.

Acquisition of HIV disease through transfusion of infected blood products has become exceedingly rare in the United States, although it is a relatively efficient mode of transmission, with rates approaching 100 percent [54]. However, the likelihood that blood components contain HIV has decreased markedly through the introduction of donor self-exclusion, HIV antibody screening of blood products, and heat treatment of coagulation factors. In 1989, Cumming and associates [55] estimated the risk of HIV transmission through blood product transfusion to be 1:153,000 per unit, attributable primarily to blood components that test HIV antibody negative during the "window period" of infection.

Health care workers have been identified as another group at potential risk for HIV infection related to exposure to blood or body fluids from patients. A recent analysis of pooled data from 21 prospective studies estimated the risk of infection following percutaneous exposure to blood or bloody body fluids to be nine infections following 3,628 exposures, or approximately 0.2 percent. However, the risk of transmission in a specific situation is likely to vary, depending on the circulating viral titer in the source case, volume of blood injected, and immune status of the exposed person [56, 57].

The risk of HIV transmission from an infected health care worker to a patient appears to be extremely low if universal precautions are implemented [58, 59]. One outbreak involving dentist-to-patient HIV transmission has been documented, although the precise factors responsible in this instance remain unclear [60, 61].

Perinatal acquisition of HIV infection is well described, and viral acquisition can occur in utero, intrapartum from blood exposure, or postpartum through breast feeding. The relative frequency of in utero compared to intrapartum transmission remains incompletely defined. HIV has been isolated from breast milk and transmitted through breast feeding, but analysis suggests that in developing countries, where alternative forms of neonatal nutrition are not available, the benefits of nursing are greater than its risks. Quantifying perinatal HIV transmission has been complicated by difficulty in diagnosing infants because of the presence of passively acquired maternal antibody.

Reported rates of perinatal HIV transmission vary widely, from 13 to 32 percent in industrialized parts of the world and from 25 to 48 percent in developing countries [62–67]. The risk of transmission is believed to correlate with disease stage of the mother, with women undergoing primary infection and those with advanced disease at highest risk. Low CD4 lymphocyte count, high CD8 lymphocyte count, and placental inflammation have also been associated with a higher risk of HIV transmission [46].

Although HIV is not transmitted by casual exposure, there have been occasional reports of transmission among household contacts [68–72]. Pooled data from 17 studies involving over 1,100 persons who had household exposure without sexual or needle-sharing contact revealed no cases of transmission [72]. Studies in which household transmission of HIV infection has occurred describe exposure to blood or bloody body fluids from symptomatic HIV-infected persons, emphasizing the importance of using appropriate precautions to minimize risk.

Human Immunodeficiency Virus, Type 2

In contrast to HIV-1, there has been little international spread of HIV-2, despite the fact that the two viruses share similar modes of transmission. Most HIV-2 infection has been reported in West Africa, and only 32 cases have been identified in the United States since 1987. Individual case reports, available for 17 of the 32 cases, indicate that the majority of HIV-2–infected persons were West Africans residing in the United States [73]. Until HIV-2–related immunodeficiency becomes significant, the viral titer as determined by culture and polymerase chain reaction appears to be lower than that of HIV-1, a finding probably responsible for HIV-2's diminished infectivity [74, 75].

References

1. Gottlieb MS, Schanker HM, Fan PT, et al. *Pneumocystis* pneumonia—Los Angeles, *MMWR* 30:25–32, 1981.
2. Gottlieb MS, Schroff R, Schanker HM, et al. *Pneumocystis carinii* pneumonia and mucosal candidiasis in previously healthy homosexual men: Evidence of a new acquired cellular immunodeficiency. *N Engl J Med* 305:425–431, 1981.
3. Centers for Disease Control. Follow-up on Kaposi's sarcoma and Pneumocystis pneumonia. *MMWR* 30:409–410, 1981.
4. Friedman-Kein L, Lauberstein L, Marmor M, et al. Kaposi's sarcoma and Pneumocystis pneumonia among homosexual men—New York City and California. *MMWR* 30:305–308, 1981.
5. Barre-Sinoussi F, Chermann JC, Rey F, et al. Isolation of a T-lymphotrophic retrovirus from a patient at risk for acquired immune deficiency syndrome (AIDS). *Science* 220:868–871, 1983.
6. Gallo RC, Salahuddin SZ, Popovic M, et al. Frequent detection and isolation of cytopathic retroviruses (HTLV-III) from patients with AIDS and at risk for AIDS. *Science* 224:500–503, 1984.
7. Broder S, Gallo RC. A pathogenic retrovirus (HTLV-III) linked to AIDS. *N Engl J Med* 311:1292–1297, 1984.
8. Tappero JW, Conant MA, Wolfe SF, et al. Kaposi's sarcoma: Epidemiology, pathogenesis, histology, clinical spectrum, staging criteria and therapy. *J Am Acad Dermatol* 28:371–395, 1993.
9. Haverkos HW, Drotman DP, Hanson D. Epidemiology of AIDS-related Kaposi's sarcoma (KS): An update. Ninth International Conference on AIDS, Berlin, June 1993.
10. Gallant JE, Moore RD, Richman DD, et al. Risk factors for Kaposi's sarcoma in patients with advanced human immunodeficiency disease treated with zidovudine. Zidovudine Epidemiology Study Group. *Arch Intern Med* 154:566–572, 1994.
11. Centers for Disease Control, Food and Drug Administration, Alcohol, Drug Abuse, and Mental Health Administration, et al. Provisional Public Health

Service inter-agency recommendations for screening donated blood and plasma for antibody to the virus causing acquired immunodeficiency syndrome. *MMWR* 34:1–5, 1985.

12. Farizo KM, Buehler JW, Chamberland ME, et al. Spectrum of disease in persons with human immunodeficiency virus infection in the United States. *JAMA* 267:1798–1805, 1992.

13. Global Program on AIDS, WHO. World AIDS Day—December 1, 1994. *MMWR* 43:825, 1994.

14. Centers for Disease Control. Update on acquired immune deficiency syndrome (AIDS)—United States. *MMWR* 31:507–508, 1982.

15. Centers for Disease Control. Classification system for human T-lymphotropic virus type III/lymphadenopathy-associated virus infections. *MMWR* 35:334–339, 1986.

16. Centers for Disease Control. Revision of the CDC surveillance case definition for acquired immunodeficiency syndrome. *MMWR* 36:1–15S, 1987.

17. Centers for Disease Control. 1993 revised classification system for HIV infection and expanded surveillance case definition for AIDS among adolescents and adults. *MMWR* 41 (RR–17):1–15, 1992.

18. Goedert JJ, Bigger RJ, Melbye M, et al. Effect of T4 count and cofactors on the incidence of AIDS in homosexual men infected with human immunodeficiency virus. *JAMA* 257:331–334, 1987.

19. Lang W, Perkins H, Anderson RE, et al. Patterns of T-lymphocyte changes with human immunodeficiency virus infection: From seroconversion to the development of AIDS. *J Acquir Immune Defic Syndr* 2:63–69, 1989.

20. Lange MA, de Wolf F, Goudsmit J. Markers for progression of HIV infection. *AIDS* 3(suppl 1):S153–S160, 1989.

21. Taylor JM, Fahey JL, Detels R, et al. CD4 percentage, CD4 numbers, and CD4:CD8 ratio in HIV infection: Which to choose and how to use. *J Acquir Immune Defic Syndr* 2:114–124, 1989.

22. Masur H, Ognibene FP, Yarchoan R, et al. CD4 counts as predictors of opportunistic pneumonias in human immunodeficiency virus (HIV) infection. *Ann Intern Med* 111:223–231, 1989.

23. Fahey JL, Taylor JMG, Detels R, et al. The prognostic value of cellular and serologic markers in infection with human immunodeficiency virus type 1. *N Engl J Med* 322:166–172, 1990.

24. Fernandez-Cruz E, Desco M, Garcia Montes M, et al. Immunological and serological markers predictive of progression to AIDS in a cohort of HIV-infected drug users. *AIDS* 4:987–994, 1990.

25. Redfield RR, Wright DC, Tramont EC. The Walter Reed staging classification for HTLV-111/LAV infection. *N Engl J Med* 314:131–132, 1986.

26. World Health Organization. Interim proposal for a WHO staging system for HIV infection and diseases. *Weekly Epidemiol Record* 65:221–224, 1990.

27. Chaisson RE, Volberding PA. Clinical Manifestations of HIV Infection. In GL Mandell, JE Bennett, R Dolin, (eds), *Principles and Practice of Infectious Diseases.* New York: Churchill Livingstone, 1995. Pp 1217–1252.

28. Haverkos HW, Goulieb MS, Killen JY, et al. Classification of HTLV III/LAV related diseases. *J Infect Dis* 152:1905, 1985.

29. Justice AC, Feinstein AR, Wells CK. A new prognostic staging system for the acquired immunodeficiency syndrome. *N Engl J Med* 320:1388–1393, 1989.

30. Centers for Disease Control. Update: Trends in AIDS diagnosis and reporting under the expanded surveillance definition for adolescents and adults—United States, 1993. *MMWR* 43:826–831, 1994.

31. Centers for Disease Control. Update: Acquired immunodeficiency syndrome—United States, 1994. *MMWR* 44:64–67, 1995.

32. Centers for Disease Control. Update: AIDS among women—United States, 1994. *MMWR* 44:81–84, 1995.

33. Selik RM, et al. HIV infection as leading cause of death among young adults in US cities and states. *JAMA* 269:2991–2994, 1993.

34. Centers for Disease Control. Update: Mortality attributable to HIV infection among persons aged 28–44 years—United States, 1991 and 1992. *MMWR* 42:869–872, 1993.

35. Centers for Disease Control. AIDS among racial/ethnic minorities—United States, 1993. *MMWR* 43:644–655, 1994.

36. Centers for Disease Control. Heterosexually acquired AIDS—United States, 1993. *MMWR* 43:155–160, 1994.

37. Carpenter CJJ, Mayer KH, Stein MD, et al. Human immunodeficiency virus infection in North American women: Experience with 200 cases and a review of the literature. *Medicine (Baltimore)* 70:307–325, 1991.

38. Centers for Disease Control. *National HIV Serosurveillance Summary: Results Through 1992.* Vol 3. Atlanta: US Department of Health and Human Services, Public Health Service, 1994.

39. Petersen LR, Gwinn M, Janssen R. HIV seroprevalence trends in the United States, 1988–1992. Tenth International Conference on AIDS, Yokohama, August 1994.

40. Withum DG, Guerena-Burgueno F, Gwinn M, et al. High HIV prevalence among female and male prisoners in the United States, 1989–1992: Implications for prevention and treatment strategies. Ninth International Conference on AIDS, Berlin, June 1993.

41. Sweeney PA, Lindegren ML, Janssen R, et al. Adolescents at risk for HIV-1 infection: Results from seroprevalence surveys in clinical settings in the United States, 1990–1992. Ninth International Conference on AIDS, Berlin, June 1993.

42. Conway GA, Epstein MR, Hayman CR, et al. Trends in HIV prevalence among disadvantaged youth. Survey results from a national job training program, 1988 through 1992. *JAMA* 269:2887–2889, 1993.

43. Hunter DJ. Aids in sub-Saharan Africa: The epidemiology of heterosexual transmission and the prospects for prevention. *Epidemiology* 4:63–72, 1993.

44. Mann JM, Chin J. AIDS: A global perspective. *N Engl J Med* 319:302–330, 1988.

45. Mantel C, Tarantolo D, Lepisto E, et al. AIDS in the world, 1992: Estimating HIV/AIDS morbidity and mortality since the beginning of the pandemic. Eighth International Conference on AIDS, Amsterdam, July 1992.

46. Chamberland ME, Ward JW, Curran JW. Epidemiology and Prevention of

AIDS and HIV Infection. In GL Mandell, JE Bennett, R Dolin (eds), *Principles and Practice of Infectious Diseases*. New York: Churchill Livingstone, 1995.

47. Coates RA, Calzavara LM, Read SE, et al. Risk factors for HIV infection in male sexual contacts of men with AIDS or an AIDS-related condition. *Am J Epidemiol* 128:729–740, 1988.

48. Padian N, Marquis L, Francis DP, et al. Male-to-female transmission of human immunodeficiency virus. *JAMA* 258:788–790, 1987.

49. Seidlin M, Vogler M, Lee E, et al. Heterosexual transmission of HIV in a cohort of couples in New York City. *AIDS* 7:1247–1254, 1993.

50. Peterman TA, Stoneburner RL, Allen JR, et al. Risk of human immunodeficiency virus transmission from heterosexual adults with transfusion-associated infections. *JAMA* 259:55–58, 1988.

51. Clumeck N, Taelman H, Hermans P, et al. A cluster of HIV infection among heterosexual people without apparent risk factors. *N Engl J Med* 321:1460–1462, 1989.

52. Fischl MA, Dickinson GM, Scott GB, et al. Evaluation of heterosexual partners, children, and household contacts of adults with AIDS. *JAMA* 257:640–644, 1987.

53. Schoenbaum EE, Hartel D, Selwyn PA, et al. Risk factors for human immunodeficiency virus infection in intravenous drug users. *N Engl J Med* 321:874–879, 1989.

54. Ward JW, Deppe DA, Samson S, et al. Risk of human immunodeficiency virus infection from blood donors who later developed the acquired immunodeficiency syndrome. *Ann Intern Med* 106:61–62, 1987.

55. Cumming PD, Wallace EL, Schoor JB, et al. Exposure of patients to human immunodeficiency virus through the transfusion of blood components that test antibody negative. *N Engl J Med* 321:941–946, 1989.

56. Gerberding JL. Management of occupational exposures to blood-borne viruses. *N Engl J Med* 332:444–451, 1995.

57. Ho DD, Moudgil T, Alam M. Quantitation of human immunodeficiency virus type I in the blood of infected persons. *N Engl J Med* 321:1621–1625, 1989.

58. von Reyn CF, Gilbert TT, Shaw FE JR, et al. Absence of HIV transmission from an infected orthopedic surgeon. A 13 year look-back study. *JAMA* 269:1807–1811, 1993.

59. Centers for Disease Control. Update: Investigations of persons treated by HIV-infected health-care workers—United States. *MMWR* 42:329–331, 1993.

60. Ou CY, Ciesielski CA, Myers G, et al. Molecular epidemiology of HIV transmission in a dental practice. *Science* 256:1165–1171, 1992.

61. Ciesielski C, Marlanos D, Ou CY, et al. Transmission of human immunodeficiency virus in a dental practice. *Ann Intern Med* 116:798–805, 1992.

62. Dabis F, Msellati P, Dunn D, et al. Estimating the rate of mother-to-child transmission of HIV. Report of a workshop on methodological issues, Ghent (Belgium), 17–20 February 1992. The Working Group on Mother-to-Child Transmission of HIV. *AIDS* 7:1139–1148, 1993.

63. European Collaborative Study. Mother-to-child transmission of HIV infection. *Lancet* 2:1039–1042, 1988.
64. Ryder RW, Nsa W, Hassig SE, et al. Perinatal transmission of the human immunodeficiency virus type 1 to infants of seropositive women in Zaire. *N Engl J Med* 320:1637–1642, 1989.
65. St. Louis ME, Kamenga M, Brown C, et al. Risk for perinatal HIV-1 transmission according to maternal immunologic, virologic, and placental factors. *JAMA* 269:2853–2859, 1993.
66. Douglas GC, King BF. Maternal-fetal transmission of human immunodeficiency virus: A review of possible routes and cellular mechanisms of infection. *Clin Infect Dis* 15:678–691, 1992.
67. Van de Perre P, Simonon A, Msellati P, et al. Postnatal transmission of human immunodeficiency virus type 1 from mother to infant: A prospective cohort study in Kigali, Rwanda. *N Engl J Med* 325:593–598, 1991.
68. Centers for Disease Control. Human immunodeficiency virus transmission in household settings—United States. *MMWR* 43:347–356, 1994.
69. Fitzgibbon JE, Gaur S, Frenkel LD, et al. Transmission from one child to another of human immunodeficiency virus type 1 with a zidovudine-resistant mutation. *N Engl J Med* 329:1835–1841, 1993.
70. Centers for Disease Control. Apparent transmission of human T-lymphotrophic virus type III/lymphadenopathy associated virus from a child to a mother providing health care. *MMWR* 35:76–79, 1986.
71. Centers for Disease Control. HIV transmission between two adolescent brothers with hemophilia. *MMWR* 42:948–951, 1993.
72. Simonds RJ, Rogers MF. HIV prevention—bringing the message home. *N Engl J Med* 329:1883–1885, 1993.
73. Centers for Disease Control. Testing for antibodies to human immunodeficiency virus type 2 in the United States. *MMWR* 41(RR–12):1–9, 1992.
74. De Cock KM, Adjorlolo G, Ekpini E, et al. Epidemiology and transmission of HIV-2: Why there is no HIV-2 pandemic. *JAMA* 270:2083–2086, 1993.
75. Marlink R, et al. Reduced rates of disease development after HIV-2 infection as compared to HIV-1. *Science* 265:1587–1590, 1994.

HIV Diagnostic Testing *3*

Peter J. Piliero, Howard Libman

In 1983, the cause of AIDS was identified as a retrovirus, which was subsequently named human immunodeficiency virus, type 1 (HIV-1). In 1985, the first laboratory test to detect antibodies to HIV-1 was licensed by the Food and Drug Administration (FDA). Based on recent data from the Centers for Disease Control (CDC), it is estimated that between 34 and 46 million HIV antibody tests are currently performed each year in the United States [WO Schalla, personal communication], although there is considerable variability of testing frequency in populations at risk for HIV infection [1].

HIV antibody testing is generally performed in persons thought to be at risk for HIV infection through sexual or drug use behaviors or through exposure to contaminated blood products (Table 3-1). In addition, under certain federal and state statutes, some employees, persons applying for a marriage license, pregnant women, prisoners, prostitutes, and sex offenders may be required to undergo HIV testing [2].

The manner in which HIV antibody tests are performed and reported varies between laboratories and can be confusing [3]. Therefore, it is important that health care providers understand the available testing modalities, when to use them, and how to interpret the results.

This chapter reviews each of the screening, confirmatory, and supplemental laboratory tests available for diagnosing HIV infection (Table 3-2). It also presents an algorithm for the management of indeterminate results and describes research modalities that may serve a clinical role in the future. The indications for, and contraindications to, HIV antibody testing are presented in Chapter 32, and issues related to pretest and post-test counseling are discussed in Chapter 35.

Over the past few years, the syndrome of idiopathic CD4+ T-lymphocytopenia (CD4 cell count < 300/mm^3 or 20% of total T cells on more than one occasion with negative HIV diagnostic tests) has been

Table 3-1 *Persons at risk for HIV infection*

Individuals who received a blood transfusion between 1978 and 1985
Homosexual/bisexual men and their sexual partners
Injection drug users
Persons with sexually transmitted diseases
Prostitutes
Prisoners
Women of childbearing age who are at risk through drug use, prostitution, or
    unprotected sex
Children born to HIV-infected mothers
Persons born in endemic areas
Heterosexuals having "unsafe sex" or multiple sexual partners

Source: Adapted from Centers for Disease Control. Perspectives in disease prevention and health promotion: Public Health Service guidelines for counseling and antibody testing to prevent HIV infection and AIDS. *MMWR* 36:509–515, 1987.

described in a limited number of patients [4]. Its epidemiology and natural history are currently under investigation by the CDC.

HIV-1 Structure

In order to understand HIV testing, one needs to have a basic knowledge of the structural antigens that comprise the HIV genome (Fig. 3-1). These antigens are identified by their estimated size in kilodaltons and are either proteins (p) or glycoproteins (gp) [5]. The major viral components to which antibodies are formed, in sequential order, are the group-specific or core antigens (*gag*) p24 and p17,

Table 3-2 *Diagnostic tests for HIV infection*

Screening
    Enzyme-linked immunoassay (EIA, ELISA) for HIV-1, HIV-2, or both
    Latex agglutination for HIV-1
    ELISA for HIV-1 detection in urine or saliva*
Confirmatory
    Western blot (WB) assay for HIV-1
    WB assay for HIV-2*
    Indirect immunofluorescence antibody assay (IFA) for HIV-1
    Radioimmunoprecipitation antibody assay (RIPA) for HIV-1*
Supplemental
    ELISA for HIV-1 p24 antigen
    HIV-1 culture*
    Polymerase chain reaction (PCR) for HIV-1*

*Not currently licensed by the Food and Drug Administration.

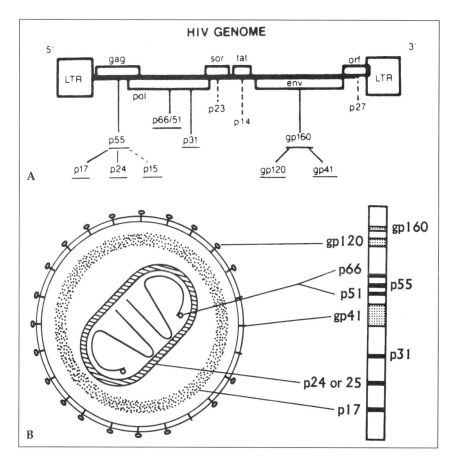

Figure 3-1. A. HIV genome. (From Human Immunodeficiency Virus [HIV] Biotech/ Du Pont HIV Western Blot Kit package insert, Du Pont Company, Wilmington, DE.) **B.** HIV and components with corresponding Western blot bands. Glycoprotein gp160 is precursor envelope glycoprotein, which is cleaved into gp120 and transmembrane gp41 envelope proteins. Proteins p66, p51, and p31 are nucleoid proteins: p66 and p51 are two active forms of reverse transcriptase; p31 is integrase protein responsible for viral integration into host cell DNA. Nucleoid shell p24 protein and p17 protein both are core proteins derived from precursor protein p55. (From A Schindzielorz. HIV-1 serology and AIDS testing: A practical approach to understanding. *South Med J* 82:1531, 1989.)

the envelope (*env*) proteins gp120/160 and gp41, and the polymerase (*pol*) proteins p31 and p66/51. Based on the presence of antibodies to these antigens, a diagnostic test will either be reactive (positive); nonreactive (negative); or, in the case of Western blot (WB), positive, negative, or indeterminate.

Screening Tests

Enzyme-Linked Immunosorbent Assay

Enzyme-linked immunosorbent assay (ELISA) is the most commonly used test to screen for the presence of antibodies to HIV-1 because of its low cost, standardized procedure, and high reliability [6]. In the ELISA, HIV antigens derived either from tissue culture (first generation) or by recombinant technology (second generation) are placed on beads or in wells. Serum is added, and, if from an HIV-infected person, the immunoglobulin G (IgG) antibodies bind to the antigen-coated beads or wells. Enzyme-labeled anti-IgG antibodies are then introduced, which bind to the HIV antibodies. Finally, in the presence of a substrate, a color reaction occurs, which is read spectrophotometrically as an optical density (OD): The more HIV antibodies present, the higher the OD. Each manufacturer's kit has an OD cutoff that determines sample status. There are nine FDA-licensed HIV-1 ELISAs, of which all but two are first-generation tests [7].

The sensitivity and specificity of the ELISA are both greater than 99 percent [8]. If the ELISA is negative, no further testing is generally performed; a positive specimen is retested to rule out a false reaction. If this repeat assay is positive, the sample is evaluated with a more specific test—WB assay, immunofluorescence assay (IFA), or radioimmunoprecipitation assay (RIPA)—to determine if it is positive, negative, or indeterminate.

Several causes of false-positive ELISAs have been reported in the literature [6, 9–11] (Table 3-3). False-positive results are usually caused by cross-reactive antibodies and are more common with first-generation tests. Second-generation ELISAs appear less affected by this problem, as they are not subject to contamination of the antigen preparation by cell culture material.

False-negative ELISAs are less common than false-positive tests but can occur if the patient has not yet seroconverted, following acquisition of HIV infection, during the so-called window period. In general, 95 percent of persons will develop viral antibody within 6 months of becoming HIV infected [12]. Two other causes of false-negative ELISAs are very advanced HIV disease, when the patient may lose the ability to make HIV antibodies, in particular p24 antibody, and a mislabeled specimen. If the ELISA is negative but HIV infection is still strongly suspected on clinical grounds, supplemental diagnostic studies should be performed.

Other Screening Tests

In addition to the ELISA kits, one FDA-approved and several experimental assays exist. The rapid latex agglutination assay is quick, inexpensive, and less technically difficult, and it has been widely used in

Table 3-3 *Causes of false-positive ELISA for HIV-1*

Human leukocyte antigen (HLA) DR antibodies (multiparous women, multiple transfusions)
Autoimmune disorders
HIV-2 infection
Multiple myeloma
Alcoholic hepatitis
Recent influenza vaccine
Hemodialysis
Positive rapid plasma reagin (RPR)
Mislabeled specimen

underdeveloped countries. Early African studies showed the sensitivity to be from 71 to 99 percent; more recently in the United States, it has ranged from 92 to 99 percent [6]. Interobserver differences in reading the agglutination reaction seem to account for the variability of test results.

Assays for detecting HIV antibodies in the urine are being studied experimentally [13, 14]. In one report, using a modified ELISA test, both the sensitivity and specificity were greater than 99 percent, and while the concentration of HIV antibodies was 10,000 to 20,000 times less than plasma, they were detectable in all 158 HIV-infected subjects [13]. ELISAs for HIV antibodies in the saliva have also been studied. Frerichs and associates [15] found a sensitivity ranging from 93.2 to 100 percent and a specificity of 98.7 to 100 percent for three different assays. Urine and saliva assays may prove to be of greatest utility in underdeveloped countries where economic and technical skills are lacking.

Johnson & Johnson has proposed the Direct Access Diagnostic Kit for home HIV antibody testing. Patients would provide a fingerstick blood sample on blot paper and send it to an FDA-licensed laboratory for ELISA; counseling and results would be available through a toll-free telephone number. The concept of home HIV testing is controversial and is currently being reviewed by the FDA [16, 17].

Confirmatory Tests

Western Blot

The WB assay is the most commonly used confirmatory test for the presence of HIV-specific antibodies [6]. Currently three different assays are licensed by the FDA [7]. In general, the test is more specific (97.8%) than the ELISA but also more time consuming and technically difficult [18].

The major HIV antigens are prepared in tissue culture and separated by weight using gel electrophoresis. They are then blotted, or transferred, onto paper. The patient's serum is added, and, if HIV antibodies are present, they adhere to the paper. Then, enzyme-linked anti-IgG antibody is introduced, which attaches to the HIV antibody-antigen complex. Finally, when substrate is added, a band appears, indicating the presence of antibody to a specific HIV antigen.

Once completed, the WB is subject to specific criteria and interpreted as positive, negative, or indeterminate. When the most stringent and specific criteria are used—requiring three bands to be positive—a test result is likely to be deemed indeterminate. Results are reported negative when no HIV-related or only non-HIV–related bands are present.

At least five different sets of criteria have been established by health care–related organizations for interpreting WB test results [19]. In 1988, when the CDC evaluated four of these by analyzing serum samples, it determined that the Association of State and Territorial Public Health Laboratory Directors (ASTPHLD) criteria resulted in the highest percentage of positive and the lowest percentage of indeterminate results [20]. Based on these findings, the CDC has recommended their use in public health and clinical practice. The ASTPHLD/CDC criteria define a WB test as positive if two of three bands—p24, gp41, or gp120/160—are present. Although laboratories are not mandated by the FDA or CDC to use these criteria, most of them do.

The false-positive rate of sequential ELISA and WB testing is estimated to be between 0.0007 and 0.01 percent [21]. Burke and associates [22] reviewed HIV antibody tests in US military recruits from low-prevalence populations and found only one false-positive result. When extrapolated to the entire recruitment, 1 of every 200 (0.5%) diagnoses of HIV infection would be inaccurate.

In contrast, the rate of indeterminate Western blot (IWB) results is much higher. Approximately 10 to 20 percent of specimens that are repeatedly reactive by ELISA are IWB. There are several possible causes of IWB, including antibody production against core (*gag*) antigens early in HIV infection, loss of core antibodies late in advanced HIV disease, cross-reactive antibody to HIV-2, and nonspecific cross-reactive antibodies [23]. IWBs have also been associated with T-cell lymphoma, multiple sclerosis, dermatologic disorders, injection drug use, alcoholic liver disease, and autoimmune diseases [8].

Because of the diagnostic uncertainty of an IWB for both patients and health care providers, several studies have been performed to examine the subsequent risk of HIV seroconversion. In a large prospective study by Celum and associates [8] of 206 subjects with repeatedly reactive ELISA and IWB, 3 percent, all of whom had recent high-risk behavior, seroconverted on subsequent testing. In women, parity and the presence of autoantibodies were significantly associated with an IWB. For men, IWBs appeared related to having had a tetanus booster in the past 2 years and a history of sex with a prostitute. There were no cross-reactive antibodies secondary to coinfection with HIV-2; human T-lymphotropic virus, type 1 (HTLV-1); bovine immunodeficiency virus; or feline leukemia virus.

In another study, Healey and associates [24] prospectively evaluated 308 subjects with an IWB and found a 7 percent rate of seroconversion. Seroconverters belonged to high-risk groups, were identified in a mean of 9 weeks, and, most importantly, had a p24 band on IWB. Other researchers have noted this same association between the presence of a p24 band and subsequent seroconversion [20].

Figure 3-2 presents an algorithmic approach to the patient with a positive ELISA and an IWB. In general, the ELISA should be repeated one month later. If it is positive and the WB is once again indeterminate, patients should be stratified based on HIV risk assessment. In persons at high risk, supplemental HIV testing should be performed (see below). In those at low risk, WB testing should be repeated at 3- and 6-month intervals. A low prior probability of HIV infection and the absence of a p24 band on WB for more than 6 months are strong evidence against the presence of HIV-1 infection [20, 23].

Other Confirmatory Tests

Indirect Immunofluorescence Antibody Assay
Indirect immunofluorescence antibody assay is another confirmatory test that has been approved by the FDA [7]. IFA shows excellent concordance with WB, is less expensive, only takes a few hours, and

Figure 3-2. Algorithm for evaluation of an indeterminate Western blot (IWB) test.

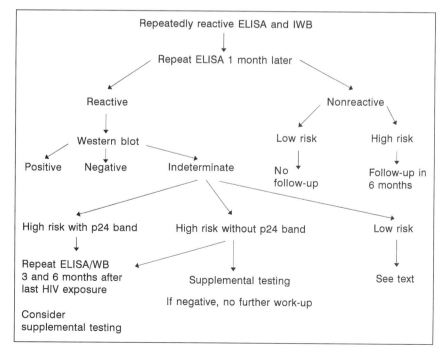

requires a small quantity of blood. HIV-infected T lymphocytes are fixed to a slide and incubated with the patient's serum. A fluorescent-labeled anti-IgG is then added, and the slide is evaluated with fluorescence microscopy to determine whether or not the sample is reactive. IFA is highly sensitive to antibodies directed at HIV envelope proteins, specifically gp120, because of their high expression on the T-cell surface.

Radioimmunoprecipitation Antibody Assay

Radioimmunoprecipitation antibody assay is currently a research test. Similar to IFA, it is more sensitive for detecting anti-envelope antibodies, but it is more costly, is technically difficult, and requires the use of radioisotopes. The viral proteins in HIV-infected cells are radiolabeled, and serum is then added. In a specimen from a person with HIV disease, antibody-antigen complexes form, which are precipitated from solution and separated by gel electrophoresis. The resulting band pattern is developed by autoradiography and then subject to interpretive criteria.

Supplemental Diagnostic Tests

HIV p24 Antigen Assay

As previously discussed, p24 is one of the HIV core proteins, and antibodies to this antigen are the first to form after infection. There is one FDA-approved ELISA for detecting HIV-1 p24 antigen (p24 Ag) [7]. This test is used either alone or in conjunction with HIV culture as a supplemental diagnostic test or determinant of virologic response to drug therapy in clinical research studies.

Technically, a well is coated with recombinant HIV p24 antibody, and the patient's serum is then added, followed by enzyme-linked anti-p24 antibody. As in the standard HIV ELISA, optical density is read spectrophotometrically, and this value is correlated to a standard curve to give a concentration of p24 Ag. Only 20 to 30 percent of HIV-infected patients have detectable p24 antigen, making this standard assay relatively insensitive despite its high specificity [25].

Recently, a modified procedure has been performed in an attempt to increase the sensitivity of the p24 antigen assay. By pretreating the serum with acid for 60 minutes, p24 antibody-antigen complexes are dissociated, allowing more p24 Ag to be detected by the ELISA. This acid pretreatment appears to cause no false-positive results but does decrease the measurable p24 Ag in HIV-infected persons with high levels of antigenemia [26].

In three reports comparing the standard p24 assay to the acid-dissociated method, a significant increase in the number of patients with detectable p24 Ag was described [25–27]. In these studies, which involved a total of 1,132 subjects, between 10.6 and 22.3 percent had detectable p24 Ag with the standard assay, whereas between 50.6 and 57.4 percent had detectable Ag by the acid-dissociated method.

As a diagnostic test, the p24 antigen assay has its greatest utility in people suspected of having acute or recent onset HIV infection. This is because in acute HIV infection there is a high level of viremia, measured as p24 antigenemia, despite the absence of HIV antibody [28, 29]. A patient with acute HIV infection will have detectable p24 Ag levels and be ELISA-negative, ELISA-positive/WB-negative, or indeterminate. Under these circumstances, the standard assay is generally adequate. Once antibodies to p24 Ag form, antibody-antigen complexes make p24 less easy to detect, and, in this setting, the acid-dissociated method may be more useful.

The role of p24 Ag as a surrogate marker of disease progression has been limited by the presence of high titers of p24 antibody and antibody-antigen complexes. This is especially true in asymptomatic HIV-infected patients with a small CD4 cell count decline, of whom only 3 to 10 percent will have detectable p24 Ag by the standard assay [25–27]. However, the reappearance of p24 Ag is associated with an increased risk of developing symptomatic disease [25].

HIV Culture

Detection of HIV in plasma was first reported in 1985 [30]. The virus is cultured by taking an infected person's plasma or peripheral blood mononuclear cells (PBMC) and coculturing them with stimulated PBMC from an HIV-seronegative donor in viral media. The supernatants of the cultures are then assayed weekly for the presence of p24 antigen by the standard p24 Ag ELISA. This provides a quantitative measure of viremia.

The sensitivity of HIV culture ranges from 10 to 100 percent, with nearly 100 percent specificity [6, 31]. However, the test is time-consuming, technically difficult, expensive, and currently available only in research settings.

HIV cultures are more frequently positive in patients with AIDS, and more than 25 percent with a positive viral culture will have a negative p24 Ag ELISA [30–33]. Baur and associates [32] studied a wide spectrum of HIV-infected patients to compare the sensitivity of p24 Ag ELISA and HIV culture. With more advanced disease, there was a significantly higher percentage of positive results for both assays [32]. In the healthiest individuals, p24 Ag and HIV culture were positive approximately 11 and 60 percent of the time, respectively; in contrast, in persons with clinically advanced disease, 59 and 100 percent of the tests were positive.

Polymerase Chain Reaction

Polymerase chain reaction (PCR) is a relatively new technique developed for in vitro amplification of the DNA or RNA of an organism [34]. PCR uses two primers that are complementary to the plus and minus strands of target DNA. With laboratory techniques of denaturization, renaturization, and elongation of the primers with a DNA polymerase, there is an exponential increase in the number of copies of the DNA region flanked by the primers [6]. This allows for the detection of as little as one copy of DNA or RNA.

In a prospective cohort study of 41 persons at risk for HIV infection in whom serial assays were performed, PCR detected virus in 97.6 percent of individuals at the time of their first positive HIV antibody test [35]. In contrast, viral culture was positive in only 65 percent of those studied. While PCR is a very sensitive test, it is prone to contamination with nucleic acids, resulting in false-positive reactions and decreased specificity. Given this limitation, the technical expertise required to perform the test, and its cost, PCR is presently available only as a research tool. The quantitative PCR assay for RNA appears promising as a means to monitor the viral load in HIV-infected patients [36].

Seroreversion

There have been a few unconfirmed reports in the medical literature describing patients who had apparently seroreverted; that is, they lost previously detectable antibodies to HIV-1. In an effort to address this issue, Roy and associates [37] examined the HIV database of the US Department of the Army, which had tested approximately 2.6 million people from 1985 to 1992, and found six potential seroreverters. By retrospective analysis of laboratory specimens and records, they demonstrated that indeed all six patients were infected with HIV. In five of the six patients, readily identifiable errors were responsible for the apparent seroreversion. They concluded that the true HIV seroreversion rate was very small and that obtaining a duplicate sample from persons who test seronegative following a positive study would eliminate most purported cases.

HIV-2 Testing

HIV-2 is a retrovirus that is antigenically similar to HIV-1 but has a different epidemiologic pattern. It is primarily seen in West Africa and parts of Europe and is spread heterosexually [38]. Only several dozen cases of HIV-2 infection have been reported to date in the United States.

There are currently two FDA-approved tests for diagnosing HIV-2 infection [7]. One is an HIV-2–specific ELISA, and the other is a combination HIV-1/HIV-2 ELISA. The latter test allows for simultaneous testing for HIV-1 and HIV-2, and, since June 1992, US blood banks have tested all donated whole blood, blood components, and source plasma for antibodies to both types of virus [38].

Both ELISAs have a sensitivity of greater than 99 percent, and HIV-2–specific WB, at this time only available as a research test, is necessary to confirm the presence of infection [38]. Each WB kit uses different viral antigens and therefore must be interpreted using criteria recommended by the manufacturer.

References

1. Berrios DC, et al. HIV antibody testing among those at risk for infection. *JAMA* 270:1576–1580, 1993.
2. Gostin LO. Public health strategies for confronting AIDS. Legislative and regulatory policy in the United States. (Published erratum appears in *JAMA* 263:950, 1990. See comments.) *JAMA* 261:1621–1630, 1989.
3. Benenson AS, Peddecord M, Hofherr LK, et al. Reporting the results of human immunodeficiency virus testing. *JAMA* 262:3435–3438, 1989.
4. Fauci AS. CD4+ T-lymphocytopenia without HIV infection: No lights, no camera, just facts. *N Engl J Med* 328:429–432, 1993.
5. Schindzielorz A. HIV-1 serology and AIDS testing: A practical approach to understanding. *South Med J* 82:1529–1533, 1989.
6. Bylund DJ, Ziegner UH, Hooper DG. Human immunodeficiency virus Western blot tests: Comparisons and considerations. *Ann Clin Lab Sci* 20:343–346, 1990.
7. FDA. FDA Licensed Retrovirus Test Kits, 1992.
8. Celum C, Coombs R, Jones M, et al. Risk factors for repeatedly reactive HIV-1 EIA and indeterminate Western blots. *Arch Intern Med* 154:1129–1137, 1994.
9. Steckelberg JM, Cockerill F, Cockerill FR. Update: Serologic testing for antibody to human immunodeficiency virus. *MMWR* 36:833–840, 1988.
10. Hsia J. False positive ELISA for human immunodeficiency virus after influenza vaccination. *J Infect Dis* 167:989–990, 1993.
11. MacKenzie W, David J, Petersen D, et al. Multiple false-positive serologic tests for HIV, HTLV-1, and hepatitis C following influenza vaccination, 1991. *JAMA* 268:1015–1017, 1992.
12. Horsburgh C, Ou CY, Lason J, et al. Duration of human immunodeficiency virus infection before detection of antibody. *Lancet* 2:637–640, 1989.
13. Connell JA, Parry JV, Mortimer PP, et al. Preliminary report: Accurate assays for anti-HIV in urine. *Lancet* 335:1366–1369, 1990.
14. Cao YZ, Friedman KA, Mirabile M, et al. HIV-1 neutralizing antibodies in urine from seropositive individuals. *J Acquir Immune Defic Syndr* 3:195–199, 1990.

15. Frerichs R, Eskes N, Htoon M. Validity of three assays for HIV-1 antibodies in saliva. *J Acquir Immune Defic Syndr* 7:522–525, 1994.
16. Bayer R, Stryker J, Smith MD. Testing for HIV infection at home. *N Engl J Med* 332:1296–1299, 1995.
17. Kingman S. Home HIV tests banned in Britain. *Br Med J* 304:864, 1992.
18. Centers for Disease Control. Update: Serologic testing for HIV-1 antibody—United States, 1988 and 1989. *MMWR* 39:380–383, 1990.
19. O'Gorman MR, Weber D, Landis SE, et al. Interpretive criteria of the Western blot assay for serodiagnosis of human immunodeficiency virus type 1 infection (Published erratum appears in *Arch Pathol Lab Med* 115:783, 1991) *Arch Pathol Lab Med* 115:26–30, 1991.
20. Centers for Disease Control. Interpretation and use of the Western blot assay for serodiagnosis of human immunodeficiency virus type 1 infections. *MMWR* 138:1–7, 1989.
21. Celum CL, Coombs RW. Indeterminate HIV-1 Western blots: Implications and considerations for widespread HIV testing. *J Gen Intern Med* 7:640–645, 1992.
22. Burke DS, Brundage JF, Redfield RR, et al. Serologic testing for human immunodeficiency virus antibodies. *Mayo Clin Proc* 63:373–380, 1988.
23. Celum CL, Coombs RW, Lafferty W, et al. Indeterminate human immunodeficiency virus type 1 Western blots: Seroconversion risk, specificity of supplemental tests, and an algorithm for evaluation. *J Infect Dis* 164:656–664, 1991.
24. Healey DS, Maskill WJ, Howard TS, et al. HIV-1 Western blot: Development and assessment of testing to resolve indeterminate reactivity. *AIDS* 6:629–633, 1992.
25. Ascher DP, Roberts C, Fowler A. Acidification modified p24 antigen capture assay in HIV seropositives. *J Acquir Immune Defic Syndr* 5:1080–1083, 1992.
26. Nishanian P, Huskins KR, Stehn S, et al. A simple method for improved assay demonstrates that HIV p24 antigen is present as immune complexes in most sera from HIV-infected individuals. *J Infect Dis* 162:21–28, 1990.
27. Bollinger RJ, Kline RL, Francis HL, et al. Acid dissociation increases the sensitivity of p24 antigen detection for the evaluation of antiviral therapy and disease progression in asymptomatic human immunodeficiency virus–infected persons. *J Infect Dis* 165:913–916, 1992.
28. Clark SJ, Saag MS, Decker WD, et al. High titers of cytopathic virus in plasma of patients with symptomatic primary HIV-1 infection. *N Engl J Med* 324:954–960, 1991.
29. Daar ES, Moudgil T, Meyer RD, Ho DD. Transient high levels of viremia in patients with primary human immunodeficiency virus type 1 infection. *N Engl J Med* 324:961–964, 1991.
30. Katzenstein DA, Holodniy M, Israelski DM, et al. Plasma viremia in human immunodeficiency virus infection: Relationship to stage of disease and antiviral treatment. *J Acquir Immune Defic Syndr* 5:107–112, 1992.
31. Ho DD, Moudgil T, Alam M. Quantitation of human immunodeficiency virus type 1 in the blood of infected persons. *N Engl J Med* 321:1621–1625, 1989.

32. Baur A, Vornhagen R, Korn K, et al. Viral culture and p24 antigenemia of human immunodeficiency virus (HIV)–infected individuals correlated with antibody profiles determined with recombinant polypeptides of all HIV-1 open-reading frames. *J Infect Dis* 165:419–426, 1992.
33. Coombs RW, Collier AC, Allain JP, et al. Plasma viremia in human immunodeficiency virus infection. *N Engl J Med* 321:1626–1631, 1989.
34. Schochetman G, Ou CY, Jones WK. Polymerase chain reaction. *J Infect Dis* 158:1154–1157, 1988.
35. Sheppard H, Busch M, Louie P, et al. HIV-1 PCR and isolation in seroconverting and seronegative homosexual men: Absence of long-term immunosilent infection. *J Acquir Immune Defic Syndr* 6:1339–1346, 1993.
36. Herman S, et al. Use of a quantitative PCR assay for measurement of HIV RNA in plasma during infection and seroconversion. Tenth International Conference on AIDS, Yokohama, August 1994.
37. Roy MJ, Damato JJ, Burke DS. Absence of true seroreversion of HIV-1 antibody in seroreactive individuals. *JAMA* 269:2876–2879, 1993.
38. Centers for Disease Control. Testing for antibodies to human immunodeficiency virus type 2 in the United States. *MMWR* 41:1–9, 1992.

Interpretation of Laboratory Studies

4

Abby Shevitz

As knowledge of HIV infection has increased, so has the availability and complexity of laboratory, radiologic, and invasive tests. Laboratory testing may be helpful in the management of HIV infection in a number of ways: (1) screening for common treatable processes, (2) staging and prognostication, (3) differential diagnosis, (4) supporting therapeutic decision, (5) monitoring disease progression, and (6) clinical research. The utility of laboratory testing is limited by cost, availability, technical skill, and diagnostic yield. The purpose of this chapter is to help the clinician interpret the results of laboratory studies used in the evaluation of HIV disease. Laboratory tests used in the initial assessment and health care maintenance of the HIV-infected patient are listed in Table 4-1.

Biochemistry and Urinalysis

Renal Function

Electrolytes and renal function often become abnormal in the course of HIV infection, especially at times of severe illness. Sodium wasting, physiologically appropriate water retention, or the syndrome of inappropriate antidiuretic hormone secretion associated with pulmonary or neurologic disease can induce hyponatremia. Potassium disorders can result from medications, intravascular volume disturbances, diarrhea, vomiting, or adrenal insufficiency. Abnormal magnesium, calcium, and phosphate values occur with renal disease, malnutrition, alcoholism, and medications (foscarnet, amphotericin B). Acute renal insufficiency occurs in 3 to 13 percent of all AIDS patients at some time during their illness and is usually associated with medications, volume deple-

Table 4-1 *Laboratory evaluation of the HIV-infected patient*

Initial
    Electrolytes
    Renal function tests
    Urinalysis
    Liver function tests
    Complete blood and differential counts
    CD4 cell count
    Glucose 6-phosphate dehydrogenase
    Syphilis serology
    Viral hepatitis screen
    Toxoplasmosis serology
    Purified protein derivative (PPD)/anergy panel
    Chest radiograph in injection drug users
    Rectal examination/stool test for occult blood
    Papanicolaou (Pap) smear in women
Health care maintenance
    Complete blood and differential counts
    Biochemistries (if indicated)
    CD4 cell count
    Syphilis serology
    PPD/anergy panel
    Stool test for occult blood
    Pap smear in women

tion, or sepsis [1–3]. Chronic renal failure generally is seen in injection drug users (IDUs) and blacks and associated with advanced HIV disease, but the severity of involvement and clinical course of renal insufficiency are more variable than originally reported [4].

Urinalysis often reveals abnormalities in HIV disease. Pyuria, microscopic hematuria, and urinary tract infection are common [1]. Although up to 50 percent of HIV-infected patients excrete over 500 mg protein in 24 hours, only 7 to 10 percent have nephrotic-range proteinuria [1–3, 5].

Hepatic Function

Although hepatic failure is unusual in AIDS, seen in 5 percent of cases, liver function tests (LFTs) become abnormal in 60 to 70 percent of patients sometime during the course of the disease [6]. Icterus is rare, and serum bilirubin usually remains normal. An increased bilirubin level has been associated with bacterial sepsis, chronic active hepatitis, and micronodular cirrhosis [7]. Serum transaminase levels often become abnormal but in no characteristic pattern. An increased alkaline phosphatase (ALP) is often a marker of serious disease. In several series, a serum ALP of greater than 200 units per liter with a normal bilirubin was present in almost every case of hepatic *Mycobacterium avium* complex (MAC) infection, cytomegalovirus (CMV) infection, histoplasmosis, drug toxicity, or Kaposi's sarcoma (KS) diagnosed by liver biopsy or at autopsy [6, 8, 9]. One study described very high values in the absence of clinical evidence of opportunistic infection or obstruction, but 4 of 5 persons were demonstrated on postmortem examination to have had hepatic MAC [10].

Hepatic involvement with lymphoma is usually reflected by increased ALP and bilirubin levels [7]. Sclerosing cholangitis, papillary stenosis, and bile duct strictures occur in patients with AIDS and usually present as severe right upper quadrant pain, fever, high ALP, normal bilirubin, and variable transaminases. Serum lactate dehydrogenase (LDH) level may be increased with other LFTs in hepatic disease or by itself in pulmonary disease (especially *Pneumocystis carinii* pneumonia [PCP]), central nervous system disorders, or lymphoma [8].

Serum albumin determination is useful in the evaluation of nutritional status, hepatic function, and renal protein wasting. A low albumin value carries a poor prognosis. Although total protein measurement usually reveals a large globulin fraction, this is rarely of clinical significance.

Endocrine Function

Endocrinologic testing is discussed only briefly here (see Chap. 16). While all endocrine glands may be affected in the course of HIV infection, the adrenal glands, pancreas, and testicles are those most frequently found to be involved at autopsy. Clinical endocrinopathy is infrequent [11]. Marked adrenal insufficiency is unusual; when it occurs, CMV infection is usually responsible. Impotence or decrease in libido may be due to testicular failure caused by infections (toxoplasmosis, *Mycobacterium tuberculosis*, CMV) or medications (ketoconazole, corticosteroids). Pancreatic disorders include asymptomatic infiltration (CMV, cryptosporidiosis, toxoplasmosis, KS, or lymphoma), and idiopathic, alcohol and drug-associated (intravenous pentamidine, didanosine, alcohol) pancreatitis. Sick euthyroid syndrome has also been described [11].

Hematology

Complete Blood Count with Differential

A complete blood count (CBC) with differential frequently reveals abnormalities such as neutropenia, anemia, and thrombocytopenia [12]. Thrombocytopenia may occur independently and at any stage of HIV infection, whereas anemia and neutropenia tend to present together and become more prevalent and severe with advancing disease [13]. Cytopenias result from primary HIV marrow suppression, peripheral destruction by antibodies, medications (zidovudine [ZDV], chemotherapeutic agents, ganciclovir, sulfonamides), or marrow invasion by my-cobacterial infection or lymphoma.

CD4 Lymphocyte Count

The CD4 lymphocyte count or percentage is the most commonly used surrogate marker for assessing the degree of immunodeficiency. The CD4 count should be obtained in the initial evaluation of all HIV-infected persons for staging purposes and rechecked at least every 6 to 12 months if it is greater than $500/mm^3$. If the count is lower, falling rapidly, or near a critical value, more frequent retesting is advised. Acute viral infections, such as herpes simplex or varicella-zoster, may transiently lower the CD4 count. While the effect of acute fungal, bacterial, and protozoal infections is less clear, CD4 counts are optimally obtained in the absence of acute illness.

When the CD4 count is less than $500/mm^3$, antiretroviral therapy may be indicated. In two studies, ZDV slowed progression to AIDS, improved CD4 cell counts, and decreased p24 antigen compared to placebo in persons with counts between 200 and $500/mm^3$ [14, 15]. However, results from the Concorde study indicated that ZDV given to patients with CD4 counts between 200 and $500/mm^3$ did not extend long-term survival, although progression to AIDS-related complex (ARC) and AIDS in the first 2 years was less frequent [16]. The therapeutic and prognostic implications of a CD4 count of less than $200/mm^3$ are much clearer, and this value is now an independent diagnostic criterion for AIDS [17]. Before the availability of ZDV, a CD4 cell count of less than $200/mm^3$ in a person without clinical criteria for AIDS indicated a 31 percent chance of development of AIDS within 1 year and an 87 percent chance in 3 years. The prognosis has since improved, presumably because of increased clinical experience and the widespread use of ZDV and PCP prophylaxis [18–20]. Survival of homosexual men with a CD4 cell count of $200/mm^3$ has lengthened from 28.4 months in the mid-1980s to 38 to 40 months in the late 1980s and early 1990s [21]. Opportunistic infections are most common for persons with CD4 cell counts of less than $200/mm^3$, and PCP prophylaxis is recommended [22]. CD4 counts of less than $50/mm^3$ in patients receiving ZDV are associated with a median survival of 12 months [23].

Other Surrogate Markers

p24 antigen (HIV viral core protein) measurements are not available in many clinical laboratories but may be prognostically useful [18]. β_2-microglobulin levels increase with disease progression. Initial studies revealed that a level of over 5 µg/ml predicted AIDS in 69 percent of patients over 3 years; no patients with values of 2.6 µg/ml or less developed AIDS at a mean of 2 years follow-up study [18, 24]. Immunoglobulin A (IgA), $ß_2$-microglobulin, and erythrocyte sedimentation rate were reported to contribute significantly to the prediction of the development of AIDS in patients with CD4 counts of less than 500/ mm^3 [25]. $ß_2$-microglobulin has been shown to be increased in injection drug users and, therefore, may not be a reliable surrogate marker in this population [26]. Quantitative methods, including p24 antigen measurement, viral culture, and polymerase chain reaction are becoming increasingly refined. Although their correlation with disease activity is better understood, they are expensive, have varying reliability because of limited experience, and are primarily research tools at this time [27, 28].

Glucose 6-Phosphate Dehydrogenase

Patients being considered for PCP prophylaxis or treatment with dapsone should be screened for glucose 6-phosphate dehydrogenase (G6PD) deficiency because of the risk of severe drug-induced hemolysis.

Erythropoietin

Serum erythropoietin levels in AIDS patients with anemia are often low, whether or not ZDV has been administered, and should be assayed to predict potential response to erythropoietin administration [13, 29]. Recombinant erythropoietin has been shown to significantly decrease transfusion dependence for persons receiving ZDV who have anemia and a serum erythropoietin level of less than 500 mU/ml [30].

Bone Marrow Examination

Bone marrow abnormalities occur throughout the course of HIV infection, even in the absence of opportunistic diseases [12, 31]. Hypocellularity is the most frequent finding associated with peripheral cytopenias. Dysplasia is common, as are atypical lymphocytic aggregates. Bone marrow aspirate/biopsy may reveal granulomas or organisms, or both, permitting a rapid presumptive diagnosis of disseminated fungal or mycobacterial disease. Isolator blood cultures, which are more sensitive and less invasive, are also useful in this setting [32, 33].

Serologies

Syphilis

Syphilis serologic testing should be performed routinely in all patients who are HIV infected or at risk for HIV infection. All persons who are rapid plasma reagin (RPR) and treponemal antibody positive should be encouraged to undergo HIV testing. Because neurosyphilis may be asymptomatic, some authorities advocate that all HIV-infected individuals with serologic evidence of syphilis should have lumbar puncture performed [34]. Most HIV-infected patients have a normal serologic response to syphilis infection, but some may have false-negative tests, and others may have extraordinarily high titers [35]. Close monitoring of HIV-infected patients with syphilis is essential because of the increased risk of treatment failure or relapse [34, 36]. Nontreponemal testing should be performed monthly for the first 3 months and at 3-month intervals thereafter [35].

Viral Hepatitis

The great majority (90%) of HIV-infected patients have serologic evidence of current or prior hepatitis B infection. Of all AIDS patients, 5 to 19 percent test positive for hepatitis B surface antigen (HBsAg), although chronic active hepatitis and cirrhosis are less common [6, 37]. At-risk HIV-infected persons who are negative for HBsAg and hepatitis B core antibody (HBcAb) should be offered hepatitis B vaccine. Antibody to hepatitis C is found in the majority of patients with non-A, non-B hepatitis, and chronic hepatitis is frequent [38]. Rates of hepatitis C in IDUs have been reported to be as high as 70 percent but are lower in homosexual men with HIV infection [39, 40].

Toxoplasmosis Serology

Toxoplasmosis has been reported to occur in 24 percent of AIDS patients who carry toxoplasmic antibodies at baseline but rarely in persons without them [41, 42]. The immunoglobulin G (IgG) antibody titer was initially thought to be almost always positive in patients with central nervous system (CNS) disease [43, 44]. However, a more recent study reports that about 20 percent of people with CNS toxoplasmosis have no detectable antibodies [45]. Serology can be used to identify those at greatest risk for toxoplasmosis who might benefit from prophylaxis with trimethoprim-sulfamethoxazole or other agents.

Cryptococcal Infection

Cryptococcal antigen level is almost always elevated in cerebrospinal fluid (CSF) from persons with cryptococcal meningitis [44]. Because of wide fluctuations, it is not as useful for determining prognosis nor for monitoring response to therapy. However, persistently high CSF titers are associated with an increased risk of relapse [46, 47].

Cytomegalovirus

While the majority of HIV-infected patients have a history of CMV infection, CMV serology may be useful as a screening test prior to blood transfusion. When possible, patients with HIV disease who are sero-negative for CMV should be given white blood cell–poor blood products in an effort to decrease the likelihood of acquiring new infection [48].

Pulmonary Studies

Purified Protein Derivative/Anergy Panel

As HIV-infected patients become progressively immunocompromised, they lose skin test reactivity to purified protein derivative (PPD) and control antigens [49]. Nonetheless, 20 to 30 percent of HIV-infected patients are PPD positive. These patients are more likely to develop active disease than are PPD-positive persons without HIV infection [50–52]. Intermediate-strength (5TU) PPD testing with a control panel should be performed in HIV-infected individuals as part of initial screening, and on a regular basis thereafter in those who test negative to detect PPD conversions or loss of skin test reactivity. Induration of 5 mm or more at 48 to 72 hours is significant in this population and requires preventive therapy with isoniazid for 12 months [52]. Anergic patients who are at high risk for tuberculosis (TB) exposure should also receive prophylaxis. A chest x-ray (CXR) should be performed on anergic and PPD-positive individuals to rule out active TB.

Chest Roentgenography

It is reasonable to obtain a baseline CXR in HIV-infected patients with a history of injection drug use so that comparison for subtle changes can be made in the event of new respiratory symptoms. PCP usually presents with an abnormal CXR, but up to 23 percent of radiographs are unremarkable [53]. In PCP, the CXR usually demonstrates bilateral perihilar infiltrates, which progress to a diffuse interstitial pattern and later to alveolar infiltrates or consolidation with air bronchograms [53–56]. The interstitial markings may be reticular or finely nodular [57]. Other less common presentations include apical infiltrates, unilateral or unilobar infiltrates, nodules greater than 10 mm, cavitary lesions, and pneumothorax [53, 54, 57–59]. In persons who have been receiving aerosol pentamidine, localized upper-lobe infiltrates may develop. As intrathoracic adenopathy is rare in PCP, this finding suggests other diseases, such as mycobacterial or cryptococcal infection, KS, or lymphoma [53, 54, 60, 61]. Pleural effusions are more likely to represent TB, KS, or bacterial or fungal infection than PCP [60, 61].

Pulmonary herpes simplex virus (HSV), CMV, nonspecific interstitial pneumonitis (NIP), and lymphocytic interstitial pneumonitis (LIP) usually present with a diffuse interstitial pattern on CXR indistinguishable from that of PCP [54, 61, 63]. MAC may show similar findings but has an upper-lobe predilection, associated intrathoracic adenopathy, and a coarsely nodular pattern [53]. Pulmonary TB usually appears as unilateral or bilateral middle- or lower-lobe infiltrates, sometimes with hilar or mediastinal adenopathy or pleural effusions. Coccidioidomycosis and histoplasmosis may be difficult to differentiate from other opportunistic infections, although calcifications and cavitation are frequent [64]. Cryptococcal infection presents with a nodular pattern, cavitation, adenopathy, and/or consolidation [53]. In evaluating pulmonary symptoms and signs, it is important to remember that often more than one pathogen is present; for example, up to 27 percent of patients with PCP have coexistent infections [53, 55, 62, 65]. Pulmonary KS may not be evident on CXR, but generally presents as large nodules, cavities, or a pleural effusion. Lymphoma may cause an interstitial pattern, intrathoracic adenopathy, mass effect, or pleural effusion [54, 56].

Arterial Blood Gases

In addition to CXR, arterial blood gases are an essential first step in the evaluation of respiratory symptoms in an HIV-infected individual. Because a change in the alveolar-arterial oxygen gradient is an important early indicator of pulmonary disease, patients with a history of smoking or chronic lung disease should have a baseline blood gas analysis performed. Of patients with active PCP, 8 to 25 percent have normal blood gases [62, 66].

Gallium and Thallium Scans

Gallium-67 citrate scanning is 95 percent sensitive for PCP, and, when lung uptake is equal to or greater than hepatic uptake, specificity approaches 90 percent [66–69]. Because the predictive value of a positive scan is so high (85–95%), it may be useful in determining the need for bronchoscopic lavage in individuals with respiratory symptoms but a normal CXR and negative induced sputum. Gallium scanning may also be helpful in diagnosing recurrent PCP. Nodal gallium uptake suggests MAC, TB, lymphoma, toxoplasmosis, or generalized lymphadenopathy [70, 71].

Gallium scanning is negative in KS, whether pulmonary, nodal, cutaneous, or visceral [67, 72]. Thallium-201 scintigraphy, however, may detect KS of the skin, mucous membranes, nodes, and viscera [73]. Therefore, nodal and pulmonary lesions that are gallium negative but thallium avid generally represent KS.

Sputum Analysis

Sputum Gram's stain, acid-fast stain, and cultures should be performed on all HIV-infected patients with pneumonia. Many centers now have the capability to induce and evaluate sputum specimens for PCP by direct fluorescent antibody staining, but the sensitivity of this technique is variable [74, 75]. Even in experienced hands, the diagnostic yield of sputum induction is somewhat less than that of bronchoalveolar lavage [76]. A positive sputum sample is indicative of PCP, but a negative examination does not exclude the diagnosis.

Bronchoscopy

While the diagnosis of PCP is sometimes made presumptively, and, increasingly, on the basis of induced sputum examination, bronchoscopy still has an important role. Bronchoalveolar lavage is diagnostic in 80 to 90 percent of patients with PCP, but, when performed on lobar or segmental bronchi or with biopsy, the yield approaches 95 to 100 percent [77, 78]. Patients with atypical CXR features or inadequate response to empiric PCP therapy may require bronchoscopy to identify or rule out other pathogens. The yield of bronchoscopic biopsy for TB or MAC is approximately 80 percent [69, 76]. Although KS lesions may be visible on bronchoscopy, biopsy yield is only 8 percent, whereas that of open thoracotomy is greater than 90 percent [77]. A diagnosis of NIP, LIP, or lymphoma may be supported by bronchoscopy, but open thoracotomy is sometimes necessary. Thus, bronchoscopy is optimally used to diagnose first episodes of PCP when reliable examination of induced sputum is unavailable or negative, and to determine the cause of an atypical CXR appearance or of poor response to empiric antimicrobial therapy.

Gastrointestinal and Hepatic Studies

Rectal Examination/Stool Occult Blood Test

Because of the increased risk of gastrointestinal KS and squamous cell carcinoma of the rectum in HIV-infected homosexual men, periodic rectal examinations and stool testing for occult blood are indicated.

Stool Studies

For evaluation of diarrhea, stool specimens should be cultured for bacterial pathogens and examined for ova and parasites. In advanced HIV disease, a modified acid-fast stain should also be performed to look for evidence of cryptosporidiosis or isosporiasis. Detection of *Microsporidia* in stool requires modified trichrome, chromotrope, or chitin-specific staining and highly trained laboratory personnel. Patients who have recently received antibiotic therapy should have a *Clostridium difficile* titer assay performed.

Upper and Lower Endoscopy

Esophageal candidiasis can be diagnosed presumptively if thrush is present in association with odynophagia or retrosternal pain with swallowing. If there is no response to empiric antifungal therapy, upper endoscopy is necessary for differentiation from CMV or HSV infection. The stomach is the least commonly involved portion of the gastrointestinal tract in AIDS, but KS, lymphoma, CMV, cryptosporidiosis, and occasionally MAC and TB may be found [72]. Biopsy of the small intestine may reveal the causative organism in patients with diarrhea. Alternatively, there may be diffuse cellular changes suggesting primary HIV enteropathy without other identifiable pathogens. Stool cultures and sigmoidoscopy with biopsy may be useful in investigating diarrhea in patients who are severely immunocompromised [79].

Liver Biopsy

Liver function test results are frequently abnormal in the AIDS population, and liver biopsy may be indicated on occasion. Biopsy sometimes reveals fulminant hepatitis or cirrhosis, but opportunistic diseases and biliary tract abnormalities may also be identified. MAC is the most common opportunistic infection involving the liver [9]. In 60 percent or more of cases, the organism is also present in other tissues, and the sensitivity of isolator blood cultures is very high, reducing the need for liver biopsy [6, 7, 35]. Patients generally have hepatomegaly and fever, significantly increased ALP, and normal bilirubin and coagulation studies [6–9]. Disseminated CMV involves the liver in 40 percent of cases and presents much like MAC [6]. Other less common causes of a high ALP with normal bilirubin include TB, histoplasmosis, coccidioidomycosis, cryptococcosis, and granulomatous drug reactions. Kaposi's sarcoma is associated with a similar LFT pattern but is rarely identifiable on biopsy. Cutaneous lesions are usually present in persons with hepatic KS [6, 7, 9]. Hepatic lymphoma is occasionally diagnosed by biopsy and can be visualized as a mass on abdominal computed tomographic (CT) scan or ultrasound. Alkaline phosphatase and bilirubin levels are generally increased [7].

Endoscopic Retrograde Cholangiopancreatography

Sclerosing cholangitis, papillary stenosis, and bile duct strictures are characterized by the same LFT pattern described for MAC but present with upper quadrant abdominal pain [80]. Abdominal radiologic studies may suggest these diagnoses, but endoscopic retrograde cholangiopancreatography (ERCP), liver biopsy, or both, are necessary for confirmation.

Neurologic Studies

Computed Tomography and Magnetic Resonance Imaging

Computed tomography and magnetic resonance imaging (MRI) of the brain are essential parts of the evaluation of the HIV-infected patient with new CNS symptoms. The most common radiologic abnormality in HIV-infected patients with neurologic symptoms is atrophy [45, 81]. A study of MRI scans performed on neurologically asymptomatic HIV-positive and HIV-negative homosexual men found similar prevalence of ventricular and sulcal enlargement as well as abnormal punctate areas [82]. The presence and size of these abnormalities could not be correlated with the severity of immunodeficiency, alcohol or drug use, or results of neuropsychological testing. On the other hand, a review of CT scans ordered from the emergency room for patients with neurologic symptoms and HIV infection or risk factors for HIV infection revealed that 21 percent had focal lesions. Abnormal findings were most common in patients with focal neurologic examinations or altered mental status, but were also present in 16 percent of those without localized complaints or findings [83].

Single or multiple contrast-enhancing nodules or rings in the white matter, corticomedullary junction, or basal ganglia are most commonly caused by toxoplasmosis [56, 84]. There is often mass effect and edema. Lesions usually show improvement after 10 to 14 days of therapy, with resolution occurring in 10 days to 6 months, but calcifications may persist [56, 84, 85]. Mycobacterial, fungal, and bacterial abscesses, as well as lymphoma, may also occasionally cause ring-enhancing lesions on head CT [86]. Lymphomatous lesions may be deeper, periventricular, or demonstrate irregular or meningeal enhancement [86, 87]. Cryptococcal infection and CMV cause nonspecific CT abnormalities [85]. Herpes simplex virus encephalitis may show unilateral or reduced attenuation in the temporal lobes [86]. Progressive multifocal leukoencephalopathy (PML) appears as low-density areas in white matter without mass effect or contrast enhancement [85, 87]. Magnetic resonance imaging is more sensitive for toxoplasmosis and PML, making this the preferred study when available [88].

Lumbar Puncture

Among asymptomatic HIV-infected persons who have CD4 lymphocyte counts over 400/mm³, 25 to 30 percent have a CSF white cell count of greater than 10/mm³, 6 to 8 percent have a CSF protein greater than 55 mg/dl, and 5 to 10 percent have a low CSF glucose level [89]. With more advanced stages of the disease, neurologically asymptomatic individuals more often have a high protein, but the other changes in CSF profile are less clearly correlated. In acute aseptic meningitis associated with primary HIV infection, lumbar puncture usually reveals mononuclear pleocytosis, low CSF glucose, and high CSF protein [44]. Three-fourths of people with HIV encephalopathy have an abnormal lumbar puncture, usually showing mild mononuclear pleocytosis, hypoglycorrhachia, and increased protein level of 50 to 100 mg/dl [44, 81, 87]. Demyelinating radiculopathy, mononeuropathy multiplex, and progressive radiculopathy are associated with a variety of abnormal CSF findings, whereas symmetric peripheral neuropathy is not [90].

Cryptococcal meningitis is characterized by CSF pleocytosis in 35 percent of patients, elevated CSF protein in 69 percent, and positive cryptococcal antigen in nearly 100 percent. India ink preparation reveals the fungus in 82 percent of cases, and fungal cultures are always positive [44]. In toxoplasmosis, the CSF protein level is often increased, but other findings are variable. Less common infections potentially diagnosed by CSF analysis include aspergillosis, coccidiodomycosis, histoplasmosis, candidiasis, TB, MAC, and bacterial meningitis [91]. A normal CSF is common with lymphoma, but occasionally mild pleocytosis, increased protein, or suspicious cytology may be present [44, 87].

Although symptomatic neurosyphilis remains unusual in HIV-infected persons, syphilis may progress more rapidly with early neurologic involvement [34, 43, 44]. Therefore, a syphilis serology should be obtained on all CSF specimens, and lumbar puncture considered in all HIV-infected persons who are RPR and treponemal antibody positive. Any CSF abnormality in this context should be interpreted as being indicative of possible neurosyphilis.

Neuropsychological Testing

HIV-infected patients without acute medical illness or evidence of neurologic disease frequently demonstrate subtle abnormalities on formal neuropsychological testing. Twelve percent of asymptomatic persons demonstrate significant impairments [88, 92]. Common abnormalities include slow information processing, impaired problem solving, visuospatial difficulty, poor abstraction ability, and impaired fine motor control and speed. A clinical diagnosis of HIV dementia is based on findings of psychomotor slowing, forgetfulness, personality change, and decreased knowledge acquisition. Whereas formal neuro-psychological testing will reliably identify these abnormalities, the "mini-mental status examination" is much less sensitive [44]. Confirming the diagnosis of HIV dementia/encephalopathy is important as a qualifying criterion for AIDS and because symptoms may improve in response to high-dose ZDV therapy [93, 94].

Tissue Biopsy

Skin

Dermatologic lesions are extremely common in HIV-infected patients. Viral, fungal, bacterial, parasitic, drug-related, malignant, and idio-pathic conditions have been described. Therefore, biopsy with special stains and cultures is often necessary for lesions that are unusual in appearance or do not respond to empiric therapy. Because syphilis serologies may be falsely negative, lesions suggestive of this diagnosis should be biopsied. Although the diagnosis of KS may be made presumptively by experienced clinicians, a decision to treat patients with chemotherapy or radiation therapy should generally be based on skin biopsy results.

Lymph Node

Because persistent generalized lymphadenopathy representing follicu-lar hyperplasia is commonly associated with HIV infection, it is not necessary to biopsy all persons with enlarged nodes. However, many other processes, including syphilis, TB, toxoplasmosis, lymphoma, and KS, may also cause adenopathy. Biopsy is appropriate for nodes that are asymmetric, rapidly growing, or associated with constitutional symptoms or cytopenia [95].

Pelvic Examination/Papanicolaou Smear

Regular pelvic examination and Pap smear are important in HIV-in-fected women because of their high rate of cervical dysplasia [96–98]. The Centers for Disease Control recommends that HIV-infected women have annual Pap smears, assuming this yields adequate cytology [98]. Some clinicians perform routine Pap smears twice a year. More frequent pelvic examinations may be necessary because of the high incidence of vaginal candidiasis, pelvic inflammatory disease, and genital ulcer disease [99–102].

References

1. Kaplan MS, Wechsler M, Benson MC. Urologic manifestations of AIDS. *Urology* 30:441–443, 1987.
2. Rao TK, Friedman EA, Nicastri AD. The types of renal disease in the acquired immunodeficiency syndrome. *N Engl J Med* 316:1062–1068, 1987.
3. Pardo V, et al. Glomerular lesions in the acquired immunodeficiency syndrome. *Ann Intern Med* 101:429–434, 1984.
4. Mazbar SA, et al. Renal involvement in patients infected with HIV: Experience at San Francisco General Hospital. *Kidney Int* 37:1325–1332, 1990.
5. Rao TK, et al. Associated focal and segmental glomerulosclerosis in the acquired immunodeficiency syndrome. *N Engl J Med* 310:669–673, 1984.
6. Glasgow BJ, et al. Clinical and pathologic findings of the liver in the acquired immunodeficiency syndrome (AIDS). *Am J Clin Pathol* 83:582–588, 1985.
7. Schneiderman DJ, et al. Hepatic disease in patients with the acquired immunodeficiency syndrome (AIDS). *Hepatology* 7: 925–930, 1987.
8. Kahn SA, et al. Hepatic disorders in the acquired immunodeficiency syndrome: A clinical and pathological study. *Am J Gastroenterol* 81:1145–1148, 1986.
9. Rodgers VD, Kagnoff MF. Acquired immunodeficiency syndrome and disease of the gastrointestinal tract. *Immunol Allergy Clin North Am* 8:451–467, 1988.
10. Payne TH, et al. Marked elevations of serum alkaline phosphatase in patients with AIDS. *J Acquir Immune Defic Syndr* 4:238–243, 1991.
11. Aron DC. Endocrine complications of the acquired immunodeficiency syndrome. *Arch Intern Med* 149:330–333, 1989.
12. Zon LI, Arkin C, Groopman JE. Hematologic manifestations of the human immune deficiency virus (HIV). *Br J Haematol* 66:251–256, 1987.
13, Doweiko JP. Hematologic aspects of HIV infection. *AIDS* 7:753–775, 1993.
14. Fischl MA, et al. The safety and efficacy of zidovudine (AZT) in the treatment of subjects with mildly symptomatic human immunodeficiency virus type 1 (HIV) infection. *Ann Intern Med* 112:727–737, 1990.
15. Volberding PA, et al. Zidovudine in asymptomatic human immunodeficiency virus infection. *N Engl J Med* 322:942–949, 1990.
16. Concorde Coordinating Committee. Concorde: MRC/ANRS randomised double-blind controlled trial of immediate and deferred zidovudine in symptom-free HIV infection. *Lancet* 343:871–881, 1994.
17. Centers for Disease Control. 1993 revised classification system for HIV infection and expanded surveillance case definition for AIDS among adolescents and adults. *MMWR* 41(RR-17):1–19, 1992.
18. Moss AR, Bacchetti P, Osmond D, et al. Seropositivity for HIV and the development of AIDS or AIDS related condition: Three year follow up of the San Francisco General Hospital cohort. *Br Med J* 296:745–750, 1988.
19. Kaplan JE, Spira TJ, Fishbein DB, et al. A six-year follow-up of HIV-infected homosexual men with lymphadenopathy: Evidence for an increased risk for developing AIDS after the third year of lymphadenopathy. *JAMA* 260:2694–2697, 1988.

20. Creagh-Kirk T, Doi P, Andrews E, et al. Survival experience among patients with AIDS receiving zidovudine. *JAMA* 260:3009–3015, 1988.
21. Osmond D, et al. Changes in AIDS survival time in two San Francisco cohorts of homosexual men, 1983 to 1993. *JAMA* 271:1083–1087, 1994.
22. Centers for Disease Control. Recommendations for prophylaxis against *Pneumocystis carinii* pneumonia for adults and adolescents infected with human immunodeficiency virus. *MMWR* 41 (RR-4):1–11, 1992.
23. Yarchoan R, et al. CD4 count and the risk for death in patients infected with HIV receiving antiretroviral therapy. *Ann Intern Med* 155:184–189, 1991.
24. Morfeldt-Manson J, et al. Elevated serum beta-2-microglobulin—a prognostic marker for development of AIDS among patients with persistent generalized lymphadenopathy. *Infection* 16:109–110, 1988.
25. Schwarlander B, et al. Improvement of the predictive value of CD4+ lymphocyte count by beta-2-microglobulin, immunoglobulin A and erythrocyte sedimentation rate. *AIDS* 7:753–775, 1993.
26. Flegg PJ, et al. Beta-2-microglobulin levels in drug users: The influence of risk behaviour. *AIDS* 5:1021–1024, 1991.
27. Schnittman SM, et al. Increasing viral burden in CD4-positive T cells from patients with HIV infection reflects rapidly progressive immunosuppression and clinical disease. *Ann Intern Med* 113:438–443, 1990.
28. Schleupner CJ. Diagnostic Tests for HIV-1 Infection. In GL Mandell, RG Douglas, JE Bennett (eds), *Principles and Practice of Infectious Diseases.* New York: Churchill Livingstone, 1990. Pp 1092–1102.
29. Rarick MU, et al. Serum erythropoietin titers in patients with human immunodeficiency virus (HIV) infection and anemia. *J Acquir Immune Defic Syndr* 4:593–597, 1991.
30. Fischl M, et al. Recombinant human erythropoietin for patients with AIDS treated with zidovudine. *N Engl J Med* 322:1488, 1990.
31. Spivak JL, et al. Hematologic abnormalities in the acquired immunodeficiency syndrome. *Am J Med* 77:224–228, 1984.
32. Norfelt DW, et al. The usefulness of diagnostic bone marrow examination in patients with human immunodeficiency virus (HIV) infection. *J Acquir Immune Defic Syndr* 4:659–666, 1991.
33. Young LS, et al. Mycobacterial infections in AIDS patients, with an emphasis on the *Mycobacterium avium* complex. *Rev Infect Dis* 8:1024–1033, 1986.
34. Johns DR, Tierney M, Felsenstein D. Alteration in the natural history of neurosyphilis by concurrent infection with the human immunodeficiency virus. *N Engl J Med 316*:1569–1572, 1987.
35. Centers for Disease Control. Recommendations for diagnosing and treating syphilis in HIV-infected patients. *MMWR* 37:600-608, 1988.
36. Berry CD, et al. Neurologic relapse after benzathine penicillin therapy for secondary syphilis in a patient with HIV infection. *N Engl J Med* 316:1587–1590, 1987.
37. Lebovics, E, et al. The hepatobiliary manifestations of human immunodeficiency virus infection. *Am J Gastroenterol* 83:1–7, 1988.
38. Alter HJ, et al. Detection of antibody to hepatitis C virus in prospectively

followed transfusion recipients with acute and chronic non-A, non-B hepatitis. *N Engl J Med* 321:1494–1500, 1989.

39. Tor J, et al. Sexual transmission of hepatitis C virus and its relation with hepatitis B virus and HIV. *Br Med J* 301:1130–1133, 1990.

40. Esteban JL, et al. Hepatitis C virus antibodies among risk groups in Spain. *Lancet* 2:295–297, 1989.

41. Grant IH, et al. *Toxoplasma gondii* serology in HIV-infected patients: The development of central nervous system toxoplasmosis in AIDS. *AIDS* 4:519–521, 1990.

42. Luft BJ, Remington JS. Toxoplasmic encephalitis. *J Infect Dis* 157:1–6, 1988.

43. Levy RM, et al. Neurological manifestations of the acquired immunodeficiency syndrome (AIDS): Experience at UCSF and review of the literature. *J Neurosurg* 62:475–495, 1985.

44. McArthur JC. Neurologic manifestations of AIDS. *Medicine (Baltimore)* 66:407–437, 1987.

45. Porter SB, Sande MA. Toxoplasmosis of the central nervous system in the acquired immunodeficiency syndrome. *N Engl J Med* 327:1643–1648, 1992.

46. Kovacs JA, et al. Cryptococcosis in the acquired immunodeficiency syndrome. *Ann Intern Med* 103:533–538, 1985.

47. Zuger A, et al. Cryptococcal disease in patients with the acquired immunodeficiency syndrome: Diagnostic features and outcome of therapy. *Ann Intern Med* 104:234–240, 1985.

48. Rabkin CS, et al. Cytomegalovirus infection and the risk of AIDS in human immunodeficiency virus-infected hemophilia patients. *J Infect Dis* 168:1260–1263, 1993.

49. Markowitz N, et al. Tuberculin and anergy testing in HIV-seropositive and HIV-seronegative persons. *Ann Intern Med* 119:185–193, 1993.

50. Stoneburner RL, et al. Tuberculosis and acquired immunodeficiency syndrome—New York City. *MMWR* 36:785–795, 1987.

51. Selwyn PA, et al. A prospective study of the risk of tuberculosis among intravenous drug users with human immunodeficiency virus infection. *N Engl J Med* 320:545–550, 1989.

52. Centers for Disease Control. Tuberculosis and human immunodeficiency virus infection: Recommendations of the Advisory Committee for the Elimination of Tuberculosis (ACET). *MMWR* 38:236–250, 1989.

53. Suster B, et al. Pulmonary manifestations of AIDS: Review of 106 episodes. *Radiology* 161:87–93, 1986.

54. Cohen BA, et al. Pulmonary complications of AIDS: Radiologic features. *Am J Radiol* 143:115–122, 1984.

55. McCauley DI, et al. Radiographic patterns of opportunistic lung infections and Kaposi sarcoma in homosexual men. *Am J Radiol* 139:653–658, 1982.

56. Barter S. Radiological features of AIDS. *Clin Immunol Allergy* 6:601–625, 1986.

57. DeLorenzo LJ, et al. Roentgenographic patterns of *Pneumocystis carinii* pneumonia in 104 patients with AIDS. *Chest* 91:323–327, 1987.

58. Milligan SA, et al. *Pneumocystis carinii* pneumonia radiographically simulating tuberculosis. *Am Rev Respir Dis* 132:1124–1126, 1985.

59. Barrio JL, et al. *Pneumocystis carinii* pneumonia presenting as cavitating

and noncavitating solitary pulmonary nodules in patients with the acquired immunodeficiency syndrome. *Am Rev Respir Dis* 134:1094–1096, 1986.

60. Afessa B, et al. *Pneumocystis carinii* pneumonia complicated by lymphadenopathy and pneumothorax. *Arch Intern Med* 148:2651–2654, 1988.

61. Freico MH, Chinoy-Acharya P. Lymphocytic interstitial pneumonia associated with the acquired immune deficiency syndrome. *Am Rev Respir Dis* 131:952–955, 1985.

62. Stover DE, et al. Spectrum of pulmonary diseases associated with the acquired immune deficiency syndrome. *Am J Med* 78:429–437, 1985.

63. Morris JC, et al. Lymphocytic interstitial pneumonia in patients at risk for the acquired immune deficiency syndrome. *Chest* 91:63–67, 1987.

64. Goodman PC, Gamsu G. Radiographic findings in the acquired immunodeficiency syndrome. *Postgrad Radiol* 7:3–15, 1987.

65. Simmons JT, et al. Nonspecific interstitial pneumonitis in patients with AIDS: Radiologic features. *Am J Radiol* 149:265–268, 1987.

66. Murray JF, et al. Pulmonary complications of the acquired immune deficiency syndrome. *N Engl J Med* 310:1682–1688, 1984.

67. Woolfenden JM, et al. Acquired immunodeficiency syndrome: Ga-67 citrate imaging. *Radiology* 162:383–387, 1987.

68. Kramer EL, et al. Diagnostic implications of Ga-67 chest-scan patterns in human immunodeficiency virus-positive patients. *Radiology* 170:671–676, 1989.

69. Tuazon CU, et al. Utility of gallium-67 scintigraphy and bronchial washings in the diagnosis and treatment of *Pneumocystis carinii* pneumonia in patients with the acquired immune deficiency syndrome. *Am Rev Respir Dis* 132:1087–1092, 1985.

70. Kramer EL, et al. Gallium-67 scans of the chest in patients with acquired immunodeficiency syndrome. *J Nucl Med* 28:1107–1114, 1987.

71. Bekerman C, Bitran J. Gallium-67 scanning in the clinical evaluation of human immunodeficiency virus infection: Indications and limitations. *Semin Nucl Med* 17:273–276, 1988.

72. Megibow AJ, Balthazar EJ, Hulnick DH. Radiology of nonneoplastic gastrointestinal disorders in acquired immune deficiency syndrome. *Semin Roentgenol* 22:31–41, 1987.

73. Lee VW, et al. AIDS-related Kaposi sarcoma: Findings on thallium-201 scintigraphy. *Am J Radiol* 151:1233–1235, 1988.

74. Kovacs JA, Ng VL, Masur H et al. Diagnosis of *Pneumocystis carinii* pneumonia: Improved detection in sputum with use of monoclonal antibodies. *N Engl J Med* 318:589–593, 1988.

75. Pitchenik AE, Ganjei P, Torres A, et al. Sputum examination for the diagnosis of *Pneumocystis carinii* pneumonia in the acquired immune deficiency syndrome. *Am Rev Respir Dis* 133:226–229, 1986.

76. Miller RF, et al. Sputum induction for the diagnosis of pulmonary disease in HIV positive patients. *J Infection* 23:5–15, 1991.

77. Murray JF, et al. Pulmonary complications of the acquired immunodeficiency syndrome: Report of a National Heart, Lung, and Blood Institute workshop. *N Engl J Med* 310:1682–1688, 1984.

78. Ognibene FP, et al. The diagnosis of *Pneumocystis carinii* pneumonia in patients with the acquired immunodeficiency syndrome using subsegmental bronchoalveolar lavage. *Am Rev Respir Dis* 129:929–932, 1984.
79. Gazzard BG, HIV disease and the gastroenterologist. *Gut* 29:1497–1505, 1988.
80. Cello JP. Acquired immunodeficiency syndrome cholangiopathy: Spectrum of disease. *Am J Med* 86:539–546, 1989.
81. Navia BA, Price RW. The acquired immunodeficiency syndrome dementia complex as the presenting or sole manifestation of human immunodeficiency virus infection. *Arch Neurol* 44:65–69, 1987.
82. Cohen WA, et al. Prospective cerebral MR study of HIV seropositive and seronegative men: Correlation of MR findings with neurologic, neuropsychologic, and cerebrospinal fluid analysis. *AJNR* 13:1231–1240, 1992.
83. Tso EL, et al. Cranial computed tomography in the emergency department evaluation of HIV-infected patients with neurologic complaints. *Ann Emerg Med* 22:1169–1176, 1993.
84. Levy RM, Rosenbloom S, Perrett LV. Neuroradiologic findings in AIDS: A review of 200 cases. *Am J Radiol* 147:977–983, 1986.
85. Elkin CM, et al. Intracranial lesions in the acquired immunodeficiency syndrome: Radiological (computed tomographic) features. *JAMA* 253:393–396, 1985.
86. Sze G, et al. The neuroradiology of AIDS. *Semin Roentgenol* 22:42–53, 1987.
87. Snider WD, et al. Neurological complications of acquired immune deficiency syndrome: Analysis of 50 patients. *Ann Neurol* 14:403–418, 1983.
88. Grant I, et al. Evidence for early central nervous system involvement in the acquired immunodeficiency syndrome (AIDS) and other human immunodeficiency virus (HIV) infections: Studies with neuropsychologic testing and magnetic resonance imaging. *Ann Intern Med* 107:828–836, 1987.
89. Marshall DW, et al. Spectrum of cerebrospinal fluid findings in various stages of human immunodeficiency virus infection. *Arch Neurol* 45:954–958, 1988.
90. Bredesen DE, et al. Human Immunodeficiency Virus Related Neurological Dysfunction. In MJ Aminoff (ed), *Neurology and General Medicine*, New York: Churchill Livingstone, 1989, Pp 673–689.
91. Elder GA, Sever JL. Neurologic disorders associated with AIDS retroviral infection. *Rev Infect Dis* 10:286–302, 1988.
92. Tross S, et al. Neuropsychological characterization of the AIDS dementia complex: A preliminary report. *AIDS* 2:81–88, 1988.
93. Yarchoan R, et al. Response of human immunodeficiency-virus-associated neurological disease to 3'-azido-3'-deoxythymidine. *Lancet* 1:132–135, 1987.
94. Schmitt FA, et al. Neuropsychological outcome of zidovudine (AZT) treatment of patients with AIDS and AIDS-related complex. *N Engl J Med* 319:1573–1578, 1988.
95. Abrams DI. AIDS-related lymphadenopathy: The role of biopsy. *J Clin Oncol* 4:126–127, 1986.
96. Maiman M, et al. Colposcopic evaluation of human immunodeficiency virus seropositive women. *Obstet Gynecol* 78:84–88, 1991.

97. Maiman M, et al. Human immunodeficiency virus and cervical neoplasia. *Gynecol Obstet* 38:377–382, 1990.
98. Centers for Disease Control. Risk for cervical disease in HIV infected women—New York City. *MMWR* 39:846–849, 1990.
99. Minkoff HL, DeHovitz JA. Care of women infected with the human immunodeficiency virus. *JAMA* 266:2253–2258, 1991.
100. Rhoads JL, et al. Chronic vaginal candidiasis in women with human immunodeficiency virus infection. *JAMA* 257:3105–3107, 1987.
101. Imam W, et al. Hierarchical pattern of mucosal candida infections in HIV seropositive women. *Am J Med* 89:142–146, 1990.
102. Hoegsberg B, et al. Sexually transmitted diseases and human immunodeficiency virus infection among women with pelvic inflammatory diseases. *Am J Obstet Gynecol* 163:1135–1139, 1990.

Clinical Syndromes

II

Fever

5

Lawrence M. Barat, Thomas W. Barber, Robert A. Witzburg

The clinician confronted with a febrile HIV-infected patient may feel overwhelmed by the potentially large differential diagnosis. A rational approach to fever in this population requires an understanding of the patient's presenting symptoms and signs in the context of his or her stage of HIV disease. A systematic search for both infectious and non-infectious etiologies is warranted for all episodes of fever.

Fever and the Natural History of HIV Disease

A self-limited febrile illness associated with seroconversion is often the first clinical manifestation of HIV infection (Table 5-1). This syndrome (Centers for Disease Control [CDC] category A1: primary HIV infection) usually occurs 8 to 12 weeks after exposure to HIV and has been well characterized [1–4]. It may present as a "mononucleosis-like" syndrome consisting of fever, constitutional symptoms, sore throat, diffuse lymphadenopathy, headache, diarrhea, and a maculopapular rash involving the trunk. Symptoms generally last 2 to 3 weeks. In some patients, seroconversion is associated with an acute, transient meningoencephalitis or peripheral neuropathy, or both. Primary HIV infection may also be asymptomatic or present as a nonspecific viral syndrome.

The progression of HIV disease after seroconversion is variable, but the patient generally remains asymptomatic for an extended period (CDC categories, A1, A2, A3: asymptomatic infection or persistent generalized lymphadenopathy). Despite the lack of clinical illness during these years, HIV continues to proliferate, resulting in damage to the immune system and a progressive decline in the CD4 lymphocyte count [5]. By definition, opportunistic infections do not occur during this period, but infections with conventional viral and bacterial pathogens may cause febrile illness [6].

Fever associated with recurrent conventional bacterial infection may be an early manifestation of HIV disease. Pneumonia, sinusitis, and skin infections are seen most frequently. The onset of symptomatic HIV disease is usually heralded by high-grade viremia, which may be associated with intermittent fevers, generalized lymphadenopathy, diarrhea, and weight loss. Previously described as AIDS-related complex (ARC), the CDC now classifies it as clinical category B. Febrile illnesses occur commonly as patients progress to CDC category C, and causes include opportunistic infections, neoplastic diseases, and other manifestations diagnostic of AIDS. Fever during advanced HIV disease may be multifactorial and requires careful evaluation.

Table 5-1 *Fever and the natural history of HIV disease*

CDC clinical category	Immune status	Causes of fever
A1	Acute illness: +p24 antigen, lymphopenia Recovery: +HIV antibody; decreased CD4:CD8 ratio	Acute HIV infection: "mononucleosis-like syndrome"
A1, A2, A3	Variable: normal → lymphopenia with decreased CD4:CD8 ratio	Fever not characteristic
B1, B2, B3	Variable: lymphopenia with decreased CD4:CD8 ratio; increased immuno-globulins; impaired humoral immunity	Increased frequency of common bacterial infections, viral infections (HSV, VZV), and tuberculosis
C1, C2, C3	Variable: lymphopenia with decreased CD4:CD8 ratio; anergy to skin tests; increased immuno-globulins; increased immune complexes; increased p24 antigen; increased β_2-microglobulin	All of above listed under category B, plus opportunistic infections (PCP, cryptococcosis, toxoplasmosis, CMV, MAC) and neoplasms (lymphoma, visceral KS)

CDC= Centers for Disease Control; HSV = herpes simplex virus; VZV = varicella-zoster virus; PCP = *Pneumocystis carinii* pneumonia; CMV = cytomegalovirus; MAC = *Mycobacterium avium* complex; KS = Kaposi's sarcoma.

Differential Diagnosis of Fever in the HIV-Infected Patient

Infections

The first consideration in differential diagnosis of fever in the HIV-positive patient is infection, as it remains the major cause of death among patients with AIDS [7]. Furthermore, many infectious complications of HIV disease respond well to appropriate antimicrobial therapy, making early, accurate diagnosis important. In two prospective case studies of febrile HIV-infected patients, infection proved to be the cause of fever in 90 and 84 percent of those in whom a source could be established [6, 8].

The list of potential infectious etiologies of fever is long and includes viral, bacterial, parasitic, and fungal pathogens. Susceptibility to these diverse infections varies with the individual patient's degree of immunodeficiency. Infections with bacteria, such as *Streptococcus pneumoniae*, *Staphylococcus aureus*, nontyphoidal strains of *Salmonella*, and other enteric pathogens, may occur early in the course of HIV disease [6, 9, 10]. *Mycobacterium tuberculosis* infection, including extrapulmonary involvement, may also be a relatively early manifestation of HIV disease, as may reactivation of herpes simplex virus (HSV) and varicella-zoster virus (VZV) infections [11, 12].

As patients become more immunocompromised (CD4 cell count < 200/mm^3), infections such as *Pneumocystis carinii* pneumonia (PCP), cryptococcal meningitis, and toxoplasmic encephalitis must be considered in the differential diagnosis of fever [13]. Also at this stage, refractory mucocutaneous HSV and multidermatomal VZV infections may be seen. In patients who are severely immunocompromised (CD4 cell count < 100/mm^3), cytomegalovirus (CMV) and *Mycobacterium avium* complex infections must also be considered [11, 13, 14]. Patients with advanced HIV disease may be even more susceptible to bacterial infections, both community-acquired and nonsocomial, than those with early disease. Except for conventional bacterial pathogens and *M. tuberculosis*, microbiologic cure of opportunistic infections is usually not possible, and relapse of symptomatic disease is common. In these instances, the goal of therapy becomes suppression of clinical disease [15–17].

HIV-infected patients who continue high-risk behaviors are at increased risk for other sexually transmitted diseases, including syphilis, gonorrhea, intestinal parasites, and mucosal viral pathogens. Coinfection with other retroviruses (e.g., HIV-2, HTLV-1) and possibly, other, as yet unidentified, viral agents may contribute to fever in some individuals [18–20].

Neoplasms

HIV-infected patients are at significantly increased risk for certain neoplastic diseases, especially non-Hodgkin's lymphoma and Kaposi's sarcoma (KS) [21]. Fever is frequently part of the clinical presentation of lymphoma; it is less commonly associated with KS, occurring only with disseminated visceral disease [22]. The clinician should be hesitant to attribute fever to diagnosed lymphoma or KS until a full evaluation has been completed to rule out concurrent infection.

Other Causes

Reactions to prescribed or illicit drugs are sometimes responsible for fever. HIV-positive patients appear to have increased sensitivity to many medications, especially antibiotics, and are often prescribed an assortment of therapeutic agents for their diverse medical problems [23]. The presence of pruritus, rash, or eosinophilia may support the diagnosis of drug fever. Injection drug users (IDUs) may present with febrile reactions to self-injected pyrogens and other non-HIV-related infectious complications [24].

Both lymphoid and nonspecific interstitial pneumonitis have been reported to cause fever in HIV-infected patients [25]. Although rare, autoimmune vasculitis has been described in some individuals and represents another possible noninfectious cause of fever [26].

Evaluation of Fever in the HIV-Infected Patient

Given an understanding of the natural history of HIV infection and the evolving differential diagnosis of fever as immunodeficiency progresses, a rational plan for evaluation of the patient can be developed (Table 5-2). Any persistent temperature greater than 100.4°F (38°C) should be considered significant. It is important to review the past medical history, list of current medications, and available baseline laboratory data. Particular attention should be given to the CD4 lymphocyte count. Recent purified protein derivative (PPD) skin test and anergy panel status, as well as prior syphilis and hepatitis serology, may also aid in the diagnostic evaluation.

The primary data collected in the history and physical examination are of critical importance in evaluating the febrile patient. The clinician should elicit from the patient a history of the duration, degree, and pattern of fever, as well as any associated symptoms. A complete review of symptoms, focusing particular attention on the respiratory, gastrointestinal, dermatologic, and neurologic systems, is also warranted. An assessment of past and current risk behaviors contributes important diagnostic clues. Whereas opportunistic infections were reported to be the most common cause of fever in a group of predominantly homosexual men, a study of a largely IDU population found that two-thirds of observed fevers were caused by infection with common bacterial pathogens [6, 8]. Finally, travel

Table 5-2 *Evaluation of fever in the HIV-infected patient*

History
    Symptoms of present illness
    Exposure to tuberculosis
    Exposure to sexually transmitted diseases
    Exposure to viral hepatitis
    Travel/hobbies
    Drug use
Physical examination
    Signs of present illness
    Focus on fundi, pharynx, lungs, abdomen, skin, and neurologic examinations
Laboratory evaluation
    Complete blood and differential counts
    Liver function tests
    Urinalysis
    Blood cultures (including isolator culture in advanced HIV disease)
    Chest x-ray
    Purified protein derivative and anergy panel
    Syphilis serology
    Viral hepatitis serologies
    Other studies as determined by clinical presentation

history, geographic region of origin, sexual practices, exposure to animals and animal products, and unusual hobbies may lead the clinician to investigate specific causes of fever.

A complete physical examination should be performed in the febrile patient, with particular attention given to the systems mentioned previously, including examination of the fundi, the oral cavity, and the skin. A dilated ophthalmologic examination is indicated in severely immunocompromised individuals to assess for CMV infection. Laboratory investigation is directed by clues obtained in the history and physical examination, but should generally include complete blood and differential counts, liver function tests, urinalysis, blood cultures, and chest x-ray. If not previously available, baseline PPD and anergy panel, as well as syphilis and viral hepatitis serologies, are indicated. In significantly immunocompromised patients, serum cryptococcal antigen and lysis-centrifugation (isolator) blood cultures for mycobacteria and fungi should be obtained, particularly if history and physical examination fail to reveal a cause of fever.

The performance of other studies should be based on presenting symptoms and signs (e.g., arterial blood gas in the patient with dyspnea). Computed tomography (CT) or magnetic resonance imaging (MRI) scan of the head and lumbar puncture are indicated in patients with new neurologic symptoms. Isotope studies, such as gallium, thallium, and indium-labeled leukocyte scans, may be useful in the diagnostic evaluation for PCP, lymphoma, and visceral KS, but should not be considered screening tests [27, 28].

The pace of the evaluation is determined by the severity of the clinical illness, likely diagnoses, degree of immunodeficiency, and probability of identifying a condition that is amenable to treatment. Empiric therapy should be initiated in acutely ill patients for the most likely diagnosis(es) and/or for those that carry the highest risk of morbidity or mortality if treatment is delayed. Final diagnosis sometimes rests on the examination of specimens obtained by invasive procedures. In individuals with advanced HIV disease, often more than one active pathologic process can be identified at a given time. Although mucosal surfaces may be colonized with many potential pathogens, any organism identified in tissue or in normally sterile body fluid is considered pathologic, even in the absence of an inflammatory response by the host.

In patients with advanced HIV disease, new symptoms associated with fever must be aggressively pursued. Mild dyspnea or cough may portend an episode of PCP and should lead to a pulmonary evaluation. Subtle complaints of headache or altered mental status and behavior should prompt the clinician to perform appropriate neurologic tests. The development of or change in degree of lymphadenopathy in one or more regions associated with constitutional symptoms may reflect the presence of lymphoma or extrapulmonary mycobacterial disease and necessitate a lymph node biopsy.

Despite careful attention to findings on history, physical examination, and laboratory studies, some febrile HIV-infected patients remain undiagnosed, even after days or weeks of intensive evaluation. A diagnosis may ultimately be made by obtaining tissue via bone marrow, liver, lymph node, or other organ biopsy, or by careful serologic evaluation for organisms that are difficult to culture. In some cases, no specific diagnosis can be made. In such instances, further evaluation can be deferred and the patient closely monitored for clinical changes.

Conclusion

Evaluation of fever in the HIV-infected patient is based on a knowledge of the natural history of the clinical and immunologic features of HIV disease and the presenting symptoms and signs of the illness. Identification of treatable infection is the first priority. Malignancy, drug reaction, and autoimmune phenomena are other potential causes of fever. Because the prevalence of opportunistic diseases in HIV infection is high and the clinical manifestations of febrile illness are often subtle early in their course, prompt evaluation is warranted.

References

1. Centers for Disease Control. 1993 revised classification system for HIV infection and expanded case definition for AIDS among adolescents and adults. *MMWR* 41(RR-17):1–19, 1992.

2. Cooper DA, Gold JW, MacLean P, et al. Acute AIDS retrovirus infection: Definition of a clinical illness associated with seroconversion. *Lancet* 1:537–540, 1985.

3. Ho DD, Sarngadharan MC, Resnick L, et al. Primary human T-lymphotropic virus type III infection. *Ann Intern Med* 103:880–883, 1985.

4. Tindall B, Bavar S, Donovan B, et al. Characterization of the acute clinical illness associated with human immunodeficiency virus infection. *Arch Intern Med* 148:945–949, 1988.

5. Margolick JB, Munoz A, Vlahov D, et al. Changes in T-lymphocyte subsets in intravenous drug users with HIV-1 infection. *JAMA* 267:1631–1636, 1992.

6. Barat LM, Gunn JE, Steger KA, et al. Bacterial infections are the most common cause of fever in HIV-infected inpatients in a municipal hospital. Eighth International Conference on AIDS, Amsterdam, July 1992.

7. Grant IH, Armstrong D. Management of infectious complications in acquired immunodeficiency syndrome. *Am J Med* 81 (Suppl 1A):59–72, 1986.

8. Sepkowitz KA, Telzak EE, Carrow M, Armstrong D. Fever among outpatients with advanced human immunodeficiency virus infection. *Arch Intern Med* 153:1909–1912, 1993.

9. Witt DJ, Craven DE, McCabe WR. Bacterial infections in adults with acquired immune deficiency syndrome (AIDS) and AIDS-related complex. *Am J Med* 82:900–906, 1987.

10. Sperber SJ, Schleupner CJ. Salmonellosis during infection with human immunodeficiency virus. *Rev Infect Dis* 9:925–934, 1987.

11. Modilevsky T, Sattler FR, Barnes PF. Mycobacterial disease in patients with human immunodeficiency virus infection. *Arch Intern Med* 149:2201–2205, 1989.

12. Melbye M, Grossman RJ, Goedert JJ, et al. Risk of AIDS after herpes zoster. *Lancet* 1:728–731, 1987.

13. Masur H, Ognibene FP, Yarchoan R, et al. CD4 counts as predictors of opportunistic pneumonias in human immunodeficiency virus infection. *Ann Intern Med* 111:223–231, 1989.

14. Palestine AG, Polis MA, De Smet MD, et al. A randomized controlled trial of foscarnet in the treatment of cytomegalovirus retinitis in patients with AIDS. *Ann Intern Med* 115:665–673, 1991.

15. Armstrong D, Gold JW, Dryjanski J, et al. Treatment of infections in patients with the acquired immunodeficiency syndrome. *Ann Intern Med* 103:738–743, 1985.

16. Kaplan LD, Wofsky CB, Volberding PA. Treatment of patients with acquired immunodeficiency syndrome and associated manifestations. *JAMA* 257:1367–1374, 1987.

17. Glatt AE, Chirgwin K, Landesman SH. Treatment of infections associated with human immunodeficiency virus. *N Engl J Med* 318:1439–1448, 1988.

18. Robert-Guroff M, Weiss SH, Giron JA, et al. Prevalence of antibodies to HTLV-I, -II, and -III in intravenous drug abusers from an AIDS endemic region. *JAMA* 255:3133–3137, 1986.

19. Centers for Disease Control. AIDS due to HIV-2 infection—New Jersey. *MMWR* 37:33–35, 1988.

20. Cortes E, Detels R, Aboulafia D, et al. HIV-1, HIV-2, and HTLV-1 infection in high-risk groups in Brazil. *N Engl J Med* 320:953–958, 1989.
21. Kaplan MH, Susin M, Pahwa S, et al. Neoplastic complications of HTLV-III infection: Lymphomas and solid tumors. *Am J Med* 82:389–396, 1987.
22. Bach MC, Bagwell SG, Fanning JP. Primary pulmonary Kaposi's sarcoma in the acquired immune deficiency syndrome: A cause of persistent pyrexia. *Am J Med* 85:274–275, 1988.
23. Bayard PJ, Berger TG, Jacobson MA. Drug hypersensitivity reactions and human immunodeficiency virus disease. *J Acquir Immune Defic Syndr* 5:1237–1257, 1992.
24. Marantz PR, Linzer M, Feiner CJ, et al. Inability to predict diagnosis in febrile intravenous drug abusers. *Ann Intern Med* 106:823–828, 1987.
25. White DA, Matthay RA. Noninfectious pulmonary complications of infection with the human immunodeficiency virus. *Am Rev Respir Dis* 140:1763–1787, 1989.
26. Kopelman RG, Zolla-Panzer S. Association of human immuno-deficiency virus infection and autoimmune phenomena. *Am J Med* 84:82–88, 1988.
27. Fineman DS, Palestro CJ, Kim CK, et al. Detection of abnormalities in febrile AIDS patients with In-III-labeled leukocyte and Ga-67 scintigraphy. *Radiology* 170:677–680, 1989.
28. Kramer EL, Sanger JJ, Garay SM, et al. Gallium-67 scans of the chest in patients with acquired immunodeficiency syndrome. *J Nucl Med* 28:1107, 1987.

Weight Loss and Malnutrition 6

James J. Heffernan, Colleen Manning Osten, Eileen Dunn

Clinical Manifestations

Substantial weight loss, generally regarded as a reduction from baseline of greater than 10 percent, occurs in an overwhelming majority (62–79%) of patients with AIDS [1, 2]. In one series, the mean weight loss among 50 men with AIDS who did not receive enteral intubation or parenteral support was 11.8 kg [3]. Primary HIV infection has been associated with some degree of weight loss in 46 percent of cases; non-AIDS symptomatic HIV disease is often characterized by tissue wasting, but the pattern and magnitude are not well defined [4]. Recognition of the frequency and importance of weight loss in AIDS resulted in the inclusion of the "HIV wasting syndrome" in the revised Centers for Disease Control surveillance case definition in 1987. This syndrome consists of serologic evidence of HIV infection and "findings of profound involuntary weight loss more than 10% of baseline body weight plus either chronic diarrhea (at least two loose stools per day for > 30 days) or chronic weakness and documented fever (intermittent or constant for > 30 days) in the absence of a concurrent illness that could explain the findings" [5].

Patients with AIDS are commonly malnourished on admission to the hospital, and their weight often drops further during hospitalization. As in those with other wasting conditions or starvation, the magnitude of weight loss seen in HIV disease, especially body cell mass depletion, predicts outcome. Death, if not caused sooner by infectious or other processes, generally occurs at 66 percent of ideal body weight or 54 percent of normal body cell mass [6]. Early in the course of the epidemic, nutritional interventions were rarely implemented [1]. While more recent data suggest better attention to nutritional support, AIDS treatment centers in the United States have been slow in adopting standard nutritional protocols [7].

The pathophysiology of weight loss associated with HIV infection is complex and multifactorial. While the mechanisms of decreased food intake or malabsorption may be readily identified and often successfully treated, concomitant derangements in metabolism are variable and poorly understood [8]. Resting energy expenditure is generally higher than normal early in the course of HIV disease and increases further with progression to AIDS [9]. In a given patient, weight loss may represent a largely appropriate adaptation to starvation, the deranged hypermetabolic state of cachexia, or both. Accelerated protein breakdown and negative nitrogen balance may also occur in the context of HIV-related opportunistic infections [9].

In otherwise normal individuals, malnutrition is associated with a number of immunologic defects: lymphopenia (especially affecting CD4 cell count), depressed cell-mediated immunity, diminished killer cell function, reduced levels of complement and secretory immunoglobulins, and depressed phagocytosis. However, it remains unclear whether malnutrition or its treatment in an HIV-infected patient alters progression of the underlying disease. Nutritional therapy clearly has beneficial effects on the clinical course and immunologic status of critically ill patients with other conditions, and most authorities consider such support to be an integral part of the management of AIDS patients [10].

Laboratory Data

The pattern of weight loss in most patients with AIDS is that of protein-calorie malnutrition, with evidence of more profound body cell mass depletion than weight reduction alone would suggest. Significant reductions in total body potassium, retinol-binding protein concentration, iron-binding capacity, and serum albumin concentration have been demonstrated in AIDS patients compared to healthy homosexual control subjects [2]. Body fat content may remain normal. Patients with AIDS also have relative overhydration in the extracellular space despite an overall decrease in body water. These findings are similar to the pattern of wasting noted in the clinical settings of burn, sepsis, trauma, and surgery. A subset of patients with AIDS, generally those with restricted protein-calorie intake but without concurrent diarrheal illness, may show a more typical pattern of starvation, with utilization of fat stores and better maintenance of body cell mass [2].

No clear pattern of endocrinologic abnormality has been identified among HIV-infected patients with weight loss. Infrequent cases of adrenal insufficiency from secondary infection or medication effects have been reported, as have decreased testosterone levels in men. Of interest is the observation that serum triiodothyronine (T3) levels are maintained in HIV disease, perhaps inappropriately in some patients, although investigators have also reported a more typical decrease in the setting of AIDS and opportunistic infections [11].

Among HIV-infected patients with weight loss, hypertriglyceridemia and evidence of high resting energy expenditure are nearly universal findings. Increased serum levels of numerous cytokines have been reported, most notably tumor necrosis factor-alpha (TNF), interleukin-1-beta (IL-1), and interferon-alpha (IFN). Tumor necrosis factor tends to rise episodically, generally in association with acute infections, where it may confer some degree of protection. Interferon-alpha is the most persistently elevated cytokine in patients with AIDS and correlates best with the serum triglyceride level [9]. It is likely that such immune modulators contribute to the anorexia and cachexia of AIDS.

Differential Diagnosis

The causes of weight loss in an HIV-infected individual are legion [12–14]. The problem is generally multifactorial (Table 6-1); identified causes of weight loss often respond to specific interventions or to the application of directed nutrition management, or both. Chronic diarrhea is quite common among patients with AIDS in the United States; not surprisingly, given broader exposure to potential gastrointestinal pathogens, severe diarrhea or wasting, or both, are even more prevalent among patients with AIDS from Haiti and Africa, contributing to the syndrome of "slim disease" [15]. North American patients with AIDS and chronic diarrhea have demonstrated more profound reductions in body cell mass and shorter survival than AIDS patients without diarrhea; pre-

Table 6-1 *Factors contributing to weight loss in HIV infection*

Problem	Etiology	Management
Food not accessible or preparation difficulties	Social or health causes	Social service Homemaker Dietary supplements
Anorexia	Intercurrent illness	Treat
	HIV infection	Megestrol acetate, dronabinol
	Depression	Antidepressant therapy
Nausea/vomiting	Medications	Discontinue
	HIV gastroparesis	Metoclopramide or cisapride
Mouth pain/dysphagia/ odynophagia	Gingivitis/periodontitis	Dental referral
	Opportunistic diseases	Specific Rx
Diarrhea/malabsorption	Opportunistic diseases	Specific Rx
	HIV infection	Antiretroviral therapy

liminary data suggest that the magnitude of depletion is more important than the cause itself in determining prognosis. The search for the cause of chronic diarrhea in patients with advanced HIV infection should proceed beyond repeated stool examinations; endoscopy with small bowel biopsy, light and electron microscopic examination, and morphometric studies have identified occult pathogens in up to 50 percent of such cases [16].

Evaluation

A complete nutritional assessment is indicated in an HIV-infected patient whenever malnutrition is suspected, especially when the individual has had an involuntary 20-lb or 10 percent reduction from usual weight. The cornerstone of nutritional assessment is an accurate diet history to evaluate and quantify the patient's past and present oral intake; to identify any difficulties with obtaining, eating, or tolerating foods; and to determine whether the patient is following nutritionally sound practices. A detailed list of medications must be obtained: Zidovudine may cause profound dysgeusia or myopathy with muscle wasting; trimethoprim-sulfamethoxazole, sulfadiazine, ketoconazole, and antimycobacterial agents commonly produce anorexia; the use of anticancer chemotherapeutic agents may be attended by severe nausea, anorexia, or mucositis; and pentamidine rarely causes diabetes mellitus. Nutritional assessment should include both anthropometric measurements and serum studies. Relevant measurements include current height, weight, and weight change over time; triceps skinfold thickness to evaluate fat reserves; and midarm circumference to assess somatic protein status. The patient's pre-illness weight is the best reference in evaluating weight changes [3]. Laboratory studies should include serum albumin, transferrin, and total protein levels. Serum albumin less than 2.5 gm/dl is associated with decreased bowel wall oncotic pressure and impaired gut function; albumin less than 2.0 gm/dl correlates with severe malnutrition and reduced survival [17]. Other studies, such as serum folate and cyanocobalamin levels, are directed by the clinical features of the case.

A patient's basal caloric requirements can be calculated using the basal energy expenditure (BEE) equation multiplied by an appropriate injury and activity factor [18, 19] (Table 6-2). Optimally, one wishes to provide 150 calories per gram nitrogen; protein needs can thus be estimated by

$$PN = EEN \times \frac{gm\ nitrogen}{150} \times \frac{6.25\ gm\ protein}{gm\ nitrogen}$$

where PN = protein needs and EEN = estimated energy needs [20].

Table 6-2 *Calculation of patient's basal caloric requirements*[a]

Basal energy expenditure = 66 + (13.7 × wt) + (5 × ht) − (6.8 × age)[b]	
(BEE) (male)	
BEE (female)	= 655 + (9.6 × wt) + (1.7 × ht) − (4.7 × age)[b]

Activity factor (AF)		Injury factor (IF)	
Confined to bed	1.2	Surgery	1.1–1.2
Ambulatory	1.3	Infection	1.2–1.6
		Trauma	1.1–1.8
		Sepsis	1.4–1.8

Estimated energy needs (EEN) = BEE × AF × IF

[a]Resting energy needs increase 13% for each degree Celsius, or 7.2% for each degree Fahrenheit.
[b]Wt = weight in kg; ht = height in cm; age = years.

Management

General Issues in Nutritional Support

The goals of nutritional support are preservation of lean body mass and provision of adequate protein, calories, and other nutrients in a formulation that minimizes side effects, especially malabsorption. Currently, there is no clinically proven superior oral, enteral, or parenteral diet for patients with symptomatic HIV disease, and, therefore, nutrition management must be individualized. Nutritional support is indicated if a patient has sustained a 20-lb or 10 percent weight loss in 6 months or is unable to meet 100 percent of his or her nutritional needs [10]. Early intervention may prevent the complications of malnutrition and maintain or improve quality of life.

In the patient with a functioning gut, oral delivery of nutrients maintains the structural and functional integrity of the gastrointestinal mucosa, minimizes costs, and decreases the risk of infection. A high-calorie, high-protein diet with a multivitamin supplement is recommended; modification of fat and lactose content is often necessary, especially in the patient with diarrhea. An enteral formula, administered orally or transnasally (and rarely per gastric tube), may supplement or replace the oral diet and should be selected with reference to fat content (< 5% or as tolerated), viscosity, cost, osmolality, caloric density, patient acceptance, feasibility for home use, protein-calorie ratio, and lactose content. Patients with weight loss may be far more receptive to the initiation of enteral feedings as a choice in an outpatient setting than when such an intervention is presented during a hospitalization for acute illness. Enteral preparations include nutritionally complete elemental or polymeric formulas and modular formulas; many such commercial products have been used successfully in patients with HIV-associated syndromes [10]. If a patient with AIDS develops diarrhea while utilizing an enteral product, one must consider the myriad of potential causes other than the product itself, including hypoalbuminemia, antibiotic therapy, bacterial contamination, or a new infection. Formula-related problems include improper rate or strength of administration, specific content (fat, lactose), and temperature of feedings.

Parenteral nutrition can be used effectively to reestablish nutritional homeostasis in malnourished HIV-infected patients, but is generally reserved for those in whom oral and enteral methods have failed or cannot be used, or for those who have a clinical indication for rapid correction of nutritional deficiencies, such as impending surgery. Many causes of gut dysfunction in AIDS, with the notable exception of severe diarrhea due to cryptosporidiosis or HIV-induced enteropathy, respond well to directed therapy. In some patients, parenteral nutrition may be required for only brief periods while specific therapy arrests or reverses gut dysfunction. A decision to implement chronic parenteral nutritional support should be made only after careful assessment of its likely effect on quality and duration of life.

Specific Nutrition Management Strategies

Anorexia is nearly universal at some point in the course of AIDS. Small frequent feedings; a high-calorie, high-protein diet; and an enteral supplement are recommended. If oral intake is inadequate, transnasal tube feedings may be required. There is increasing experience with megestrol acetate, which has been shown to be effective in promoting improved appetite, perception of well-being, and weight gain among cachectic AIDS patients [21–22]. However, no improvement in survival has been demonstrated with the use of megestrol, and weight gain, while substantial, reflects primarily an expansion of fat stores. Based on early reports of elevations of TNF in HIV-infected patients with wasting syndrome, a number of agents that decrease or block its action have been tested in vitro and employed in a number of small, uncontrolled case series. These drugs include pentoxifylline, thalidomide, and corticosteroids [11, 23–25]. To date, there is no compelling evidence that any of them is effective in ameliorating weight loss or prolonging life, and concern remains over the potential risk in enhancing susceptibility to a variety of opportunistic infections. Dronabinol (delta-9-tetrahydro-cannabinol), the principal psychoactive substance in marijuana, has also been used as an appetite enhancer in HIV-infected individuals [26]. While appetite has improved in most patients and weight gain is observed in some, neuropsychiatric side effects have been frequent [8]. Depressed patients may respond to tricyclic antidepressant therapy, with improvements in mood, appetite, and oral intake, although there are no published data demonstrating reversal of weight loss with these agents. Cyproheptadine may also enhance appetite but at the expense of sedation.

In patients with disorders of the oral cavity and esophagus, modifications in the acidity, temperature, texture, consistency, and seasoning of food may improve tolerance. If a patient's intake is compromised for more than 3 inpatient days, tube feedings should be considered. When esophageal ulcers preclude the use of nasogastric tube feedings, short-term (7–10 days) parenteral nutrition may be considered. Thrush, hairy leukoplakia, and herpetic infection occasionally pose barriers to oral intake, but generally respond to appropriate therapy. Symptomatic relief from painful mucosal lesions may be obtained with a mixture of Kaopectate and diphenhydramine oral suspension, viscous lidocaine, or sucralfate in suspension. Thalidomide has also been used for painful aphthous ulcers in AIDS patients. Instruction and encouragement in good oral hygiene may pay dividends in retarding the development of accelerated caries and periodontal disease. With long-term dysfunction of the upper digestive tract, placement of a gastrostomy or jejunostomy feeding tube is an option. Nausea and vomiting can be managed through the use of antiemetics and postprandial timing of drug therapy. A low-fat, soft, bland diet with an enteral supplement is best tolerated. Patients should maintain an upright or semi-upright posture for such feedings. Tube feedings, especially nasojejunostomy feedings, may be indicated for refractory nausea and vomiting; one should always consider the possibility of a central nervous system lesion as the cause of such symptoms. Early satiety from HIV gastroparesis may respond to metoclopramide or cisapride; mechanical obstruction from bulky abdominal or retroperitoneal tumors or adenopathy may be relieved with chemotherapy. It is also important to recognize that emotional stress and psychosocial issues may contribute to nausea and early satiety. Relaxation exercises before meals and institution of a regimen of small frequent feedings may be extremely helpful in this regard.

Diarrhea is the most common gastrointestinal manifestation of AIDS and often the most problematic to treat. The pattern of diarrhea may be enteropathic (frequent, large-volume, nonbloody stools without tenesmus), resulting in electrolyte abnormalities and profound wasting, colitic (painful bowel movements, with small-volume mucoid and/or bloody stools, abdominal pain, and often fever), or a combination. Patients with AIDS who have diarrhea manifest greater weight loss, lower CD4 lymphocyte counts, and a higher incidence of extraintestinal opportunistic infections than those without diarrhea. In the majority of such patients, enteric pathogens can be identified and treated successfully [27]. Diarrhea and other bowel problems arising from pathogenic bacteria, cytomegalovirus (CMV), herpes simplex virus, and most protozoan and helminthic infestations generally respond to antimicrobial therapy. Unfortunately, the most severe diarrhea often occurs in the setting of cryptosporidiosis, which may be resistant to therapy. The possibility of iatrogenic diarrhea, such as *Clostridium difficile*–associated colitis, should always be considered. Sometimes investigation does not reveal a specific cause of diarrhea in HIV-infected patients, and the syndrome is attributed to the enteropathogenic effects of HIV. A somatostatin analogue, octreotide, has shown promise in several case reports of severe secretory diarrhea in patients with AIDS, with or without cryptosporidial colonization [28, 29].

Several nutrition regimens have been espoused for use in the HIV-infected individual with diarrhea predicated on pattern of gut dysfunction and independent of the specific cause [7, 30, 31]. In the setting of severe small bowel disease and profound malabsorption, nutrition can only be effectively delivered parenterally. If the underlying cause of severe small bowel dysfunction can be ameliorated, an elemental enteral diet may promote gut function. With less profound small bowel dysfunction, frequent small feedings with low fat, low lactose, low fiber, low residue, and no caffeine should be administered. A similar diet in those with large bowel disease may be effective in reducing the frequency of bowel movements. Nonspecific mild enteropathy may respond to the addition of a bulking agent [31]. Most patients with AIDS and moderate or severe diarrhea require adjunctive therapy with an antidiarrheal agent. Institution of a "BRAT" (bananas, rice, apples, and tea or toast) diet may also be helpful in gaining control of diarrhea but is nutritionally incomplete and inappropriate for extended use [7]. One should add an isotonic supplement, multivitamins, and appropriate fluids to the BRAT diet after a patient has followed it successfully for several days.

Weight loss and malnutrition are concomitant with systemic infections and malignancies associated with HIV infection. Antimicrobial therapy may readily control the fever and weight loss associated with *Salmonella* or *Shigella* bacteremia, *Mycobacterium tuberculosis* infection, or systemic fungal infection. Body mass repletion has also been accomplished with ganciclovir treatment of CMV infection [32]. The most common disseminated infection resulting in weight loss and fever in patients with AIDS is *Mycobacterium avium* complex; symptomatic improvement may occur with multidrug antimycobacterial regimens. Antineoplastic therapy for non-Hodgkin's lymphoma or Kaposi's sarcoma may reverse the fever and wasting that accompany these malignancies.

Conclusion

Involuntary weight loss occurs in virtually all patients with AIDS and is seen frequently in earlier stages of HIV infection. At the time of death, most patients exhibit protein-calorie malnutrition with profound body cell mass depletion. There are numerous potential causes of weight loss in patients with HIV infection, many of which respond to specific therapy. Therefore, a complete nutritional assessment should be carried out in any patient who has lost 20 lbs or 10 percent of usual weight. Nutritional management is individualized, with the goals of preservation of lean body mass and the provision of adequate protein, calories, and nutrients. While there is no definite evidence that nutritional support alters the course of HIV disease, such therapy has become an established part of management.

References

1. O'Sullivan P, Linke RA, Dalton S. Evaluation of body weight and nutritional status among AIDS patients. *J Am Diet Assoc* 85:1483–1484, 1985.
2. Kotler DP, Wang J, Pierson RN. Body composition studies in patients with the acquired immunodeficiency syndrome. *Am J Clin Nutr* 42:1255–1265, 1985.
3. Garcia ME, Collins CL, Mansell PWA. The acquired immune deficiency syndrome: Nutritional complications and assessment of body weight status. *Nutr Clin Prac* 2:108–111, 1987.
4. Tindall B, Barker S, Donovan B, et al. Characterization of the acute clinical illness associated with human immunodeficiency virus infection. *Arch Intern Med* 148:945–949, 1988.
5. Centers for Disease Control. Revision of the CDC surveillance case definition for acquired immunodeficiency syndrome. *MMWR* 36 (suppl):3–15, 1987.
6. Kotler DP, Tierney AR, Wang J, Pierson RN, Jr. Magnitude of body-cell-mass depletion and the timing of death from wasting in AIDS. *Am J Clin Nutr* 50:444–447, 1989.
7. Ysseldyke LL. Nutritional complications and incidence of malnutrition among AIDS patients. *J Am Diet Assoc* 91:217–218, 1991.
8. Nerad JL, Gorbach SL. Nutritional aspects of HIV infection. *Infect Dis Clin North Am* 8:499–515, 1994.
9. Grunfeld C, Feingold KR. Metabolic disturbances and wasting in the acquired immunodeficiency syndrome. *N Engl J Med* 327:329–337, 1992.
10. Hickey MS, Weaver KE. Nutritional management of patients with ARC or AIDS. *Gastroenterol Clin North Am* 17:545–561, 1988.
11. Coodley GO, Loveless MO, Merrill TM. The HIV wasting syndrome: A review. *J Acquir Immune Defic Syndr* 7:681–694, 1994.
12. Greene JB. Clinical approach to weight loss in the patient with HIV infection. *Gastroenterol Clin North Am* 17:573–586, 1988.
13. Kotler DP. Intestinal and hepatic manifestations of AIDS. *Adv Intern Med* 34:43–72, 1989.
14. Resler SS. Nutrition care of AIDs patients. *J Am Diet Assoc* 88:828–832, 1988.
15. Serwadda D, Sewankambo NK, Carswell JW, et al. Slim disease: A new

disease in Uganda and its association with HTLV-III infection. *Lancet* 2:849–852, 1985.

16. Greenson JK, Belitsos PC, Yardley JH, Barlett JG. AIDS enteropathy: Occult enteric infections and duodenal mucosal alterations in chronic diarrhea. *Ann Intern Med* 114:366–372, 1991.
17. Justice AC, Feinstein AR, Wells CK. A new prognostic staging system for the acquired immunodeficiency syndrome. *N Engl J Med* 320:1388–1393, 1989.
18. Harris JA, Benedict FG. A biometric study of basal metabolism in man. Washington, DC: Carnegie Institution of Washington, 2:227, 1919.
19. Jan J, Van Lanschot B, Feenstra B, et al. Calculation versus measurement of total energy expenditure. *Crit Care Med* 14:982, 1986.
20. Krause MV, Mahan LK. *Food, Nutrition and Diet Therapy.* Philadelphia: Saunders, 1979.
21. Von Roenn JH, Armstrong D, Kotler DP, et al. Megestrol acetate in patients with AIDS-related cachexia. *Ann Intern Med* 121:393–399, 1994.
22. Oster MH, Enders SR, Samuels S, et al. Megestrol acetate in patients with AIDS and cachexia. *Ann Intern Med* 121:400–408, 1994.
23. Landman D, Sarai A, Sathe SS. Use of pentoxifylline therapy for patients with AIDS-related wasting: Pilot study. *Clin Infect Dis* 18:97–99, 1994.
24. De Zube BJ. Pentoxifylline for the treatment of infection with human immunodeficiency virus. *Clin Infect Dis* 18:285–287, 1994.
25. Moreira AL, Sampaio EP, Zmuidzinas A, et al. Thalidomide exerts its inhibitory action on tumor necrosis factor alpha by enhancing mRNA degradation. *J Ex Med* 177:1675–1680, 1993.
26. Beal JE, et al. Dronabinol as a treatment for anorexia associated with weight loss in patients with AIDS. *J Pain Sympt Manag* 10:89–97, 1995.
27. Smith PD, Lane HC, Gill VJ, et al. Intestinal infections in patients with the acquired immunodeficiency syndrome (AIDS). *Ann Intern Med* 108:328–333, 1988.
28. Cook DJ, Kelton JG, Andrzej MS, Collins SM. Somatostatin treatment for cryptosporidial diarrhea in a patient with the acquired immunodeficiency syndrome (AIDS). *Ann Intern Med* 108:708–709, 1988.
29. Robinson EN, Fogel R. SMS 201–995, a somatostatin analogue, and diarrhea in the acquired immunodeficiency syndrome (AIDS). *Ann Intern Med* 108:680–681, 1988.
30. O'Neill L. Acquired immune deficiency syndrome and nutrition. *Dietitians Nutr Support* 13:13–16, 1988.
31. Task Force on Nutrition Support in AIDS. Guidelines for nutrition support in AIDS. *Nutrition* 5:39–46, 1989.
32. Kotler DP, Tierney AR, Altilio D, et al. Body mass repletion during ganciclovir treatment of cytomegalovirus infections in patients with acquired immunodeficiency syndrome. *Arch Intern Med* 149:901–905, 1989.

Oral Manifestations 7

David L. Battinelli, Edward S. Peters

Oral manifestations can be identified in 40 percent of all HIV-infected patients and in over 90 percent of AIDS patients [1–3]. While many different types of lesions have been described, a small number predominate [4]. Most HIV-related oral lesions are fungal, viral, bacterial, or neoplastic [5] (Table 7-1). Even though many are not specific to HIV disease, their presentation, natural history, and response to therapy are affected by the patient's degree of immunodeficiency [6]. Their course is also dependent on the presence of systemic disease and the individual's state of oral hygiene. Diagnosis of HIV-related oral disease is based primarily on clinical presentation in conjunction with routine smears and cultures; biopsy is rarely indicated.

Fungal Diseases

Oral Candidiasis

Candidiasis is the most common oral manifestation of HIV infection and often the initial symptom. In one study, over 90 percent of patients with AIDS experienced oral candidiasis sometime during their course [7]. Oral candidiasis is seen with advancing immunodeficiency, generally first occurring when the CD4 cell count falls below $400/mm^3$ [5]. *Candida albicans*, part of the normal oral flora, is the most frequent pathogen, but other species have also been identified [8].

The clinical variants of oral candidiasis include pseudomembranous (thrush), hyperplastic, and atrophic forms, and angular cheilitis [8]. Candidal infection may be asymptomatic or associated with pain, burning, or irritation of the mouth [8]. The presence of odynophagia or retrosternal pain with swallowing suggests esophageal involvement. Pseudomembranous candidiasis, the most common variant, is characterized by white or cream-colored plaques, which, when scraped

Table 7-1 *Oral manifestations of HIV infection*

Fungal diseases
  Candidiasis
Viral diseases
  Herpes simplex virus
  Varicella-zoster virus
  Hairy leukoplakia
  Human papillomavirus
  Cytomegalovirus
Bacterial diseases
  Gingivitis
  Periodontitis
  Syphilis
  Gram-negative infection
  Mycobacterium avium complex infection
Neoplastic diseases
  Kaposi's sarcoma
  Lymphoma
  Squamous cell carcinoma
Miscellaneous conditions
  Aphthous ulcerations
  Xerostomia
  Salivary gland enlargement

by a tongue blade, reveal reddened or bleeding mucosa (Plate 1). Multiple lesions may involve the buccal mucosa, dorsal tongue, gingiva, and hard and soft palates. Hyperplastic candidiasis, most often found on the buccal mucosa, manifests as white plaques (leukoplakia), which cannot be removed by scraping. Atrophic candidiasis is characterized by erythematous macular lesions of the buccal mucosa, hard palate, and dorsal surface of the tongue. Angular cheilitis presents as erythema, cracking, fissuring, and ulceration of the corners of the mouth.

Initial diagnosis of oral candidiasis is based on the clinical features and demonstration of budding yeast and pseudohyphae on smears examined with Gram's stain or potassium hydroxide. Diagnosis of recurrent episodes can be made clinically and by response to empiric therapy.

Oral candidiasis responds to topical or systemic antifungal agents. Topical preparations include clotrimazole oral troches, 10 mg, dissolved slowly three to five times a day, and nystatin tablets (100,000 units) or oral pastilles (200,000 units), one to two dissolved by mouth slowly three to five times a day. Nystatin suspension, swished and swallowed three to five times a day, is less effective because of shortened contact time with the oral mucosa. Ketoconazole, an oral imidazole, 200 mg once or twice a day with food, is generally reserved for patients with refractory thrush or esophageal involvement; fluconazole,

50 to 100 mg orally once a day, is also effective but considerably more expensive [9]. Itraconazole, 200 mg orally once a day, has been shown comparable to clotrimazole and ketoconazole therapies [10]. Topical azole creams can be used to treat angular cheilitis. Oral candidiasis generally improves within a few days of initiation of treatment. Reduced doses of topical or systemic agents are effective as maintenance therapy to prevent disease recurrence, which is common as immunodeficiency progresses. Antimicrobial resistance or infection with other candidal species may emerge in patients treated with chronic antifungal therapy [11].

Other Fungi

Other fungal diseases that less frequently cause oral lesions in HIV-infected patients include histoplasmosis, cryptococcosis, and geotrichosis [4, 12]. They generally manifest as persistent ulcerations, and their diagnosis is made by biopsy and culture.

Viral Infections

Herpesvirus infections are especially prevalent in HIV disease. Herpes simplex virus (HSV), varicella-zoster virus (VZV), Epstein-Barr virus (EBV), and, less commonly, cytomegalovirus (CMV) have been associated with a variety of acute and chronic oral lesions.

Herpes Simplex Virus

Herpes simplex virus produces painful ulcerations involving the oral mucosa (gingivostomatitis), lips (herpes labialis), or both (Plate 2). Lesions appear abruptly as solitary or multiple small vesicles on an erythematous base, and the vesicles may rupture, forming ulcerations [13]. Herpes simplex virus infection frequently affects the hard and soft palate but may also involve the gingiva, floor of the mouth, and tongue. Labial lesions typically form large ulcerations that extend onto the facial skin. HIV-infected patients may have lesions that are atypical in appearance, aggressive, and persistent. Mucocutaneous HSV disease lasting longer than 4 weeks in the setting of HIV infection meets the Centers for Disease Control (CDC) case definition for AIDS.

Diagnosis of HSV infection is made presumptively on clinical grounds and is confirmed by culture or Tzanck smear, which shows multinucleated giant cells and viral inclusion bodies. Management consists of oral acyclovir, 200 to 400 mg five times a day; topical acyclovir is ineffective. Lesions generally clear within several days of initiation of therapy [13]. If response to oral therapy is inadequate, intravenous acyclovir, 5 to 10 mg/kg every 8 hours for one week, is indicated. Maintenance therapy at lower doses can be given in an effort to reduce the frequency of recurrent disease. Herpes simplex virus resistance to acyclovir has been described, and topical trifluridine or systemic foscarnet may be effective in this setting [9, 14].

Varicella-Zoster Virus

When VZV, the cause of shingles, involves the second (maxillary) or third (mandibular) branches of the trigeminal nerve, the oral mucosa may be affected. VZV infection of the mouth produces unilateral pain and a vesicular eruption that leads to mucosal ulceration [13, 15]. Diagnosis of VZV infection is made clinically. Oral acyclovir, 800 mg five times a day, is used to expedite healing and prevent dissemination. While recurrent VZV infection has been described in HIV-infected patients, maintenance therapy is generally not recommended.

Hairy Leukoplakia

Hairy leukoplakia (HL), which is caused by EBV, was originally thought to be unique to HIV infection in that it had not been described before the AIDS epidemic [16,17]. However, there have since been case reports of HL in immunosuppressed heart, kidney, and bone marrow transplant recipients [18].

Hairy leukoplakia typically manifests as leukoplakia involving the lateral borders of the tongue that is corrugated or folded in appearance (Plate 3). The folds run vertically and have hair-like or "hairy" projections, which are best appreciated when the tongue is protruded and stretched to one side [19]. In severe HL, the entire dorsal surface of the tongue may be involved, and lesions are sometimes located on the buccal or labial mucosa. Hairy leukoplakia has negative prognostic implications; in over 50 percent of patients diagnosed with the condition, AIDS develops within 30 months of presentation [20].

Presumptive diagnosis of HL is based on its clinical appearance, and biopsy is generally not necessary. On histologic examination, hyperparakeratosis, acanthosis, and vacuolation of epithelial cells with minimal subepithelial inflammation are seen. A number of other white lesions can appear on the tongue in HIV-infected patients. Differential diagnosis includes candidiasis, tobacco-associated leukoplakia, lichen planus, traumatic mucositis, restorative dental material (galvanic lesion), and geographic tongue.

Hairy leukoplakia is asymptomatic, benign, and generally requires no specific treatment. Temporary regression of HL has been observed in patients receiving antiviral therapy, including acyclovir, ganciclovir, and zidovudine [21–23]. Clinical improvement may be related to immunologic or antiviral effects [23].

Human Papillomavirus

Human papillomavirus is the agent responsible for skin and mucosal warts, which may be more frequent and less responsive to treatment in HIV-infected patients [24–26]. Lesions are often multiple and located throughout the oral cavity. Diagnosis is made by recognition of the typical sessile or "cauliflower-like" papular lesions [8]. Some oral warts are well circumscribed, have a flat surface, and may disappear completely with stretching of the mucosa [27]. Treatment is by surgical excision, cryosurgery, or laser therapy, but recurrence is common.

Cytomegalovirus

Cytomegalovirus infection is most often associated with retinitis, and mucosal involvement is uncommon. Intraoral CMV infection may manifest as nonspecific mucositis, large well-demarcated shallow ulcerations, or salivary gland enlargement and xerostomia. Severe oral disease generally occurs in the context of systemic CMV infection. Diagnosis of oral CMV disease is made by biopsy. Treatment consists of systemic ganciclovir or foscarnet [15].

Bacterial Diseases

Gingivitis and Periodontal Disease

Human immunodeficiency virus infection is associated with severe gingival and periodontal disease differing from that seen in normal hosts in its atypical appearance and rapid progression [28–30]. While HIV-related gingivitis (HIV-G) and periodontitis (HIV-P) often involve the entire mouth, they can also present as discrete lesions adjacent to areas of healthy tissue.

HIV-G is a disease of the gingival margin, gingiva, and occasionally, the alveolar mucosa, occurring in approximately 20 percent of HIV-infected patients [31]. It is characterized by marked erythema of the gingiva, which may extend several millimeters away from the margin. Spontaneous or easy bleeding, ulceration, or necrosis of the interdental gingiva may be observed [30]. HIV-G often responds poorly to conventional therapy and may progress to HIV-P.

HIV-related periodontitis presents with gingival erythema and ulceration, soft tissue necrosis, and rapid destruction of the periodontal attachment (Plate 4). Deep pain, bleeding, and exposure of the underlying bone may also be observed, with loss of more than 90 percent of the alveolar bone occurring within a few weeks. Significant tooth mobility is a common finding. HIV-P is usually seen as a localized lesion surrounded by areas of gingivitis. Untreated HIV-P is rapidly progressive and results in tooth loss [16, 28].

The management of HIV-G and HIV-P consists of removal of

plaque and calculus by scaling and root planing and debridement of necrotic tissue. Povidone-iodine solution and chlorhexidine may be useful adjunctively, as may antibiotic therapy with penicillin, metronidazole, or clindamycin. Extraction of involved teeth is often necessary [28].

Other Bacteria

There have been a few case reports of oral lesions caused by gram-negative organisms, including *Klebsiella pneumoniae* and *Enterobacter cloacae* [2]. In addition, *Mycobacterium avium* complex infection presenting as mouth ulcerations has also been described [32]. Both of these diseases are managed with systemic antimicrobial therapy.

Neoplastic Diseases

Kaposi's Sarcoma

Kaposi's sarcoma (KS) is the most common neoplasm in AIDS, and more than 50 percent of patients with KS have oral involvement [33]. Intraoral lesions may occur alone or in conjunction with skin, visceral, and lymph node disease. In 10 percent of patients with KS, mouth lesions may be the only finding [33]. Oral KS presents as red or purple, nonblanching macules, papules, or nodules. Lesions are especially common on the hard palate and gingival margins, and are frequently asymptomatic [33]. Early oral KS may be only minimally different in color from normal mucosa, but, as lesions progress, they often ulcerate and bleed. Kaposi's sarcoma of the gingiva produces diffuse swelling and may be mistaken for gingivitis or periodontitis [33] (Plate 5). Diagnosis of oral KS is by biopsy. Therapy consists of cryosurgery, laser or radiation therapy, or intralesional or systemic chemotherapy, depending on the number and size of the lesions and presence of visceral disease. Lesions may recur following treatment.

Non-Hodgkin's Lymphoma

Occasionally HIV-related non-Hodgkin's lymphoma involves the oral mucosa, presenting as a firm, painless swelling, with or without ulceration, anywhere in the mouth but especially on the gingiva or palate [34]. Any oral nodule or mass should be biopsied to rule out lymphoma. Non-Hodgkin's lymphoma is a systemic disease that requires chemotherapy.

Carcinoma

Squamous cell carcinoma, usually on the lateral and undersurface of the tongue, has also been described in HIV-infected patients [3]. Treatment consists of local excision and radiation therapy.

Miscellaneous Oral Conditions

Aphthous Ulcerations

Recurrent aphthous ulcerations are frequently associated with HIV infection [3]. While their etiology is unclear, trauma, systemic illness, and viruses have been implicated as contributing factors. Small, painful, shallow ulcers on an erythematous base, with a raised white, glistening margin are observed. These lesions may enlarge and become necrotic over time (Plate 6). Symptomatic ulcers that do not heal spontaneously should be treated with topical steroids. Fluocinonide ointment 0.05% mixed with Orabase applied three to six times a day is effective. Dexamethasone elixir swished around the mouth and expectorated has also been useful in some patients. Severe ulcers that do not respond to topical therapy can be treated with a short course of oral prednisone or thalidomide [35]. Differential diagnosis of mouth ulcers includes HSV infection, CMV infection, syphilis, and lymphoma; ulcers have also been associated with zalcitabine (formerly dideoxcytidine or ddC) therapy. Lesions that do not respond to empiric therapy should be biopsied.

Xerostomia

Xerostomia, or dry mouth, has been described with or without parotid gland enlargement in patients with HIV disease. The syndrome is characterized by failure to express saliva from Wharton's or Stensen's ducts. Viral and autoimmune causes appear responsible for some cases, but the syndrome may also result from drug toxicity, particularly tricyclic antidepressants. The presence of parotid enlargement may necessitate salivary gland biopsy to rule out lymphoma, Sjögren's syndrome, or sarcoidosis [3, 36, 37].

References

1. Murray HW, Hillman JK, Rubin BY, et al. Patients at risk for AIDS-related opportunistic infections. *N Engl J Med* 313:1504, 1985.
2. Klein RS, Harris CA, Small CR, et al. Oral candidiasis in high-risk patients as the initial manifestations of the acquired immunodeficiency syndrome. *N Engl J Med* 311:354–358, 1984.
3. Silverman S, Migliorati CA, Lozada-Nur F, et al. Oral findings in people with or at high risk for AIDS: A study of 375 homosexual males. *J Am Dent Assoc* 112:187, 1986.
4. Phelan JA, Saltzman BR, Friedland GH, Klein RS. Oral findings in patients with acquired immunodeficiency syndrome. *Oral Surg Oral Med Oral Pathol* 64:50–56, 1987.
5. Barr C, Lopez M, Rau-Dobles A, et al. HIV-associated oral lesions: Immu-

nologic, virologic and salivary parameters. *J Oral Pathol Med* 21:295–298, 1992.

6. Glick M, Muzyka BC, Lurie D, Salkin LM. Oral manifestations associated with HIV-related disease as markers for immune suppression and AIDS. *Oral Surg Oral Med Oral Pathol* 77:344–347, 1994.

7. Greenspan JS, Greenspan D, Winkler JR. Diagnosis and management of the oral manifestations of HIV infection and AIDS. *Infect Dis Clin North Am* 2:373–383, 1988.

8. Reichart PA, et al. AIDS and the oral cavity. The HIV infection: Virology, etiology, origin, immunology, precautions and clinical observations in 100 patients. *Int J Oral Maxillofac Surg* 16:129–153, 1987.

9. Scully C, McCarthy G. Management of oral health in persons with HIV infection. *Oral Surg Oral Med Oral Pathol* 73:215–225, 1992.

10. Smith DE, Midgley J, Allan M, et al. Itraconazole versus ketoconazole in the treatment of oral and oesophageal candidosis in patients infected with HIV. *AIDS* 5:1367–1371, 1991.

11. Leen CLS, Brettle RP, Willocks LJ, Milne LJR. Fluconazole-resistant candidiasis in patients with AIDS. Seventh International Conference on AIDS, Florence, Italy, June 1991.

12. Lynch DP, Naftolin LZ. Oral *Cryptococcus neoformans* infection in AIDS. *Oral Surg Oral Med Oral Pathol* 64:449, 1987.

13. Quinnan GV, Masur H, Rook AH, et al. Herpes virus infections in the acquired immunodeficiency syndrome. *JAMA* 252:72, 1984.

14. Kessler H, et al. ACTG 172: Treatment of acyclovir-resistant (ACV-R) mucocutaneous herpes simplex virus (HSV) infection in patients with AIDS: Open label pilot study of topical trifluridine (TFT). Eighth International Conference on AIDS, Amsterdam, July 1992.

15. Eversole L. Viral infections of the head and neck among HIV-seropositive patients. *Oral Surg Oral Med Oral Pathol* 73:155–163, 1992.

16. Winkler JR, Grassi M, Murray PA. Clinical Description and Etiology of HIV-Associated Periodontal Diseases. In PB Robertson, JS Greenspan (eds), *Perspectives on Oral Manifestations of AIDS*. Littleton, MA: PSG, 1988. Pp 49–70.

17. Greenspan D, Greenspan J. Significance of oral hairy leukoplakia. *Oral Surg Oral Med Oral Pathol* 73:151–154, 1992.

18. Greenspan JS, Greenspan D, Lennette ET, et al. Replication of Epstein-Barr virus within the epithelial cells of oral "hairy" leukoplakia, an AIDS-associated lesion. *N Engl J Med* 313:1564–1571, 1985.

19. Schiodt M, Greenspan D, Daniels TE, et al. Clinical and histologic spectrum of oral hairy leukoplakia. *Oral Surg Oral Med Oral Pathol* 64:716–720, 1987.

20. Greenspan D, Greenspan JS, Hearst N, et al. Relation of oral hairy leukoplakia to infection with the human immunodeficiency virus and the risk of developing AIDS. *J Infect Dis* 155:475, 1987.

21. Newman C, Polk BF. Resolution of oral hairy leukoplakia during therapy with 9-(1,3-dihydroxy-2-propoxymethyl) guanine (DHPG). *Ann Intern Med* 107:348–350, 1987.

22. Resnick L, Herbst JS, Ablashi DV, et al. Regression of oral hairy leukoplakia after orally administered acyclovir therapy. *JAMA* 259:384–388, 1988.

23. Kessler HA, Benson CA, Urbanski P. Regression of oral hairy leukoplakia during zidovudine therapy. *Arch Intern Med* 148:2496–2497, 1988.
24. Scully C, Laskaris G, Pindborg J, et al. Oral manifestations of HIV infection and their management. I. More common lesions. *Oral Surg Oral Med Oral Pathol* 71:158–166, 1991.
25. Owen WF. Sexually transmitted disease and traumatic problems in homosexual men. *Ann Intern Med* 92:805, 1980.
26. Scully C, Prime S, Maitland N. Papillomaviruses: Their possible role in oral disease. *Oral Surg Oral Med Oral Pathol* 60:166, 1985.
27. Greenspan D. Oral Manifestations of HIV Infection. In PB Robertson, JS Greenspan (eds), *Perspectives on Oral Manifestations of AIDS*. Littleton, MA: PSG, 1988. Pp 38–48.
28. Winkler JR, Robertson P. Periodontal disease associated with HIV infection. *Oral Surg Oral Med Oral Pathol* 73:145–150, 1992.
29. Winkler JR, Murray PA. AIDS update: Periodontal disease. *J Calif Dent Assoc* 15:20–24, 1987.
30. Winkler JR, Murray PA. Periodontal disease: A potential intraoral expression of AIDS may be rapidly progressive periodontitis. *J Calif Dent Assoc* 12:20, 1987.
31. Laskaris G, Potouridou I, Laskaris M, Stratigos J. Gingival lesions of HIV infection in 178 Greek patients. *Oral Surg Oral Med Oral Pathol* 74:168–171, 1992.
32. Volpe F, Schimmer A, Barr C. Oral manifestations of disseminated *Mycobacterium avium-intracellulare* in a patient with AIDS. *Oral Surg Oral Med Oral Pathol* 60:567, 1985.
33. Lozada F, Silverman S, Migliorati CA, et al. Oral manifestations of tumor and opportunistic infections in the acquired immunodeficiency syndrome (AIDS): Findings in 53 homosexual men with Kaposi's sarcoma. *Oral Surg Oral Med Oral Pathol* 56:491, 1983.
34. Ziegler JL, Miner RC, Rosenbaum E, et al. Outbreak of Burkitt's-like lymphoma in homosexual men. *Lancet* 2:261, 1982.
35. Silverman S, Jr, Lozada-Nur F, Migliorati C. Clinical efficacy of prednisone in the treatment of patients with oral inflammatory ulcerative diseases: A study of fifty-five patients. *Oral Surg Oral Med Oral Pathol* 59:360–363, 1987.
36. Ulirsch RC, Jaffe ES. Sjögren's syndrome–like illness associated with the acquired immunodeficiency syndrome–related complex. *Hum Pathol* 18:1063–1068, 1987.
37. Schidt M, Dodd CL, Greenspan D, et al. Natural history of HIV-associated salivary gland disease. *Oral Surg Oral Med Oral Pathol* 74:326–331, 1992.

Ocular Manifestations *8*

David L. Battinelli, Mariel Brittis

Nowhere is the importance of a multidisciplinary approach to the care of HIV-infected individuals more evident than in the management of eye disease. Careful evaluation of ocular symptoms by the primary care provider and referral for ophthalmologic examination are essential for early diagnosis and treatment of complications. This chapter provides an overview of the common ocular manifestations of HIV infection (Table 8-1). Comprehensive reviews of the subject are also available [1–4].

Noninfectious Etiologies

Conjunctivitis and Keratitis

Nonspecific conjunctivitis, keratitis, and keratoconjunctivitis sicca have been reported in up to 10 percent of AIDS patients. The patient should be asked about conjunctival and corneal irritation, as well as symptoms related to dry eyes. Examination reveals inflammation of the affected part of the eye without pain or change in visual acuity. Treatment of conjunctivitis and keratitis consists of topical antibiotics; artificial tears are used in the management of keratoconjunctivitis sicca [1].

Ocular Hemorrhages

Multiple subconjunctival, scleral, and retinal hemorrhages may indicate the presence of thrombocytopenia related to HIV disease or drug toxicity.

Cotton-Wool Spots

Cotton-wool spots (CWS) are the most common ocular abnormality in HIV disease, occurring in up to 50 percent of patients [3]. Cotton-wool

Table 8-1 *Ocular manifestations of HIV infection*

Noninfectious	Infectious
Nonspecific conjunctivitis	Conjunctivitis
Nonspecific keratitis	Keratitis
Keratoconjunctivitis sicca	Iridocyclitis
Hemorrhages	Uveitis
Cotton-wool spots	Vitreitis
Papilledema	Retinitis
Kaposi's sarcoma	Multifocal choroiditis
Lymphoma	
Ocular palsies	

spots are asymptomatic, white, fluffy, superficial retinal lesions with feathered edges generally distributed near the large vessels of the posterior retinal vascular arcade adjacent to the optic nerve [4] (Plate 7). Histologically they represent infarction of the nerve fiber layer of the retina. HIV-related CWS can be distinguished from those occurring with diabetes mellitus and hypertension by the absence of associated vascular retinopathy.

Diagnosis of CWS is made by their typical appearance on ophthalmoscopic examination. Differential diagnosis includes early retinitis caused by cytomegalovirus (CMV) and, less commonly, other opportunistic pathogens. Unlike retinitis, CWS regress spontaneously in about 2 months, are rarely associated with hemorrhage, and do not produce visual impairment. No specific treatment is indicated.

Cotton-wool spots, retinal hemorrhages, and other microvascular anomalies are collectively referred to as HIV retinopathy, the etiology of which is uncertain [5]. It has been suggested that CMV enters the retina at CWS, but evidence supporting this hypothesis is inconclusive [6, 7]. One report described isolation of *Pneumocystis carinii* from CWS [8]. Others have suggested that CWS results directly from HIV infection of the retina with immune complex deposition [9]. Increased serum viscosity secondary to high fibrinogen levels with resultant "sludging" and retinal infarction has also been proposed as the pathogenesis [5].

Papilledema

Papilledema reflects increased intracranial pressure. In HIV-infected patients, this is often an indication of an expanding infectious or neoplastic mass lesion of the central nervous system. Toxoplasmosis and lymphoma are the two most frequent causes.

Kaposi's Sarcoma

Ocular Kaposi's sarcoma (KS) occurs in up to 20 percent of AIDS patients who have systemic KS but is rarely the initial site of involvement

[1]. Presenting signs include proptosis, ptosis, eyelid edema, conjunctival injection, and diplopia resulting from ocular nerve palsies. The characteristic deep-red or violaceous lesion is most often found along the eyelid margins or bulbar conjunctivae and can be easily confused with a conjunctival hemorrhage [2]. Diagnosis is made by biopsy of an associated mucocutaneous lesion.

Lymphoma

Aggressive non-Hodgkin's lymphoma associated with HIV infection may rarely involve ocular structures. Symptoms and signs, similar to those of KS, are related primarily to local infiltration of the tumor. Computed tomography (CT) or magnetic resonance imaging (MRI) scans together with biopsy are used to diagnose retroorbital mass lesions; vitrectomy permits cytologic sampling for intraocular involvement.

Ocular Palsies

Abnormalities of extraocular movements may be an early manifestation of retroorbital and intracranial mass lesions or lymphomatous meningitis.

Infectious Etiologies

A variety of bacterial, fungal, viral, and parasitic organisms are responsible for many of the ocular complications of HIV disease.

Conjunctivitis and Keratitis

Herpes simplex virus (HSV) keratitis in HIV-infected patients tends to be difficult to treat and prone to relapse [1]. Symptoms include eye pain and blurred vision. Diagnosis is by clinical examination, scrapings, and culture. Treatment is with topical trifluridine; prognosis is variable [10]. Varicella-zoster virus (VZV) ophthalmicus may be the initial manifestation of HIV infection. It presents as severe eye pain associated with keratitis, anterior uveitis, and cutaneous vesicles in a dermatomal distribution. Diagnosis is made clinically, and treatment consists of systemic acyclovir [1]. In addition to keratoconjunctivitis, both HSV and VZV are causes of necrotizing retinitis, which is discussed later in this section.

Iridocyclitis and Anterior Uveitis

Symptoms of iridocyclitis and anterior uveitis include pain and photophobia, and the eyes may appear glossy and red. Slit-lamp examination is necessary for evaluation. Syphilis is an important consideration in the differential diagnosis of eye disease in HIV-infected patients. It may present atypically, be more aggressive, and relapse more frequently than in immunocompetent hosts [11–13]. While relatively uncommon, secondary syphilis may manifest as ocular disease, including iridocyclitis, anterior uveitis, retinitis, and vitreitis. Serologically false-negative cases of syphilis have been reported in HIV disease but are probably unusual [14]. HIV-infected patients with ocular syphilis should be treated with an antibiotic regimen appropriate for neurosyphilis, and close clinical and serologic follow-up study is essential [15].

Vitreitis

Inflammation of the vitreous occurs in many retinal infections. Symptoms include "floaters" and blurred vision, and, with marked inflammation, the vitreous appears cloudy on funduscopic examination.

Retinitis

Cytomegalovirus

The most common cause of retinitis and visual loss associated with HIV disease is CMV infection [2, 3, 16]. The incidence of CMV retinitis ranges from 15 to 46 percent, the vast majority of cases occurring when the CD4 cell count is below $100/mm^3$ [2, 3, 17, 18]. Despite antiviral therapy, approximately 40 percent of patients lose central vision in both eyes by the time of death [6, 19, 20]. Cytomegalovirus retinitis is probably the result of hematogenous spread of the virus to the retina after reactivation of latent infection [19]. Cytomegalovirus spreads along the retinal nerve fiber layer at a rate of 250 μm per week, with proliferating virus found in the leading edge, advancing in a "brush fire" manner [20].

Symptoms of CMV infection depend on its location in the retina [16, 21]. The disease generally starts in one eye, with the onset gradual over a period of weeks. If retinitis does not involve the macula or optic nerve, the patient may have no symptoms, or the only symptoms may be floaters or peripheral visual field loss. If the lesion lies closer to the posterior retina, near the macula or optic nerve, a corresponding scotoma or defect in the visual field may occur [16]. Ocular pain, photophobia, and erythema of the eye are unusual [1, 2, 22].

Untreated unilateral CMV infection becomes bilateral in up to 80 percent of cases. Visual loss results from retinal necrosis, edema, and detachment. Involvement of the optic nerve results in visual loss regardless of disease in the surrounding retina [19]. With resolution of edema and necrosis, the retina is left as an atrophic, thin tissue susceptible to breaks or tears [1]. Sudden onset of multiple floaters, flashing lights, visual field defects, and decreased vision portends retinal detachment. The surgical treatment of retinal detachment associated with CMV disease is difficult, and early results were disappointing [23]. However, more recent reports, reflecting careful patient selection and earlier intervention, have been encouraging [24, 25].

Ophthalmologic examination is somewhat variable [3, 20]. Early CMV retinitis is often subtle and characterized by one or two small white granular lesions, similar to CWS, often without hemorrhage. Early lesions are more commonly seen in the anterior or peripheral retina. More advanced CMV retinitis is characterized by perivascular, fluffy, yellow-white infiltrates accompanied by hemorrhage ("scrambled eggs and ketchup" or "pizza pie" pattern) (Plate 8). Late lesions are often found in the posterior retina near the major vascular arcade, macula, and optic nerve.

Diagnosis of CMV retinitis relies on funduscopic examination [16]. Serology and blood and urine cultures are nondiagnostic, and vitreal aspiration is not specific. Retinal biopsy, although possible, is impractical and should be reserved for progressive retinitis of uncertain etiology [1]. Lesions suspicious for, but not diagnostic of, CMV infection should be followed closely, by serial funduscopic examinations and retinal photographs.

Two antiviral agents, ganciclovir and foscarnet, offer effective treatment but not cure for CMV retinitis. Ganciclovir is a nucleotide analogue of acyclovir that is 10 to 100 times more effective against CMV. Approximately 85 percent of patients respond to a 2-week course of ganciclovir given at the dose of 5 mg/kg intravenously every 12 hours [22, 26]. Maintenance therapy with ganciclovir at 5 mg/kg/day intravenously five to seven times per week is required to prevent relapse [21]. Eventually, progressive retinitis may occur in up to 50 percent of patients despite institution of therapy [1]. Neutropenia is the major toxicity of ganciclovir, occurring in up to 40 percent of patients and often requiring a dose reduction, the addition of granulocyte colony stimulating factor, or substitution of foscarnet. The concurrent use of ganciclovir and zidovudine is generally not recommended [27]. Intravitreal ganciclovir injection and implants designed to avoid systemic toxicity are currently under investigation [28, 29]. Oral ganciclovir has recently been approved by the Food and Drug Administration for maintenance therapy in patients with CMV retinitis; the dose is 1 gram orally 3 times per day. Its role in primary prophylaxis has not been established.

Foscarnet also has antiviral activity against CMV, and response and relapse rates are similar to those of ganciclovir [30–32]. Primary therapy consists of 60 mg/kg intravenously every 8 hours for 2 to 3 weeks. Renal dysfunction and metabolic abnormalities, including hypocalcemia and hypomagnesemia, are common [33]. Maintenance therapy with 90 to 120 mg/kg/day intravenously is necessary to prevent relapse. A trial comparing foscarnet and ganciclovir showed that they were equally effective in the treatment of CMV retinitis, but that patients who received foscarnet lived a median of 4 months longer [34]. This survival advantage has been postulated to be due to inherent antiretroviral activity of foscarnet.

The combination of ganciclovir and foscarnet has recently been proposed for primary therapy of CMV infection, with the use of alternating agents for maintenance therapy [35]. While this regimen appears to be effective and well tolerated, it has not yet been compared to conventional treatments.

Toxoplasma gondii

Toxoplasma gondii is the second most common cause of retinitis, identified in approximately 3 percent of patients with AIDS [36, 37]. It may occur during the course of primary infection or from relapse of latent extraocular infection with dissemination to the retina. Ten percent of patients with toxoplasmic encephalitis have retinitis, and over 50 percent of those with retinitis are diagnosed with encephalitis [36]. Symptoms include photophobia, floaters, and decreased vision; physical findings consist of anterior uveitis, vitreitis, and necrotizing retinitis [37]. Although toxoplasmic retinitis may be confused with CMV disease, it is seldom associated with hemorrhage and frequently causes a marked vitreitis or anterior uveitis [37, 38]. Diagnosis is clinical; central nervous system involvement should be ruled out by CT or MRI scanning. Serologic tests are generally not useful. Treatment with pyrimethamine-sulfadiazine or pyrimethamine-clindamycin is effective, with regression of lesions occurring in 2 to 3 weeks [36, 37]. Maintenance therapy is required to prevent relapse.

Herpes Simplex and Varicella-Zoster

Although acute retinal necrosis caused by these viruses has been reported with HIV infection, it is much less frequent than CMV disease [39]. Symptoms include photophobia, floaters, and decreased vision. Funduscopic examination reveals confluent areas of necrotizing retinitis, frequently with retinal arteritis and optic neuritis. One third of cases are bilateral, with the disease progressing to severe visual loss in most cases. Therapy with high-dose intravenous acyclovir may be helpful [40]. Multiple viral pathogens have been isolated in some patients with acute retinal necrosis, leading authorities to recommend combination antiviral treatment [41, 42].

Candida albicans

Fungal retinitis is unusual in AIDS [1–3]. Candidal involvement produces one or more fluffy, yellow-white, deep retinal lesions, which may be associated with significant vitreitis but not hemorrhage. Positive blood cultures may support the diagnosis. Treatment consists of systemic, and sometimes intravitreal, amphotericin B and removal of the primary source of infection, such as an intravascular catheter.

Bacteria

Bacterial retinitis and endophthalmitis are also uncommon but should be considered in differential diagnosis, especially if the patient uses injection drugs or has concomitant endocarditis. Diagnosis is made by blood or vitreous cultures, or both. Treatment consists of systemic antibiotics.

Other Pathogens

Pneumocystis carinii, Mycobacterium avium complex, *Cryptococcus neoformans, Histoplasma capsulatum,* and other opportunistic organisms can cause ocular disease in HIV-infected patients, presenting as a multifocal choroiditis, although less commonly than CMV and toxoplasmosis. Vitrectomy with culture establishes the specific diagnosis. Newer techniques, such as retinal biopsy by pars plana vitrectomy and polymerase chain reaction testing of ocular fluids, are increasingly important in the diagnosis of retinal manifestations of AIDS [43, 44].

References

1. Freeman WR, Gross JG. Management of ocular disease in AIDS patients. *Ophthalmol Clin North Amer* 1:91–100, 1988.
2. Freeman WR, Lerner CW, Mines JA, et al. A prospective study of the ophthalmologic findings in the acquired immune deficiency syndrome. *Am J Ophthalmol* 97:133–142, 1984.
3. Holland GN, Pepose JS, Pettit TH, et al. Acquired immune deficiency syndrome: Ocular manifestations. *Ophthalmology* 90:859–873, 1983.
4. Mansour AM, Jampol IM, Logani S, Reed J. Cotton wool spots in acquired immunodeficiency syndrome compared with diabetes mellitus, systemic hypertension, and central retinal vein occlusion. *Arch Ophthalmol* 106:1074–1077, 1988.
5. Engstrom RE, Holland GN, Hardy WD, Meiselman HG. Hemorrheologic abnormalities in patients with human immunodeficiency virus infection and ophthalmic microvasculopathy. *Am J Ophthalmol* 109:153–161, 1990.
6. Mill J, Jacobson MA, O'Donnell JJ, et al. Treatment of cytomegalovirus retinitis in patients with AIDS. *Rev Infect Dis* 10(suppl 3):5522–5531, 1988.
7. Newsome DA, Green RW, Miller ED, et al. Microvascular aspects of acquired immune deficiency syndrome retinopathy. *Am J Ophthalmol* 98:590–601, 1984.
8. Kwok S, O'Donnell JJ, Wood I. Retinal cotton wool spots in a patient with *Pneumocystis carinii* infection. *N Engl J Med* 307:184–185, 1982.
9. Pomerantz RJ, Kuritzkes DR, de la Monte SM, et al. Infection of the retina by human immunodeficiency virus type I. *N Engl J Med* 317:1643–1647, 1987.

10. Young TL, Robin JB, Holland GN, et al. Herpes simplex keratitis in patients with acquired immune deficiency syndrome. *Ophthalmology* 96:1476–1479, 1989.

11. Tramont EC. Syphilis in the AIDS era. *N Engl J Med* 316:1600–1601, 1987.

12. Johns DR, Tierney M, Felsenstein D. Alteration in the natural history of neurosyphilis by concurrent infection with the human immunodeficiency virus. *N Engl J Med* 316:1569–1572, 1987.

13. Passo MS, Rosanbaum JT. Ocular syphilis in patients with human immunodeficiency virus infection. *Am J Ophthalmol* 106:1–6, 1988.

14. Hicks CB, Benson PM, Lupton GP, et al. Seronegative secondary syphilis in a patient with the human immunodeficiency virus (HIV) with Kaposi's sarcoma. *Ann Intern Med* 107:492–495, 1987.

15. Berry CD, Hooten TM, Collier AC, Lukehart SA. Neurologic relapse after benzathine penicillin therapy for secondary syphilis in a patient with HIV infection. *N Engl J Med* 316:1587–1589, 1987.

16. Bloom JN, Palestine AG. The diagnosis of cytomegalovirus retinitis. *Ann Intern Med* 109:963–969, 1988.

17. Henderly DE, Freeman WR, Smith RE, et al. Cytomegalovirus as the initial manifestation of the acquired immune deficiency syndrome. *Am J Ophthalmol* 103:316–320, 1987.

18. Kuppermann BD, Petty JG, Richman DD, et al. Correlation between CD4+ counts and prevalence of cytomegalovirus retinitis and human immunodeficiency virus–related non-infectious retinal vasculopathy in patients with acquired immunodeficiency syndrome. *Am J Ophthalmol* 115:572–582, 1993.

19. Grossniklaus HE, Frank KE, Tomsak RL. Cytomegalovirus retinitis optic neuritis in acquired immune deficiency syndrome. *Ophthalmology* 94:1601–1604, 1987.

20. Pepose JS, Holland GN, Nestor MS, et al. Acquired immune deficiency syndrome. Pathogenic mechanisms of ocular disease. *Ophthalmology* 92:472–484, 1985.

21. Henderly DE, Freeman WR, Causey DM, Rao NA. Cytomegalovirus retinitis and response to therapy with ganciclovir. *Ophthalmology* 94:425–434, 1987.

22. Collaborative DHPG Study Group. Treatment of serious cytomegalovirus infections with 9-(1,3-dihydroxy-2-propoxymethyl) guanine in patients with AIDS and other immunodeficiencies. *N Engl J Med* 314:801–805, 1986.

23. Jabs DA, Enger C, Haller J, de Bustros S. Retinal detachments in patients with cytomegalovirus retinitis. *Arch Ophthalmol* 109:794–799, 1991.

24. Lim JI, Enger C, Haller JA, et al. Improved visual results after surgical repair of cytomegalovirus-related retinal detachments. *Ophthalmology* 101:264–269, 1994.

25. Kuppermann BD, Flores-Aguilar M, Quiceno JI, et al. A masked prospective evaluation of outcome parameters for cytomegalovirus-related retinal detachment surgery in patients with acquired immune deficiency syndrome. *Ophthalmology* 101:46–55, 1994.

26. Culbertson WW. Discussion of DE Henderly, WR Freeman, DM Casey, NA Rao. Cytomegalovirus retinitis and response to therapy with ganciclovir. *Ophthalmology* 94:432–434, 1987.

27. Hochster H, Dieterich D, Bozzette S, et al. Toxicity of combined ganciclovir and zidovudine for cytomegalovirus disease associated with AIDS. *Ann Intern Med* 113:111–117, 1990.
28. Ussery F, Gibson S, Conklin R, et al. Intravitreal ganciclovir in the treatment of AIDS associated with cytomegalovirus retinitis. *Ophthalmology* 95:640–648, 1988.
29. Heinemann M-H. Long-term intravitreal ganciclovir therapy for cytomegalovirus retinopathy. *Arch Ophthalmol* 107:1767–1772, 1989.
30. Farthing CF, Dalgleish AG, Clark A, et al. Phosphonoformate (foscarnet): A pilot study in AIDS and AIDS-related complex. *AIDS* 1:21–25, 1987.
31. Walmsley S, Chew E, Fanning MM, et al. Treatment of cytomegalovirus retinitis with trisodium phosphonoformate hexahydrate (foscarnet). *J Infect Dis* 157:569–572, 1988.
32. Palestine AG, Polis MA, DeSmet MD, et al. A randomized, controlled trial of foscarnet in the treatment of cytomegalovirus retinitis in patients with AIDS. *Ann Intern Med* 115:665–673, 1991.
33. Foscarnet. *Med Lett* 34:3–4, 1992.
34. Studies of Ocular Complications of AIDS Research Group, in collaboration with the AIDS Clinical Trials Group. *N Engl J Med* 23:213–220, 1992.
35. Malte P, Bergmann F, Grunewald T, et al. Safety and efficacy of combined and alternating ganciclovir and foscarnet in acute and maintenance therapy for CMV infection in HIV positive patients. Eighth International Conference on AIDS, Amsterdam, July 1992.
36. Holland GN, Engstrom RE, Glasgow BJ, et al. Ocular toxoplasmosis in patients with the acquired immunodeficiency syndrome. *Am J Ophthalmol* 106:653–667, 1988.
37. Weiss A, Margo CE, Ledford DK, et al. Toxoplasmic retinochoroiditis as an initial manifestation of the acquired immune deficiency syndrome. *Am J Ophthalmol* 101:248–249, 1986.
38. Parke DW, Font RL. Diffuse toxoplasmic retinochoroiditis in a patient with AIDS. *Arch Ophthalmol* 104:571–575, 1986.
39. Duker JS, Blumenkranz MS. Diagnosis and management of the acute retinal necrosis (ARN) syndrome. *Surv Ophthalmol* 35:327–343, 1991.
40. Blumenkranz MS, Culbertson WW, Clarkson JG, Dix R. Treatment of the acute retinal necrosis syndrome with intravenous acyclovir. *Ophthalmology* 93:296–300, 1986.
41. Rummelt V, Rummelt C, Jahn G, et al. Triple retinal infection with human immunodeficiency virus type 1, cytomegalovirus, and herpes simplex virus type 1: Light and electron microscopy, immunohistochemistry, and in situ hybridization. *Ophthalmology* 101:270–279, 1994.
42. Engstrom RE, Holland GN, Margolis TP, et al. The progressive outer retinal necrosis syndrome: A variant of necrotizing herpetic retinopathy in patients with AIDS. *Ophthalmology* 101:1488–1502, 1994.
43. Freeman WR, Stern WH, Gross JG, et al. Pathologic observation made by retinal biopsy. *Retina* 10:195–204, 1990.
44. Fox GM, Crouse CA, Chuang EL, et al. Detection of herpesvirus DNA in vitreous and aqueous specimens by the polymerase chain reaction. *Arch Ophthalmol* 109:266–271, 1991.

Dermatologic Manifestations 9

Howard K. Koh, Bret E. Davis

Dermatologic disorders may be the first or most prominent signs of HIV infection (Table 9-1). In this chapter, we present an overview of the assessment and management of these conditions. The reader is referred to additional references for further discussion [1–4].

Approach to the Patient

One should consider HIV infection when encountering patients with skin disease that is severe or atypical, or does not respond to routine treatment. In addition to performing an HIV risk assessment, the physician should ask about local skin symptoms (such as burning, pain, or itch), the length of time a lesion has been present, its distribution, and its initial appearance. Dermatologic examination should be an organized regional survey, which includes inspection and palpation.

Viral Infections

HIV Exanthem

Approximately 75 percent of patients symptomatic from primary HIV infection will have an exanthem in addition to fever, lethargy, malaise, and lymphadenopathy [5].

Clinical Manifestations

The exanthem appears much like that seen in other acute viral infections. Asymptomatic, oval, erythematous macules or urticarial plaques, usually 0.5 to 2.0 cm in diameter, may be generalized, involving the

Table 9-1 *Dermatologic manifestations of HIV infection*

Disease	Clinical manifestations	Diagnosis	Treatment
		Viral infections	
Acute HIV exanthem (primary HIV infection)*	Fever, myalgias, uticaria Truncal, palmar, plantar maculopapules	HIV antibodies usually within 12 wk of infection Low white blood cell count, thrombocytopenia, hypergammaglobulinemia	Symptomatic treatment
Herpes simplex*	May be widely disseminated, persistent erosions and perirectal ulcers (see Plate 9)	HSV culture Tzanck smear for multinucleated giant cells	Acyclovir, 200–400 mg PO 5 ×/day Topical trifluridine or systemic foscarnet for acyclovir-resistant strains
Varicella-zoster*	May be severe, persistent, dermatomal (see Plate 10), disseminated, or deeply scarring Intractable herpetic pain	Herpesvirus culture Tzanck smear for multinucleated giant cells	Acyclovir, 800 mg PO 5 ×/day for dermatomal
Molluscum contagiosum*	Clusters of white umbilicated papules (see Plate 11)	Biopsy or KOH preparations of soft central material show large viral inclusions	Cryosurgery
Oral hairy leukoplakia	Whitish, nonremovable verrucous plaques on sides of tongue	Biopsy	None generally necessary
Warts (human papillomavirus)	Increased number, size of verrucous lesions	Biopsy or clinical appearance	Topical agents Surgical excision Cryosurgery

Fungal infections

*Candida albicans**	Oral mucosal white plaques, sore throat, dysphagia, deep tongue erosions Intractable vaginal infection Nail infection	Culture KOH slide prepartion	Topical: nystatin suspension, clotrimazole troche Systemic: oral ketoconazole or fluconazole
Tinea versicolor	Thick, scaly hypopigmented or light-brown plaques on trunk	KOH slide shows numerous short hyphae and spores Wood's light accentuates lesions	Topical: selenium sulfide, miconazole, clotrimazole, sodium thiosulfate
Dermatophytes (tinea corporis, pedis, cruris)	Extensive involvement, especially groin and feet	KOH slide preparation shows branched, septated hyphae	Topical: miconazole Oral: griseofulvin, ketoconazole

Bacterial infections

Staphylococcal*	Superficial and subcutaneous infections Impetigo (see Plate 12)	Culture	Dicloxacillin First-generation cephalosporin
Syphilis*	Painless chancre (primary, see Fig. 23-1) Generalized plaques and papulosquamous lesions (secondary, see Plate 13) Incubation period for neurosyphilis may be very short (mo)	VDRL or RPR *and* FTA-abs or MHA-TP Skin biopsy	Standard recommended treatment may not be sufficient to prevent central nervous system involvement

Table 9-1 *Continued*

Disease	Clinical manifestations	Diagnosis	Treatment
Bacterial infections			
Bacillary angiomatosis*	Dome-shaped or pedunculated solitary or multiple papules and nodules (4 mm–2 cm) Visceral angiomatosis	Biopsy	Erythromycin, 250–500 mg PO q6h Chronic suppressive therapy may be necessary
Arthropod infestations			
Scabies	Generalized crusted papules and eczematous lesions	KOH or oil preparation shows mites	Lindane Pyrethrin Permethrin
Miscellaneous disorders			
Seborrheic dermatitis*	Red scaling plaques (see Plate 14) with yellow greasy scales and distinct margins, on the face and scalp	Biopsy KOH to rule out tinea	Ketoconazole cream Oral ketoconazole, 200–400 mg/day Low-potency topical steroids
Psoriasis	Activation of prior disease or no previous history	Biopsy	Treatment-resistant cases may respond to etretinate or zidovudine
Xeroderma	Severe dry skin, possible erythroderma	Clinical presentation	Lactic acid emollients Lac-Hydrin
Papular eruption	2–5 mm skin-colored papules on head, neck, upper trunk Pruritic, chronic	Biopsy shows lymphocytic perivascular infiltrate	Low-potency topical steroids Antipruritic lotions Antihistamines

Eosinophilic and bacterial folliculitis*	Groups of small vesicles and pustules that can become confluent EF: Polycyclic plaques with central hypopigmentation Severe, intractable pruritus	Biopsy Negative culture for atypical organisms	Ultraviolet B phototherapy for EF Topical/systemic antibiotics for bacterial folliculitis
Thrombocytopenic purpura	Petechiae	Complete blood count	Antiretroviral therapy
Yellow nails	Yellow discoloration of nail plate May be associated with *Pneumocystis carinii* pneumonia	Clinical examination	None
Darkened nails	Dark blue appearance at bases of fingernails	Recent history of zidovudine treatment	None
Premature hair graying, long eyelashes	Usually with advanced HIV disease	Physical examination	None
Drug reactions*	Most commonly sulfonamides, ampicillin Widespread maculopapular eruption	Clinical examination	Alternative drugs
Neoplastic disorders			
Kaposi's sarcoma*	Pale to deep violaceous, oval plaques (see Plate 15) and papules (see Plate 16) Oral lesions (usually palate) Visceral lesions	Biopsy	Localized disease: intralesional chemotherapy, cryotherapy, radiation therapy Systemic disease: chemotherapy, interferon

*Discussed in text.
Source: Modified from TP Habif, *Clinical Dermatology: A Color Guide to Diagnosis and Therapy* (2nd ed). St. Louis: Mosby, 1990; some data also from *Med Lett Drugs Ther* 35:75–86, 1993.

palms and soles, or affect the trunk and upper body only. The lesions may be centrally hemorrhagic, and desquamation may occur. Patients may also have an oral enanthem, with superficial ulcerations or candidiasis extending into the esophagus.

Laboratory Data
Patients may have leukopenia, lymphopenia with reversed CD4:CD8 lymphocyte ratio, thrombocytopenia, and p24 antigenemia. The HIV antibody test, initially negative, usually becomes positive within 6 to 12 weeks.

Differential Diagnosis
Viral infections (including mononucleosis and aseptic meningitis); rickettsial, *Mycoplasma*, and bacterial infections; toxoplasmosis; and strongyloidiasis must be distinguished from primary HIV infection. Secondary syphilis is another important diagnostic consideration, especially when lesions involve the palms and soles.

Evaluation
The clinical impression should be confirmed by demonstration of HIV seroconversion, p24 antigenemia, or HIV viremia. Skin biopsy findings are nonspecific, showing a lymphocytic perivascular infiltrate in the papillary dermis.

Management
The exanthem and symptoms usually resolve with supportive care over a period of several weeks.

Herpesviruses

Chronic herpes simplex virus (HSV) and varicella-zoster virus (VZV) lesions may be early indicators of HIV disease. These infections usually reflect reactivation of latent disease. Herpesvirus infections in HIV-infected patients can cause severe morbidity, and genital ulcerations increase the risk of transmitting and acquiring HIV infection.

Clinical Manifestations
Classic HSV type 1 and 2 infections present as self-limited, grouped vesicles, often with an erythematous base, affecting the lips of genitalia. However, in patients with advanced HIV disease, nonhealing HSV erosions may enlarge into severe, painful ulcers that can reach up to 20 cm in diameter (Plate 9). Any ulcerative lesion should be considered herpetic until proven otherwise. Herpes simplex virus infection may occasionally affect the oropharynx and esophagus, with resultant dysphagia and odynophagia. An ulceration demonstrated to harbor HSV and present for over one month in an individual known to be HIV-infected is an AIDS-defining condition.

Varicella-zoster virus infection occurs seven times more frequently in HIV-infected persons than in the general population. Typically, zoster appears as a painful, unidermatomal vesicular eruption on an erythematous base (Plate 10). However, in the context of HIV infection, it is sometimes multidermatomal or disseminated, with hemorrhagic and necrotic lesions. Painful, hyperkeratotic nodules may persist for months. Serious eye complications, including visual loss, may follow zoster ophthalmicus.

Laboratory Data
For immediate diagnosis, Tzanck stain of scrapings from the base of a lesion may show multinucleated giant cells. A rapid assay can demonstrate VZV antigen from vesicular smears. Viral culture of vesicular fluid can differentiate HSV from VZV and provide drug sensitivity information. Skin biopsy is rarely necessary.

Differential Diagnosis
In most cases, grouped vesicles for HSV or dermatomal vesicles for VZV will lead to an accurate diagnosis. On occasion, contact dermatitis can be confused with herpetic infection, as can chancroid, cellulitis, and mycobacterial or fungal disease.

Evaluation
Cutaneous HSV and VZV infections are usually diagnosed clinically.

Management
For HSV, the treatment is oral acyclovir, 200–400 mg five times a day, or, if necessary, intravenously 5 to 10 mg/kg every 8 hours until lesions heal. Maintenance therapy may be necessary in patients with advanced HIV disease. Ulcerative HSV lesions that fail to respond to acyclovir may indicate resistant virus, and topical trifluridine or foscarnet is indicated in such instances. For VZV infection, the treatment is oral acyclovir, 800 mg five times a day, or, if necessary, 10 to 12 mg/kg intravenously every 8 hours for 7 to 14 days. Topical soaks (Domeboro Solution) can be used to help dry wet lesions.

Molluscum Contagiosum

Approximately 20 percent of symptomatic HIV-infected patients develop these pox virus–associated lesions.

Clinical Manifestations
Classic lesions are pearly, dome-shaped, 2- to 4-mm papules with central umbilication (Plate 11). In immunocompetent adults, papules typically appear on the thigh or genital regions after intimate contact. However, in patients with advanced HIV disease, lesions may disseminate widely and are especially common on the face. Individual lesions

can be quite small and lack classic umbilication, or can enlarge to one centimeter or more.

Laboratory Data
Pathognomonic "molluscum bodies" (large viral inclusion formations) can be demonstrated by both potassium hydroxide touch preparations and skin biopsy.

Differential Diagnosis
The most common differential diagnosis is warts caused by human papillomavirus. Disseminated fungal disease, such as cryptococcosis, histoplasmosis, or coccidioidomycosis, may mimic molluscum, but tends to have a more acute onset. Large lesions, especially of the face and head, may be confused with basal cell carcinoma, keratoacanthoma, or squamous cell carcinoma.

Evaluation
The diagnosis of molluscum contagiosum is usually made clinically. However, the presence of atypical lesions in the patient with fever, headache, confusion, or pulmonary infiltrate requires biopsy to rule out systemic fungal infection. Biopsy may also be necessary to exclude malignancy.

Management
Liquid nitrogen applications every 2 weeks may be helpful. Patients can prevent spread of mollusca by discontinuing blade shaving. Electrodesiccation, while effective, is painful, potentially scarring, and has raised concerns about potential aerosolization of HIV.

Fungal Infections

Candidiasis

Mucocutaneous candidal infection is common in HIV-infected patients. Vaginitis and thrush are often seen with early disease. Esophageal, and rarely, tracheal, bronchial, and pulmonary involvement are associated with advanced immunodeficiency and constitute AIDS-defining criteria.

Clinical Manifestations
Candida species are historically known for involving moist intertriginous skin regions with tender, erythematous patches and satellite pustules. Although candidal intertrigo is uncommon in HIV-infected patients, severely immunocompromised individuals may have balanitis, distal urethritis, or paronychia.

Laboratory Data
Potassium hydroxide preparations of smears from affected areas show diagnostic pseudohyphae and budding yeast.

Differential Diagnosis
Thrush must be distinguished from oral hairy leukoplakia, lichen planus, and lichenoid drug eruption. Dermatophyte infections and intertrigo occur in similar locations but do not have satellite lesions.

Evaluation
Clinical appearance and smear are diagnostic. Biopsy is generally unnecessary.

Management
Thrush can be treated topically with nystatin tablets or clotrimazole troches, or systemically with oral ketoconazole or fluconazole. Management of cutaneous lesions includes topical antifungal cream, such as clotrimazole, and local preventive measures to maintain a dry surface, effective both for treatment and prevention of recurrence. Drying macerated skin with twice-daily soaks may also decrease pain.

Bacterial Infections

Staphylococcal Disease

Staphylococcus aureus is a common cutaneous pathogen in HIV-infected patients. There is increased risk for *S. aureus* skin infection and bacteremia associated with disruptions of the skin barrier, such as dermatitis or the presence of an intravascular catheter, qualitative and quantitative neutrophil defects, and increased nasal carriage.

Clinical Manifestations
Cutaneous presentations of *S. aureus* infection include folliculitis, impetigo (Plate 12), ecthyma, furuncles, carbuncles, cellulitis, pyomyositis, and toxic shock syndrome. *Staphylococcus aureus* may secondarily infect other skin lesions, such as those caused by herpesvirus infections and eczema.

Folliculitis is the most common manifestation of staphylococcal skin infection. Follicular pustules may affect the trunk, face, or groin, and usually heal without scarring. Other types of folliculitis include *Pityrosporum* disease (a fungal process confirmed by potassium hydroxide [KOH] scraping) and eosinophilic folliculitis (EF), which is culture negative and of unknown etiology. EF is generally an acneiform, pruritic, papular, or pustular eruption. EF lesions may coalesce to form keratotic, lichenified, or indurated plaques that are bordered by active papular, vesicular areas. Severe pruritus is a cause of significant morbidity in many patients with EF.

With warmer weather, the blisters or erosions of bullous impetigo frequently involve the axilla or groin. Ecthyma, a pyoderma formed of "punched out" firm ulcerations with a purulent base, is sometimes seen in HIV-infected injection drug users. Staphylococcal abscesses at sites of needle entry are also common in this population.

Laboratory Data
Leukocytosis may be present. Cultures in bacterial folliculitis generally grow *S. aureus*, *Streptococcus pneumoniae*, and, less commonly, diphtheroids or gram-negative organisms. Bacterial cultures in EF yield no growth; histologic findings on skin biopsy include diagnostic follicular destruction with striking eosinophilic infiltration.

Differential Diagnosis
Follicular inflammation is ordinarily seen with acne, local shaving, and topical steroid withdrawal. In the setting of HIV infection, acneiform papules may occur with histoplasmosis, cryptococcosis, and mycobacterial infection. Differential diagnosis also includes dermatophytosis, pustular psoriasis, superficial pemphigus, *Demodex* or scabies infestations, and dermatitis herpetiformis. Candidal folliculitis usually appears with characteristic satellite lesions. Ecthyma gangrenosum presents with a distinctive dark discoloration.

Evaluation
Gram's stain and culture of swab of biopsy specimens, or both, comprise the initial evaluation of suspected staphylococcal skin infection. EF is diagnosed by skin biopsy.

Management
Treatment of folliculitis may prevent progression to furuncles, carbuncles, abscess, or cellulitis. Uncomplicated folliculitis is treated with topical antibacterial agents such as clindamycin or mupirocin and antibacterial soap (chlorhexidine). For more advanced lesions, any areas of enclosed infection should be incised and drained. Oral antistaphylococcal penicillins (e.g., dicloxacillin) and first-generation cephalosporins are useful. Some authors recommend the addition of rifampin or topical mupirocin in an attempt to clear staphylococcal nasal carriage and augment clinical response. Occasionally, HIV-infected patients require chronic low-dose oral antibiotics, but most staphylococcal pyodermas are curable. In EF, remissions have occurred with the use of ultraviolet B light treatments (290-320 nm) [6]. Progressively increasing doses three times per week has been associated with significant relief of pruritus.

Syphilis

The incidence of syphilis rose in the late 1970s and early 1980s, concomitant with onset of the HIV epidemic. Persons with primary syphilis have disruption of normal skin integrity and are at increased risk for HIV transmission. Any patient diagnosed with syphilis is a candidate for HIV counseling and testing, and all patients with HIV disease should be routinely screened for syphilis. HIV-infected patients with *Treponema pallidum* infection may have false-negative serologic tests, severe or atypical clinical presentations, poor response to antibiotic therapy, and accelerated progression to meningovascular syphilis.

Clinical Manifestations
Most HIV-infected patients with syphilis have typical skin lesions. These include the painless chancre of primary syphilis (see Fig 23-1) and the diffuse copper-colored papulosquamous eruption of secondary syphilis, which has predilection to palms, soles, and mucocutaneous surfaces (Plate 13). However, atypical presentations, such as painful ulcers and slowly growing isolated papules or nodules, are also common.

Laboratory Data
Serologic tests are generally positive in primary and secondary syphilis. Skin biopsy shows typical findings of perivascular lymphocytic and plasma cell infiltrates. Multinucleated giant cells and vascular degenerative changes are seen with more chronic lesions. Warthin-Starry silver stains and immunofluorescent staining may demonstrate the pathogenic spirochete.

Differential Diagnosis
The differential diagnosis of primary syphilis includes chancroid, HSV infection, and trauma. Secondary syphilis should be considered in the differential diagnosis of generalized maculopapular eruptions, especially those with palmar or plantar involvement.

Evaluation
Serologic tests are used to confirm the clinical diagnosis. Nontreponemal tests (RPR, VDRL) are used both to screen for the disease and to follow response to treatment. Treponemal tests (FTA-abs, MHA-TP) are employed to confirm positive nontreponemal tests. Nontreponemal tests may be falsely negative in secondary syphilis because of the prozone effect, in which extreme titers yield such antibody excess that the cross-linking necessary for agglutination is absent. Testing of progressively diluted samples eliminates this problem. Both nontreponemal and treponemal serologies may be falsely negative in primary syphilis.

Management

Penicillin continues to be the drug of choice for patients with primary and secondary syphilis. In patients without neurologic involvement, treatment consists of 2.4 to 4.8 million units of intramuscular benzathine penicillin G with clinical and serologic monitoring of response. Controversy exists as to whether HIV-infected patients with early syphilis require lumbar puncture as part of their evaluation. This and other issues pertaining to diagnosis and management of syphilis are discussed in Chapter 23.

Bacillary Angiomatosis

Bacillary angiomatosis (BA) is a vascular proliferative disorder of the skin, lymph nodes, and viscera [7–9]. Associated organisms include the rickettsia-like species, *Rochalimaea quintana*, the cause of body louse–transmitted trench fever, and *Rochalimaea henselae* [10, 11].

While the cutaneous lesion is asymptomatic, hematogenous or lymphatic spread may result in weight loss, nausea, vomiting, and hepatosplenomegaly; untreated BA can be fatal. Environmental sources for the bacillus remain unclear, although in some patients domestic cats may serve as a reservoir.

Clinical Manifestations

Moderately firm lesions (approximately 1 cm in diameter) are most often red to purple, dome-shaped, friable papules. Scale and erythematous border may be present. Superficial lesions, which may be single or number 100 or more, may ulcerate and crust. Distribution frequently includes face, trunk, and extremities but usually spares palms, soles, and mouth. Other manifestations include subcutaneous lesions, and plaques or masses with erythema resembling cellulitis. Atypical presentations with generalized or zosteriform patterns may also occur.

Laboratory Data

Skin biopsy shows increased endothelial-lined vascular spaces in the dermis, with large cuboidal cells containing gram-negative rods. The fastidious, motile, curved organisms stain by the Warthin-Starry method and can be grown in culture with blood cell lysis technique.

Differential Diagnosis

Kaposi's sarcoma (KS) is the lesion most difficult to distinguish from BA both clinically and histologically. Less frequently, dermatofibroma, cherry angioma, or pyogenic granuloma (PG) appears similar to BA. Because superficial thinning and ulceration are often present in BA, shave biopsy may suggest PG, but full-thickness biopsy should distinguish between the two conditions. BA may occasionally be confused with angiosarcoma.

Evaluation

Full-thickness biopsy is the diagnostic method of choice. Lesions bleed profusely after sharp instrumentation.

Management

Oral erythromycin is the treatment of choice. Recommended doses range from 250 to 500 mg every 6 hours until lesions resolve (generally 2 weeks to one month). Less consistent success has been obtained with trimethoprim-sulfamethoxazole, isoniazid, rifampin, or doxycycline. Chronic suppressive therapy may be necessary to prevent relapse.

Miscellaneous Disorders

Seborrheic Dermatitis

Seborrheic dermatitis (SD), a common skin disease of the face and scalp, may occur as a severe variant in HIV-infected patients, afflicting 50 to 80 percent of this population [12]. The etiology of SD is unknown, although *Pityrosporum* is thought by some authorities to have a causative role.

Clinical Manifestations

In normal hosts, SD typically appears as a mildly erythematous scaly eruption involving the scalp, forehead, eyebrows, cheeks, and nose. In HIV-infected patients, there is often sudden production of markedly erythematous, inflammatory, papular, or even psoriasiform lesions (Plate 14). Lesions may have adherent yellow scales with a greasy appearance, crusts, and distinct margins. Distribution is often symmetric and may include facial, posterior auricular, neck, and back regions; less frequently the trunk, groin, and extremities are involved. With chronic disease, there may be central atrophy, with hypopigmentation and loss of skin lines.

Laboratory Data

Biopsy of HIV-related SD may reveal unusual histologic features, including plasma cells, leukocytoclasis, focal obliteration of the dermoepidermal interface by lymphoid clusters, psoriasiform hyperplasia of the epidermis, widespread nuclear retention in the outer epidermal layers, overproduction of keratin, and dilated, thick-walled vessels of the upper dermis. *Pityrosporum* may be present.

Differential Diagnosis

More severe SD cases resemble psoriasis, but do not exhibit extensor surface extremity or gluteal cleft involvement. Also, the yellow scale and associated crusting are distinct from the usual silvery psoriatic scale. Other considerations in differential diagnosis include contact or exfoliative dermatitis, parapsoriasis, drug eruption, ichthyosis, and tinea faciale.

Evaluation
Diagnosis is generally made by clinical appearance. Potassium hydroxide preparation of scrapings should be done to rule out tinea infection. Skin biopsy is generally not necessary.

Management
Low-potency topical steroids result in improvement of mild SD. For resistant cases, antifungal agents, such as topical ketoconazole cream, or oral ketoconazole in doses of 200 to 400 mg per day can be used.

Kaposi's Sarcoma

Kaposi's sarcoma is a multifocal endothelial cell-derived tumor that primarily affects the skin but may involve other tissues as well [13, 14]. There is ongoing debate about the precise cell of origin, the potential causative role of a herpesviruslike agent, and whether KS represents a true malignancy. Classic KS is a rare tumor involving the lower extremities of men from well-defined ethnic groups, including Central European Jews, Poles, Russians, and Italians, in their sixth and seventh decades. HIV-infected patients have a 20,000-fold increased rate of KS.

Clinical Manifestations
In the early (patch or macular) stage, cutaneous lesions are irregular, reddish-blue, or purple to violaceous macules. Some have a bruise-like or "contusiform" appearance. Macules may become papular or nodular, or coalesce to form enlarging patches, plaques, and fusiform and oval tumors (Plates 15 and 16). Individual lesions may be asymptomatic, although pain, itching, and burning are frequently noted. Lymphadenopathy, both reactive and neoplastic, is common, as are oral and mucous membrane involvement. Gastrointestinal tract lesions, while generally asymptomatic, may cause abdominal pain, bowel obstruction, or bleeding. The lungs, and, less frequently, liver, abdominal lymph nodes, spleen, adrenal glands, and heart may also be involved. AIDS-related KS lesions differ from those of classic KS by their smaller size (commonly < 1 cm in diameter), their tendency to follow the lines of cutaneous cleavage, and their generalized distribution.

Laboratory Data
In early KS, histopathologic differentiation from granulation tissue may be difficult. Biopsy of these lesions shows the upper half of the dermis to contain irregular, thin-walled vascular channels with jagged and dilated lumina lined by flattened to slightly plump endothelial cells. As lesions evolve, capillary-sized vascular channels and spindle-shaped

cell components proliferate. Intertwining fascicles and aggregates of spindle-shaped cells lining erythrocyte-filled vascular slits allow a definitive histologic diagnosis of KS.

The histogenesis of KS has been debated for years, but recent studies involving factor VIII-related antigen and *Ulex europaeus* agglutinin suggest an endothelial cell of origin. Whether these endothelial cells are of lymphocytic or blood vessel derivation, or both, is unclear.

Differential Diagnosis

Although cutaneous lesions of KS usually have distinctive coloration, differential diagnosis includes other vascular lesions, such as pyogenic granuloma, BA, hemangioma, or glomus tumor; granulomatous diseases, such as sarcoidosis; and cancers, such as malignant melanoma and lymphoma. Parasitic and fungal infections should also be considered when ulcerated lesions are present.

Evaluation

Diagnosis of initial or atypical KS lesions is made by skin biopsy. Recognition of new lesions in a patient with established KS is generally based on clinical experience.

Management

Localized disease can be treated with intralesional agents, such as vinblastine sulfate, cryotherapy, or radiation therapy. Experimental approaches with tumor necrosis factor and antiangiogenesis factors are currently being explored. Treatment options for more widespread disease are addressed in Chapter 29.

Cutaneous Drug Reactions

HIV-infected patients are estimated to have drug-related eruptions approximately 10 times more often than the general population. Agents frequently associated with skin rash include sulfonamides and aminopenicillins. Morbilliform and urticarial presentations are most common [15]. Bullous drug reactions, including toxic epidermal necrolysis, may also be more frequent in HIV disease [16].

References

1. James W, Thiers BH (eds). AIDS: A ten-year perspective. *Dermatol Clin* 9:465–501, 1991.
2. Habif TP. *Clinical Dermatology: A Color Guide to Diagnosis and Therapy* (2nd ed). St. Louis: Mosby, 1990.
3. Friedman-Kien AE. *Color Atlas of AIDS*. Philadelphia: Saunders, 1989.

4. Dover JS, Johnson RA. Cutaneous manifestations of human immunodeficiency virus infection. *Arch Dermatol* 127:1383–1391 and 1549–1558, 1991.

5. Hulsebosch HJ, Claessen FAP, van Ginkel CJW, et al. Human immunodeficiency virus exanthem. *J Am Acad Dermatol* 23:483–486, 1990.

6. Buchness MR, Lim HW, Hatcher VA, et al. Eosinophilic pustular folliculitis in the acquired immunodeficiency syndrome: Treatment with ultraviolet B phototherapy. *N Engl J Med* 318:1183–1186, 1988.

7. Relman DA, Loutit JS, Schmidt TM, et al. The agent of bacillary angiomatosis: An approach to the identification of uncultured pathogens. *N Engl J Med* 323:1573–1580, 1990.

8. Slater LN, Welch DF, Hensel D, et al. A newly recognized fastidious gram-negative pathogen as a cause of fever and bacteremia. *N Engl J Med* 323:1587–1593, 1990.

9. Cockerell CJ, LeBoit PE. Bacillary angiomatosis: A newly characterized, pseudoneoplastic, infectious, cutaneous vascular disorder. *J Am Acad Dermatol* 22:501–512, 1990.

10. Koehler JE, Quinn FD, Berger TG, et al. Isolation of *Rochalimaea* species from cutaneous and osseous lesions of bacillary angiomatosis. *N Engl J Med* 327:1625–1631, 1992.

11. Koehler JA, et al. *Rochalimaea henselae* infection: A new zoonosis with the domestic cat as reservoir. *JAMA* 271:531–535, 1994.

12. Soeprono FF, Schinella RA, Cockerell CJ, et al. Seborrheic-like dermatitis of acquired immunodeficiency syndrome. *J Am Acad Dermatol* 14:242–248, 1986.

13. Rutherford GW, Schwarcz SK, Lemp GF, et al. The epidemiology of AIDS-related Kaposi's sarcoma in San Francisco. *J Infect Dis* 159:3:569–571, 1989.

14. Chachoua A, Krigel R, Lafleur F, et al. Prognostic factors and staging classification of patients with epidemic Kaposi's sarcoma. *J Clin Oncol* 7:774–780, 1989.

15. Coopman SA, Johnson RA, Platt R, Stern RS. Cutaneous disease and drug reactions in HIV infection. *N Engl J Med* 328:1670–1674, 1993.

16. Saiag P, Caumes E, Chosidow O, et al. Drug-induced toxic epidermal necrolysis (Lyell syndrome) in patients infected with the human immunodeficiency virus. *J Am Acad Dermatol* 26:567–574, 1992.

Cardiac Manifestations *10*

Sheilah A. Bernard

The epidemic of HIV infection has resulted in a low but significant cardiac morbidity (6–7%) and mortality (1–6%) based on reports from the United States and Europe [1]. Cardiac disease may occur at any stage of HIV infection, but important manifestations are more frequent with advanced immunodeficiency.

The first reports documenting cardiac involvement in AIDS were published in 1983. In their review of pathologic findings in 10 patients with AIDS, Reichert and associates [2] reported one case of Kaposi's sarcoma (KS) adjacent to the right coronary artery. The following year, Welch and colleagues [3] described cardiac involvement at autopsy in 11 of 36 AIDS patients; findings included myocardial infiltrates and necrosis, KS of the epicardium and myocardium, and cytomegalovirus (CMV) infection of the myocardium. In 1989, Lewis [4] identified cardiac disease in 59 of 115 postmortem examinations, including pericardial effusion, secondary right ventricular hypertrophy, KS of the pericardium and myocardium, nonbacterial thrombotic endocarditis, myocardial infiltrates, congestive cardiomyopathy, and focal abscess.

Human immunodeficiency virus infection can affect all parts of the heart, including the pericardium, myocardium, and endocardium (Table 10-1).

Pericardial Disease

Clinical Manifestations

Significant pericardial effusion has been identified in up to 46 percent of AIDS patients by echocardiography or autopsy [5]. While generally an incidental finding not associated with symptoms, it can sometimes present as or progress to cardiac tamponade, especially in the setting of advanced HIV disease. Acute pericarditis can be silent or present

Table 10-1 *Cardiac manifestations of HIV infection*

Pericardial disease
    Viral infection: cytomegalovirus, herpes simplex virus
    Bacterial infection: tuberculosis, *Mycobacterium avium* complex
    Disseminated fungal infection
    Neoplasia: Kaposi's sarcoma, lymphoma
Myocardial disease
    HIV myocarditis/cardiomyopathy
    Disseminated opportunistic infections
    Neoplasia: Kaposi's sarcoma, lymphoma
    Medications: pentamidine, alpha-interferon, antiretroviral therapy
Endocardial disease
    Bacterial endocarditis
    Nonbacterial thrombotic endocarditis
    Disseminated fungal infection

with fever, cough, dyspnea, and chest pain. Patients with a prior history of pericarditis may develop chronic pericarditis with recurrent pericardial effusion.

Physical findings of pericardial disease include tachypnea, friction rub, and Ewart's sign (dullness to percussion with tubular breath sounds between the left scapula and spine associated with large effusions). The manifestations of tamponade include tachypnea, hypotension with pulsus paradoxus, elevated jugular venous pressure with absent y descent, and remote heart sounds. Of note is the phenomenon of "low-pressure tamponade," which is sometimes observed in HIV-infected patients. Severe volume depletion or cachexia may cause reduced right ventricular filling pressures, and minimal pericardial effusion may increase intrapericardial pressures sufficiently to exceed right atrial pressure at low levels. In this setting, jugular venous pressure or pulsus paradoxus may be absent despite hemodynamic tamponade.

Laboratory Data

Chest x-ray may be nondiagnostic with a small pericardial effusion (< 200 ml). As the effusion increases, the cardiac silhouette develops a classic "water bottle" appearance. Cardiomegaly with a straightened left heart border and absence of pulmonary vascular redistribution should also raise the question of pericardial effusion. Electrocardiography (ECG) may demonstrate ST-T wave changes of pericarditis. With large effusions, loss of QRS voltage and electrical alternans may appear.

Differential Diagnosis

Most pericardial effusions are idiopathic. Once non–HIV-related conditions, such as renal failure, trauma, radiation effect, drug toxicity, and hypothyroidism, are excluded, differential diagnosis includes viral, bacterial, fungal, and neoplastic etiologies.

Cytomegalovirus has been reported to cause cardiac tamponade in a patient with cryptococcal meningitis [6]. While pericardial fluid analysis was not diagnostic, the pericardium revealed characteristic intranuclear inclusion bodies. Herpes simplex virus pericarditis has also been reported in AIDS patients [7, 8]. It remains unclear whether HIV can independently cause pericarditis. Both *Mycobacterium tuberculosis* and *Mycobacterium avium* complex (MAC) have been identified in pericardial fluid or tissue of HIV-infected patients with disseminated infection [9, 10]. *Nocardia asteroides* has been cultured from pericardial fluid in two patients with AIDS [11]. Bacterial pericarditis remains rare in HIV disease. *Staphylococcus aureus* pericarditis has been reported in AIDS-related complex and AIDS [12, 13]. Pneumococcal pericarditis with tamponade developed in two HIV-seropositive patients with acute left-sided pneumococcal empyemas, the result of local spread of infection [14]. Disseminated fungal infections may involve the pericardium. *Cryptococcus neoformans* pericarditis has been diagnosed by pericardial fluid stain and culture, and increased antigen titer [15]. Aspergillus pericarditis with mycotic plaques has been described in an immunocompromised patient [16].

Kaposi's sarcoma can involve the pericardium as well as the epicardium [17] (Fig. 10-1). Silver and associates [18] reported 5 of 18 AIDS necropsies with cutaneous and subepicardial KS. Kaposi's sarcoma of the pericardium has caused sanguineous pericarditis and tamponade [19]. Isolated cardiac KS has been described in one patient [20]. Cardiac involvement with AIDS-related lymphoma has been reported in several patients, with evidence of pericardial effusion or fibrinous pericarditis [21–23].

Evaluation

The evaluation of pericardial disease in the HIV-infected patient is directed at diagnosis of the underlying pathology. A CD4 lymphocyte count and skin testing for tuberculosis should be performed. As pericardial disease is sometimes associated with bacteremia, blood cultures should be obtained in all patients.

Echocardiography is highly sensitive and specific for detecting pericardial effusion and cardiac tamponade. An echo-free space with or without fibrinous strands is diagnostic of pericardial effusion. Right ventricular compression or prolonged right atrial collapse indicates cardiac tamponade. In this setting, Doppler study demonstrates inspiratory augmentation of right-sided flow with simultaneous reduction of left-sided flow, representing the pulsus paradoxus of tamponade physiology. Tamponade physiology may be confirmed by Swan-Ganz monitoring, which reveals increased and equalized right atrial, right ventricular, and pulmonary artery end-diastolic pressures. Intraperi-

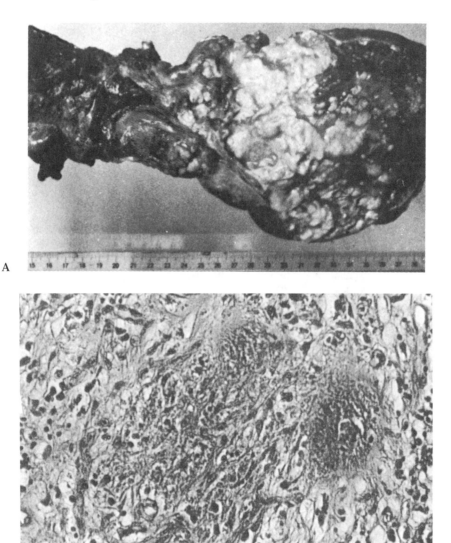

Figure 10-1. Kaposi's sarcoma in an AIDS patient. **A.** Nodular neoplastic infiltration of the anterior surface of the heart. **B.** Hemorrhagic necrosis typical of Kaposi's sarcoma. (Reprinted with permission from the American College of Cardiology. G Baroldi, S Corallo, M Moroni, et al. Focal lymphocytic myocarditis in acquired immunodeficiency syndrome (AIDS): A correlative morphologic and clinical study in 26 consecutive total cases. *J Am Coll Cardiol* 12:463–469, 1988.)

cardial pressure at the time of pericardiocentesis is increased and equal to right atrial pressure. Pericardial thickening associated with KS can be identified echocardiographically, but computed tomography and magnetic resonance imaging may provide more accurate assessment of neoplastic cardiac disease.

Management

Small asymptomatic pericardial effusions that require only serial evaluation and no specific therapy occur in up to 10 percent of HIV-infected patients. Nonsteroidal antiinflammatory agents have been used with success in larger asymptomatic effusions [24]. Corticosteroid therapy is generally avoided. The diagnostic utility of aspirating an asymptomatic pericardial effusion is low. Febrile patients often have an etiology identified from blood cultures or biopsy of other involved organs; pericardiocentesis is performed only when presumed infectious pericarditis fails to respond to appropriate antibiotics.

Pericardiocentesis can be used as a therapeutic procedure. In cases of tamponade, it offers immediate resolution of hemodynamic compromise. Pericardial fluid should be stained and cultured for bacteria, mycobacteria, and fungi. Draining pericardiotomy or pericardiectomy may be appropriate for recurring effusion or when pericardial tissue is necessary to diagnose KS or tuberculous pericarditis.

The prognosis of pericardial involvement in AIDS depends on the etiology. It appears that tuberculous pericarditis is less likely to respond to therapy than extracardiac tuberculosis [25].

Myocardial Disease

Clinical Manifestations

Myocardial disease in the context of HIV infection takes three forms. The first is myocarditis, with pathologic specimens revealing opportunistic pathogens, lymphocytic myocarditis (with or without myocardial fiber necrosis), and noninflammatory myocardial necrosis [26]. The second form, dilated cardiomyopathy, reflects severe cardiac dysfunction, which may be either primary or secondary to systemic disease. Finally, the myocardium can be replaced or infiltrated with neoplastic disease.

Myocarditis is a biopsy or postmortem finding that is generally clinically silent. Cardiac symptoms may be obscured by underlying opportunistic infection or neoplasm. Baroldi and associates [17] found lymphocytic infiltrates in 20 of 26 hearts in AIDS patients without cardiac symptoms [27] (Fig. 10-2). Reilly and colleagues [28] noted that 6 of 26 AIDS patients with myocarditis had symptoms of congestive heart failure. Neoplastic involvement may present as heart failure, chest pain, or dysrhythmia [29]. Patients with symptomatic myocarditis or cardiomyopathy complain of dyspnea and fatigue, and biventricular

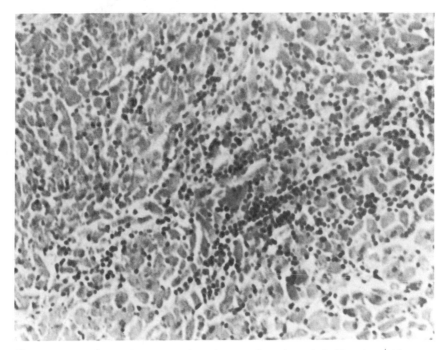

Figure 10-2. Lymphocytic myocarditis showing lymphocytic infiltration with myocardial degeneration. (From M Klima, SM Escudier. Pathologic findings in the hearts of patients with acquired immunodeficiency syndrome. *Tex Heart Inst J* 18:116–121, 1991.)

dysfunction may result in peripheral edema and ascites. Symptoms of dysrhythmia, include palpitations, dizziness, and syncope.

Vital signs may show relative hypotension, tachypnea, tachycardia, and ectopy. Physical examination may reveal elevated neck veins, diminished pulses, and rales on auscultation of the lungs. The cardiac examination may show a displaced point of maximal impulse. The S1 and S2 may be quiet, and an S3 gallop may be present. Mitral and tricuspid regurgitant murmurs secondary to biventricular dilatation may be heard. Hepatomegaly with hepatojugular reflex, ascites, and peripheral edema may be present.

Laboratory Data

Chest x-ray commonly shows cardiomegaly, with left atrial and ventricular dilatation and pulmonary vascular redistribution. Electrocardiography may reveal dysrhythmias, including premature ventricular contractions or atrioventricular block. A pseudoinfarct pattern may occur if focal infiltrates or neoplasm are present. Left ventricular hypertrophy or nonspecific ST-T wave changes may be associated with ventricular dilatation.

Differential Diagnosis

Non–HIV-related etiologies for myocarditis or cardiomyopathy must be excluded. These include hypertension, diabetes mellitus, ischemia, and alcoholic or valvular heart disease. In injection drug users (IDUs), consideration should also be given to hypersensitivity reactions. Geographic variability in rates of myocarditis in HIV disease has been noted, possibly the result of the different patient populations studied. Institutions with mostly HIV-infected IDUs describe an incidence of myocarditis of 34 to 52 percent, whereas series of patients with homosexually acquired HIV disease report an incidence of 2 to 10 percent [4, 26, 28, 30–32]. Cocaine has been shown to produce a myocarditis as well as a myopathy resulting from coronary spasm and ischemia [33].

Multiple pathogens have been found in the myocardium at postmortem or biopsy. Cytomegalovirus has been identified in the myocardium, both with and without inflammatory infiltrate [28]. Neidt and Schinella [34] reported that 43 of 56 AIDS postmortem examinations had evidence of CMV infection, but only four patients had myocarditis with clinical heart failure, dysrhythmia, or ECG changes. The frequency of *Toxoplasma gondii* infection of the heart in AIDS necropsy studies has ranged from 12 to 14 percent [30, 35]. *Mycobacterium tuberculosis*, MAC, *C. neoformans* (Fig. 10-3), *Candida albicans*, *Aspergillus fumigatus*, *Histoplasma capsulatum*, and *Pneumocystis carinii* have all been associated with myocarditis in the presence of underlying systemic disease [4, 17, 31, 36]. Homosexual patients have myocarditis related to protozoal and fungal pathogens, KS, and mycobacteria, while IDUs have fungal, viral, and protozoal causes [17, 31].

Not all myocarditis associated with AIDS is the result of opportunistic infections. Anderson and associates [31] reported myocarditis in 37 of 71 necropsies of AIDS patients; in only 7 was there an identified etiologic agent. The Dallas criterion for the diagnosis of myocarditis—inflammatory infiltrate with focal myocyte damage or necrosis—may not be appropriate in HIV-infected patients [37]. The AIDS virus may cause myocytic degeneration without inflammation [38]. RNA probes have identified HIV nucleic acid sequences in the myocardium at autopsy in 6 of 22 AIDS patients who did not have cardiac symptoms [39]. Possible immune-mediated mechanisms of myocarditis include anti-HIV antibodies cross-reacting with myocardium, autoantibodies directed against damaged myocardium, cytotoxic T lymphocytes lysing HIV-infected myocytes that express viral antigen on their surface, and natural killer cells lysing uninfected myocytes [40]. Nutritional defi-

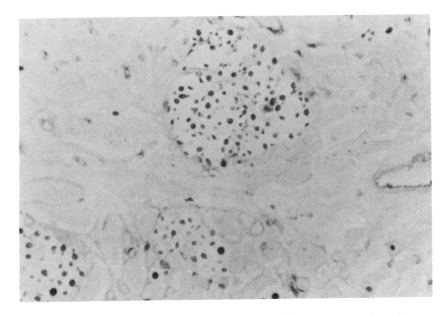

Figure 10-3. *Cryptococcus* myocarditis showing intact myocytes with foci of necrosis and clumps of periodic acid–Schiff positive capsules. An inflammatory reaction is notably absent. (Reprinted with permission from the American College of Cardiology. C Cammarosano, W Lewis. Cardiac lesions in acquired immune deficiency syndrome (AIDS). *J Am Coll Cardiol* 5:703–706, 1985.)

ciencies and malnutrition are probably not as important contributing factors as was originally thought [41].

Evaluation

Echocardiography remains the single best noninvasive procedure to assess chamber size and left ventricular function. Infiltration of myocardium by lymphoma or subepicardial KS may also be seen echocardiographically. Right ventricular hypertrophy and pulmonary hypertension are commonly identified in patients with concomitant pulmonary disease [26]. Holter monitoring is valuable in detecting dysrhythmias, such as bradycardias or ventricular ectopy, caused by patchy infiltration of the conduction system. Signal-averaged ECGs, which reveal late potentials in patients prone to ventricular tachycardia, may be abnormal in HIV-infected patients [42]. Computed tomography or magnetic resonance imaging is helpful in the detection of cardiac tumors. Gallium scanning is nonspecific but may be useful in selected patients [43, 44]. Increased serum immunoglobulin levels and cardiac antibodies may be associated with myocarditis [45]. Endomyocardial biopsy is of limited utility because blood contamination of specimens may give spurious immunocytochemistry results. Biopsy underestimates the prevalence of myocarditis, found to be 50 percent on post-mortem studies, because of sampling error due to focal inflammation [46]. Rarely, it may prove useful in diagnosing unusual cases such as isolated cardiac lymphoma [47].

Management

Infectious myocarditis is treated with appropriate antibiotic therapy. Steroids are not recommended as therapy for myocarditis. One patient with HIV-associated lymphocytic myocarditis was successfully treated with zidovudine (ZDV), as documented by serial biopsies [48]. Recent data also suggest fewer cardiac abnormalities by noninvasive testing in ZDV-treated subjects [42]. Conventional treatment of congestive heart failure with bed rest, inotropic agents, vasodilators, diuretics, and where indicated, antidysrhythmics and anticoagulants should be implemented, although it is not clear that regimen improves survival. Although spontaneous regression of dilated cardiomyopathy may occur rarely, the prognosis of this condition is generally poor [49].

While lymphomatous cardiac involvement is rare and usually fatal, a case report has been published of complete remission of a large-cell lymphoma in an HIV-infected patient following combination chemotherapy with cyclophosphamide, doxorubicin, vincristine, and prednisone [29]. Kaposi's sarcoma of the heart is generally a pathologic diagnosis, and there is no evidence that chemotherapy or radiotherapy is beneficial.

Of concern recently is the appearance of cardiac disease as a result of HIV-related therapies. Pentamidine, both intravenous and intramuscular, has been associated with torsades de pointes, with or without potassium, calcium, and magnesium deficiency [50]. This is treated by drug termination and repletion of electrolytes, with a possible role for type IB antidysrhythmics, overdrive atrial or ventricular pacing, or isoproterenol administration. Alpha-interferon, used in the treatment of KS, may act synergistically with HIV to produce a reversible cardiomyopathy [51]. There have been case reports of cardiomyopathy associated with ZDV and didanosine (ddI), and ZDV has been implicated in the exacerbation of preexisting cardiac disease [52]. Amphotericin B may cause dysrhythmias and cardiac arrest.

Endocardial Disease

Clinical Manifestations

Endocardial disease in HIV-infected patients takes the form of bacterial endocarditis and marantic (nonbacterial thrombotic) endocarditis. It is curious that endocarditis in AIDS has been relatively infrequent, despite the fact that IDUs account for the second largest patient population with HIV infection. It is possible that HIV-infected IDUs with endocarditis die from bacterial infection before they become significantly immunocompromised or that they succumb prematurely to other diseases related to substance abuse. Alternatively, IDUs may be using needle-cleansing practices that protect them from bacterial infection but not from HIV transmission [53].

Clinical features of bacterial endocarditis include the acute or insidious onset of fever, malaise, anorexia, and weight loss. In IDUs, right-sided valvular lesions may present with chest pain, cough, and dyspnea. Left-sided involvement may be evident from peripheral embolization or symptoms of heart failure related to aortic or mitral regurgitation.

Marantic endocarditis, associated with other severe chronic illnesses, has been infrequently reported in AIDS (Fig. 10-4). It is characterized by large, friable vegetations that may embolize or become secondarily infected. Marantic endocarditis may cause systemic embolization and disseminated intravascular coagulation [32, 54, 55].

Physical examination may reveal fever; peripheral stigmata of endocarditis, such as petechiae, splinter hemorrhages, Osler's nodes, or Janeway lesions; splenomegaly; and abnormalities on cardiac examination. Although up to 15 percent of patients with subacute bacterial endocarditis may not have a murmur when they are initially exam-

Figure 10-4. Nonbacterial thrombotic endocarditis showing large, friable vegetations on the atrial surface of both mitral valve leaflets. No organisms are demonstrated histologically. (Reprinted with permission from the American College of Cardiology. C Cammarosano, W Lewis. Cardiac lesions in acquired immune deficiency syndrome (AIDS). *J Am Coll Cardiol* 5:703–706, 1985.)

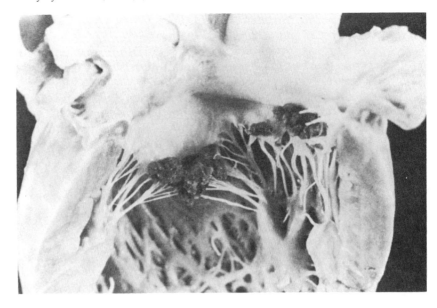

ined, evidence of mitral, tricuspid, or aortic regurgitation will develop over time in the majority [56]. Signs of congestive heart failure are most often present with left-sided cardiac involvement.

Laboratory Data

Anemia is a common laboratory finding in infective endocarditis, but the white blood cell count may not be increased in HIV disease. The urinary sediment may show hematuria or proteinuria, or both. Bacteremia is present in 90 percent of patients; recent use of antibiotics may cause negative culture results. Fungal and other nonbacterial pathogens are infrequently identified. Chest x-ray may reveal pulmonary infiltrates from right-sided septic emboli, pulmonary venous congestion, and/or vascular redistribution with overt heart failure. Electrocardiography may show progressive heart block from ring abscess formation involving the conduction system.

Differential Diagnosis

Endocarditis in the immunocompromised host may be more virulent than in the normal host. Bacterial endocarditis in the HIV-infected IDU is most commonly caused by *S. aureus* (> 75% of cases), *Streptococcus pneumoniae*, and *Haemophilus influenzae* [57]. Fungal endocarditis is often the result of systemic spread from an extracardiac source; pathogens include *Aspergillus* and *Candida* species and *C. neoformans* [26, 36, 58].

Evaluation

Although endocarditis is often a clinical diagnosis, echocardiography remains an important diagnostic test. Weisse and colleagues [53] advise blood cultures and empiric antibiotic coverage as initial management in febrile IDUs, reserving echocardiography only for patients with positive blood cultures, pulmonary or systemic embolism, or other cardiac complications. The sensitivity of transthoracic echocardiography in the detection of vegetations is approximately 75 percent, and that of transesophageal echocardiography is 96 percent [59]. Transesophageal technique is superior to transthoracic in the detection of ring abscesses (sensitivity 84% vs. 19%) [60]. Echocardiography and Doppler studies can also provide information on ventricular function and degree of valvular insufficiency. Computed tomography is useful in the evaluation of cerebral embolic events. Cardiac catheterization, which can be performed safely during active endocarditis, is recommended for patients over the age of 40 when valvular surgery is anticipated [61].

Management

Bacterial endocarditis should be presumed in the HIV-infected IDU with fever and a new regurgitant murmur or peripheral stigmata. After blood cultures are obtained, empiric antibiotic therapy directed against the most likely pathogens should be initiated. Once the etiologic agent has been identified, treatment can be made specific. Duration of intravenous therapy is generally 4 weeks. When available, peak and trough levels of antibiotics should be monitored. Measurement of serum bactericidal titer may be helpful clinically when the organism or antibiotic regimen is unusual or when treatment appears to be failing.

Patients with advanced HIV disease in whom endocarditis develops have a poor prognosis. In one study, endocarditis patients with advanced HIV disease had a 40 percent mortality compared to 10 percent in asymptomatic HIV-infected individuals [55]. It appears that most HIV-infected patients can undergo successful valve replacement, but those with continued bacteremia at the time of surgery do poorly [62]. There is no evidence that cardiac anesthesia or valve replacement has an adverse effect on the natural history of HIV disease [63].

References

1. Anderson DW, Virmani R. Emerging patterns of heart disease in human immunodeficiency virus infection. *Hum Pathol* 21:253–259, 1990.
2. Reichert CM, O'Leary TJ, Levens DL, et al. Autopsy pathology in the acquired immune deficiency syndrome. *Am J Pathol* 112:357–382, 1983.
3. Welch K, Finkbeiner W, Alpers CE, et al. Autopsy findings in the acquired immunodeficiency syndrome. *JAMA* 252:1152–1159, 1984.
4. Lewis W. AIDS: Cardiac findings from 115 autopsies. *Prog Cardiovasc Dis* 32:207–215, 1989.
5. Fink L, Reichek N, St John Sutton M. Cardiac abnormalities in acquired immune deficiency syndrome. *Am J Cardiol* 54:1161–1163, 1984.
6. Nathan PE, Arsura EL, Zappi M. Pericarditis with tamponade due to cytomegalovirus in the acquired immunodeficiency syndrome. *Chest* 99:765–766, 1991.
7. Freedberg RS, Gindea AJ, Dietrich DT, et al. Herpes simplex pericarditis in AIDS. *NY State J Med* 87:304–306, 1987.
8. Toma E, Poisson M, Claessens MR, et al. Herpes simplex type 2 pericarditis and bilateral facial palsy in a patient with AIDS (letter). *J Infect Dis* 160:553–554, 1989.
9. Dalli E, Quesada A, Juan A, et al. Tuberculous pericarditis as the first manifestation of acquired immunodeficiency syndrome. *Am Heart J* 114:905–906, 1987.
10. Woods GL, Goldsmith JC. Fatal pericarditis due to *Mycobacterium avium-intracellulare* in acquired immunodeficiency syndrome. *Chest* 95:1355–1357, 1989.

11. Holtz HA, Lavery DP, Kapila R. Actinomycetales infection in the acquired immunodeficiency syndrome. *Ann Intern Med* 102:203–205, 1985.
12. Stechel RP, Cooper DJ, Greenspan J, et al. Staphylococcal pericarditis in a homosexual patient with AIDS-related complex. *NY State J Med* 86:592–593, 1986.
13. Decker CF, Tuazon CU. *Staphylococcus aureus* pericarditis in HIV-infected patients. *Chest* 105:615–616, 1994.
14. Karve MM, Murali MR, Shah HM, et al. Rapid evolution of cardiac tamponade due to bacterial pericarditis in two patients with HIV-1 infection. *Chest* 101:1461–1463, 1992.
15. Schuster M, Valentine F, Holtzman R. Cryptococcal pericarditis in an IVDA. *J Infect Dis* 152:842, 1985.
16. Schwartz DA. Aspergillus pancarditis following bone marrow transplantation for chronic myelogenous leukemia. *Chest* 95:1338–1339, 1989.
17. Baroldi G, Corallo S, Moroni M, et al. Focal lymphocytic myocarditis in acquired immunodeficiency syndrome (AIDS): A correlative morphologic and clinical study in 26 consecutive fatal cases. *J Am Coll Cardiol* 12:463–469, 1988.
18. Silver MA, Macher AM, Reichert CM, et al. Cardiac involvement by Kaposi's sarcoma in acquired immune deficiency syndrome (AIDS). *Am J Cardiol* 53:983–985, 1984.
19. Stotka JL, Good CB, Downer WR, et al. Pericardial effusion and tamponade due to Kaposi's sarcoma in acquired immunodeficiency syndrome. *Chest* 95: 1359–1361, 1989.
20. Autran B, Gorin I, Leibowitch M, et al. AIDS in a Haitian woman with cardiac Kaposi's sarcoma and Whipple's disease. *Lancet* 1:767–768, 1983.
21. Gill PS, Chandraratna AN, Meyer PR, et al. Malignant lymphoma: A clinicopathologic study. *Cancer* 49:944–951, 1982.
22. Ioachim HL, Cooper MC, Hillman GC. Lymphoma in men at high risk for acquired immune deficiency syndrome (AIDS). *Cancer* 56:2831–2842, 1985.
23. Balasubramanyam A, Waxman M, Kazal HL, et al. Malignant lymphoma of the heart in acquired immune deficiency syndrome. *Chest* 90:243–246, 1986.
24. Himelman RB, Chung WS, Chernoff DN, et al. Cardiac manifestations of human immunodeficiency virus infection: A two dimensional echocardiographic study. *J Am Coll Cardiol* 13:1030–1036, 1989.
25. Kinney EL, Monsuez JJ, Kitzis M, et al. Treatment of AIDS-associated heart disease. *Angiology* 40:970–976, 1989.
26. Acierno LJ. Cardiac complications in acquired immunodeficiency syndrome (AIDS): A review. *J Am Coll Cardiol* 13:1144–1154, 1989.
27. Klima M, Escudier SM. Pathologic findings in the hearts of patients with acquired immunodeficiency syndrome. *Tex Heart Inst J* 18:116–121, 1991.
28. Reilly JM, Cunnion RE, Anderson DW, et al. Frequency of myocarditis, left ventricular dysfunction and ventricular tachycardia in the acquired immune deficiency syndrome. *Am J Cardiol* 62:289–293, 1988.
29. Kelsey RC, Saker A, Morgan M. Cardiac lymphoma in a patient with AIDS. *Ann Intern Med* 115:370–371, 1991.
30. Hofman P, Drici MD, Gribelin P, et al. Prevalence of toxoplasma

myocarditis in patients with the acquired immunodeficiency syndrome. *Br Heart J* 70:376–381, 1993.

31. Anderson DW, Virmani R, Reilly JM, et al. Prevalent myocarditis at necropsy in the acquired immunodeficiency syndrome. *J Am Coll Cardiol* 11:792–799, 1988.

32. Cammarosano C, Lewis W. Cardiac lesions in acquired immune deficiency syndrome (AIDS). *J Am Coll Cardiol* 5:703–706, 1985.

33. Isner JM, Chokski SK. Cardiovascular complications of cocaine. *Curr Probl Cardiol* 16:95–123, 1991.

34. Neidt GW, Schinella RA. Acquired immunodeficiency syndrome: Clinicopathologic study of 56 autopsies. *Arch Pathol Lab Med* 109:727–734, 1985.

35. Roldan EO, Moskowitz L, Hensley GT. Pathology of the heart in acquired immunodeficiency syndrome. *Arch Pathol Lab Med* 111:94–946, 1987.

36. Cox JN, diDio F, Pizzolato GP, et al. Aspergillus endocarditis and myocarditis in a patient with the acquired immunodeficiency syndrome (AIDS): A review of the literature. *Virchows Arch A Pathol Anat Histopathol* 417:255–259, 1990.

37. Aretz HT, Billingham ME, Edwards WD, et al. Myocarditis: A histopathologic definition and classification. *Am J Cardiovasc Pathol* 1:1–14, 1986.

38. Calabrese LH, Proffitt MR, Yen-Lieberman B, et al. Congestive cardiomyopathy and illness related to the acquired immunodeficiency syndrome (AIDS) associated with isolation of retrovirus from myocardium. *Ann Intern Med* 107:691–692, 1987.

39. Grody WW, Cheng L, Lewis W. Infection of the heart by the human immunodeficiency virus. *Am J Cardiol* 66:203–206, 1990.

40. Herskowitz A, Willoughby S, Wu TC, et al. Immunopathogenesis of HIV-1-associated cardiomyopathy. *Clin Immunol Immunopathol* 68:234–241, 1993.

41. Fisher LL, Fisher EA. Myocarditis associated with human immunodeficiency virus infection. *Prim Cardiol* 16:49–60, 1990.

42. Hsia J, Adams S, Ross AM. Natural history of human immunodeficiency virus (HIV) associated with heart disease (abstract). *Circulation* 84:11–3, 1991.

43. Cregler LL, Sosa I, Ducey S, et al. Myopericarditis in acquired immunodeficiency syndrome diagnosed by gallium scintigraphy. *J Natl Med Assoc* 82:511–513, 1990.

44. Constantino A, West TE, Gupta M, et al. Primary cardiac lymphoma in a patient with acquired immune deficiency syndrome. *Cancer* 60:2801–2805, 1987.

45. Hershowitz A, de Oliveria M, Willoughby S, et al. Cardiomyopathy: An initial presentation of human immunodeficiency virus (HIV) infection (abstract). *Circulation* 82:111–118, 1990.

46. Dittrich H, Chow L, Denaro F, et al. Human immunodeficiency virus, coxsackievirus, and cardiomyopathy. *Ann Intern Med* 108:308–309, 1988.

47. Andress JD, Polish LB, Clark DM, et al. Transvenous biopsy diagnosis of cardiac lymphoma in an AIDS patient. *Am Heart J* 118:421–423, 1989.

48. Wilkins CE, Sexton DJ, McAllister HA. HIV-associated myocarditis treated with zidovudine (AZT). *Tex Heart Inst J* 16:44–45, 1989.

49. Hakas JF Jr, Generalovich T. Spontaneous regression of cardiomyopathy in a patient with the acquired immunodeficiency syndrome. *Chest* 99:770–772, 1992.
50. Grogin H, Liem LB. Pentamidine-induced torsades de pointes. *Cardiology* 2:114–115, 1991.
51. Deyton LR, Walker RE, Kovacs JA, et al. Reversible cardiac dysfunction associated with interferon alpha therapy in AIDS patients with Kaposi's sarcoma. *N Engl J Med* 321:1246–1249, 1989.
52. Herskowitz A, et al. Cardiomyopathy associated with antiretroviral therapy in patients with HIV infection: A report of six cases. *Ann Intern Med* 116:311–313, 1992.
53. Weisse AB, Heller DR, Schimenti RJ, et al. The febrile parenteral drug users: A prospective study in 121 patients. *Am J Med* 94:274–280, 1993.
54. Guarda LA, Luna MA, Smith LJ, et al. Acquired immune deficiency syndrome: Postmortem findings. *Am J Clin Pathol* 81:549–557, 1984.
55. Kaul S, Fishbein MC, Siegel RJ. Cardiac manifestations of acquired immune deficiency syndrome: A 1991 update. *Am Heart J* 122:535–544, 1991.
56. Durack DT. Endocarditis. In JW Hurst (ed), *The Heart, Arteries and Veins* 7th ed. New York: McGraw-Hill, 1990. Pp 1230–1255.
57. Nahass RG, Weinstein MP, Bartels J, et al. Infective endocarditis in intravenous drug users: A comparison of human immunodeficiency virus type 1–negative and –positive patients. *J Infect Dis* 162:967–970, 1990.
58. Francis CK. Cardiac involvement in AIDS. *Curr Probl Cardiol* 15:572–639, 1990.
59. Mugge A, Daniel WG, Frank G, et al. Echocardiography in infective endocarditis: Reassessment of prognostic implications of vegetation size determined by the transthoracic and the transesophageal approach. *J Am Coll Cardiol* 14:631–638, 1989.
60. Daniel WG, Mugge A, Martin RP, et al. Improvement in the diagnosis of abscesses associated with endocarditis by transesophageal echocardiography. *N Engl J Med* 324:795–800, 1991.
61. Welton DE, Young JB, Raizner AE, et al. Value and safety of cardiac catheterization during active infective endocarditis. *Am J Cardiol* 44:1306–1310, 1977.
62. Frater RWM, Sisto D, Condit D. Cardiac surgery in human immunodeficiency virus (HIV) carriers. *Eur J Cardiothorac Surg* 3:146–151, 1989.
63. Brau N, Espositi RA, Simberkoff MS. Cardiac valve replacement in patients infected with the human immunodeficiency virus. *Ann Thorac Surg* 54:552–554, 1992.

Pulmonary Manifestations *11*

Randall P. Wagner, Harrison W. Farber

The pulmonary manifestations of HIV disease are a major cause of morbidity and mortality. More than 80 percent of patients with AIDS have pulmonary disorders, of which 90 percent are infectious in origin [1–4]. In addition, the prevalence of noninfectious pulmonary disorders is increasing, perhaps as a result of improved survival. Autopsy studies have documented significant pathology in the lower respiratory tract of most AIDS patients [5].

The spectrum of pulmonary diseases associated with HIV infection continues to broaden. Table 11-1 presents a list of common conditions that are caused or exacerbated by HIV infection.

Infectious Pulmonary Disorders

Infections involving the respiratory tract are the result of a failure of one or more components of the immune system to protect against a nearly continuous assault of infectious agents. In early HIV disease, when the CD4 lymphocyte count is relatively preserved, patients have an increased incidence of the same pulmonary infections that afflict the general population [6–8]. When the CD4 cell count falls below $200/mm^3$, or 20 percent of total lymphocytes, the patient is also at significant risk for opportunistic infections [9]. Although *Pneumocystis carinii* is still the most frequently recognized opportunistic pathogen, other protozoans, fungi, nontuberculous mycobacterial species, viruses, and unusual bacteria can also cause illness in patients with advanced HIV disease. The probability of infection with specific pathogens depends on the patient's geographic residence, travel history, medical history, and to some extent, socioeconomic status.

Table 11-1 *Common etiologies of pulmonary disease in the HIV-infected patient*

Infectious diseases
    Bacterial: *Streptococcus pneumoniae, Haemophilus influenzae,* tuberculosis,
        Mycobacterium avium complex*
    Protozoal: *Pneumocystis carinii**
    Viral: Cytomegalovirus*
    Fungal: Cryptococcosis,* histoplasmosis,* coccidioidomycosis*
Neoplastic diseases
    Kaposi's sarcoma*
    Non-Hodgkin's lymphoma*
Miscellaneous
    Lymphoid interstitial pneumonitis

*Conditions generally associated with advanced HIV disease.

Bacterial Infections

Recurrent pneumonia is now included in the AIDS case definition in recognition of the clear association between HIV disease and conventional bacterial infection of the lung. Community-acquired pneumonia is the most frequent pulmonary manifestation of HIV infection, with the annual incidence of pneumococcal pneumonia being as high as five times that of the general population [7, 8, 10]. Pneumonias caused by *Haemophilus influenzae, Mycobacterium tuberculosis, Staphylococcus aureus, Legionella* species, *Chlamydia pneumoniae,* and *Klebsiella* species are also more common [11]. Bacterial pneumonias in HIV-infected patients are often associated with bacteremia and may recur after appropriate antibiotic therapy.

A syndrome of persistent *Pseudomonas aeruginosa* pulmonary disease, similar to that which occurs in cystic fibrosis, recently was described in patients with advanced HIV disease [12, 13]. In the majority of cases, *Pseudomonas* infection is community acquired and has an indolent course. Although responsive to antimicrobial therapy, the infection recurs in more than 80 percent of patients, suggesting that prolonged suppressive therapy may be necessary [12].

Nocardia asteroides infection has become increasingly common in patients with advanced HIV disease. Patients generally present with fever, cough, dyspnea, and chest pain. The chest x-ray (CXR) typically shows an upper lobe process with cavitation, consolidation, or interstitial infiltrate; pleural effusions, hilar adenopathy, or both, also occur [14]. Diagnosis is made by demonstrating branching, beaded, filamentous, gram-positive, weakly acid-fast organisms in respiratory secretions, in transbronchial biopsy specimens, or in biopsy specimens of skin lesions or lymph nodes. Treatment with sulfonamides or ampicillin for at least 6 months is necessary; the choice of antibiotics should be guided by culture and sensitivity results since resistant organisms have been identified [15]. Because CXR findings often mimic those of reactivation tuberculosis, broncho-

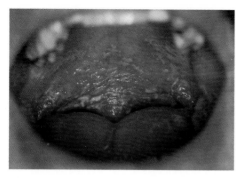

Plate 1. Pseudomembranous candidiasis of the palate. (Courtesy of Dr. ES Peters, Brigham and Women's Hospital and Dana Farber Cancer Institute.)

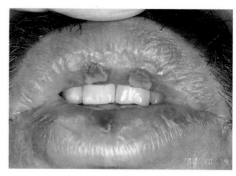

Plate 2. Herpes simplex virus infection of the lip. (Courtesy of Dr. SB Woo, Brigham and Women's Hospital and Dana Farber Cancer Institute.)

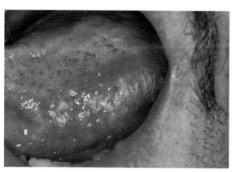

Plate 3. Hairy leukoplakia. (Courtesy of Dr. ES Peters, Brigham and Women's Hospital and Dana Farber Cancer Institute.)

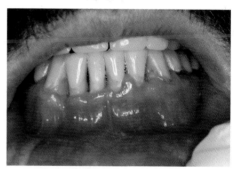

Plate 4. HIV-related periodontitis. (Courtesy of Dr. ES Peters, Brigham and Women's Hospital and Dana Farber Cancer Institute.)

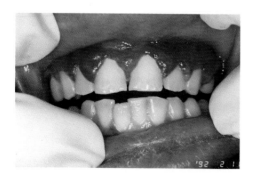

Plate 5. Kaposi's sarcoma of the gingiva. (Courtesy of Dr. SB Woo, Brigham and Women's Hospital and Dana Farber Cancer Institute.)

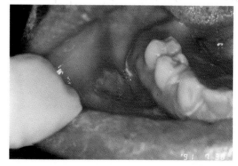

Plate 6. Aphthous ulceration of the buccal mucosa. (Courtesy of Dr. SB Woo, Brigham and Women's Hospital and Dana Farber Cancer Institute.)

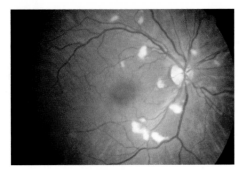

Plate 7. Cotton-wool spots.

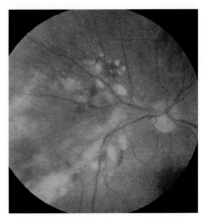

Plate 8. Cytomegalovirus retinitis. (From JN Bloom, AG Palestine. The diagnosis of cytomegalovirus retinitis. *Ann Intern Med* 109:963-969, 1988.)

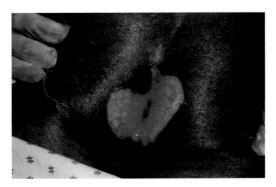

Plate 9. Perianal ulcerative herpes simplex infection.

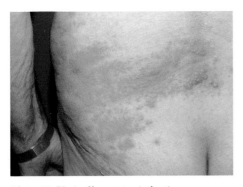

Plate 10. Varicella-zoster infection (shingles).

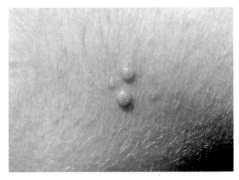

Plate 11. Molluscum contagiosum.

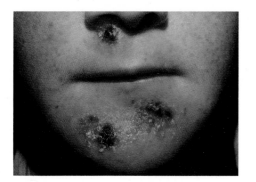

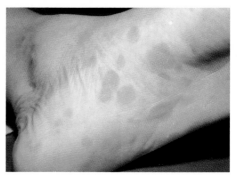

Plate 12. Impetigo. (From JJ O'Connell, J Groth (eds). *The Manual of Common Communicable Diseases*. Boston: Boston Health Care for the Homeless Program, 1991.)

Plate 13. Secondary syphilis. (From JJ O'Connell, J Groth (eds). *The Manual of Common Communicable Diseases*. Boston: Boston Health Care for the Homeless, 1991.)

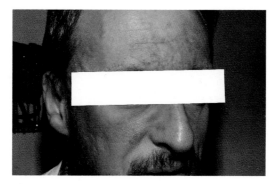

Plate 14. Seborrheic dermatitis.

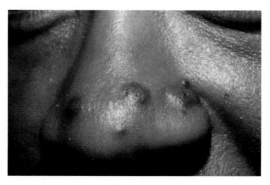

Plate 15. Kaposi's sarcoma (plaque-like lesions).

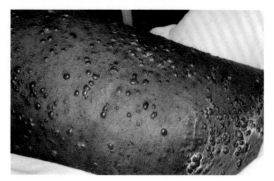

Plate 16. Kaposi's sarcoma (papular lesions).

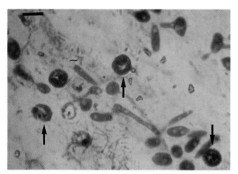

Plate 17. Cryptosporidial cysts in stool. (Courtesy of Dr. S Nikulasson, Pathology Department, Boston University School of Medicine.)

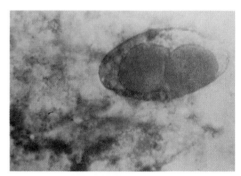

Plate 18. *Isospora belli* cyst in stool. (From JA DeHovitz, et al. Clinical manifestations and therapy of *Isospora belli* infection in patients with AIDS. *N Engl J Med* 315:87-90, 1986. Reprinted by permission of the *New England Journal of Medicine*.)

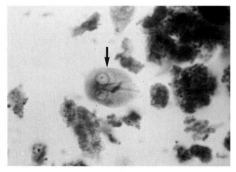

Plate 19. *Giardia lamblia* trophozoite in stool. (Courtesy of Dr. S Nikulasson, Pathology Department, Boston University School of Medicine.)

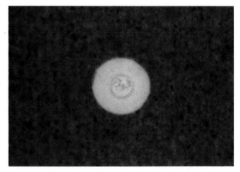

Plate 20. *Cryptococcus neoformans* demonstrated on India ink preparation.

scopy should be performed if expectorated sputum fails to yield a diagnosis.

Rhodococcus equi infection generally develops in HIV-infected patients who have been exposed to farm animals or to soil where such animals have been kept. Pneumonia usually occurs in patients with advanced immunodeficiency, presenting as fever, cough, fatigue, pleuritic chest pain, and progressive dyspnea evolving over 2 to 3 weeks [16, 17]. The CXR usually shows dense consolidation with cavitation; pleural effusions are common. Although cultures of sputum and blood are often diagnostic, bronchoscopy, biopsy, and/or thoracentesis may be required. Therapy is individualized based on culture and sensitivity results; surgical resection of abscess is occasionally required [18, 19]. The optimal duration of treatment is unknown, but lifelong suppressive therapy may be necessary.

Nosocomial pneumonia is common in HIV-infected patients. Frequent hospitalization and impaired local and systemic immune function magnify the risk of pulmonary infections with *S. aureus*, *P. aeruginosa*, and enteric gram-negative organisms [20].

Pneumocystis carinii

P. carinii pneumonia (PCP) is the most commonly diagnosed AIDS-related infection in the United States [1, 21]. It occurs at least once in approximately 70 percent of HIV-infected patients and, despite early recognition and aggressive therapy, still carries a 10 to 20 percent mortality per episode [22]. Because the clinical and roentgenographic features of PCP are nonspecific, diagnosis requires a high index of suspicion.

Pneumonitis often develops more gradually than in other immunosuppressed patients but may present abruptly. Usual symptoms include fever, dyspnea, malaise, and a nonproductive cough; chills, chest pain, and sputum production may also occur. Physical examination is notable for fever and tachypnea; auscultation of the lungs is generally normal.

The CXR typically shows diffuse, bilateral interstitial infiltrates, although they may be subtle early in the course; cavitary lesions, focal infiltrates, and nodular densities have also been described (Fig. 11-1). Apical infiltrates have become more common, particularly in patients receiving aerosol pentamidine (AP) prophylaxis. The CXR appears normal in a minority of patients [1, 21, 23]. Enlarged hilar or mediastinal lymph nodes and pleural effusions are unusual and suggest another diagnosis or a copathogen [24].

Pneumothorax, pleural-based blebs, and cystic lesions are increasingly recognized as manifestations of PCP. It is now understood that pulmonary destruction is related to the duration of *P. carinii* infection [25–28]. However, AP may predispose to the development of chronic pneumonitis in regions of poor ventilation by inhibiting, but not eliminating, growth of the pathogen.

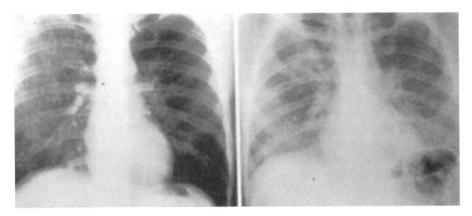

Figure 11-1. Chest x-ray showing the development of *Pneumocystis carinii* pneumonia. (From J Golden. Pneumocystis lung disease in homosexual men. *West J Med* 137:400–407, 1982.)

Arterial blood gas determination usually reveals hypoxemia and an abnormal alveolar-arterial oxygen gradient, but the results may be normal in patients with mild or early PCP. Exercise-induced oxygen desaturation is common and often occurs with normal or near-normal arterial blood gas levels. Pulmonary function testing usually demonstrates a diminished diffusing capacity for carbon monoxide; gallium scintigraphy reveals diffuse parenchymal uptake [29]. Several investigators noted increased serum lactic dehydrogenase (LDH) levels at the time of diagnosis that correlate with disease severity [30, 31].

Diagnosis of PCP has traditionally depended on the identification of the organism on methenamine silver or Giemsa staining of lung tissue or respiratory secretions. The development of fluorescent antibody staining (sensitivity 60–80%) has made sputum induction the initial diagnostic test of choice [32, 33]. In facilities that lack the capacity to perform induced sputum analysis or in patients with negative results on sputum analysis and a high clinical suspicion of PCP, fiberoptic bronchoscopy with bronchalveolar lavage (BAL) remains the diagnostic mainstay. Overall, the sensitivity of BAL for the diagnosis of PCP is approximately 90 percent. The sensitivity is somewhat less in the first episode of PCP in patients receiving AP prophylaxis; transbronchial biopsy or upper lobe lavage improves the yield in this population [34, 35].

Empiric therapy can be initiated without affecting the ability to establish a definitive diagnosis. Trimethoprim-sulfamethoxazole (TMP-SMX) is the drug of choice, with therapeutic serum levels attainable with 15 to 20 mg/kg/day (dose based on the trimethoprim content) administered in four divided doses. Treatment is continued for 21 days. Although TMP-SMX is available in both intravenous and oral preparations, there is no advantage to intravenous administration for patients with normal gastrointestinal function, since absorption is complete and equivalent serum drug levels are achievable [36]. HIV-infected patients treated with TMP-SMX have an unusually high incidence of adverse effects, including fever, rash, leukopenia, thrombocytopenia, and renal dysfunction. If the patient has no clinical response after 5 to 7 days or if drug toxicity develops, pentamidine is used as an alternative agent.

Pentamidine isethionate is given in a dose of 3 to 4 mg/kg/day intravenously. Intramuscular administration should be avoided because injections are painful and sterile abscesses are common. Intravenous pentamidine may cause severe hypotension if the drug is given too rapidly. Neutropenia, renal impairment, and hepatic dysfunction are frequent complications. Hypoglycemia is common, and glucose intolerance or frank diabetes mellitus may occur following completion of therapy [37]. Combination therapy with TMP-SMX and pentamidine offers no additional benefit and should be avoided because of cumulative toxicity [1, 21].

The combination of dapsone and trimethoprim has also been shown to be highly effective for the treatment of mild to moderate PCP. Both components are given orally: dapsone, 100 mg once a day, and trimethoprim, 15 to 20 mg/kg/day in four divided doses. Glucose 6-phosphate dehydrogenase deficiency is a contraindication to the use of this regimen [38]. Side effects have been milder with this regimen than with TMP-SMX but are of a similar nature. Methemoglobinemia has been described but is rarely of clinical significance [39]. Initial success of AP prophylaxis has led to its use as a treatment of mild to moderate PCP. Although systemic side effects are minimal, AP is not as effective as TMP-SMX, and early relapses are common. Given these limitations, AP should be reserved for patients with mild disease who are intolerant to other forms of therapy [40, 41].

An oral hydroxynaphthoquinone, atovaquone, is now available for the treatment of mild to moderate PCP. Studies demonstrated that, although atovaquone achieved fewer complete responses than TMP-SMX, it was as effective on an intent-to-treat basis because of its improved tolerance [42, 43]. The recommended dose is 750 mg three times a day with food. Toxicities include rash and gastrointestinal intolerance.

Several other alternative regimens have been evaluated as rescue therapy for patients who fail to improve with, or who are intolerant to, conventional treatment. In these settings, intravenous or oral clindamycin (600 mg four times a day) with oral primaquine (15–30 mg base daily) has resulted in a response rate of approximately 90 percent [44]. Trimetrexate, an analogue of methotrexate, has been effective in approximately 70 percent of patients [45]. However, the lack of an oral trimetrexate preparation, the expense of the required adjuvant therapy with folinic acid, and high early relapse rates have limited its use.

Adjuvant systemic corticosteroids are now the standard of care in patients with PCP and respiratory compromise [46, 47]. Prednisone, 40 mg, or its equivalent, twice daily for 5 days, followed by 40 mg daily for 5 days and 20 mg daily for an additional 11 days, is now recommended for patients with moderate to severe PCP (room air arterial oxygen tension < 70 mm Hg, or alveolar-arterial oxygen gradient > 35 mm Hg) [48]. Currently, no data are available to justify the use of steroids in mild PCP, as rescue therapy, or in children.

Clinical response of PCP to antimicrobial therapy usually becomes evident between the second and sixth day of treatment [49]. If no improvement is noted by the seventh day, the diagnosis of PCP should be confirmed (if therapy was empiric) or a second diagnosis should be considered. Concurrent bacterial pneumonia, which may be difficult to diagnose, is a frequent cause for poor response to therapy. Patients treated initially with TMP-SMX have a survival rate of higher than 80 percent. Patients who are started on TMP-SMX but switched to pentamidine have lower survival rates: 70 percent if pentamidine is used because of TMP-SMX toxicity and 30 percent if there is no clinical response to TMP-SMX [1, 21]. Subsequent episodes of PCP, the need for assisted mechanical ventilation, and concurrent bacterial pneumonia are associated with a poorer prognosis [1–4, 21, 50, 51] (Table 11-2).

Because of the high incidence of relapse, numerous regimens of secondary PCP chemoprophylaxis have been devised, including TMP-SMX, aerosol pentamidine, and dapsone (see Chap. 19). The use of these agents for primary prophylaxis of PCP delays its occurrence by 6 to 12 months [52]. An updated review of recommendations for PCP prophylaxis was published recently [53].

Table 11-2 *Predictors of poor outcome in* Pneumocystis carinii *pneumonia*

Prolonged history of dyspnea/dry cough (> 4 wk)
Admission respiratory rate > 30/min
Recurrent *Pneumocystis carinii* pneumonia
Copathogens in BAL fluid
Poor oxygenation on admission (PaO_2 < 55 mm Hg or alveolar-arterial oxygen gradient > 30 mm Hg)
Low serum albumin on admission (< 3.5 mg/dl)
Severe radiographic abnormalities (diffuse bilateral interstitial infiltrates with or without alveolar consolidation)
Increased white blood cell count on admission (> 10,900/mm³)
Increased serum lactate dehydrogenase (> 300 IU/L)
Severe interstitial edema in transbronchial biopsy specimens

Source: Adapted from RF Miller, DM Mitchell. Management of respiratory failure in the acquired immune deficiency syndrome and *Pneumocystis* pneumonia. *Thorax* 45:140–146, 1990.

Mycobacterial Infections

Tuberculosis

The rise in the incidence of tuberculosis (TB) in the United States, which began in 1986, is largely due to cases occurring in the HIV-infected population [54–57]. The symptoms and signs of TB in HIV disease vary significantly depending on the degree of immunodeficiency [58]. Presenting symptoms include cough, fever, weight loss, and night sweats. Extrapulmonary disease is common, and symptoms resulting from liver, bone marrow, central nervous system, or lymphatic involvement may predominate [59–61]. Chest x-rays frequently do not reveal cavities, apical scarring, or pleural effusions and may be normal in up to 10 percent of patients [60–63]. In severely immunocompromised patients, the most common abnormalities are diffuse or miliary infiltrates, focal infiltrates, and mediastinal or hilar adenopathy (Fig. 11-2). Patients with closer to normal CD4 cell counts have radiographic findings more typical of TB in immunocompetent hosts [58]. The wide variety of clinical and roentgenographic findings makes the diagnosis of TB problematic in the HIV-infected population [64].

Figure 11-2. Pulmonary tuberculosis presenting as a localized right middle lobe infiltrate in an HIV-infected patient.

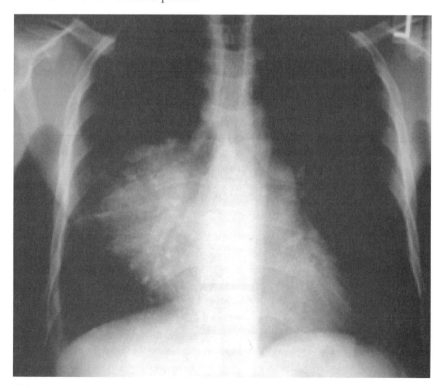

All HIV-infected patients with suspected mycobacterial disease should receive a treatment regimen effective against *M. tuberculosis*, as untreated TB is both transmissible and potentially fatal [55]. Pending culture results, initial therapy should consist of isoniazid (INH; 300 mg/day) and rifampin (600 mg/day); pyrazinamide (25 mg/kg/day) should be added for the first 2 months. Ethambutol (15 mg/kg/day) or streptomycin (15 mg/kg/day) should be added if there is suspicion of INH resistance and in regions where the prevalence of INH resistance is higher than 4 percent [65]. Therapy should be adjusted when culture results are available, and continued for 9 to 12 months for INH-sensitive organisms and 18 months for INH-resistant organisms. The key to success in the treatment of TB is adherence of the patient to the prescribed regimen. Directly observed therapy is strongly recommended since there is a reduced margin of safety in treating HIV-infected patients. Outbreaks of multidrug-resistant tuberculosis (MDR-TB) have been reported in health care facilities in Miami and New York City [66, 67]. Despite the use of multidrug regimens, MDR-TB has been uniformly fatal in patients with advanced HIV disease.

Tuberculosis is a largely preventable disease, and chemoprophylaxis should be considered for all patients with documented HIV infection. All HIV-infected patients with induration greater than or equal to 5 mm on an intermediate-strength (5-TU) purified protein derivative (PPD) test should receive prophylaxis, regardless of age, once active disease has been excluded [55, 65]. Patients who are anergic on skin testing but at high risk for TB (> 10% prevalence in the population), such as drug users, alcoholics, the homeless, past or current prison inmates, and patients from an endemic area, should also receive prophylaxis [55, 65]. In addition, patients with a history of a positive reaction to PPD who have never received treatment, patients with CXR abnormalities suggestive of previous untreated TB, and close contacts of patients with active TB should receive preventive therapy [55, 65]. Prophylaxis consists of INH or rifampin (in patients intolerant to INH or in whom INH resistance is suspected) for a minimum of 12 months [65].

Mycobacterium avium Complex

Mycobacterium avium complex (MAC) infection occurs most often in patients with advanced HIV disease. *M. avium* complex infection is generally disseminated even in its early stages. However, because the lungs are frequently colonized, they may be the initial site from which the organism is isolated [68]. Evidence of pulmonary MAC infection is usually lacking on CXR, and recovery of the organism from the lungs does not seem to affect prognosis. In some studies, the rate of recovery of MAC by bronchoscopy is approximately 50 percent but increases to 80 percent with the addition of transbronchial biopsy [1].

Patients prescribed combination therapy with ethambutol, rifampin, clofazimine, and ciprofloxacin, with or without amikacin, often have improvement of MAC-related symptoms, but drug toxicity is common and bacteriologic cure unusual [69–71]. Recently, newer macrolide antibiotics, such as clarithromycin and azithromycin, have been used with ethambutol as part of a multidrug regimen [72].

Rifabutin has been shown effective in preventing MAC bacteremia in HIV-infected patients with CD4 cell counts of $200/mm^3$ or lower [73]. However, its widespread use has been tempered by concerns of selecting for rifampin-resistant strains of *M. tuberculosis* and reports of uveitis when it is used in combination with the macrolide agents for treatment of MAC. In addition, rifabutin prophylaxis has not been shown to alter the overall prognosis in patients with advanced HIV disease. Clarithromycin has recently been reported to be effective for MAC prevention and may confer a survival benefit [74].

Nontuberculous Mycobacteria Other Than *Mycobacterium avium* Complex

Several species of atypical mycobacteria have been isolated from the respiratory tract of patients with AIDS. *Mycobacterium kansasii* is the second most common nontuberculous mycobacterial pathogen after MAC in HIV disease, with dissemination reported in patients with severe immunodeficiency [75]. The illness usually presents with fever, cough, and dyspnea. Chest x-ray frequently shows thin-walled cavities and reticular nodular infiltrates, with radiologic features reminiscent of TB. Regimens containing INH, rifampin, and ethambutol are generally effective and may provide a bacteriologic cure [76].

Viral Infections

Disseminated cytomegalovirus (CMV) infection commonly occurs in patients with advanced HIV disease. Clinical manifestations include chorioretinitis, encephalitis, esophagitis, hepatitis, colitis, adrenalitis, and pneumonitis [77]. Pulmonary symptoms and signs, as well as CXR findings of a diffuse interstitial infiltrate, are nonspecific. Definitive diagnosis requires demonstration of characteristic intranuclear inclusions on histologic examination of lung parenchyma obtained by fiberoptic bronchoscopy with transbronchial biopsy [78]. Cytomegalovirus pneumonitis is often associated with other pulmonary infections such as PCP. There appears to be no relationship between pulmonary CMV infection and survival in patients with a first episode of PCP [79]. Evidence of pulmonary involvement should prompt a careful ophthalmologic examination, since treatment for CMV retinitis can prevent blindness [80]. Antiviral therapy may not be effective for pulmonary CMV infection [81].

Herpesvirus infections are an infrequent cause of pneumonia in patients with HIV disease, but isolation of the virus from respiratory tract specimens is not unusual. Herpes simplex pneumonitis should only be considered when there is histologic evidence of pulmonary infection and no other pathogen is isolated [6]. The diagnosis of varicella-zoster pneumonia is generally less difficult; CXR reveals diffuse, bilateral infiltrates in patients with widely disseminated varicella infection [82]. Acyclovir is the drug of choice for both herpes simplex and varicella-zoster pneumonitis; foscarnet can be used to treat resistant organisms [83]. Human herpesvirus type 6 (HHV-6) recently was reported as a cause of fatal pneumonitis in severely immunocompromised patients. Although ganciclovir and foscarnet are active against HHV-6, their role in the treatment of pneumonitis must be evaluated [84].

Fungal Infections

Cryptococcal infection generally presents as meningitis, with evidence of coexisting pneumonitis in 10 to 30 percent of patients [85]. Chest x-ray studies usually demonstrate a focal or diffuse interstitial infiltrate, but cavitary lesions, adenopathy, and pleural effusions may also be seen. Identification of this organism in sputum or BAL specimens should prompt a lumbar puncture to rule out meningeal involvement. Cryptococcal pneumonitis, like meningitis, is treated with either amphotericin B or fluconazole followed by lifelong suppressive therapy [86].

Disseminated histoplasmosis has emerged as a common diagnosis in HIV-infected patients from endemic areas, such as the Ohio and Mississippi River valleys, Haiti, Puerto Rico, and South and Central America [87]. Histoplasmosis in patients who have not visited endemic areas for many years likely represents reactivation of latent infection. Chest x-ray generally shows bilateral nodular infiltrates with or without adenopathy; dissemination may occur in the absence of pulmonary involvement. In the presence of pulmonary infiltrates, the diagnostic yield of bronchoscopy is approximately 80 percent. However, in disseminated disease, bone marrow biopsy or blood culture has a sensitivity of approximately 90 percent [88, 89]. Amphotericin B is the drug of choice, but even with therapy the initial episode has a mortality rate of 20 to 50 percent; relapse is common and lifelong suppressive therapy is required [88]. Itraconazole has also been successfully used for the treatment and suppression of histoplasmosis [90].

Coccidioidomycosis with dissemination is a relatively frequent diagnosis in AIDS patients living in endemic areas [91]. The CXR appears abnormal in approximately 70 percent of patients, with diffuse reticulonodular infiltrates or focal infiltrates with hilar adenopathy and pleural effusions [92, 93]. The organism may be isolated from lymph nodes, blood, urine, and skin, in addition to pulmonary specimens. Despite severe immunosuppression, tube precipitins or complement-fixing antibodies are present in more than 90 percent of patients. Patients with a diffuse nodular pattern on CXR have a poor prognosis, with 50 percent dying within 1 month of diagnosis despite aggressive therapy with amphotericin B [92]. Ketoconazole and fluconazole may be useful for treatment as well as prophylaxis.

Pulmonary aspergillosis has only recently been recognized as a complication of HIV infection [94–96]. Pulmonary infection with aspergillus occurs as an invasive parenchymal process or as obstructing bronchial disease. The majority of patients have significant neutropenia, and almost all have had a prior AIDS-defining disorder. The clinical picture consists of cough and fever; many patients also have chest pain. In patients with invasive aspergillosis, CXR studies demonstrate unilateral or bilateral reticulonodular infiltrates with cavities or pleural-based lesions. Diffuse interstitial infiltrates may be seen in patients with obstructing bronchial disease, as well as in those with invasive aspergillosis [94, 95]. Despite aggressive therapy with amphotericin B, the median survival time has been approximately 3 months. Itraconazole may be useful in patients who cannot tolerate amphotericin.

Although cultures obtained at bronchoscopy frequently grow *Candida* species, the diagnosis of pulmonary candidiasis rests on the demonstration of fungal forms invading the lung parenchyma. Pulmonary candidiasis is exceedingly uncommon and rarely occurs except in gravely ill patients with disseminated candidiasis. Patients may respond to treatment with amphotericin B, ketoconazole, or fluconazole, but the mortality rate is high [93].

Protozoal Infections

Toxoplasmosis occurs in only 1 to 3 percent of AIDS patients in the United States but is more common in patients from Spain, Haiti, and other endemic areas. It usually presents a necrotizing encephalitis with multiple ring-enhancing lesions on computed tomographic scans or magnetic resonance images [97]. Pneumonitis may occur alone or as a complication of central nervous system disease. The CXR generally shows a nodular infiltrate or irregular consolidation. Demonstration of the parasite by Wright or Giemsa staining of biopsy material is required for diagnosis [93]. Treatment with sulfadiazine and pyrimethamine is generally effective, but lifelong suppressive therapy is required.

Species of the intestinal parasites *Strongyloides* and *Cryptosporidium* may cause pulmonary symptoms in patients with gastrointestinal infestation. Identification of *Strongyloides* organisms in the sputum denotes pulmonary infection [98]. Patients with respiratory cryptosporidiosis complain of unremitting cough. Examination of tissue specimens usually demonstrates localization of the organism to bronchial epithelial cells; identification of the pathogen in alveoli is rare, and invasion of the lung parenchyma has not been reported [99, 100]. Isolated pulmonary cryptosporidial disease does not appear to alter survival [101]. In contrast to *Strongyloides* infection, there is no effective therapy for disseminated cryptosporidiosis, and patients usually succumb to overwhelming gastrointestinal infestation.

Pulmonary microsporidial disease is now recognized as a complication of gastrointestinal infection with *Encephalitozoon hellem* and *Septata intestinalis* [102, 103]. Although microsporidia can be detected in BAL material using light microscopy, electron microscopy is required for speciation. A therapeutic trial with albendazole is appropriate for patients with documented symptomatic respiratory infestation [104].

Noninfectious Pulmonary Disorders

Kaposi's Sarcoma

Kaposi's sarcoma (KS) in the setting of AIDS generally presents as a multicentric disease involving the skin and oral mucosa. Internal organ involvement, particularly of the lymphatic system and gastrointestinal tract, occurs in 50 percent of patients with cutaneous KS [105, 106]. Thirty percent of patients with KS have symptomatic lung disease, which accounts for 8 to 12 percent of the pulmonary complications of AIDS [107]. Pulmonary KS most often occurs in the context of disseminated disease, although isolated pulmonary involvement has been reported [108, 109]. While nonspecific systemic symptoms such as fever and weight loss are most common, patients may also complain of wheezing, hemoptysis, pleuritic chest pain, or stridor [110]. Physical examination is usually not revealing, although stridor suggests bulky lesions of the upper airway [111]. Chest x-ray findings include bilateral interstitial or alveolar infiltrates, or both, often with poorly defined nodularity and accompanying pleural effusions [108] (Fig. 11-3).

Definitive diagnosis of pulmonary KS may require open lung biopsy. However, visualization of the typical macular or plaque-like cherry-red lesions of KS in the trachea or endobronchial tree during bronchoscopy is considered adequate in patients with established disease. Endobronchial biopsy, transbronchial biopsy, or bronchial brushing with cytology is generally not diagnostic [1, 24, 107, 108]. Pleural biopsy occasionally provides useful specimens. Therapy for pulmonary KS is palliative and consists of radiation therapy, combination chemotherapy, or both.

Lymphoma

Unlike non-Hodgkin's lymphoma in the seronegative population, HIV-associated lymphoma is composed of multiple clones with highly malignant histology, and is usually disseminated and extranodal at the time of presentation [112]. The central nervous system, gastrointestinal tract, and liver are most commonly involved; lung disease is less frequent. In patients with thoracic involvement, CXR reveals mediastinal nodes, in-

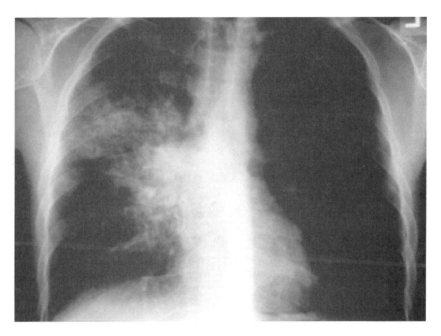

Figure 11-3. Pulmonary Kaposi's sarcoma. Radiologic findings generally include nodular parenchymal infiltrates.

terstitial and nodular infiltrates, solitary parenchymal nodules, or pleural thickening with effusions [110]. Transbronchial biopsy is rarely diagnostic, and open lung biopsy is generally required.

Hodgkin's lymphoma is also more frequent in HIV-infected patients, but thoracic involvement is less common than with non-Hodgkin's lymphoma. Similar to non-Hodgkin's lymphoma, advanced disease at the time of presentation is common, and open lung biopsy is required for diagnosis. In the few cases of HIV-related pulmonary Hodgkin's lymphoma that have been reported, the CXRs demonstrated either mediastinal involvement or bilateral infiltrates [113, 114].

Lymphoid Interstitial Pneumonitis

Lymphoid interstitial pneumonitis (LIP) is an immunologic disorder of unknown etiology; it typically occurs in pediatric AIDS patients but is also seen in adults [110]. The mononuclear infiltrate of LIP is composed of CD8 lymphocytes and plasma cells, which is phenotypically suggestive of a response to chronic antigenic stimulation. Although the antigen has not been defined, direct infection of the pulmonary parenchyma with HIV or Epstein-Barr virus has been suggested [115, 116]. The syndrome is highly dependent on the human leukocyte antigen (HLA) type of the patient and occurs most frequently in blacks with HLA-DR5 and whites with HLA-DR6 [117].

Patients typically present with slowly progressive dyspnea and non-productive cough; fever and weight loss may also be present. Physical examination often reveals adenopathy, hepatosplenomegaly, uveitis, or parotid gland enlargement. Although examination of the chest may be normal, crackles at the bases are frequently noted on auscultation [118]. The CXR demonstrates bilateral lower lobe interstitial or reticulonodular infiltrates with occasional areas of alveolar filling defects, similar to the pattern seen with PCP [119]. Hypergammaglobulinemia and lymphocytosis may occur [118, 119].

Diagnosis of LIP in adults is difficult. The clinical presentation is nonspecific, and because of its rarity, LIP is usually not considered early in the evaluation of dyspnea. Recurrent bacterial pneumonia is strongly associated with LIP and may further hinder diagnosis. Patients with LIP may respond to treatment of pathogens recovered from sputum, and the CXR appearance may improve but rarely return to normal. Histologic study of transbronchial or open lung biopsy specimens shows alveolar and interstitial infiltration of lymphocytes and plasma cells [120].

Therapeutic benefit has been attributed to zidovudine or corticosteroid therapy, or both [117]. Abnormalities demonstrated on CXR show considerable improvement, and oxygenation may return to normal or near normal. In many patients, no recurrence of symptoms occurs after discontinuation of corticosteroid treatment [117, 118]. However, in some individuals, clinical and radiologic deterioration follows within days of stopping therapy, and steroids must be continued for the long term [121].

Nonspecific Interstitial Pneumonitis

Nonspecific interstitial pneumonitis is a histologic entity characterized in biopsy specimens by a mild mononuclear cell infiltrate, with varying degrees of interstitial edema, fibrin deposition, alveolar cell hyperplasia, septal thickening, and fibrosis [4, 122]. Patients usually have nonspecific respiratory symptoms but may be asymptomatic [123]. Diagnosis relies on demonstration of typical histologic abnormalities and the exclusion of another underlying process. The clinical course usually stabilizes or improves without specific therapy. Steroids may be useful in symptomatic patients [4, 122].

Bronchogenic Carcinoma

Several patients with HIV infection have been described with bronchogenic carcinoma [124–126]. Whether bronchogenic carcinoma should be considered a complication of HIV disease has not yet been clarified. Patients with concurrent HIV infection and bronchogenic carcinoma are, in general, tobacco users but present at an earlier age and at a more advanced stage of disease than do immunocompetent individuals. Few patients survive longer than 2 months after diagnosis [125, 126].

Pulmonary Hypertension

The etiology of HIV-associated pulmonary hypertension remains unknown [127]. Even though pulmonary hypertension occurs 10 to 100 times more often in the setting of HIV infection, it is still a relatively infrequent finding. The presentation of HIV-associated pulmonary hypertension is remarkably similar to that of primary pulmonary hypertension, although the disorder appears to progress more rapidly. Patients may present early in the course of HIV disease. Complaints of rapidly progressive dyspnea on exertion are usual, but evaluation yields no evidence of infection or malignancy [127, 128]. The CXR typically shows normal pulmonary parenchyma with right-sided cardiac enlargement and pruning of the pulmonary vasculature. Echocardiography with Doppler evaluation of the tricuspid valve documenting a high gradient is suggestive of pulmonary hypertension, but direct measurement of the pulmonary artery pressure is required to confirm the diagnosis [128, 129]. There is currently no effective therapy.

Pleural Disease

The insidious onset of PCP allows significant pulmonary parenchymal destruction, leading to the development of cysts, cavities, bullae, and pneumothorax [26, 28]. The risk of pneumothorax is increased in patients with recurrent PCP and in those receiving AP prophylaxis [27]. Treatment of pneumothorax with chest tube suction is adequate in fewer than 50 percent of patients; air leaks are slow to resolve, and sclerotherapy or thoracotomy, or both, are frequently required [27, 130]. Treatment of PCP in AIDS patients with pneumothorax should be considered because of the common association of these two conditions.

Pleural effusions are relatively common in HIV disease, with infection, frequently bacterial, the cause in two-thirds of patients [131]. Massive effusions are most often indicative of TB, KS, or lymphoma.

Lymphadenopathy

Persistent generalized lymphadenopathy is a common finding in patients with HIV disease. Hilar and mediastinal adenopathy is not, however, part of the syndrome [132, 133]. Consequently, patients with radiographic evidence of thoracic adenopathy should be evaluated carefully for infectious or neoplastic diseases. Extrathoracic lymph node biopsy will often identify the cause; when nondiagnostic, open biopsy of the chest should be considered.

Diagnostic Approach for Respiratory Symptoms

A physician caring for an HIV-infected patient with respiratory symptoms faces a lengthy differential diagnosis that requires a rational management plan. In 1984, the National Heart, Lung, and Blood Institute, in a report of its workshop on pulmonary complications of AIDS, presented a series of algorithms designed to facilitate the diagnosis of pulmonary problems [3]. These algorithms, with a few modifications, have withstood the test of time. The following diagnostic approach, modified by more recent information, is recommended.

1. Patients with fever, cough, dyspnea, or weight loss should have chest roentgenography performed. Differential diagnosis and evaluation of commonly observed CXR patterns are presented in Table 11-3 and Figure 11-4.
2. If CXR appears normal, one should measure the alveolar-arterial oxygen gradient, determine the diffusing capacity for carbon monoxide, and/or perform gallium scanning of the lungs.

Table 11-3 *Differential diagnosis of chest x-ray (CXR) patterns in the HIV-infected patient*

CXR pattern	Differential diagnosis
Diffuse reticulonodular infiltrate	*Pneumocystis carinii* pneumonia Tuberculosis Disseminated histoplasmosis Disseminated coccidioidomycosis Lymphoid interstitial pneumonitis
Focal air space consolidation	Bacterial pneumonia Kaposi's sarcoma Cryptococcosis Bronchogenic carcinoma
Normal	*Pneumocystis carinii* pneumonia Disseminated MAC infection Disseminated histoplasmosis Pulmonary hypertension
Lymphadenopathy	Tuberculosis Kaposi's sarcoma Disseminated MAC infection Non-Hodgkin's lymphoma
Pleural effusion	Kaposi's sarcoma Tuberculosis Non-Hodgkin's lymphoma Pyogenic empyema

Source: Adapted from JF Murray, J Mills. Pulmonary infectious complications of human immunodeficiency virus infection (part 1). *Am Rev Respir Dis* 141:1356–1372, 1990.

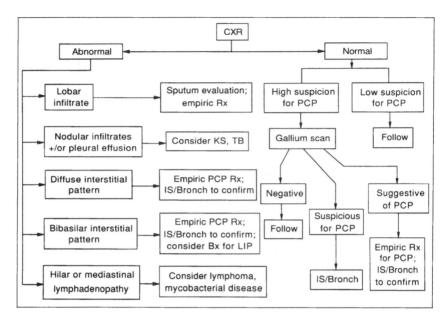

Figure 11-4. Algorithm for the evaluation of pulmonary disease associated with HIV infection based on chest x-ray (CXR) appearance. IS/Bronch = induced sputum/bronchoscopy; Bx = biopsy; LIP = lymphoid interstitial pneumonitis; Rx = treatment; KS = Kaposi's sarcoma; TB = tuberculosis; PCP = *Pneumocystis carinii* pneumonia. (Courtesy of Dr. Jon Fuller, Boston City Hospital.)

If the results of all three studies are unremarkable, pulmonary disease is highly unlikely.

3. If CXR reveals a focal abnormality, an attempt should be made to identify a conventional infection. Staining and culturing of sputum for bacteria and acid-fast bacilli should be included in this evaluation. If CXR shows diffuse infiltrates, an empiric trial of therapy for PCP is reasonable in patients previously diagnosed with AIDS who have only mild to moderate gas exchange abnormalities.

4. A firm diagnosis should be pursued for patients who lack an AIDS-defining illness. Induced sputum studies for *P. carinii*, acid-fast bacilli, and other pathogens should be the first step in such evaluation. In institutions that lack the capacity to perform this procedure, flexible fiberoptic bronchoscopy with BAL is appropriate. A similar approach is warranted in patients whose CXR abnormalities are focal, mild, or otherwise atypical of PCP after conventional pneumonia has been excluded.

5. If examination of induced sputum or initial fiberoptic bronchoscopy with BAL is nondiagnostic, fiberoptic bronchoscopy with BAL, bronchial brushing, and multiple trans-

bronchial biopsies should be performed. The biopsy and lavage specimens should be processed with appropriate stains or cultures, or both, for bacterial pathogens, including *Legionella* species, *P. carinii*, acid-fast bacilli, fungi, and CMV. Specimens should also undergo routine cytologic and histologic analysis.

6. If fiberoptic bronchoscopy with transbronchial biopsy is nondiagnostic and the patient's clinical condition is deteriorating, either repeat bronchoscopy with transbronchial biopsy or open lung biopsy should be performed.

7. If fiberoptic bronchoscopy with transbronchial biopsy is nondiagnostic and the patient's clinical condition is stable, diffusing capacity and alveolar-arterial oxygen gradients should be measured, and/or gallium scanning performed. If the results of these tests show that the patient's condition is stable or improving, clinical observation is appropriate. If the results show a worsening condition, either repeat bronchoscopy or open lung biopsy should be considered.

References

1. White DA, Stover DE. Pulmonary effects of AIDS. *Clin Chest Med* 9:363–535, 1988.
2. Hopewell PC, Luce JM. Pulmonary involvement in the acquired immunodeficiency syndrome. *Chest* 87:104–112, 1985.
3. Murray JF, Felton CP, Garay SM, et al. Pulmonary complications of the acquired immunodeficiency syndrome: Report of a National Heart, Lung, and Blood Institute workshop. *N Engl J Med* 320:1682–1688, 1984.
4. Stover DE, White DA, Roman PA, et al. Spectrum of pulmonary diseases associated with the acquired immune deficiency syndrome. *Am J Med* 78:429–437, 1985.
5. McKenzie R, Travis WD, Dolan SA, et al. The causes of death in patients with human immunodeficiency virus infection: A clinical and pathologic study with emphasis on the role of pulmonary diseases. *Medicine (Baltimore)* 70:326–343, 1991.
6. Murray JF, Mills J. Pulmonary infectious complications of human immunodeficiency virus infection (part 1). *Am Rev Respir Dis* 141:1356–1372, 1990.
7. Magnenat J-L, Nicod LP, Auckenthaler R, Funod AF. Mode of presentation and diagnosis of bacterial pneumonia in human immunodeficiency virus-infected patients. *Am Rev Respir Dis* 144:917–922, 1991.
8. Wallace JM, Rao AV, Glassroth J, et al. Respiratory illness in persons with human immunodeficiency virus infection: The Pulmonary Complications of HIV Infection Study Group. *Am Rev Respir Dis* 148:1523–1529, 1993.
9. Masur H, Ognibene FP, Yarchoan R, et al. CD4 counts as predictors of opportunistic pneumonias in human immunodeficiency virus (HIV) infection. *Ann Intern Med* 111:223–231, 1989.

10. Polsky B, Gold JWM, Whimbey E, et al. Bacterial pneumonia in patients with the acquired immunodeficiency syndrome. *Ann Intern Med* 104:38–41, 1986.

11. Blasi F, Boschini A, Costentini R, et al. Outbreak of *Chlamydia pneumoniae* infection in former injection-drug users. *Chest* 105:812–815, 1994.

12. Baron AD, Hollander H. *Pseudomonas aeruginosa* bronchopulmonary infection in late human immunodeficiency virus disease. *Am Rev Respir Dis* 148:992–996, 1993.

13. Nelson MR, Shanson DC, Barter GJ, et al. *Pseudomonas* septicemia associated with HIV. *AIDS* 5:761–763, 1991.

14. Kramer MR, Uttamchandani RB. The radiographic appearance of pulmonary nocardiosis associated with AIDS. *Chest* 98:382–385, 1990.

15. Joshi N, Hamory BH. Drug resistant *Nocardia asteroides* infection in a patient with acquired immunodeficiency syndrome. *South Med J* 84:1155–1156, 1991.

16. Harvey RL, Suntrum JC. *Rhodococcus equi* infection in patients with and without human immunodeficiency virus infection. *Rev Infect Dis* 13:139–145, 1991.

17. Verville RD, Huycke MM, Greenfield RA, et al. *Rhodococcus equi* infections of humans: 12 cases and a review of the literature. *Medicine (Baltimore)* 73:119–132, 1994.

18. Emmons W, Reichwein B, Winslow DL. *Rhodococcus equi* infection in the patient with AIDS: Literature review and report of an unusual case. *Rev Infect Dis* 13:91–96, 1991.

19. Scannell KA, Portoni EJ, Finkle HI, Rice M. Pulmonary malacoplakia and *Rhodococcus equi* infection in a patient with AIDS. *Chest* 97:1000–1001, 1990.

20. Tucker KJ, Anton B, Tucker HJ. The effect of human immunodeficiency virus infection on the distribution and outcome of pneumonia in intensive care units. *West J Med* 157:637–640, 1992.

21. Catterall JR, Potasman I, Remington JS. *Pneumocystis carinii* pneumonia in the patient with AIDS. *Chest* 88:758–762, 1985.

22. Freedberg KA, Tosteson ANA, Cohen CJ, Cotton DJ. Primary prophylaxis for *Pneumocystis carinii* pneumonia in HIV-infected people with CD-4 counts below 200/mm^3: A cost effectiveness analysis. *J Acquir Immune Defic Syndr* 4:521–531, 1991.

23. Opravil M, Marincek B, Fuchs WA, et al. Shortcomings of chest radiography in detecting *Pneumocystis carinii* pneumonia. *J Acquir Immune Defic Syndr* 7:39–45, 1994.

24. Weissler JC, Mootz AR. Southwestern Internal Medicine Conference: Pulmonary disease in AIDS patients. *Am J Med Sci* 300:330–343, 1990.

25. Tung KT. Cystic pulmonary lesions in AIDS. *Clin Radiol* 45:149–152, 1992.

26. Feurerstein IM, Archer A, Pluda JM, et al. Thin walled cavities, cysts, and pneumothorax in *Pneumocystis carinii* pneumonia: Further observations with histopathologic correlation. *Radiology* 177:697–702, 1990.

27. Sepkowitz KA, Telzak EE, Gold JWM, et al. Pneumothorax in AIDS. *Ann Intern Med* 114:455–459, 1991.

28. Joe L, Gordin F, Parker RH. Spontaneous pneumothorax with *Pneumocystis carinii* infection. *Arch Intern Med* 146:1816–1817, 1986.

29. Stover D, Greeno R, Gagliardi A. The use of a simple exercise test for the

diagnosis of *Pneumocystis carinii* pneumonia in patients with AIDS. *Am Rev Respir Dis* 139:1343–1346, 1989.

30. Garay SM, Green J. Prognostic indicators in the initial presentation of *Pneumocystis carinii* pneumonia. *Chest* 95:769–772, 1989.

31. Zaman MK, White DA. Serum lactate dehydrogenase levels and *Pneumocystis carinii* pneumonia: Diagnostic and prognostic significance. *Am Rev Respir Dis* 137:796–800, 1988.

32. Kovacs JA, Ng VL, Masur H, et al. Diagnosis of *Pneumocystis carinii* pneumonia: Improved detection in sputum with use of monoclonal antibodies. *N Engl J Med* 318:589–593, 1988.

33. Pitchenik AE, Ganjei P, Torres A, et al. Sputum examination for the diagnosis of *Pneumocystis carinii* pneumonia in the acquired immunodeficiency syndrome. *Am Rev Respir Dis* 133:226–229, 1986.

34. Jules-Elysee K, Stover D, Zaman M, et al. Aerosolized pentamidine: Effect on diagnosis and presentation of *Pneumocystis carinii* pneumonia. *Ann Intern Med* 112:750–757, 1990.

35. Yung RC, Weinacker AB, Steiger DJ, et al. Upper and middle lobe bronchoalveolar lavage to diagnose *Pneumocystis carinii* pneumonia. *Am Rev Respir Dis* 148:1563–1566, 1993.

36. Satter FR, Cowan R, Nielsen DM, Ruskin J. Trimethoprim-sulfamethoxazole compared with pentamidine for treatment of *Pneumocystis carinii* pneumonia in the acquired immunodeficiency syndrome: A prospective, non-crossover study. *Ann Intern Med* 109:280–287, 1988.

37. Sands M, Kron MA, Brown RB. Pentamidine: A review. *Rev Infect Dis* 7:625–637, 1985.

38. Leoung G, Mills J, Hopewell P, et al. Dapsone-trimethoprim for *Pneumocystis carinii* pneumonia in the acquired immunodeficiency syndrome. *Ann Intern Med* 105:45–48, 1986.

39. Gallant JE, Hoehn-Saric E, Smith MD. Respiratory insufficiency from dapsone induced methemoglobinemia. *AIDS* 5:1392–1393, 1991.

40. Montgomery AB, Debs R, Luce J, et al. Aerosolized pentamidine as sole therapy for *Pneumocystis carinii* pneumonia in patients with acquired immunodeficiency syndrome. *Lancet* 2:480–483, 1987.

41. Conte J, Hollander H, Golden J, et al. Selective delivery of pentamidine to the lung by aerosol. *Am Rev Respir Dis* 137:477–478, 1988.

42. Hughes W, Leoung G, Kramer F, et al. Comparison of atovaquone (566C80) with trimethoprim-sulfamethoxazole to treat *Pneumocystis carinii* pneumonia in patients with AIDS. *N Engl J Med* 32:1521–1527, 1993.

43. Falloon J. Treatment of *Pneumocystis carinii* pneumonia. *Ann Intern Med* 120:946–947, 1994.

44. Toma E, Fournier S, Poisson M, et al. Clindamycin with primaquine for *Pneumocystis carinii* pneumonia. *Lancet* 1:1046–1048, 1989.

45. Allegra CJ, Chabner BA, Tuazon CU, et al. Trimetrexate for the treatment of *Pneumocystis carinii* pneumonia in patients with acquired immunodeficiency syndrome. *N Engl J Med* 317:978–985, 1987.

46. Gagnon S, Booth AM, Fischl MA, et al. Corticosteroids as adjunctive therapy for severe *Pneumocystis carinii* pneumonia in the acquired immunodeficiency syndrome. *N Engl J Med* 323:1444–1450, 1990.

47. Bozzette SA, Sattler FR, Chui J, et al. A controlled trial of early adjunctive treatment for *Pneumocystis carinii* pneumonia in the acquired immunodeficiency syndrome. *N Engl J Med* 323:1451–1457, 1990.

48. NIH-UC Expert Panel for Corticosteroids as Adjunctive Therapy for *Pneumocystis* Pneumonia. Consensus statement for use of corticosteroids as adjunctive therapy for *Pneumocystis* pneumonia in AIDS. *N Engl J Med* 323:1500–1504, 1990.

49. Mitchell DM, Johnson MA. Treatment of lung disease in patients with the acquired immune deficiency syndrome. *Thorax* 45:219–224, 1990.

50. Miller RF, Mitchell DM. Management of respiratory failure in the acquired immune deficiency syndrome and *Pneumocystis* pneumonia. *Thorax* 45:140–146, 1990.

51. Wachter RM, Luce JM, Turner J, et al. Intensive care of patients with the acquired immunodeficiency syndrome: Outcome and changing patterns of utilization. *Am Rev Respir Dis* 134:891–896, 1986.

52. Hoover DR, Saah AJ, Bacellar H, et al. Clinical manifestations of AIDS in the era of *Pneumocystis* prophylaxis. Multicenter AIDS Cohort Study. *N Engl J Med* 329:1922–1926, 1993.

53. Centers for Disease Control. USPHS/IDSA guidelines for the prevention of opportunistic infections in persons infected with human immunodeficiency virus: A summary. *MMWR* 44(RR-8):1–34, 1995.

54. Centers for Disease Control. Update: Tuberculosis elimination—United States. *MMWR* 39:153–156, 1990.

55. Centers for Disease Control. Tuberculosis and human immunodeficiency virus infection: Recommendations of the Advisory Committee for the Elimination of Tuberculosis (ACET). *MMWR* 38:236–250, 1989.

56. Rieder HL, et al. Tuberculosis and acquired immunodeficiency syndrome—Florida. *Arch Intern Med* 149:1268–1273, 1989.

57. Chaisson RE, Slutkin G. Tuberculosis and human immunodeficiency virus infection. *J Infect Dis* 159:96–99, 1989.

58. Jones BE, Young SMM, Antoniskis D, et al. Relationship of the manifestations of tuberculosis to CD4 cell counts in patients with human immunodeficiency virus infection. *Am Rev Respir Dis* 148:1292–1297, 1993.

59. Chaisson RE, Schecter GF, Theuer CP, et al. Tuberculosis in patients with the acquired immunodeficiency syndrome: Clinical features, response to therapy, and survival. *Am Rev Respir Dis* 136:570–574, 1987.

60. Theuer CP, Hopewell PC, Elias D, et al. Human immunodeficiency virus infection in tuberculosis patients. *J Infect Dis* 1623:8–12, 1990.

61. Pitchenik AE, Cole C, Russell BW, et al. Tuberculosis, atypical mycobacteriosis, and the acquired immunodeficiency syndrome among Haitian and non-Haitian patients in south Florida. *Ann Intern Med* 101:610–615, 1984.

62. Pitchenik AE, Rubinson A. The radiographic appearance of tuberculosis in patients with the acquired immune deficiency syndrome (AIDS and pre-AIDS). *Am Rev Respir Dis* 131:393–396, 1985.

63. Coleblunders RE, Ryder RW, Nzilambi N, et al. HIV infection in patients with tuberculosis in Kinshasa, Zaire. *Am Rev Respir Dis* 139:1082–1085, 19889.

64. Kramer F, Modilevsky T, Waliany AR, et al. Delayed diagnosis of tuber-

culosis in patients with human immunodeficiency virus infection. *Am J Med* 89:451–456, 1990.

65. American Thoracic Society. Treatment of tuberculosis and tuberculosis infection in adults and children. *Am J Respir Crit Care Med* 149:1359–1374, 1994.

66. Fischl M, Uttamchandani R, Daikos G, et al. Outbreak of multiple drug resistant tuberculosis (MDR-TB) among patients with HIV infection (abstract). Eighth International Conference on AIDS, Amsterdam, July 1992.

67. Edlin BR, et al. An outbreak of multi-drug resistant tuberculosis among hospitalized patients with the acquired immunodeficiency syndrome. *Ann Intern Med* 104:184–188, 1986.

68. Hawkins C, Gold J, Whimbley E, et al. *Mycobacterium avium* complex in patients with acquired immunodeficiency syndrome. *Ann Intern Med* 105:184–188, 1986.

69. Hoy J, Mitch A, Sandland M, et al. Quadruple drug therapy for *Mycobacterium avium-intracellulare* bacteremia in AIDS patients. *J Infect Dis* 161:801–805, 1990.

70. Chiu J, Nussbaum J, Bozzette S, et al. Treatment of disseminated *Mycobacterium avium* complex infection in AIDS with amikacin, ethambutol, rifampin, and ciprofloxacin. *Ann Intern Med* 113:358–361, 1990.

71. Agins BC, Berman DS, Spicehandler D, et al. Effect of combined therapy with ansamycin, clofazamine, ethambutol and isoniazid for *Mycobacterium avium* infection in patients with AIDS. *J Infect Dis* 159:784–787, 1989.

72. Masur H, the Public Health Service Task Force on Prophylaxis and Therapy for *Mycobacterium avium* complex. Recommendations on prophylaxis and therapy for disseminated *Mycobacterium avium* complex disease in patients infected with the human immunodeficiency virus. *N Engl J Med* 329:989–904, 1993.

73. Cameron W, Sparti P, Pietroski N, et al. Rifabutin therapy for the prevention of MAC bacteremia in patients with AIDS and CD4<200 (abstract). Eighth International Conference on AIDS, Amsterdam, July 1992.

74. Second National Conference on Human Retroviruses and Related Infections. Washington DC, January 1995.

75. Shafer RW, Sierra MF. *Mycobacterium xenopi, Mycobacterium fortuitum, Mycobacterium kansasii,* and other non-tuberculous mycobacteria in an area of endemicity for AIDS. *Clin Infect Dis* 15:161–162, 1992.

76. Davey RT. Mycobacterial disease in HIV-1 infection: Recent therapeutic advances. *Ann Intern Med* 120:949–951, 1994.

77. Wallace JM, Hannah J. Cytomegalovirus pneumonitis in patients with AIDS: Findings in an autopsy series. *Chest* 92:198–203, 1987.

78. Jacobson MA, Mills J. Cytomegalovirus infection. *Clin Chest Med* 9:443–448, 1988.

79. Jacobson MA, Mills J, Rush J, et al. Morbidity and mortality of patients with AIDS and first-episode *Pneumocystis carinii* pneumonia unaffected by concomitant pulmonary cytomegalovirus infection. *Am Rev Respir Dis* 144:6–9, 1991.

80. Jacobson MA, Mills J. Serious cytomegalovirus disease in the acquired immunodeficiency syndrome (AIDS). *Ann Intern Med* 108:585–594, 1988.

81. Collaborative DHPG Treatment Study Group. Treatment of serious cytomegalovirus infection with 9-(1,3-dihydroxy-2-propoxymethyl) guanine in patients with AIDS and other immunodeficiencies. *N Engl J Med* 314:801–805, 1986.

82. Cohen PR, Belltrani VP, Grossman ME. Disseminated herpes-zoster in patients with human immunodeficiency virus infection. *Am J Med* 84:1076–1080, 1988.

83. Erlich K, Jacobson MA, Loehler J, et al. Foscarnet therapy for severe acyclovir resistant herpes simplex virus infections in patients with acquired immunodeficiency syndrome. *Ann Intern Med* 110:710–713, 1989.

84. Knox KK, Carrigan DR. Disseminated active HHV-6 infections in patients with AIDS. *Lancet* 343:578, 1994.

85. Cameron ML, Bartlett JA, Gallos HA, Waskin HA. Manifestations of pulmonary cryptococcosis in patients with acquired immunodeficiency syndrome. *Rev Infect Dis* 13:64–67, 1991.

86. Saag MA, Powderly WG, Cloud GA, et al. Comparison of amphotericin B with fluconazole in the treatment of acute AIDS-associated cryptococcal meningitis. *N Engl J Med* 326:83–89, 1992.

87. Mandell W, Goldberg DM, Neu HC. Histoplasmosis in patients with the acquired immune deficiency syndrome. *Am J Med* 81:974–978, 1986.

88. Wheat LJ, Connolly-Stringfield PA, Baker RL, et al. Disseminated histoplasmosis in the acquired immune deficiency syndrome: Clinical findings, diagnosis and treatment, and review of the literature. *Medicine (Baltimore)* 69:361–374, 1990.

89. Pretcher GC, Prakash UBS. Bronchoscopy in the diagnosis of pulmonary histoplasmosis. *Chest* 95:1033–1036, 1989.

90. Wheat J, et al. Prevention of relapse of histoplasmosis with itraconazole in patients with the acquired immunodeficiency syndrome. *Ann Intern Med* 118:610–616, 1993.

91. Sobonya RE, Barbee RA, Wiens J, Trego D. Detection of fungi and other pathogens in immuno-compromised patients by bronchoalveolar lavage in an area endemic for coccidioidomycosis. *Chest* 97:1349–1355, 1990.

92. Fish DG, Ampel NM, Calgiani JN, et al. Coccidioidomycoses during HIV infection: A review of 77 patients. *Medicine (Baltimore)* 69:384–391, 1990.

93. Murray JF, Mills J. Pulmonary infectious complications of HIV infection (part 2). *Am Rev Respir Dis* 131:1582–1598, 1990.

94. Denning DW, Follansbee SE, Scolaro M, et al. Pulmonary aspergillosis in the acquired immunodeficiency syndrome. *N Engl J Med* 324:654–662, 1991.

95. Klapholz A, Salomon N, Perlman DC, Talavera W. Aspergillosis in the acquired immunodeficiency syndrome. *Chest* 100:1614–1618, 1991.

96. Lortholary O, et al. Invasive aspergillosis in patients with acquired immunodeficiency syndrome: Report of 33 cases. *Am J Med* 95:177–187, 1993.

97. McCabe RE, Remington JS. *Toxoplasma gondii*. In GL Mandell, RG Douglas, JE Bennett (eds), *Principles and Practices of Infectious Diseases* (3rd ed). New York: Churchill Livingstone, 1989. Pp 2093–2094.

98. Armignacco O, Capecchi A, DeMori P. *Strongyloides stercoralis* hyperinfection and the acquired immunodeficiency syndrome. *Am J Med* 86:258, 1989.

99. Brady EM, Margolis ML, Korzeniowski OM. Pulmonary cryptosporidiosis in acquired immunodeficiency syndrome. *JAMA* 252:89–90, 1984.
100. Ma P, Villaneuva TG, Kaufman D, Gillooley JF. Respiratory cryptosporidiosis in the acquired immunodeficiency syndrome. *JAMA* 252:1298–1301, 1984.
101. Hojlyng N, Jenson BN. Respiratory cryptosporidiosis in HIV-positive patients. *Lancet* 1:590–591, 1988.
102. Orenstein JM, Dieterich DT, Kotler DP. Systemic dissemination by a newly recognized microsporidia in AIDS. *AIDS* 6:1143–1150, 1992.
103. Weber R, Kuster H, Visvesvara GS, et al. Disseminated microsporidiosis due to *Encephalitozoon hellem*: Pulmonary colonization, microhematuria, and mild conjunctivitis in a patient with AIDS. *Clin Infect Dis* 17:415–419, 1993.
104. Orenstein JM, Dieterich DT, Lew EA, Kotler DP. Albendazole as a treatment for intestinal and disseminated microsporidiosis due to *Septata intestinalis* in AIDS patients: A report of four patients. *AIDS* 7(suppl 3):S40–S42, 1993.
105. Safai B, Johnson KG, Myskowski PL, et al. The natural history of Kaposi's sarcoma in the acquired immunodeficiency syndrome. *Ann Intern Med* 102:471–475, 1985.
106. Friedman SL, Wright TL, Altman DF. Gastrointestinal Kaposi's sarcoma in patients with the acquired immune deficiency syndrome. Endoscopic and autopsy findings. *Gastroenterology* 890:102–108, 1985.
107. Garay S, Belenko M, Fazzini E, Schinella R. Pulmonary manifestations of Kaposi's sarcoma. *Chest* 91:39–43, 1987.
108. Meduri GU, Stover DE, Lee M, et al. Pulmonary Kaposi's sarcoma in the acquired immune deficiency syndrome. *Am J Med* 81:11–18, 1986.
109. Zibrak JD, Silvestri RC, Costello P, et al. Bronchoscopic and radiologic features of Kaposi's sarcoma involving the respiratory system. *Chest* 90:476, 1986.
110. White DA, Matthay RA. Non-infectious complications of infection with the human immunodeficiency virus. *Am Rev Respir Dis* 140:1763–1787, 1989.
111. Malabonga VM, Smith PR. Upper airway obstruction due to Kaposi's sarcoma in the acquired immunodeficiency syndrome. *NY State J Med* 90:613–614, 1990.
112. Kaplan LD, Abrams DI, Feigal E, et al. AIDS-associated non-Hodgkin's lymphoma in San Francisco. *JAMA* 261:719–724, 1989.
113. Knowles LD, Chamulak GA, Subar M, et al. Lymphoid neoplasia associated with the acquired immunodeficiency syndrome (AIDS). *Ann Intern Med* 108:744–753, 1988.
114. Scheib RG, Seigal RS. Atypical Hodgkin's disease and the acquired immunodeficiency syndrome. *Ann Intern Med* 102:554, 1985.
115. Resnick L, Pitchenik AE, Fisher E, Croney R. Detection of HTLV-III/LAV specific IgG and antigen in bronchoalveolar lavage fluid from two patients with lymphocytic interstitial pneumonitis associated with AIDS-related complex. *Am J Med* 82:553–556, 1987.
116. Lin RY, Gruber PJ, Saunders R, Perla EN. Lymphocytic interstitial pneumonitis in adult HIV infection. *NY State J Med* 88:273–276, 1988.

117. Itescu S, Winchester R. Diffuse infiltrative lymphocytosis syndrome: A disorder occurring in human immunodeficiency virus-1 infection that may present as a sicca syndrome. *Rheum Dis Clin North Am* 18:683–697, 1992.
118. Oldham SAA, Castillo M, Jacobson FL, et al. HIV associated lymphocytic interstitial pneumonia: Radiologic manifestations and pathology correlation. *Radiology* 170:83–87, 1989.
119. Rubinstein A, Morecki R, Silverman B, et al. Pulmonary disease in children with the acquired immunodeficiency syndrome and AIDS-related complex. *J Pediatr* 108:498–503, 1986.
120. Barrio JL, Harcup C, Baier HJ, Pitchenik AE. Value of repeat fiberoptic bronchoscopies and significance of non-diagnostic bronchoscopy results in patients with the acquired immunodeficiency syndrome. *Am Rev Respir Dis* 135:422–425, 1987.
121. Morris JC, Rosen MJ, Marchevsky A, Tierstein AS. Lymphocytic interstitial pneumonitis in patients at risk for the acquired immunodeficiency syndrome. *Chest* 91:63–67, 1987.
122. Suffredini AF, Ognibene FP, Lack EE, et al. Nonspecific interstitial pneumonitis: A common cause of pulmonary disease in the acquired immunodeficiency syndrome. *Ann Intern Med* 107:7–13, 1987.
123. Ognibene FP, Masur H, Rogers P, et al. Nonspecific interstitial pneumonitis without evidence of *Pneumocystis carinii* in asymptomatic patients with human immunodeficiency virus (HIV). *Ann Intern Med* 109:874–879, 1988.
124. Scott WW Jr, Kuhlman JE. Focal pulmonary lesions in patients with AIDS: Percutaneous transthoracic needle biopsy. *Radiology* 180:419–421, 1991.
125. Karp J, Profeta G, Marantz PR, Karpel JP. Lung cancer in patients with immunodeficiency syndrome. *Chest* 103:410–413, 1993.
126. Tenholder MF, Jackson HD. Bronchogenic carcinoma in patients seropositive for human immunodeficiency virus. *Chest* 104:1049–1053, 1993.
127. Mette SA, Palevsky HI, Pietra GG, et al. Primary pulmonary hypertension associated with human immunodeficiency virus infection. *Am Rev Respir Dis* 145:1196–1200, 1992.
128. Coplan NL, Shimony RY, Ioachim HL, et al. Primary pulmonary hypertension associated with human immunodeficiency viral infection. *Am J Med* 89:96–99, 1990.
129. Goldsmith GH, Baily RG, Brettler DB, et al. Primary pulmonary hypertension in patients with classic hemophilia. *Ann Intern Med* 108:797–799, 1988.
130. Fleisher AG, McElvaney G, Lawson L, et al. Surgical management of spontaneous pneumothorax in patients with acquired immunodeficiency syndrome. *Ann Thorac Surg* 45:21–23, 1988.
131. Joseph J, et al. Pleural effusions in hospitalized patients with AIDS. *Ann Intern Med* 118:856–859, 1993.
132. Stern RG, Gamsu G, Golden JA, et al. Intrathoracic adenopathy: Differential features of AIDS and diffuse lymphadenopathy syndrome. *Am J Radiol* 142:689–692, 1984.
133. Suster B, Akerman M, Orenstein M, Wax MR. Pulmonary manifestations of AIDS; review of 106 episodes. *Radiology* 161:87–93, 1986.

Gastrointestinal Manifestations   *12*

Michael S. Karasik, Nezam H. Afdhal

Gastrointestinal (GI) involvement in AIDS is almost universal, and clinically significant disease occurs in 50 to 90 percent of patients [1, 2]. Common and opportunistic infections, malignancies, and specific HIV-related syndromes all affect the GI tract. Symptoms include diarrhea with associated weight loss and wasting, odynophagia, and abdominal pain. Hepatobiliary disease, although common, is often asymptomatic. Prompt diagnosis and treatment of HIV-related GI disorders are necessary to prevent significant morbidity from weight loss and malnutrition.

Diarrhea

Diarrhea is experienced by nearly all patients with HIV disease at some time. It is considered significant when the stool output is greater than 500 gm per day. Over 70 percent of cases of diarrhea are caused by infection [3]. The diarrhea may be mild and intermittent, or severe and disabling; spontaneous exacerbations and remissions are common. The history can prove useful in localizing the site of diarrhea to the small or large bowel. Large-volume diarrhea, frequently pale and bulky, is generally associated with small bowel disease such as that seen with cryptosporidiosis. Frequent small-volume stools with tenesmus, hematochezia, or rectal discharge may suggest perianal disease, such as herpes simplex proctitis, or an invasive viral or bacterial colitis. Epidemiologic features may be useful in differential diagnosis. For example, patients from the Caribbean are at increased risk for infection with parasites such as *Isospora belli* and *Strongyloides stercoralis*.

The initial evaluation of diarrhea is similar to that performed in an immunocompetent patient. Examination of the stool is essential and should include (1) wet preparation for leukocytes and motile trophozoites; (2) test for occult blood; (3) bacterial culture for common pathogens, such as *Salmonella*, *Campylobacter*, and *Shigella*; and (4) three samples for ova and parasites. An acid-fast or Kinyoun stain for *Mycobacterium avium* complex (MAC), modified acid-fast stains for cryptosporidial and *I. belli* oocysts, and a chromotrope-based stain for microsporidia should also be included, especially in patients with advanced HIV disease (CD4 count < 200/mm^3). Patients receiving antimicrobial therapy should have their stool assayed for *Clostridium difficile* cytotoxin.

If results of these studies are negative and significant diarrhea persists, further investigations should include colonoscopy or flexible sigmoidoscopy with biopsy. Upper GI endoscopy with biopsy and duodenal fluid aspiration may also be helpful in some cases. Small bowel biopsy and aspiration can be useful in excluding parasites that are intermittently shed in stool. Tissue obtained at colonoscopy or endoscopy should be sent for histopathologic examination, as well as viral, fungal, and mycobacterial cultures.

The differential diagnosis for HIV-associated diarrhea is presented in Table 12-1. Gastroenteritis may result from bacterial, viral, and parasitic infections. Diarrhea may also be the result of neoplasms, HIV enteropathy, or drug toxicity.

Bacterial Infections

Salmonella Species
HIV-infected patients have a 20-fold increased risk of salmonellosis, usually nontyphoidal, which is associated with bacteremia in 50 to 80 percent of patients [4, 5]. Bacteremia may occur in the presence of negative stool cultures. Recurrent *Salmonella* infection may be the first manifestation of AIDS and has also been described with HIV-2 infection. *Salmonella* species are resistant to ampicillin in 50 percent of patients, and trimethoprim-sulfamethoxazole (TMP-SMX) or a quinolone (ciprofloxacin or ofloxacin) is recommended [6]. Parenteral therapy is necessary for patients with evidence of sepsis. In patients with chronic relapsing disease, long-term suppressive therapy with a quinolone antibiotic is indicated.

Shigella Species
Shigella flexneri is the usual pathogen, and bacteremia is uncommon. Blood and leukocytes are frequently identified in the stool. A quinolone antibiotic is the treatment of choice.

Table 12-1 *Differential diagnosis of diarrhea in the HIV-infected patient*

Infections
  Bacterial
    Mycobacterium avium complex
    Salmonella species
    Shigella species
    Campylobacter species
    Clostridium difficile
  Viral
    Cytomegalovirus
    Rotavirus
    Norwalk agent
  Fungal
    Candida species
    Histoplasma capsulatum
  Parasitic
    Cryptosporidium species
    Isospora belli
    Microsporidia
    Giardia lamblia
    Entamoeba histolytica
Neoplasms
  Lymphoma
  Kaposi's sarcoma
HIV enteropathy
Drug toxicity

Campylobacter Species

Infection may present with diarrhea, cholecystitis, or a Crohn's disease–like terminal ileitis. Treatment is with erythromycin; or a quinolone antibiotic can be used for resistant cases.

Viral Infections

Cytomegalovirus

Disseminated cytomegalovirus (CMV) infection is associated with advanced HIV disease and can affect any part of the GI tract [7]. Frequent bloody bowel movements are common [8]. Colonic disease is characterized endoscopically by patchy inflammation with vasculitis and histologically by intranuclear inclusions. Enteritis manifested by abdominal pain may also occur, and fistula formation with perforation is not unusual. Inflammatory masses that mimic tumors— "CMVomas"—have been described in the cecum, colon, and small bowel. Treatment with ganciclovir or foscarnet for 2 to 4 weeks results in clinical improvement in a majority of patients. Maintenance therapy may be necessary, and CMV colitis is associated with a poor long-term prognosis.

Herpes Simplex Virus

Herpes simplex virus (HSV), usually type 2, proctitis is common in patients who practice receptive anal intercourse and manifests as severe anorectal pain with tenesmus. Constipation is more common than diarrhea, and sacral nerve involvement may result in local paresthesias and urinary retention. Diagnosis is based on flexible sigmoidoscopic biopsy and culture. Oral acyclovir is the treatment of choice; intravenous administration is reserved for severe infection. Foscarnet is used for acyclovir-resistant HSV strains.

Parasitic Infections

Cryptosporidium Species

Cryptosporidiosis in the severely immunocompromised host is characterized by chronic, voluminous small bowel diarrhea (up to 20 liters per day) associated with cramping abdominal pain and weight loss [9]. In early HIV disease, its course may be self-limited [10]. Diagnosis is made by identification of the oocyst in stool (Plate 17). Spiramycin, erythromycin, and clindamycin have proved to be ineffective, but paromomycin, azithromycin, and immune bovine dialyzable leukocyte extract may be useful in some patients [11, 12].

Isospora belli

This sporozoan is frequently seen in patients from the Caribbean and causes a clinical syndrome similar to cryptosporidiosis [13] (Plate 18). Treatment with TMP-SMX (double-strength tablet four times a day for 10 days, then twice a day for 3 weeks) is effective, but relapse rates as high as 50 percent have been described following initial therapy. Pyrimethamine plus folinic acid is an alternative regimen for patients who cannot tolerate TMP-SMX.

Strongyloides stercoralis

This nematode helminth is endemic to the tropics and can be transmitted sexually. Latent infection has been reported to last for as long as 30 years. Diarrhea is watery with few leukocytes. A hyperinfection syndrome with larvae invading the bowel wall has been reported in AIDS, presenting as respiratory symptoms, meningitis, and polymicrobial sepsis [14]. Stool and duodenal juice aspirates are frequently required for diagnosis. Thiabendazole is the treatment of choice.

Entamoeba histolytica

Cyst carriage is seen in 5 percent of the US population and in 20 to 30 percent of homosexuals. Active infection is indicated by bloody stools containing the trophozoites with ingested red cells (hemophagocytosis).

Treatment is with metronidazole, 750 mg orally three times a day for 10 days, followed by iodoquinol, 650 mg orally three times a day for 20 days.

Giardia lamblia

This flagellated protozoan is a common cause of traveler's diarrhea, and 3 to 7 percent of the US population are asymptomatic cyst carriers. Giardiasis can cause diarrhea, flatulence, abdominal cramps, and bloating; the illness appears to be no more severe in HIV-infected patients than in immunocompetent persons. The syndrome may be acute or chronic, and diagnosis depends on demonstration of trophozoites in stool or duodenal fluid (Plate 19). Metronidazole, 250 mg orally three times a day for 5 to 10 days, is the treatment of choice.

Microsporidia

This unicellular protozoan, which is sometimes associated with nonbloody diarrhea, has been shown in the small bowel of AIDS patients by Giemsa stain and electron microscopy [15]. Albendazole therapy may be effective in some patients.

HIV Enteropathy

In 20 to 30 percent of HIV-infected patients with diarrhea, no specific pathogen can be isolated [16]. There is evidence of malabsorption, and small bowel biopsy demonstrates partial villous atrophy, with evidence of tissue injury and increased intraepithelial lymphocytes (Fig. 12-1). The etiology of this syndrome is unclear, but may include a direct enterocytopathic effect of HIV or other viral pathogens. Immunologic injury induced by these agents is also a possibility. Treatment is supportive, and octreotide administration may be useful in some patients.

"Gay Bowel Syndrome"

A syndrome of perianal pain with diarrhea and rectal discharge has been described in homosexual men [17, 18]. It appears most commonly to be caused by sexually transmitted diseases, including syphilis, gonorrhea, and chlamydia and HSV infection. Rectal Kaposi's sarcoma (KS) and squamous cell carcinoma of the anus may produce a similar syndrome. In addition to stool examination, a high rectal swab and culture should be performed. Sigmoidoscopy is recommended if the diagnosis is uncertain.

General Management of Diarrhea

Diarrhea in HIV-infected patients can be associated with severe dehydration and weight loss; appropriate fluid and electrolyte management

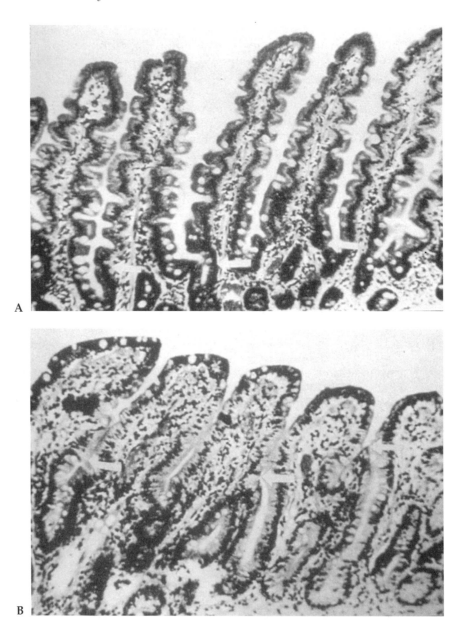

Figure 12-1. **A**. Normal small intestinal villi. **B**. Abnormal villi in HIV enteropathy. (From DP Kottler, HP Gaetz, M Lange, et al. Enteropathy associated with the acquired immunodeficiency syndrome. *Ann Intern Med* 101:421–428, 1984.)

is vital. For patients who do not require hospitalization, oral rehydration therapy with fluids containing electrolytes and glucose (juice, soda, soup) may be sufficient. In the absence of *Salmonella* infection or antibiotic-associated colitis, antidiarrheal agents, such as diphenoxylate hydrochloride (Lomotil), loperamide hydrochloride (Imodium), or deodorized tincture of opium (DTO), can be safely given and are often effective. In resistant cases in which no treatable pathogen is identified, therapy with a somatostatin analogue, octreotide (doses of 50–500 µg three times a day subcutaneously), has proved useful [19, 20]. Nutritional support in patients with chronic diarrhea is important since severe weight loss may adversely affect immune function. Enteral or parenteral nutrition may be required in severe cases.

Odynophagia

Odynophagia, or pain on swallowing, a manifestation of esophageal disease, is described in up to 90 percent of patients with AIDS. Infectious esophagitis, either fungal or viral, is the usual cause. Esophageal candidiasis, which can occur in the absence of oral involvement, is characterized by white plaque-like lesions with associated erythema and ulceration [21] (Fig. 12-2A). Viral infections, such as with CMV or HSV, usually manifest as discrete or giant ulcers of the esophagus; esophageal perforation or severe GI bleeding may ensue [22, 23]. In about 10 percent of patients, multiple pathogens can be identified. Esophageal ulceration may also occur as a direct result of HIV infection. Primary HIV infection has been associated with multiple, small esophageal ulcers that resolve within 3 to 7 days in most patients [24]. Retrovirus particles resembling HIV have also been identified in giant esophageal ulcers in patients with advanced HIV disease. In contrast to HIV seroconversion–related ulcers, these are usually very large and deep, with remarkably little surrounding erythema or edema (Fig. 12-2B). In addition, they are extremely painful and generally do not improve spontaneously. Unusual causes of odynophagia include tumors, such as lymphoma or KS, and MAC infection.

Definitive diagnosis of esophagitis requires endoscopy with biopsy and brushings for histology, as well as viral and fungal culture [25]. When endoscopic findings are negative, computed tomography of the thorax may identify disease in the submucosa or mediastinum.

Treatment of odynophagia is initially empiric and usually targeted against candidal infection. A trial of ketoconazole, 200 to 400 mg orally daily, or fluconazole, 50 to 100 mg orally daily, can be given, but if improvement is not seen within 1 week, endoscopy with biopsy and cultures should be performed. Esophageal candidiasis may be refractory to treatment with ketoconazole because of fungal resistance or impaired GI absorption secondary to achlorhydria. HSV infection is managed with acyclovir, and CMV ulcerations with ganciclovir or foscarnet. Giant ulcers associated with advanced HIV disease may respond to oral, topical, or submucosally injected corticosteroids.

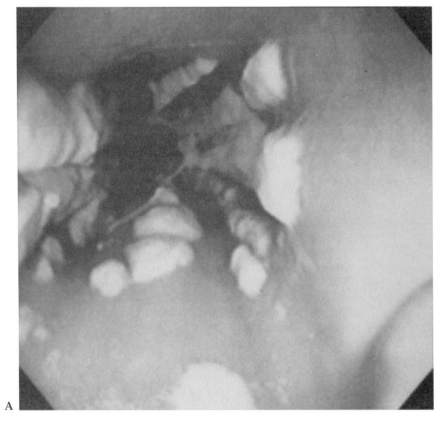

A

Figure 12-2. A. Endoscopic view of candidal plaques in the esophagus of a patient with AIDS. Initially linear, these plaques can become diffuse and confluent along the esophageal wall.

Abdominal Pain

HIV-infected patients are susceptible to common causes of abdominal pain, such as appendicitis and cholecystitis, seen in immunocompetent persons. These should be excluded by careful clinical evaluation and appropriate diagnostic tests. Opportunistic diseases may also cause abdominal pain. Cytomegalovirus and MAC enterocolitis may result in deep ulcers, fistulas, and bowel perforation. Nodal involvement by MAC and lymphoma can give rise to severe postprandial pain secondary to mesenteric compression. Pancreatitis may be related to drug therapy (pentamidine, didanosine, sulfa drugs) or opportunistic diseases; CMV infection, toxoplasmosis, candidiasis, lymphoma, and KS have all been implicated. Typhlitis, a clinical syndrome described in patients receiving chemotherapy for hematologic malignancy, has also

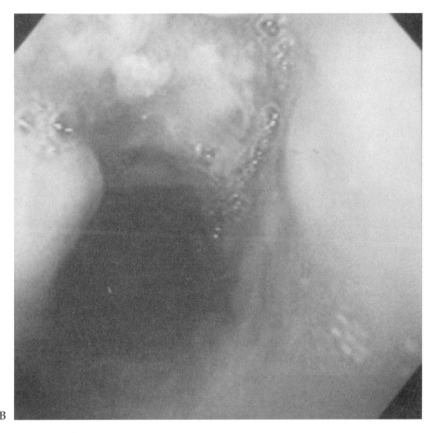

B

Figure 12-2. B. Endoscopic view of a 7-cm idiopathic ulcer of the distal esophagus in a patient with advanced AIDS. No evidence of infection was present despite the examination of numerous biopsy specimens. Although the lesion did not respond to an empiric 2-week trial of ganciclovir, it completely resolved with prednisone therapy.

been associated with HIV infection [26]. It presents as fever and right lower quadrant pain and is characterized by cecal wall thickening on computed tomographic scan. Treatment consists of bowel rest and intravenous antibiotics.

Hepatic Disease

The clinical and histologic spectrum of hepatobiliary disease in HIV infection is extremely diverse [27, 28] (Table 12-2).

Table 12-2 *Hepatobiliary disease in HIV infection*

Hepatic parenchymal disease
  Viral pathogens
    Hepatitis B
    Hepatitis C
    Hepatitis D (delta)
    Cytomegalovirus
    Herpes simplex virus
  Mycobacterial pathogens
    Mycobacterium avium complex
    Mycobacterium tuberculosis
  Fungal pathogens
    Cryptococcus neoformans
    Candida species
    Histoplasma capsulatum
  Neoplastic
    Lymphoma
    Kaposi's sarcoma
  Drug-related
    Sulfonamides
    Ketoconazole
    Isoniazid
    Rifampin
    Rifabutin
    Zidovudine
    Didanosine
    Stavudine
    Pentamidine
Biliary tract disease
  Acalculous cholecystitis
  Papillary stenosis
  Sclerosing cholangitis
  Vanishing bile duct syndrome

Viral Hepatitis

Evidence of past or present hepatitis is seen in 90 percent of HIV-infected patients [29, 30]. Careful serologic and biochemical evaluation is necessary to determine its significance.

Hepatitis A
The course of hepatitis A appears unaffected by HIV serostatus, and there is no evidence for loss of immunity to hepatitis A virus in coinfected patients.

Hepatitis B
Serologic evidence of prior self-limited hepatitis B virus (HBV) infection is seen frequently, but only 10 percent of patients have detectable hepatitis B surface antigen (HBsAg) and markers of active viral

replication. Following HBV infection, the risk of chronic antigenemia in HIV-infected patients is three to six times that seen in HIV-seronegative individuals [31]. However, the impaired immunity associated with HIV disease may result in active HBV replication without significant evidence of biochemical or histologic injury. Serum transaminase levels are frequently normal, and progression to either severe chronic active hepatitis or fulminant liver failure is unusual, although paradoxically it may occur with antiretroviral therapy. The clinical response to treatment of chronic HBV infection with alpha-interferon in HIV-infected patients has been disappointing.

The antigenic response to HBV vaccination in HIV-infected patients appears to be impaired. In one study, less than 25 percent of patients with CD4 cell counts above $700/mm^3$ responded to the vaccine and even fewer of those with lower counts [32]. These rates compare to a response rate higher than 95 percent in HIV-negative patients. Because of such findings, the effectiveness of vaccinating HIV-infected patients at high risk of contracting HBV is uncertain.

Hepatitis C
Hepatitis C virus (HCV) is a common cause of chronic hepatitis in injection drug users and appears to be directly hepatotoxic. In approximately 10 percent of HIV-infected patients, HCV-induced hepatic injury may be accelerated, with a rapid progression from chronic active hepatitis to cirrhosis. The efficacy of alpha-interferon therapy for chronic HCV infection associated with HIV disease is uncertain.

Hepatitis D
As with HCV, the damage to the liver from hepatitis delta virus is presumed to result from direct viral cytotoxicity and has been associated with more aggressive hepatic disease in patients with HIV infection.

Hepatitis E
No information is currently available on coinfection with HIV.

Opportunistic Infections

The liver is susceptible to the many opportunistic infections seen in AIDS. Patients may present with a variety of symptoms and signs, including fever, abdominal pain, and hepatomegaly. If noninvasive diagnostic testing is unhelpful, liver biopsy for histology and culture may be necessary.

Mycobacteria
Tuberculosis and MAC are the most common bacterial liver infections in AIDS patients [33]. Hepatic involvement is often associated with

widely disseminated disease. Liver function test abnormalities include a mixed picture of both hepatitis and cholestasis (increased levels of transaminases and alkaline phosphatase). Hepatic imaging is not useful, and definitive diagnosis is made by liver biopsy. Patients with positive acid-fast staining on liver biopsy specimens should be placed on antituberculous therapy pending culture results.

Cytomegalovirus

Clinically significant hepatitis is surprisingly uncommon in HIV-infected patients with disseminated CMV infection. Treatment consists of ganciclovir or foscarnet.

Fungal Infections

Candidiasis, cryptococcosis, and histoplasmosis can involve the liver, and each of these infections is associated with granuloma formation. Definitive diagnosis requires liver biopsy.

Peliosis Hepatitis

Peliosis is a histologic diagnosis characterized by multiple small blood-filled cysts throughout the liver. Similar lesions are seen in the lymph nodes, spleen, and bones. This condition appears to be caused by the agent responsible for bacillary angiomatosis, *Rochalimaea henselae*, a rickettsial organism transmitted by the fleas of infested cats [34, 35]. Treatment with erythromycin has been successful.

Drug-Induced Liver Injury

Many of the common therapeutic drugs used in HIV-infected patients are potentially hepatotoxic. If significantly abnormal liver function or clinical hepatitis develops, hepatotoxic agents should be discontinued and the patient's clinical course observed. Drugs frequently associated with hepatotoxicity include isoniazid, rifampin, rifabutin, sulfa agents, and ketoconazole.

Fatty Liver

Severe hepatic dysfunction and hepatomegaly of unclear etiology have been described in some HIV-infected patients, with liver biopsy showing considerable steatosis [36].

Role of Liver Biopsy

Liver biopsy seldom influences therapy or survival in HIV-infected patients. However, it should be considered in the following clinical situations: (1) fever, hepatomegaly, and/or abnormal liver function of undetermined cause; (2) suspected drug-induced hepatotoxicity where discontinuation of the agent may be harmful; and (3) chronic cholestasis with negative findings on ultrasound and endoscopic retrograde cholangiopancreatography (ERCP). Anecdotal reports suggest a higher morbidity and mortality associated with liver biopsy in patients with AIDS.

Biliary Tract Disease

Disorders of the intrahepatic and extrahepatic ducts and gallbladder have been reported in HIV disease. Biliary tract disease is manifested by right upper abdominal quadrant pain with or without fever or jaundice.

Acute Cholecystitis

Acute acalculous cholecystitis has been reported in AIDS patients, sometimes with systemic toxicity [37]. Etiologic agents include CMV, *Candida* species, and *Cryptosporidium* species. Diagnosis is by hepatic 2,6-dimethyliminodiacetic acid (HIDA) scan. Urgent cholecystectomy may be necessary to prevent rupture of the gallbladder and peritonitis.

Papillary Stenosis

Papillary stenosis is a syndrome characterized by recurrent episodes of right upper quadrant pain accompanied by transient liver function abnormalities with or without common bile duct (CBD) dilatation on ultrasonography [38]. Diagnosis is confirmed by ERCP, which reveals an edematous and swollen ampulla; biopsy may reveal CMV infection or cryptosporidiosis. Sphincterotomy may relieve the pain and fever and provide adequate biliary drainage.

Sclerosing Cholangitis

Sclerosing cholangitis can involve the CBD alone, CBD and ampulla, CBD and intrahepatic ducts, or intrahepatic ducts alone [39, 40] (Fig. 12-3). Patients generally present with right upper quadrant pain and an increased alkaline phosphatase level. Diagnosis is made by ERCP, and any significant strictures can be bypassed with an endoprosthesis at the time of the procedure. Cytomegalovirus and cryptosporidiosis are often detected on biopsy. Recent data suggest that microsporidia may also play a role in some patients [41]. Intrahepatic disease appears to progress rapidly and is relatively inaccessible to interventional therapy.

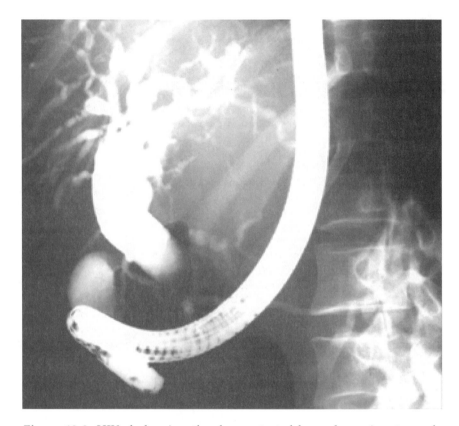

Figure 12-3. HIV cholangiopathy demonstrated by endoscopic retrograde cholangiopancreatography (ERCP) in a patient with AIDS. Two areas of the biliary system are involved. Papillary stenosis has resulted in significant dilatation of the extrahepatic biliary tree. Additionally, intrahepatic ducts demonstrate areas of stricture and ectasia resulting in the classic "beads on a string appearance" of sclerosing cholangitis.

Vanishing Bile Duct Syndrome

Chronic progressive cholestasis with normal extrahepatic ducts has been anecdotally described in HIV-infected patients. Liver biopsy reveals a paucity of intrahepatic ducts similar to that seen in primary biliary cirrhosis or liver allograft rejection. Treatment with ursodeoxycholic acid may be effective in slowing progression of this disease to end-stage biliary cirrhosis.

References

1. Dworkin B, et al. Gastrointestinal manifestations of the acquired immunodeficiency syndrome. *Am J Gastroenterol* 80:774, 1985.

2. Malenbranche R, et al. AIDS with severe gastrointestinal manifestations in Haiti. *Lancet* 2:873, 1983.
3. Smith PD, et al. Intestinal infections in patients with the acquired immunodeficiency syndrome. *Ann Intern Med* 108:328, 1988.
4. Glaser JB, et al. Recurrent *Salmonella typhimurium* bacteremia associated with the acquired immunodeficiency syndrome. *Ann Intern Med* 102:189, 1985.
5. Jacobs JL, et al. *Salmonella* infections in patients with AIDS. *Ann Intern Med* 102:186, 1985.
6. Rolston KVI, et al. Antimicrobial therapy for *Salmonella* infections in the acquired immunodeficiency syndrome. *Ann Intern Med* 108:309, 1988.
7. Jacobsen MA, et al. Serious cytomegalovirus infection in AIDS. *Ann Intern Med* 108:585, 1988.
8. Meiselman MS, et al. Cytomegalovirus colitis: Report of the clinical, endoscopic and pathological findings in 2 patients with the acquired immunodeficiency syndrome. *Gastroenterology* 88:171, 1984.
9. Soave R, et al. *Cryptosporidium* and *Isospora belli* infections. *J Infect Dis* 157:225, 1988.
10. Flanigan T, et al. *Cryptosporidium* infection and CD4 counts. *Ann Intern Med* 116:840–842, 1992.
11. Portnoy D, et al. Treatment of intestinal cryptosporidiosis with spiramycin. *Ann Intern Med* 101:202, 1984.
12. McMeeking A, et al. A controlled trial of bovine dialyzable leukocyte extract for cryptosporidiosis in patients with AIDS. *J Infect Dis* 161:108, 1990.
13. DeHovitz JA, et al. Clinical manifestations and therapy of *Isospora belli* infection in patients with AIDS. *N Engl J Med* 315:87, 1986.
14. Maayan S, et al. *Strongyloides stercoralis* hyperinfection in a patient with the acquired immunodeficiency syndrome. *Am J Med* 83:945, 1987.
15. Modigliani R, et al. Diarrhea and malabsorption in acquired immunodeficiency syndrome. *Gut* 26:179, 1985.
16. Ullrich R, et al. Small intestinal structure and function in patients infected with HIV: Evidence for HIV induced enteropathy. *Ann Intern Med* 111:15, 1989.
17. Weller IVD. The gay bowel. *Gut* 26:869, 1985.
18. Laughon BE, et al. Prevalence of enteric pathogens in homosexual men with and without AIDS. *Gastroenterology* 94:984, 1988.
19. Robinson EW, et al. SMS 201-995, a somatostatin analogue and diarrhea in AIDS. *Ann Intern Med* 111:15, 1989.
20. Cello JP, et al. Effect of octreotide on refractory AIDS-associated diarrhea. *Ann Intern Med* 115:705, 1991.
21. Tavitian A, et al. Oral candidiasis as a marker for esophageal candidiasis in AIDS. *Ann Intern Med* 104:54, 1986.
22. Balthazar EJ, et al. Cytomegalovirus esophagitis in AIDS; radiographic features in 16 patients. *Am J Radiol* 149:919, 1987.
23. Agha FP, et al. Herpetic esophagitis: A diagnostic challenge in immunocompromised patients. *Am J Gastroenterol* 81:246, 1986.

24. Rabeneck L, et al. Acute HIV infection presenting with painful swallowing and esophageal ulcers. *JAMA* 263:2318, 1990.
25. McBane RD, et al. Herpes esophagitis: Clinical syndrome, endoscopic appearance and diagnosis in 23 patients. *Gastrointest Endosc* 37:600, 1991.
26. Till M, et al. Typhlitis in patients with HIV infection. *Ann Intern Med* 116:998, 1992.
27. Lebovics E, et al. The liver in AIDS: A clinical and histological study. *Hepatology* 5:293, 1985.
28. Schneiderman DJ, et al. Hepatic disease in patients with AIDS. *Hepatology* 7:925, 1987.
29. Rustgi VK, et al. Hepatitis B virus infection in AIDS. *Ann Intern Med* 101:795, 1984.
30. Ravenholt RT. Role of hepatitis B virus in AIDS. *Lancet* 2:885, 1983.
31. Horvath J, Raffanti S. Clinical aspects of the interactions between human immunodeficiency virus and the hepatotropic viruses. *Clin Infect Dis* 18:339, 1994.
32. Bruguera M, et al. Impaired response of recombinant hepatitis B vaccine in HIV-infected persons. *J Clin Gastroenterol* 14:27, 1992.
33. Hawkins CC, et al. *Mycobacterium avium* complex infection in patients with AIDS. *Ann Intern Med* 105:184, 1986.
34. Koehler JE, et al. *Rochalimaea henselae* infection. A new zoonosis with the domestic cat as reservoir. *JAMA* 271:531, 1994.
35. Perkocha LA, et al. Clinical and pathological features of bacillary peliosis hepatitis in association with HIV infection. *N Engl J Med* 23:1581, 1990.
36. Frieman JP, et al. Hepatomegaly with severe steatosis in HIV-seropositive patients. *AIDS* 7:379, 1993.
37. Blumberg RS, et al. Cytomegalovirus and cryptosporidium associated acalculous gangrenous cholecystitis. *Am J Med* 76:1118, 1984.
38. Schneiderman DJ, et al. Papillary stenosis and sclerosing cholangitis in AIDS. *Ann Intern Med* 106:546, 1987.
39. Margulis SJ, et al. Biliary tract obstruction in AIDS. *Ann Intern Med* 105:207, 1986.
40. Cello JP. Acquired immunodeficiency syndrome cholangiopathy; spectrum of disease. *Am J Med* 86:539, 1989.
41. Pol S, et al. Microsporidia infection in patients with the human immunodeficiency virus and unexplained cholangitis. *N Engl J Med* 328:95, 1993.

Hematologic Manifestations

13

Paul E. Berard, Timothy P. Cooley

The hematologic consequences of HIV infection are dominated by peripheral blood cytopenias. These have become more common with the advent of antiretroviral therapy and treatments for HIV-related infections and malignancies [1]. Anemia occurs in approximately 60 to 70 percent of AIDS patients, neutropenia in 50 percent, and thrombocytopenia in 40 percent [2]. Current research efforts are focused on better understanding the pathophysiology and treatment of these hematologic complications.

In general, the incidence and severity of low cell counts increase with advancing HIV disease. An exception is thrombocytopenia, which may be an early manifestation of HIV infection, occurring in 3 to 12 percent of asymptomatic patients [3]. Whereas thrombocytopenia is most often the result of immune-mediated peripheral destruction, present data suggest that the anemia and neutropenia of HIV infection reflect an abnormally maturing, hypoproliferative bone marrow. Myelosuppressive therapies or marrow-infiltrating opportunistic diseases may further contribute to the development of cytopenias.

Bone Marrow Findings in HIV Infection

Bone marrow cellularity in the presence of HIV infection is decreased in 5 to 20 percent of patients [3–5]. A dry tap or difficult aspiration is observed in up to 40 percent of patients; however, this does not correlate with the presence of increased marrow reticulin [4]. Increased plasma cells are frequently seen and, together with a polyclonal gammopathy, may reflect an immune response to unusual antigenic stimulation or dysregulation of B-lymphocyte activity [2]. Increased eosinophils may also be present, as well as a slight increase in reticulin, the latter often associated with granulomas or lymphoid aggregates [3, 5]. Megakaryocytes are normal or increased in most patients [3, 5, 6]. Mild to moderate megaloblastic erythrocytic changes are commonly present, reflecting abnormal erythroid maturation [6]. Dysplasia of the megakaryocytic and myeloid cell lines is also observed and appears to correlate with the presence of peripheral blood cytopenias, concurrent infection, and/or drug therapy [3, 6]. Granulomas related to mycobacterial or fungal infection, or infiltration by B-cell lymphoma are common findings. Kaposi's sarcoma rarely involves the bone marrow [7].

Pathophysiology of Hematologic Complications

Multiple defects in hematopoiesis have been reported, consistent with the described changes in bone marrow morphology. These include (1) decreased numbers of bone marrow progenitors, (2) HIV infection of bone marrow progenitors with resulting abnormal maturation and proliferation, (3) deficient production of hematopoietic growth factors by bone marrow accessory cells, and (4) HIV-induced factors that inhibit normal hematopoiesis.

Several investigators reported decreased erythrocyte and granulocyte/monocyte colony formation in vitro using bone marrow progenitor cells from HIV-infected individuals [8]. However, other researchers using sera from subjects without HIV infection and growth factors from different sources demonstrated no differences in colony formation [9, 10]. Interpretation of these studies is difficult because of variability in cell culture media and techniques.

Human immunodeficiency virus infection of hematopoietic progenitor cells both in vitro and in vivo has been documented using techniques such as in situ hybridization and immunohistochemistry [11–13]. Interpretation of these results is difficult due to the potential contamination in vitro of myeloid colonies by differentiated HIV-infected monocytes [2]. A recent study using a polymerase chain reaction technique was unable to demonstrate HIV DNA within colonies derived from hematopoietic progenitor cells of HIV-infected individuals [10].

Within the bone marrow environment, T lymphocytes, monocytes-macrophages, and stromal cells produce growth factors that stimulate proliferation and differentiation of normal hematopoietic tissue. T cells and macrophages are infected in vivo with HIV, and this may affect their ability to produce these factors. Sera from individuals with certain hematologic disorders characterized by peripheral cytopenias, such as aplastic anemia, are able to support colony growth of normal bone marrow progenitor cells, even in the absence of exogenous stimulating factors. Sera from cytopenic patients with advanced HIV disease do not promote colony formation, raising the possibility of deficient growth factor production [9]. This view is supported by the ability of progenitor cells from HIV-infected patients to respond normally in vitro to exogenous growth factors [10].

Additionally, there is evidence to suggest that HIV may induce factors that inhibit normal hematopoietic activity. Stella and associates [8] demonstrated that depleting the bone marrow of T cells before culture resulted in increased colony growth. Molina and coworkers [10] observed inhibition of colony formation by sera from HIV-infected patients. As this inhibitor activity was isolated to the antibody fraction, it was thought to be immune mediated. Leiderman and colleagues [14] described a unique glycoprotein isolated from bone marrow cultures of AIDS patients that specifically inhibited granulopoiesis. This glycoprotein did not react with HIV antibodies and was believed to represent an induced, rather than direct, product of HIV infection. In addition, the increased production of cytokines, such as tumor necrosis factor (TNF) and interleukin-1 (IL-1), by HIV-infected monocytes is a potential cause of hematopoiesis inhibition [2].

Anemia

Anemia is a common manifestation of HIV disease [3, 15]. The anemia is consistent with a chronic disease state and is typically normochromic and normocytic. Reticulocyte counts are low or inappropriately normal. Microcytosis is uncommon and has been found to correlate poorly with bone marrow iron stores [16]. Macrocytosis occurs in more than 90 percent of patients receiving zidovudine (ZDV) but does not correlate with the development of anemia [17, 18].

Anti–red blood cell antibodies cause a positive Coombs' test in approximately 20 percent of HIV-infected patients with hypergammaglobulinemia [19]. These antibodies appear to behave as polyagglutinins and may be induced by infections associated with HIV disease. McGinniss and associates [20] observed autoantibodies of anti-u and anti-i specificity in most of the AIDS patients in their study, but in none of their seronegative control subjects. Despite this high incidence of positive Coombs' test results, immunohemolysis in nonbacteremic patients is rare [21].

Burkes and associates [22] reported that 20 percent of HIV-infected patients have low vitamin B_{12} levels. However, these patients all had normal folate levels and mean corpuscular volumes and neutrophil lobe counts, and bone marrow biopsies did not show megaloblastic changes. Furthermore, no patients had clinical manifestations of B_{12} deficiency, and parenterally administered B_{12} did not lead to hematologic improvement. Other studies showed an abnormal Schilling test result in up to

75 percent of AIDS patients, but clinically significant B_{12} deficiency appears to be rare [23].

When the HIV-infected patient with anemia is evaluated, special consideration should be given to the possibility of gastrointestinal bleeding, hypersplenism, liver disease, and bone marrow infiltration. Drug-related hemolysis, such as that caused by dapsone in glucose 6-phosphate dehydrogenase (G6PD)–deficient patients, may also occur.

Perhaps of greatest significance is the progressive anemia that often accompanies ZDV therapy. Richman and associates [24] reported that 31 percent of ZDV-treated patients had reductions in hemoglobin level to less than 7.5 gm/dl compared to only 2.7 percent of those given placebo. These patients required red blood cell transfusions, and approximately 20 percent became transfusion dependent. Despite the current use of lower ZDV doses, anemia remains an important clinical problem [25].

In the past, management of ZDV-induced anemia included discontinuation of the agent or chronic transfusion therapy. Presently, multiple therapeutic options are available, including (1) substitution of a nonmyelosuppressive drug such as didanosine (ddI), zalcitabine (formerly dideoxycytidine or ddC), or stavudine (d4T); (2) addition of a nonmyelosuppressive drug to a reduced-dose ZDV regimen; and (3) treatment with recombinant erythropoietin (r-EPO) [26–30].

Many HIV-infected patients with anemia have low levels of erythropoietin [31, 32]. In a randomized, double-blind controlled trial of r-EPO, 63 patients treated with ZDV were randomized to receive either placebo or r-EPO [30]. Patients received r-EPO at a dose of 100 IU/kg intravenously three times a week, and a statistically significant decrease in the number of patients requiring transfusion was observed in the r-EPO–treated group. Retrospective analysis showed that an entry serum erythropoietin level of less than 500 mU/ml was predictive of a response to r-EPO [30].

The majority of patients who are intolerant of ZDV because of anemia and not candidates for other antiretroviral agents may be managed effectively with r-EPO [30, 33]. A starting dose of 100 IU/kg may be given intravenously or subcutaneously three times a week. If no reticulocyte response is seen after 2 weeks of therapy, the dose can be increased to 150 IU/kg and then to 200 IU/kg after an additional 2 weeks if there still is no response.

Neutropenia

In addition to evidence for abnormal granulopoiesis, antigranulocyte antibodies have been described in 30 to 67 percent of HIV-infected patients [34, 35]. The significance of this finding is unclear, but some investigators believe that it may contribute to neutropenia [34].

Qualitative defects in neutrophil function have also been described in HIV disease, and these may predispose to bacterial infection [36]. Similar to the anemia of HIV infection, the major clinical significance of the HIV-induced neutropenia is that it often precludes therapy with ZDV and some drugs used for the treatment of opportunistic diseases.

Granulocyte macrophage colony stimulating factor (GM-CSF) is a cytokine produced by T cells that is known to stimulate the proliferation and function of myeloid cells. It has been produced in bacteria, yeast, and human cells by recombinant technology. Baldwin and associates [36] showed that GM-CSF may reverse the neutrophil phagocytic and killing defects in patients with HIV infection.

The first clinical study of GM-CSF in 1987 included 16 neutropenic AIDS patients and demonstrated a rapid increase in granulocytes and monocytes [37]. However, several in vitro studies demonstrated stimulation of HIV replication in peripheral blood monocytes-macrophages [38, 39]. Other clinical trials reported little or no effect on HIV expression by GM-CSF, although a recent trial conducted at the National Cancer Institute found a statistically significant increase in HIV p24 antigen when GM-CSF was used as a single agent [37, 40–42]. In vitro studies combining GM-CSF and ZDV showed an increased inhibition of certain monocytotrophic HIV strains and human monocytes-macrophages. This has been ascribed to the increase in monocyte cellular thymidine kinase activity induced by GM-CSF, resulting in increased intracellular levels of the nucleoside triphosphate [39]. Presently, it is anticipated that the beneficial myeloproliferative effects of GM-CSF will more than offset any viral-enhancing effect [43]. Granulocyte colony stimulating factor (G-CSF), another cytokine, does not stimulate monocyte proliferation/differentiation and has not been shown to have a stimulatory effect on HIV replication in macrophages [38].

GM-CSF has had more extensive clinical testing than G-CSF to date. It has potential benefits in HIV-infected patients in whom neutropenia develops secondary to treatment with ZDV, ganciclovir, alpha-interferon, or chemotherapy for Kaposi's sarcoma and non-Hodgkin's lymphoma [41–52]. The major toxicities of GM-CSF are pain or erythema at the injection site, fever, bone pain, and myalgias. When combined with alpha-interferon, it may potentiate the typical "flu-like" symptoms described with that agent [41, 47, 48].

G-CSF has also shown potential in ameliorating neutropenia resulting from ZDV therapy [53]. Within the population studied, all who required concurrent ganciclovir therapy were able to receive it without dose modification, and little toxicity was experienced. G-CSF may eventually prove more clinically useful than GM-CSF, given its low toxicity and lack of stimulatory effect on HIV. The starting dose of G-CSF is 1 µg/kg given subcutaneously each day.

Thrombocytopenia

The most common cause of HIV-related thrombocytopenia is immune-mediated peripheral destruction. Thrombocytopenia in heroin users was described at Boston City Hospital in 1978 [54]. In retrospect, this may have represented the first report of idiopathic thrombocytopenic purpura (ITP) in HIV-infected persons. Thrombocytopenia is also sometimes the result of drug therapy with agents such as trimethoprim-sulfamethoxazole. Transient thrombocytopenia has been described in primary HIV infection [55]. Thrombotic thrombocytopenic purpura has also been reported in HIV-infected patients [56].

The peripheral blood smear in HIV-related ITP shows decreased numbers of platelets that are increased in size. As in classic ITP, the spleen is not enlarged, and the bone marrow biopsy specimen reveals normal to increased numbers of megakaryocytes. Initially, it was thought that asymptomatic HIV-infected men with thrombocytopenia were more likely to advance to AIDS; this has not been borne out in other studies [57]. Hemorrhagic complications were first described as unusual, although recently, clinically significant bleeding with severe thrombocytopenia has been reported [58–60].

Much controversy exists regarding the pathogenesis of HIV-associated ITP. There is evidence to support both autoantibody-mediated and antigen-containing immune complex mechanisms [61]. Immune complexes containing HIV antibody have been demonstrated on the platelet surfaces of homosexual men and drug users [62]. An autoantibody that binds to a membrane glycoprotein of 25 kilodaltons (gp25) in seropositive thrombocytopenic homosexual men has also been identified [63]. This antibody was not detected in sera from hemophiliacs, drug users, or patients with transfusion-acquired HIV infection who had ITP. These discrepancies may be explained by different mechanisms of ITP in sexually acquired versus parenterally acquired HIV infection. Alternatively, an immune complex consisting of an autoantibody and a second anti-F(ab)$_2$ antibody might be involved [64].

The optimal management of HIV-associated ITP has not been clearly defined (Table 13-1). Zidovudine has an established role in managing ITP, although its action is poorly understood [65, 66]. Most patients respond with a long-term remission. A recent report suggests that alpha-interferon may be useful in treating severe ZDV-resistant thrombocytopenia [67]. Prednisone produces an initial response in approximately 50 percent of patients, but its effect is often short-lived [59, 68]. The risks of corticosteroid therapy in HIV-infected patients include further immunosuppression and progression of Kaposi's sarcoma [69]. Intravenous immunoglobulin is effective initially in 70 to 90 percent of patients, although the response is durable in fewer than 10 percent [70, 71]. Likewise, anti-Rh immunoglobulin therapy results in few long-term responses [72]. Splenectomy is generally

Table 13-1 *Management of HIV-related ITP*

Modality	Initial response (%)	Durable response (%)
Zidovudine	30–90	Unknown
Prednisone	40–60	10–20
Intravenous immunoglobulin	70–90	< 10
Anti-Rh (D)	64	< 10
Splenectomy	70–100	40–60

Source: Data from [65, 66, 68–74].

effective, and in approximately 50 percent of patients the response is maintained [73, 74]. Low-dose splenic irradiation has been used successfully in some patients as an alternative to surgery [75]. Before splenectomy, all patients should have cultures performed for *Mycobacterium avium* complex (MAC), as the clinical course of patients with disseminated MAC infection following splenectomy is uniformly poor [76].

In general, ZDV should be considered the drug of choice for significant thrombocytopenia. If ZDV therapy fails, alpha-interferon therapy should be considered or splenectomy performed. Intravenous immunoglobulin is reserved for the management of acute hemorrhagic episodes or for preoperative use.

Coagulation Abnormalities

The presence of antiphospholipid antibodies similar to the lupus anticoagulant has been documented in HIV-infected patients [77–83]. This abnormality is characterized by a prolonged partial thromboplastin time not corrected by the addition of normal plasma in simple mixing studies. The prothrombin time is generally normal. High titers of anticardiolipin antibodies are also commonly found in this setting [84, 85]. A relationship may exist between major opportunistic infections such as *Pneumocystis carinii* pneumonia and the development of this lupus-like anticoagulant [77, 79]. However, some investigators found no such association [83, 84]. Thrombotic events have only rarely been described in HIV-infected patients with the lupus-like anticoagulant [78].

Thrombopathy has also been reported in HIV disease, although its clinical significance is not clear [77]. Prolonged bleeding times and abnormal results on platelet aggregation tests with adenosine diphosphate, collagen, and epinephrine have been described [77, 85]. Dilution studies suggest that this abnormality is related to an unidentified serum factor [85].

References

1. Pluda JM, Mitsuya H, Yarchoan R. Hematologic effects of AIDS therapies. *Hematol Oncol Clin North Am* 5:229–248, 1991.
2. Scadden DT, Zon LI, Groopman JE. Pathophysiology and management of HIV-associated hematologic disorders. *Blood* 74:1455–1463, 1989.
3. Zon LI, Arkin C, Groopman JE. Haematologic manifestations of the human immune deficiency virus (HIV). *Br J Haematol* 66:251–256, 1987.
4. Treacy M, Lai L, Costello D, Clark A. Peripheral blood and bone marrow abnormalities in patients with HIV related disease. *Br J Haematol* 65:289–294, 1987.
5. Castella A, Croxson TS, Mildvan D, et al. The bone marrow in AIDS: A histologic, hematologic and microbiologic study. *Am J Clin Pathol* 84:425–431, 1985.
6. Schneider DR, Picker LJ. Myelodysplasia in the acquired immune deficiency syndrome. *Am J Clin Pathol* 84:144–152, 1984.
7. Little BJ, Spivak JL, Quin TC, et al. Case report: Kaposi's sarcoma with marrow involvement–occurrence in a patient with AIDS. *Am J Med Sci* 292:44–46, 1986.
8. Stella CC, Ganser A, Hoelzer D. Defective in vitro growth of the hemopoietic progenitor cells in the acquired immunodeficiency syndrome. *J Clin Invest* 80:286–293, 1987.
9. Donahue RE, Johnson MM, Zon LI, et al. Suppression of *in vitro* haematopoiesis following human immunodeficiency virus infection. *Nature* 326:200–203, 1987.
10. Molina J-M, Scadden DT, Sakaguchi M, et al. Lack of evidence for infection of or effect on growth of hematopoietic progenitor cells after *in vivo* or *in vitro* exposure to human immunodeficiency virus. *Blood* 76:2476–2482, 1990.
11. Busch M, Beckstead J, Gantz D, et al. Detection of human immunodeficiency virus infection of myeloid precursors in bone marrow samples from AIDS patients (abstract). *Blood* 68:122a, 1986.
12. Zucker-Franklin D, Cao Y. Megakaryocytes of human immunodeficiency virus–infected individuals express viral RNA. *Proc Natl Acad Sci USA* 86:5595, 1989.
13. Folks TM, Kessler SW, Orenstein JM, et al. Infection and replication of HIV-1 in purified progenitor cells of normal human bone marrow. *Science* 242:919–922, 1988.
14. Leiderman IZ, Greenberg ML, Adelsberg BR, et al. A glycoprotein inhibitor of *in vitro* granulopoiesis associated with AIDS. *Blood* 70:1267–1272, 1987.
15. Spivak JL, Bender BS, Quinn TC. Hematologic abnormalities in the acquired immune deficiency syndrome. *Am J Med* 77:224–228, 1984.
16. Osborne BM, Guarda LA, Butler JJ. Bone marrow biopsies in patients with AIDS. *Hum Pathol* 15:1048–1053, 1984.
17. Fischl MA, Richman DD, Hansen N, et al. The safety and efficacy of zidovudine (AZT) in the treatment of patients with mildly symptomatic

HIV infection. A double-blind, placebo-controlled trial. *Ann Intern Med* 112:437–443, 1992.

18. Volberding PA, Lagakos SW, Koch MA, et al. Zidovudine in asymptomatic human immunodeficiency virus infection. A controlled trial in persons with fewer than 500 CD4+ cells/mm³. *N Engl J Med* 322:941–949, 1990.
19. Aboulafia D, Mitsuyasu R. Hematologic abnormalities in AIDS. *Hematol Oncol Clin North Am* 5:195–214, 1992.
20. McGinniss MH, Macher AM, Rook AH, et al. Red cell autoantibodies in patients with acquired immune deficiency syndrome. *Transfusion* 26:405–409, 1986.
21. Perkocha LA, Rodgers GM. Hematologic aspects of human immunodeficiency virus infection: Laboratory and clinical considerations. *Am J Hematol* 29:94–105, 1988.
22. Burkes RL, Colten H, Krailo M, et al. Low serum cobalamin levels occur frequently in the acquired immunodeficiency syndrome and related disorders. *Eur J Haematol* 38:141–147, 1987.
23. Harriman GR, Smith PD, Horne MK, et al. Vitamin B12 malabsorption in patients with acquired immunodeficiency syndrome. *Arch Intern Med* 149:2039–2041, 1989.
24. Richman DD, Fischl MA, Grieco MH, et al. The toxicity of azidothymidine (AZT) in the treatment of patients with AIDS and AIDS-related complex. *N Engl J Med* 317:192–197, 1987.
25. Fischl MA, Parker CD, Pettinelli C, et al. A randomized controlled trial of a reduced daily dose of zidovudine in patients with the acquired immunodeficiency syndrome. *N Engl J Med* 323:1009–1014, 1990.
26. Yarchoan R, Mitsuya H, Thomas RV, et al. In vivo activity against HIV and favorable toxicity profile of 2'3'-dideoxyinosine. *Science* 245:412–415, 1989.
27. Lambert JS, Seidlin M, Reichman RC, et al. 2'3'-Dideoxyinosine (ddI) in patients with the acquired immunodeficiency syndrome or AIDS-related complex. *N Engl J Med* 322:1333–1340, 1990.
28. Cooley TP, Kunches LM, Saunders CA, et al. Once daily administration of 2'3'-dideoxyinosine (ddI) in patients with the acquired immunodeficiency syndrome or AIDS-related complex. *N Engl J Med* 322:1340–1345, 1990.
29. Meng TC, et al. Combination therapy with zidovudine and dideoxycytidine in patients with advanced human immunodeficiency virus infection. *Ann Intern Med* 116:13–20, 1992.
30. Fischl M, Galpin JE, Levine JD, et al. Recombinant human erythropoietin for patients with AIDS treated with zidovudine. *N Engl J Med* 322:1488–1493, 1990.
31. Spivak JL, Barnes DC, Fuchs E, et al. Serum immunoreactive erythropoietin in HIV-infected patients. *JAMA* 261:3104–3107, 1989.
32. Rarick MV, Loureiro C, Grosus S, et al. Serum erythropoietin levels in patients with human immunodeficiency virus infection and anemia. *J Acquir Immune Defic Syndr* 4:593–597, 1991.
33. Henry DH, Beall GN, Benson CA, et al. Recombinant human erythropoietin in the treatment of anemia associated with human immunodeficiency

virus (HIV) infection and zidovudine therapy. *Ann Intern Med* 117:739–748, 1992.

34. Murphy MF, Metcalfe P, Waters AH, et al. Incidence and mechanism of neutropenia and thrombocytopenia in patients with human immunodeficiency virus infection. *Br J Haematol* 66:337–340, 1987.

35. van der Lelie J, Lange JMA, Vos JJE, et al. Autoimmunity against blood cells in human immunodeficiency virus (HIV) infection. *Br J Haematol* 67:109–114, 1987.

36. Baldwin GC, Gasson JC, Quan SG, et al. Granulocyte-macrophage colony-stimulating factor enhances neutrophil function in acquired immunodeficiency syndrome patients. *Proc Natl Acad Sci USA* 85:2763–2766, 1988.

37. Groopman JE, Mitsuyasu RT, DeLeo MS, et al. Effect of recombinant human granulocyte-macrophage colony stimulating factor on myelopoiesis in the acquired immunodeficiency syndrome. *N Engl J Med* 317:593–598, 1987.

38. Koyanagi Y, O'Brien WA, Zhao JQ, et al. Cytokines alter production of HIV-1 from primary mononuclear phagocytes. *Science* 241:1673–1675, 1988.

39. Perno C-F, Yarchoan R, Cooney DA, et al. Replication of human immunodeficiency virus in monocytes: Granulocyte/macrophage colony stimulating factor (GM-CSF) potentiates viral production yet enhances the antiviral effect mediated by 3'-azido-2'3'-dideoxythymidine and other dideoxynucleoside cogeners of thymidine. *J Exp Med* 169:933, 1988.

40. Mitsuyasu R, Levine J, Miles SA, et al. Effect of long term subcutaneous (SC) administration of recombinant granulocyte-macrophage colony stimulating factor (GM-CSF) in patients with HIV-related leukopenia (abstract). *Blood* 72:357, 1988.

41. Krown SE, Paredes J, Bundow D. Interferon-alpha, zidovudine and granulocyte-macrophage colony stimulating factor: A phase I AIDS Clinical Trials Group study in patients with Kaposi's sarcoma associated with AIDS. *J Clin Oncol* 10:1344–1351, 1992.

42. Pluda JM, Yarchoan R, Smith PD, et al. Subcutaneous recombinant granulocyte-macrophage colony-stimulating factor used as a single agent and in an alternating regimen with azidothymidine in leukopenic patients with severe human immunodeficiency virus infection. *Blood* 76:463–472, 1990.

43. Folks TM. Human immunodeficiency virus in bone marrow: Still more questions than answers. *Blood* 77:1625–1626, 1991.

44. Levine SD, Allan JD, Testitore SH, et al. Recombinant human granulocyte-macrophage colony stimulating factor ameliorates zidovudine-induced neutropenia in patients with acquired immunodeficiency syndrome (AIDS)/AIDS-related complex. *Blood* 78:3148–3154, 1991.

45. Hardy WD. Combined ganciclovir and recombinant human granulocyte-macrophage colony-stimulating factor in the treatment of cytomegalovirus retinitis in AIDS patients. *J Acquir Immune Defic Syndr* 4:S22-S28, 1991.

46. Grossberg HS, Bonnem EM, Buhles WC. GM-CSF with ganciclovir for the treatment of CMV retinitis in AIDS (letter). *N Engl J Med* 320:1560, 1989.

47. Scadden DT, Bering HA, Levine JD, et al. GM-CSF as an alternative to dose modification of the combination of zidovudine and interferon-alpha in the treatment of AIDS-associated Kaposi's sarcoma. *Am J Clin Oncol* 14:S40-S44, 1991.

48. Scadden DT, Bering HA, Levine JD, et al. Granulocyte-macrophage colony-stimulating factor mitigates the neutropenia of combined interferon-alpha and zidovudine treatment of acquired immunodeficiency syndrome-associated Kaposi's sarcoma. *J Clin Oncol* 9:2215–2217, 1991.

49. Gill PS, Bernstein-Singer M, Espina BM, et al. Adriamycin, bleomycin and vincristine chemotherapy with recombinant granulocyte-macrophage colony-stimulating factor in the treatment of AIDS-related Kaposi's sarcoma. *AIDS* 6:477–481, 1992.

50. Walsh C, Werna J, Laubenstein L, et al. Phase I study of m-BACOD and GM-CSF in AIDS associated non-Hodgkin's lymphoma. *J Acquir Immune Defic Syndr* 6:265–271, 1993.

51. Kaplan LD, Kahn JO, Crowe S, et al. Clinical and virologic effects of recombinant human granulocyte-macrophage colony stimulating factor in patients receiving chemotherapy for human immunodeficiency virus-associated non-Hodgkin's lymphoma: Results of a randomized trial. *J Clin Oncol* 9:929–940, 1991.

52. Davey RT Jr, Davey VJ, Metcalf JA, et al. A phase I/II trial of zidovudine, interferon-alpha and granulocyte-macrophage colony stimulating factor in the treatment of human immunodeficiency type-1 infection. *J Infect Dis* 164:43–52, 1991.

53. Miles SA, Mitsuyasu RT, Moreno J. Combined therapy with erythropoietin decreases hematologic toxicity from zidovudine. *Blood* 77:2109–2117, 1991.

54. Adams WH, Rufo RA, Talarico L, et al. Thrombocytopenia and intravenous heroin use. *Ann Intern Med* 84:2207–2211, 1978.

55. Goldman R, Lang W, Lyman D. Acute AIDS viral infection. *Am J Med* 81:1122–1123, 1986.

56. Nair JMG, Bellevue R, Bertrant M, et al. Thrombotic thrombocytopenic purpura in patients with the acquired immunodeficiency syndrome (AIDS)-related complex. *Ann Intern Med* 109:204–212, 1988.

57. Holzman RS, Walsh CM, Karputkin S. Risk for acquired immunodeficiency syndrome among thrombocytopenic and non-thrombocytopenic homosexual men seropositive for the human immunodeficiency virus. *Ann Intern Med* 106:383–386, 1987.

58. Goldsweig HG, Grossman R, Williams D. Thrombocytopenia in homosexual men. *Am J Hematol* 21:243–247, 1986.

59. Landmio G, Galli M, Nosari A, et al. HIV-related severe thrombocytopenia in intravenous drug users: Prevalence, response to therapy in a medium-term follow up and pathogenic evaluation. *AIDS* 4:24–34, 1990.

60. Brusamolino E, Malfitano A, Pagnullo O, et al. HIV-related thrombocytopenic purpura: A study of 24 cases. *Haematologica* 74:51–56, 1989.

61. Karpatkin S. Immunologic thrombocytopenic purpura in HIV-seropositive homosexuals, narcotic addicts and hemophiliacs. *Semin Hematol* 25:219–224, 1988.

62. Karpatkin S, Nardi M, Lannette ET, et al. Anti human immunodeficiency virus type 1 antibody complexes on platelets of seropositive thrombocytopenic homosexuals and narcotic addicts. *Proc Natl Acad Sci USA* 85:9763–9767, 1988.

63. Stricker RB, Abrams DI, Corash L, et al. Target platelet antigen in homo-

sexual men with immune thrombocytopenia. *N Engl J Med* 313:1375–1380, 1985.

64. Stricker RB. Hemostatic abnormalities in HIV disease. *Hematol Oncol Clin North Am* 5:249–266, 1991.

65. Hynes KB, Green JB, Karpatkin S. The effect of azidothymidine in HIV-related thrombocytopenia. *N Engl J Med* 318:516–517, 1988.

66. Oksenhendler E, Bierling P, Brossard Y, et al. Zidovudine for thrombocytopenic purpura related to human immunodeficiency virus (HIV) infection. *Ann Intern Med* 110:365–368, 1989.

67. Marroni M, et al. Interferon-alpha is effective in the treatment of HIV-1-related, severe, zidovudine-resistant thrombocytopenia. *Ann Intern Med* 121:423–429, 1994.

68. Rosenfelt FP, Rosenbloom BE, Weinstein IH. Immune thrombocytopenia in homosexual men. *Ann Intern Med* 106:911–912, 1987.

69. Gill PS, Loureiro C, Bernstein-Singer M, et al. Clinical effect of glucocorticoids on Kaposi sarcoma related to the acquired immunodeficiency syndrome (AIDS). *Ann Intern Med* 110:937–940, 1989.

70. Bussel JB, Haimi JS. Isolated thrombocytopenia in patients infected with HIV: Treatment with intravenous gammaglobulin. *Am J Hematol* 28:79–84, 1988.

71. Pollack AT, Janinis J, Green D. Successful intravenous immune globulin therapy for human immunodeficiency virus–associated thrombocytopenia. *Arch Intern Med* 148:695–697, 1988.

72. Oksenhendler E, Bierling P, Brossard Y, et al. Anti-Rh immunoglobulin therapy for human immunodeficiency virus–related immune thrombocytopenic purpura. *Blood* 71:1499–1502, 1988.

73. Landonio G, Nosari AM, Barbarano L, et al. Splenectomy for severe HIV-related thrombocytopenia in heroin abusers. *Br J Haematol* 69:290, 1988.

74. Ravikumar TS, Allen JD, Bothe A Jr, et al. Splenectomy: The treatment of choice for human immunodeficiency virus–related immune thrombocytopenia. *Arch Surg* 124:625–628, 1989.

75. Needleman SW, Sorace J, Poussin-Rosillo K, et al. Low-dose splenic irradiation in the treatment of autoimmune thrombocytopenia in HIV-infected patients. *Ann Intern Med* 116:310–311, 1992.

76. Mathew A, Raviglione MC, Niranjan U, et al. Splenectomy in patients with AIDS. *Am J Hematol* 32:184–189, 1989.

77. Cohen AJ, Philips TM, Kessler CM. Circulating coagulation inhibitors in the acquired immunodeficiency syndrome. *Ann Intern Med* 104:175–180, 1986.

78. Bloom EJ, Abrams DI, Rodgers G. Lupus anticoagulant in the acquired immunodeficiency syndrome. *JAMA* 256:491–493, 1986.

79. Gold JE, Haubenstock A, Zulusky R. Lupus anticoagulant and AIDS (letter). *N Engl J Med* 314:1252–1253, 1986.

80. Haire WD. The acquired immunodeficiency syndrome and lupus anticoagulant (letter). *Ann Intern Med* 105:301, 1986.

81. LeFrere J-J, Gozin D, Modai J, et al. Circulating anticoagulant in the acquired immunodeficiency syndrome (letter). *Ann Intern Med* 108:429–430, 1987.

82. LeFrere J-J, Gozin D, Leratte J. Circulating anticoagulant in asymptomatic persons seropositive for human immunodeficiency virus (HIV). *Ann Intern Med* 108:771, 1988.
83. Brien W, Inwood M, Denome G. Antiphospholipid antibodies in haemophiliacs. *Br J Haematol* 68:270–271, 1988.
84. Canoso RT, Zon LI, Groopman JE. Anticardiolipin antibodies associated with HTLV-III infection. *Br J Haematol* 65:495–498, 1988.
85. Berstein Z, Cappacino A, Cappacino H. Platelet function and bound antibodies in AIDS-ARC patients with thrombocytopenia (abstract). *Blood* 70:118a, 1987.

Renal Manifestations 14

Steven C. Borkan

Epidemiology

HIV-associated nephropathy (HIVAN) is characterized by the onset of proteinuria and progressive renal dysfunction associated with focal, segmental glomerulosclerosis (FSGS) [1–5]. Distinguishing HIVAN from other treatable causes of renal dysfunction is important [1, 4, 6, 7].

The disease now recognized as HIVAN was first described in patients with AIDS in 1984 [8, 9]. The absence of confirmatory studies initially supported speculation that HIVAN either was unrelated to HIV infection or resulted from host-specific factors such as injection drug use (IDU) or race [2]. Further confusing the issue were early reports that homosexual men with AIDS had no discernible renal pathology, and the existence of common epidemiologic and pathologic features delayed the distinction of HIVAN from heroin-associated nephropathy (HAN) [10]. The hypothesis that HIV is associated with a distinct nephropathy is now widely accepted [1, 4, 7].

The prevalence of HIVAN in HIV-infected patients is estimated to be 10 percent; men comprise 80 to 90 percent of cases [1, 2, 7, 11]. Approximately 50 percent of patients with HIVAN have a history of drug use, and the remainder are either homosexual or originate from regions where HIV infection is endemic [1, 2, 7, 11, 12]. In approximately 10 percent of patients, no specific risk factor for HIV can be identified [11]. Black men appear to be at increased risk for development of HIVAN, but they also have a twofold to fivefold increased risk for renal dysfunction associated with other systemic diseases, as well as for idiopathic FSGS [2, 13, 14].

HIVAN is recognized throughout the spectrum of HIV disease, although in one study 57 percent of patients with HIVAN fulfilled Centers for Disease Control criteria for AIDS [7, 15]. HIVAN can be the first manifestation of HIV infection or even precede detection of HIV antibodies [1, 16]. HIVAN has also been reported as the presenting feature of HIV infection in infants born to seropositive mothers [17].

Clinical Manifestations

The onset of HIVAN is heralded by the appearance of heavy proteinuria, often with renal insufficiency. Azotemia, proteinuria, or both were the presenting features in more than 90 percent of HIV-infected patients reported by inpatient renal consultation services [15, 18] (Table 14-1). Gross or microscopic hematuria and electrolyte abnormalities comprised the other abnormalities. Most patients (89%) excreted 1 gm or more of protein per day [15].

Some of the clinical and epidemiological features of HIVAN overlap with HAN, leading to diagnostic confusion [19] (Table 14-2). Fortunately, several clinical features permit the distinction of HIVAN from HAN (Table 14-3). Features consistent with the diagnosis of HIVAN include the absence of hypertension, a characteristic urine sediment, normal or large kidneys, hypoalbuminemia disproportionate to the degree of proteinuria, and rapidly progressive renal insufficiency. The absence of hypertension in patients with HIVAN is striking and unexplained, given the high prevalence of essential hypertension in black men and the presence of advanced renal failure with reduced salt and water clearance. Examination of the urine sediment in HIVAN often reveals evidence of severe proteinuria with oval fat bodies and frank lipiduria. Large numbers of broad (giant) waxy casts (Fig. 14-1A) have also been observed in patients whose renal biopsy specimens showed HIVAN (E Alexander, Boston City Hospital, personal communication, 1994).

Renal ultrasound in patients with HIVAN typically shows a normal or enlarged renal silhouette with increased echogenicity, even with advanced renal failure. In one series of patients with HIVAN, renal size averaged 12.3 cm [20]. Renal enlargement may be the result of (1) insufficient time for global sclerosis and fibrosis given the rapid progression of renal disease; (2) marked dilatation of the tubules with numerous microcysts, in contrast to the tubular collapse frequently seen in other forms of chronic renal injury; and (3) interstitial edema [2, 4, 21]. The dramatic decline observed in serum albumin concentration (to ≤ 1 gm/dl) with moderate albuminuria (< 10 gm per day) may be caused by malnutrition or a defect in hepatic albumin synthesis, or both. HIVAN is a rapidly progressive form of renal failure; in one series of 55 patients, progression to end-stage disease occurred in an average of 10.9 weeks from the onset of mild azotemia [21].

Table 14-1 *Clinical presentation of HIVAN*

Presentation	% of patients
Azotemia	63
Proteinuria	19
Azotemia and proteinuria	9
Electrolyte imbalances	6
Gross hematuria	3

Source: Adapted from JJ Bourgoignie, R Meneses, C Ortiz, et al., The clinical spectrum of renal disease associated with the acquired immunodeficiency syndrome. *Am J Kidney Dis* 12:131–137, 1988.

Table 14-2 *Similar features of HIVAN and HAN*

Age at presentation, 20–40 yr
Gender, > 90% men
IDU, 40–50% (HIVAN) vs. 100% (HAN)
Race at risk, 90% black
Renal insufficiency
Proteinuria (≥ 3 gm) in most patients

Source: Adapted from [2] and [19].

Table 14-3 *Features that distinguish HIVAN from HAN*

Feature	HIVAN	HAN
Clinical		
Hypertension	< 7%	Usual
Broad waxy casts	Yes	No
Renal size (late)	Large (12.3 cm)	Small
Severe hypoalbuminemia*	Yes	Unusual
Rate of progression to ESRD	4–16 wk	2–4 yr
Histologic		
Light microscopy	Microcystic tubules	Normal tubules
Electron microscopy	No inclusions	No inclusions
Tissue HIV	Yes	No
Prognosis	Poor	Good

ESRD = end-stage renal disease.
*Disproportionate to the degree of proteinuria.
Source: Adapted from [2], [19], and [21].

Pathology

HIVAN is predominantly a glomerular disease with FSGS. *FSGS* is a term that describes a pattern of renal response to a variety of insults and is not specific for HIVAN [2]. Autopsy data demonstrate that 90 percent of patients with the clinical diagnosis of HIVAN have focal and

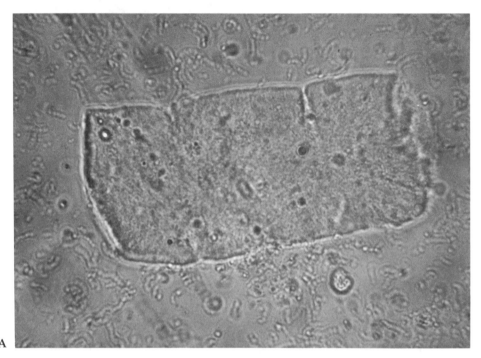

A

Figure 14-1. Renal histopathology in HIVAN. **A.** Giant waxy cast with the characteristic rectangular shape, "squared-off" ends, and twists (rectangular indentations) along the longitudinal axis. Note the broad width of the cast compared to the diameter of the degenerating cell (polarized light at 400X magnification; kindly donated by Dr. Edward A. Alexander, Boston City Hospital).

segmental glomerulosclerosis [4, 7]. Of 160 renal biopsies in patients with HIV infection reviewed by Rao and Friedman [2], 90 percent showed either FSGS or mesangial hyperplasia, a probable precursor lesion to FSGS.

Renal biopsy can confirm the clinical diagnosis of HIVAN. The light microscopic features include FSGS (Figs. 14-1B, -1C) or mesangial hyperplasia with (1) severe epithelial cell injury; (2) interstitial infiltration by lymphocytes or monocytes; (3) dilated, degenerating proximal tubules filled with eosinophilic material, possibly representing cast formation in situ (Fig. 14-1D); (4) marked tubular microcyst accumulation (see Fig. 14-1D); and (5) mesangial hyperplasia [2, 18, 22]. The presence of numerous tubuloreticular inclusions (TRIs) within endothelial cells (Fig. 14-1E) is another important finding in HIVAN [16, 23]. Tubuloreticular inclusions are more common and more numerous in HIVAN than in either HAN or idiopathic FSGS. D'Agati and colleagues [22] observed TRIs in 92 percent (23/25) of patients with HIVAN but in only 23 percent (3/13) of those with HAN. A more than 10-fold

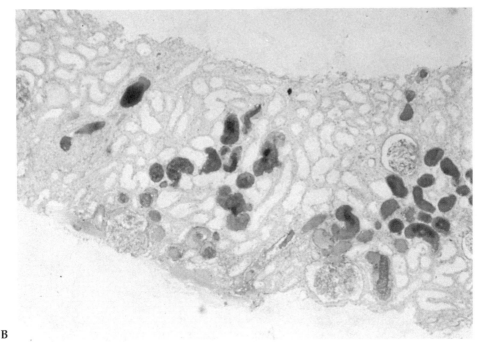

B

Figure 14-1 (continued). B. Renal biopsy specimen demonstrating regions of focal, segmental glomerulosclerosis (FSGS) in six glomeruli with partial collapse and expansion of Bowman's space. Markedly dilated tubules are noted, many containing eosinophilic material. The interstitium is moderately expanded by edema and cellular infiltrates (200X magnification).

increase in the number of TRIs per glomerular capillary was noted in HIVAN (86%) compared to HAN (6%) and idiopathic FSGS (2%) [22]. Finding numerous TRIs in capillary endothelial cells in a patient with FSGS prompts some pathologists to request HIV antibody testing (H Rennke, Brigham and Women's Hospital, personal communication, 1994).

In contrast, the absence of TRIs in black men presenting with rapidly progressive renal failure, hypertension, and severe proteinuria is also an important finding. Prominent glomerular collapse without TRIs recently was observed in a series of HIV-seronegative patients who had no prior history of IDU. Detweiler and colleagues [24] termed this lesion *collapsing glomerulopathy*.

Tubuloreticular inclusions do not represent particles of HIV, since other diseases such as lupus nephritis are associated with similar findings, and exposure of cultured cells to exogenous interferon may result in the appearance of identical inclusions [25]. Rather, TRIs may be a component of interferon or reflect a cellular response to in-

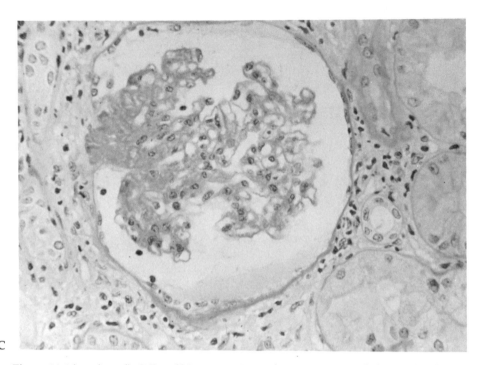

C

Figure 14-1 (continued). C. Renal biopsy specimen showing segmental glomerulosclerosis, partial collapse of the glomerular tuft, and expansion of Bowman's space (400X magnification).

terferon. Although renal tissue may stain for immunoglobulin M (IgM), C1q, C3, and kappa or lambda light chains in areas of focal sclerosis, immunologic mechanisms are probably not central to the genesis of HIVAN [22]. Both immunoglobulins and complement can be trapped nonspecifically by sclerosing glomeruli. In addition, similar glomerular deposits of immunoglobulins and complement occur in the majority of HIV-infected patients without nephropathy, and serum complement levels are normal in patients with HIVAN [26].

The finding of IgA nephropathy in two patients with serum antibodies to HIV recently prompted investigation of a causal link between the viral infection and renal deposition of immune complexes containing IgA [27]. The patients presented with proteinuria, red blood cell casts, and increased serum levels of IgA. IgA antibodies directed against immunoglobulins that reacted with anti-HIV IgG or IgM antibodies to HIV surface proteins were found in intracapillary immune complexes. These cases suggest that immune complex–mediated IgA nephritis may complicate the humoral response to circulating viral antigens.

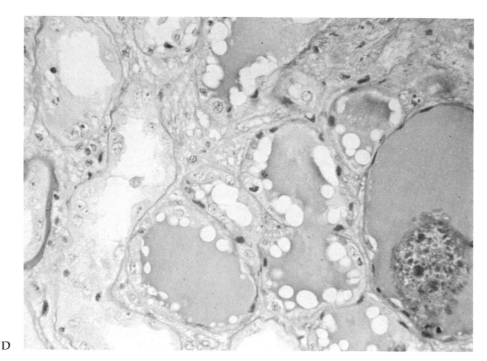

D

Figure 14-1 (continued). D. Renal biopsy specimen illustrating microcystic dilatation of proximal tubules with severe degeneration of tubular epithelial cells. Tubular lumina are filled with eosinophilic staining material. Moderate interstitial infiltration with mononuclear cells is apparent (400X magnification).

Pathogenesis

Human immunodeficiency virus appears to be trophic for specific cell types, including lymphocytes (T cells) and epithelial cells of the colon, central nervous system, and kidney. The basis of this tropism is complex and is not simply related to the presence of a surface CD4 receptor on susceptible cells [28, 29]. Regardless of the mechanism of viral entry, proliferation of HIV is generally associated with cytotoxicity. Within the kidney, tubular epithelial and glomerular epithelial cells undergo the most severe injury. Damage to renal epithelial cells probably accounts for leakage of filtered protein (nephrotic syndrome) and renal failure.

Although a direct causal link between HIV and HIVAN has yet to be established, several lines of evidence indicate a strong association. Viral DNA and protein markers specific for HIV have been localized within tubular and glomerular epithelial cells in renal biopsy specimens from HIV-infected patients with nephrotic syndrome [30, 31]. A study using

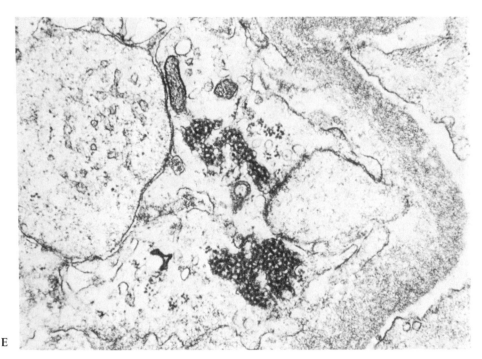

E

Figure 14-1 (continued). E. Electron micrograph of an endothelial cell with the characteristic intracellular accumulation of electron-dense tubuloreticular structures (TRI). (Micrographs of the renal biopsy tissue (**B–E**)were donated by Dr. Helmut Rennke, Brigham and Women's Hospital.)

the transgenic murine model of HIV infection suggested a critical role of HIV in the pathogenesis of HIVAN; severe proteinuria, renal failure, and specific expression of HIV markers within the kidney were associated with FSGS in the offspring of parents in whom an HIV provirus had been introduced [32].

One of the most striking features of HIVAN is the generally prolonged period of dormancy between the detection of antiretroviral antibodies and the onset of renal disease. Since proliferation of HIV appears to be the major determinant of cytotoxicity, factors that precipitate viral replication within the kidney could explain the sudden onset of disease. Several mechanisms for rapid HIV proliferation have been suggested. HIV proliferation is regulated by at least two genes, *nef* and *vif*, with opposing actions. Minor diversification (mutation) in either of these could lead to rapid viral reproduction and death of the host cell. Concomitant infection with viral hepatitis, syphilis, or cytomegalovirus (CMV), all common in the HIV-infected population, could induce HIV replication. Recent in vitro studies showed that susceptibility to HIV infection can be conferred to fibroblasts by a CMV-induced Fc receptor [33]. Cytomegalovirus infection may also promote viral proliferation through a mechanism that is dependent on tumor necrosis factor (TNF) [34]. Lastly, concomitant viral infection might remove inhibition to HIV replication by depleting CD4 lymphocytes, further depressing the immune system. The susceptibility of blacks, men, and persons with a history of IDU suggests that both genetic and environmental factors may modulate the development of HIV-associated renal disease.

Prognosis and Management

HIV-associated nephropathy rapidly evolves from mild renal insufficiency to end-stage renal disease (ESRD) and is associated with shortened survival [6, 11, 13, 21, 35]. AIDS patients with HIVAN have increased mortality compared to AIDS patients without nephropathy (50% survival rate at 10 vs. 15 months) [35]. In a series of patients with HIVAN who were receiving maintenance hemodialysis, 75 percent died within 3 months and 100 percent died within 9 months of the onset of ESRD [6]. Two subsequent reports confirmed the poor prognosis for HIVAN patients on maintenance hemodialysis [13, 21]. Unrelenting cachexia, progressive neurologic deterioration, and opportunistic infections were the most common causes of death. In a study of patients with HIVAN who were undergoing dialysis, asymptomatic HIV-infected patients lived longer than those with symptomatic disease, and patients with AIDS had the shortest survival time [13].

Treatment of early HIVAN to reverse or retard progression of renal insufficiency and proteinuria is based on anecdotal information. Oral prednisone decreased proteinuria in a patient with mesangial hyperplasia and intense, diffuse IgM deposition [36]. In a second case report, zidovudine (ZDV) restored renal function but did not decrease proteinuria in a patient with a clinical and histologic diagnosis of HIVAN [37]. Whether antiretroviral drug therapy can avert ESRD in patients with early HIVAN or prolong survival once ESRD develops remains to be determined.

The role of renal transplantation in patients with HIV disease is controversial. HIV infection shortens life expectancy, and the requirement for chronic immunosuppressive therapy to prevent allograft rejection may have detrimental effects on HIV proliferation. A National Institutes of Health task force concluded that HIV infection should not be a contraindication to transplantation given the paucity of data regarding the outcome of asymptomatic HIV carriers with renal allografts [11]. Rarely, seronegative organ and tissue donors have transmitted HIV infection [38]. In patients who have undergone renal transplantation for non–HIV-related disease and have identifiable risk factors for HIV infection, the diagnosis of AIDS should be considered when atypical opportunistic infections occur [39].

Patients with HIVAN and ESRD can be managed by either hemodialysis or peritoneal dialysis. Theoretically, peritoneal dialysis has several advantages compared to hemodialysis in patients who are equally suited for either modality (Table 14-4), but no controlled trials comparing the two types of dialysis have been reported [11]. Because of the relatively poor prognosis for HIV-infected patients with ESRD, the decision to provide dialysis support should be individualized.

Incidental HIV Infection in the ESRD Patient

Seronegative patients with ESRD are susceptible to HIV infection. The occurrence of AIDS from drug use or sexual contact in patients receiving chronic dialysis is often associated with rapid demise from opportunistic infection [13]. Routine testing for HIV is not recommended in the ESRD population when no risk factors are identified [11].

Other Renal and Electrolyte Abnormalities in the HIV-Infected Patient

The HIV-infected population is at increased risk for renal and electrolyte abnormalities apart from HIVAN. Conditions such as diarrhea, volume depletion, malnutrition, loss of muscle mass (leading to diminished generation of creatinine and overestimation of renal function), and opportunistic infections treated with potentially nephrotoxic agents all predispose to a spectrum of renal and electrolyte disorders. Reversible causes of renal insufficiency associated with HIV infection include kidney infection, exposure to nephrotoxic antibiotics or radiologic contrast agents, endotoxemia, and hypoperfusion (Table 14-5). Although rare, progressive renal insufficiency may result from parenchymal infiltration with Kaposi's sarcoma or lymphoma.

Of the electrolyte abnormalities observed in HIV-infected patients,

Table 14-4 *Advantages of peritoneal dialysis for ESRD in HIVAN*

Reduced T-cell activation and cytokine release (mediators of HIV proliferation) attributed to hemodialysis membranes
Enhanced humoral immune function
Improved nitrogen balance from glucose absorption
Permits larger doses of antiretroviral agents in patients with membrane-associated leukopenia
Higher average hematocrit
Lower risk of transmitting HIV infection

ESRD = end-stage renal disease; HIVAN = HIV-associated nephropathy.
Source: Adapted from P Schoenfeld, NJ Feduska. Acquired immunodeficiency syndrome and renal disease: Report of the National Kidney Foundation–National Institutes of Health Task Force on AIDS and Kidney Disease. *Am J Kidney Dis* 16:14–25, 1990.

Table 14-5 *Etiologies of acute renal failure in the HIV-infected patient*

Prerenal azotemia
    Volume depletion (diarrhea, bleeding, decreased intake)
    Early obstructive uropathy
Acute tubular necrosis
    Ischemia/hypoperfusion
    Sepsis/endotoxemia
    Nephrotoxic antibiotics
    Radiocontrast exposure
Infiltrative lesions
    Kaposi's sarcoma
    Renal cell carcinoma
    Lymphoma
    Amyloidosis
Allergic interstitial nephritis
    Nephrotoxic antibiotics
    Nonsteroidal agents
Systemic infections
    Mycobacterium species
    Candida species
    Cryptococcus species
    Aspergillosis
    Cytomegalovirus
    Bacterial endocarditis
    Renal microabscess formation
Vasculitis
    Hemolytic-uremic syndrome
    Thrombotic thrombocytopenic purpura
    Renal cortical infarction
Miscellaneous
    Heroin (HAN)
    "Nephrosarca" (renal edema with severe hypoalbuminemia)
    Primary glomerulonephropathies
    Chemical interference with the creatinine assay
        Trimethoprim-sulfamethoxazole
        Cephalosporins
        Cimetidine

Source: Adapted from [1], [2], and [4].

two—hyponatremia and hyperkalemia—are of most significance. Hyponatremia has been reported in 40 to 50 percent of hospital admissions of patients with symptomatic HIV infection or AIDS, and severe hyponatremia may be associated with decreased survival [4, 40]. Excess total body water was attributed either to hypovolemia with physiologic stimulation of antidiuretic hormone (ADH), administration of hypotonic fluids, or the syndrome of inappropriate ADH secretion (SIADH). SIADH in HIV-infected patients is usually associated with central nervous system or pulmonary disease. Hyperkalemia and mild metabolic acidosis may be the presenting features of adrenal insufficiency. In addition, hyporeninemic hypoaldosteronism with hyperkalemia has been reported in patients with AIDS [41]. Hypoadrenalism with hyperkalemia has been associated with ketoconazole therapy [42]. A recent report suggested that idiopathic lactic acidosis can accompany advanced HIV disease in the absence of hypoxemia, sepsis, malignancy, or other obvious causes [43]. Of note, six of seven patients died within 5 weeks of the recognition of this condition.

Drug Therapy in the HIV-Infected Patient with Renal Insufficiency

Dosage adjustment of agents that are nephrotoxic, undergo significant renal metabolism, or depend on glomerular filtration for their elimination is frequently necessary in the HIV-infected patient with renal insufficiency [44]. Potentially nephrotic agents commonly used in the management of HIV disease include acyclovir, amikacin, amphotericin B, foscarnet, pentamidine, sulfadiazine, and trimethoprim-sulfamethoxazole (TMP-SMX). When available, drug levels should be used to monitor treatment. TMP-SMX and pentamidine cause acute renal insufficiency in 15 and 60 percent of patients, respectively [45]. Drug therapy can also produce relatively unusual renal complications. In one patient, sulfadiazine treatment for toxoplasmosis resulted in acute obstructive uropathy from renal stone formation [46]. Table 14-6 shows dosage adjustments for commonly used agents at various levels of renal dysfunction.

Conclusion

Patients with HIV infection may develop a form of renal disease characterized by severe proteinuria, profound hypoalbuminemia, rapid deterioration of renal function, and FSGS. HIVAN is found throughout the clinical spectrum of HIV disease. Renal disease may be the first manifestation of HIV infection, occasionally preceding the detection of HIV antibodies. HIVAN is most common in urban centers, with a prevalence of about 10 percent. Most patients with HIVAN in the United States are black, are male, or use injection drugs. The prognosis for patients with HIVAN is poor and may depend on the clinical status of the HIV infection, the presence of ESRD, or both. Although FSGS represents a nonspecific pattern of renal injury, HIVAN is associated with characteristic histologic changes. Severe glomerular and tubular epithelial cell injury, markedly dilated tubules with microcysts, and moderate interstitial inflammation are observed on light microscopy. Electron microscopy reveals abundant TRIs in glomerular and vascular endothelial cells. Clinical presentation and histopathologic findings can

Table 14-6 *HIV drug dosage adjustments for renal insufficiency*

Drug	Glomerular filtration rate (GFR)					
	> 50 ml/min	25–50 ml/min	10–25 ml/min	< 10 ml/min	HD	PD
Sulfadiazine	1.0–1.5 gm q6h	0.50–0.75 gm q6h or 1.0–1.5 gm q8–12h	0.50–0.75 gm q12h or 1.0–1.5 gm q24h	Avoid or use 1.0–1.5 gm q48–72h[a]	No Δ	No Δ
TMP-SMX[b]						
TMP	5 mg/kg q6h	2.5 mg/kg q6h or 5 mg/kg q12h	1.7 mg/kg q6h or 5 mg/kg q18h	1.25 mg/kg q6h or 5 mg/kg q24h	No Δ	No Δ
SMX	25 mg/kg q6h	12.5 mg/kg q6h or 25 mg/kg q12h	8 mg/kg q6h or 25 mg/kg q18h	6.25 mg/kg q6h or 25 mg/kg q24h	Add 6.25 mg/kg post-HD	No Δ
Acyclovir[c]	5–10 mg/kg q8h	5–10 mg/kg q12h	5–10 mg/kg q24h	2.5–5.0 mg/kg q24h	5–10 mg/kg q48h post-HD or 2.5–5.0 mg/kg 24h	2.5–5.0 mg/kg q24h
Ganciclovir	2.5 mg/kg q8h or 5 mg/kg q12h	3 mg/kg q12h	3 mg/kg q24h	1.5 mg/kg q24h	Add 1.25–2.50 mg/kg post-HD	(U)
Ethambutol	15–25 mg/kg/day	No Δ	15–25 mg/kg q24–36h or 7.5–15.0 mg/kg q24h	15–25 mg/kg q48h or 3–10 mg/kg q24h	No Δ	No Δ

Table 14-6 Continued

| | Glomerular filtration rate (GFR) | | | | | |
Drug	> 50 ml/min	25–50 ml/min	10–25 ml/min	< 10 ml/min	HD	PD
Fluconazole	50–400 mg/day	No Δ	25–200 mg/day	12.5–100 mg/day	FDD after each HD	50–100 mg/day
Foscarnet	60 mg/kg q8h (B) or 9–20 mg/kg (L) then 0.16–0.19 mg/kg/min (C)	Decrease dose for each ml/min loss of GFR (B): reduce by 3.5 mg/kg for each 0.1 ml/min/kg loss in GFR < 1.6 ml/min/kg (C): reduce dose by 0.02 mg/kg/min for each 20 μmole/ L^d rise in serum Cr > 70 μmole/ L^e Stop drug if GFR < 0.6 ml/min/kg or serum Cr > 250 μmole/ L^f			Removed, check serum level[g]	(U)

HD = hemodialysis; PD = peritoneal dialysis; h = hours, d = days; no Δ = no change; (U) = unknown; (B) = bolus dose; (L) = loading dose; (C) = continuous infusion; Cr = creatinine; FDD = full daily dose.

[a] If essential.

[b] Can be given by oral or intravenous routes at equivalent dosage.

[c] Oral dose of acyclovir with renal insufficiency is 200 mg twice daily.

[d] 20 μmole/L creatinine = 0.2 mg/dl.

[e] 70 μmole/L creatinine = 0.8 mg/dl.

[f] 250 μmole/L creatinine = 2.8 mg/dl.

[g] Foscarnet clearance by HD estimated to be 80 ml/min.

Note: When available, drug levels should be followed, especially in patients with renal insufficiency. To convert serum creatinine in μmole/L to mg/dl, divide by 88.40.

Source: Adapted from JS Berns, RM Cohen, RJ Stumacher, et al. Renal aspects of therapy for immunodeficiency virus and associated opportunistic infections. J Am Soc Nephrol 1:1061–1080, 1991.

be used to distinguish HIVAN from HAN. Until the factors that pre-cipitate HIVAN are identified and randomized drug trials performed, its therapy will remain empiric and be limited to suppression of viral proliferation.

References

1. Rao TKS. Clinical features of human immunodeficiency virus associated nephropathy. *Kidney Int* 40 (suppl):13–18, 1991.
2. Rao TKS, Friedman EA. AIDS (HIV)-associated nephropathy; does it exist? *Am J Nephrol* 9:441–453, 1989.
3. Bourgoignie JJ, Pardo V. The nephropathology in human immunodeficiency virus (HIV-1) infection. *Kidney Int* 40:S19–S23, 1991.
4. Glassock RJ, Cohen AH, Danovitch G, Parsa P. Human immunodeficiency virus (HIV) infection and the kidney. *Ann Intern Med* 112:35–49, 1990.
5. Langs C, Gallo GR, Schacht RG, et al. Rapid renal failure in AIDS-associated focal glomerulosclerosis. *Arch Intern Med* 150:287–292, 1990.
6. Rao TKS, Friedman EA, Nicastri AD. The types of renal disease in the acquired immuno-deficiency syndrome. *N Engl J Med* 316:1062–1068, 1987.
7. Bourgoignie JJ, Jacques J. Renal complications of human immunodeficiency virus type 1. *Kidney Int* 37:1571–1584, 1990.
8. Rao TKS, Fillippone EJ, et al. Associated focal and segmental glomerulosclerosis in AIDS. *N Engl J Med* 310:669–673, 1984.
9. Pardo V, Aldana M, Colton RM, et al. Glomerular lesions in AIDS. *Ann Intern Med* 101:429–434, 1984.
10. Mazbar S, Humphreys MH. AIDS-associated nephropathy is not seen at San Francisco General Hospital. *Kidney Int* 33:202, 1988.
11. Schoenfeld P, Feduska NJ. Acquired immunodeficiency syndrome and renal disease: Report of the National Kidney Foundation–National Institutes of Health Task Force on AIDS and Kidney Disease. *Am J Kidney Dis* 16:14–25, 1990.
12. Frasetto L, Schoenfeld PY, Humphreys MH. Increasing incidence of human immunodeficiency virus–associated nephropathy at San Francisco General Hospital. *Am J Kidney Dis* 18:655–659, 1991.
13. Ortiz C, Meneses R, Jaffe D, et al. Outcome of patients with immunodeficiency virus on maintenance hemodialysis. *Kidney Int* 34:248–253, 1988.
14. Cantor ES, Kimmel PL, Bosch JP. Effect of race on expression of acquired immunodeficiency syndrome–associated nephropathy. *Arch Intern Med* 151:125–128, 1991.
15. Bourgoignie JJ, Meneses R, Ortiz C, et al. The clinical spectrum of renal disease associated with the acquired immunodeficiency syndrome. *Am J Kidney Dis* 12:131–137, 1988.
16. Chander P, Agarwal A, Soni A, et al. Renal cytomembranous inclusions in idiopathic renal disease as predictive markers for the acquired immunodeficiency syndrome. *Hum Pathol* 19:1060–1064, 1988.
17. Pardo V, Meneses R, Ossa L, et al. AIDS-related glomerulopathy: Occurrence in specific risk groups. *Kidney Int* 31:1167–1173, 1987.

18. Gardenschwartz MH, Lerner CW, Seligson GR, et al. Renal disease in patients with AIDS: A clinicopathologic study. *Clin Nephrol* 21:197–204, 1984.
19. Cunningham EE, Brentjens JR, Zielenzy MA, et al. Heroin nephropathy: A clinical and epidemiologic study. *Am J Med* 68:47–53, 1980.
20. Schaffer RM, Schwartz GE, Becker JA, et al. Renal ultrasound in acquired immunodeficiency syndrome. *Radiology* 153:511–513, 1984.
21. Carbone L, D'Agati V, Cheng JT, Appel GB. Course and prognosis of human immunodeficiency virus–associated nephropathy. *Am J Med* 87:389–395, 1989.
22. D'Agati V, Suh JI, Carbone L, et al. Pathology of HIV-associated nephropathy: A detailed morphologic and comparative study. *Kidney Int* 35:1358–1370, 1989.
23. Alpers CE, Harawi S, Rennke HG. Focal glomerulosclerosis with tubuloreticular inclusions: Possible predictive value for acquired immunodeficiency syndrome (AIDS). *Am J Kidney Dis* 12:240–242, 1988.
24. Detweiler R, Falk R, Hogan S, Jennette J. Collapsing glomerulonephropathy: A clinically and pathologically distinct variant of focal segmental glomerulosclerosis. *Kidney Int* 45:1416–1424, 1994.
25. Grimley PM, Kang Y-H, Frederick W, et al. Interferon-related leukocyte inclusions in acquired immunodeficiency syndrome: Localization in T-cells *Am J Clin Pathol* 81:147–155, 1984.
26. Bourgoignie JJ, Meneses R, Pardo V. The nephropathy related to acquired immunodeficiency syndrome. *Adv Nephrol* 17:113–126, 1988.
27. Kimmel P, Phillips T, Ferreira-Centeno A, et al. Idiotypic IgA nephropathy in patients with human immunodeficiency virus infection. *N Engl J Med* 327:702–706, 1992.
28. Edelman AS, Zolla-Pazner S. AIDS: A syndrome of immune dysregulation, dysfunction and deficiency. *FASEB J* 3:22–30, 1989.
29. Camerini D, Seed B. A CD4 domain important for HIV-mediated syncytium formation lies outside the virus binding site. *Cell* 60:747–754, 1990.
30. Cohen AH, Sun NCJ, Shapshak P, et al. Demonstration of human immunodeficiency virus in renal epithelium in HIV-associated nephropathy. *Mod Pathol* 2:125–128, 1989.
31. Farkas-Szallasi T, Fereira-Centeno A, Abraham AA, et al. Viral DNA in biopsy material from HIV infected patients with nephrotic syndrome (abstract). *J Am Soc Nephrol* 2:306, 1991.
32. Dickie P, Felser J, Eckhaus M, et al. HIV-associated nephropathy in transgenic mice expressing HIV-1 genes. *Virology* 185:109–119, 1991.
33. McKeating JA, Griffiths PD, Weiss RA. HIV susceptibility conferred to human fibroblasts by cytomegalovirus-induced Fc receptor. *Nature* 343:659–661, 1990.
34. Peterson PK, Gekker G, Chao CC, et al. Human cytomegalovirus-stimulated peripheral blood mononuclear cells induce HIV-1 replication via a tumor necrosis factor-a–mediated mechanism. *J Clin Invest* 89:574–580, 1992.
35. Valeri A, Neusy AJ. Acute and chronic renal disease in hospitalized AIDS patients. *Clin Nephrol* 35:110–118, 1991.

36. Appel RG, Neill J. A steroid responsive nephrotic syndrome in a patient with human immunodeficiency virus (HIV) infection. *Ann Intern Med* 113:892–893, 1990.
37. Lam M, Park MC. HIV-associated nephropathy: Beneficial effect of zidovudine therapy. *N Engl J Med* 323:1775–1776, 1990.
38. Simonds RJ, Holmberg SD, Hurwitz RL, et al. Transmission of human immunodeficiency virus type I from a seronegative organ and tissue donor. *N Engl J Med* 326:726–732, 1992.
39. Carbone LG, Cohen DJ, Hardy MA, et al. Determination of acquired immunodeficiency syndrome (AIDS) after renal transplantation. *Am J Kidney Dis* 11:387–392, 1988.
40. Vitting KE, Gardenschwartz MH, Zabetakis PM, et al. Frequency of hyponatremia and nonosmolar vasopressin release in the acquired immunodeficiency syndrome. *JAMA* 263:973–978, 1990.
41. Kalin MF, Poretsky L, Seres DS, Zumoff B. Hyporeninemic hypoaldosteronism associated with acquired immune deficiency syndrome. *Am J Med* 82:1035–1038, 1987.
42. Best TR, Jenkins JK, Nicks SA, et al. Persistent adrenal insufficiency secondary to low-dose ketoconazole therapy. *Am J Med* 82:676–680, 1988.
43. Chattha G, Arieff A, Cummings C, Tierney L. Lactic acidosis complicating the acquired immunodeficiency syndrome. *Ann Intern Med* 118:37–39, 1993.
44. Berns JS, Cohen RM, Stumacher RJ, et al. Renal aspects of therapy for immunodeficiency virus and associated opportunistic infections. *J Am Soc Nephrol* 1:1061–1080, 1991.
45. Sattler FR, Cowan R, Nielsen DM, Ruskin J. Trimethoprim-sulfamethoxazole compared with pentamidine for treatment of *Pneumocystis carinii* pneumonia in the acquired immunodeficiency syndrome. *Ann Intern Med* 109:280–287, 1988.
46. Carbone LG, Bendixen B, Appel GB. Sulfadiazine-associated obstructive uropathy in a patient with the acquired immunodeficiency syndrome. *Am J Kidney Dis* 2:72–75, 1988.

Rheumatologic Manifestations

15

Robert W. Simms

The spectrum of HIV disease includes a number of rheumatologic disorders, ranging from relatively benign arthralgia and fibromyalgia to potentially life-threatening conditions such as septic arthritis and systemic vasculitis [1–12] (Table 15-1). A variety of noninfectious articular syndromes, including Reiter's syndrome, psoriatic arthritis, and non-specific oligoarthritis, have also been associated with HIV infection, as has the development of autoantibodies [13–17]. The precise relationship of these conditions to HIV itself remains to be determined.

Clinical Manifestations

Arthralgia

Arthralgia is the most common rheumatic manifestation of HIV infection, with a prevalence ranging from 10 to 35 percent of unselected patients [1, 18]. A particularly disabling, severe, painful articular syndrome has also been identified [1]. Transient arthralgias may occur at the time of HIV seroconversion or become part of a more chronic syndrome without the development of actual arthritis [1, 3]. Most often arthralgia is intermittent and involves large joints such as the shoulders and knees [1].

Fibromyalgia Syndrome

Two studies identified fibromyalgia syndrome (FMS) in patients with HIV infection [2, 3]. Fibromyalgia syndrome is a common cause of chronic musculoskeletal pain, manifested by widespread pain and characteristic sites of muscle tenderness ("trigger points"), as defined

213

Table 15-1 *Rheumatologic manifestations of HIV infection*

Arthralgia
Fibromyalgia syndrome
Reiter's syndrome
Psoriatic arthritis
Infectious arthritis
Myositis
Sjögren's-like syndrome
Vasculitis
Autoantibody production

by American College of Rheumatology (ACR) criteria [19]. The etiology of FMS is unknown, but it has been linked to depression and possibly chronic viral infection [20, 21]. The reported prevalence of FMS in the setting of HIV infection ranges between 10 and 20 percent [2, 3]. Patients with chronic musculoskeletal pain should be carefully evaluated for FMS; symptoms are sometimes confused with other conditions, such as myositis or arthritis, for which the treatment is quite different. Fibromyalgia syndrome in HIV-infected patients is often associated with fatigue, sleep disturbance, and depressive symptoms [3].

Arthritis

Several arthritis syndromes have been described in the setting of HIV infection, including Reiter's syndrome, psoriatic arthritis, nonspecific oligoarthritis, and septic arthritis.

Reiter's Syndrome

Reiter's syndrome, one of the seronegative spondyloarthropathies, is classically described as a triad of arthritis, conjunctivitis, and urethritis [22]. ACR criteria do not require the presence of all three components of the triad simultaneously [22]. Reiter's syndrome in patients with and without HIV infection has been strongly associated with the presence of HLA-B27 [22]. Both enteric and sexually transmitted infections are important risk factors for the development of this condition [22]. It has been estimated that approximately 20 percent of HLA-B27–positive individuals (5–8% of the adult white population) who experience bacterial gastroenteritis will subsequently develop Reiter's syndrome [23].

The relative risk of Reiter's syndrome in HIV-infected patients is 144- to 312-fold greater than that of the general population, and a particularly aggressive form of Reiter's syndrome has been described [1, 13]. The majority of patients report unprotected homosexual contact as their risk behavior, and a specific infectious precipitant is often identified [13]. The arthritis is characteristically a large-joint, lower-extremity, asymmetric oligoarthritis, frequently associated with Achilles tendonitis and dactylitis or "sausage digits." Radiographic evidence of joint destruction is reported in approximately 50 percent of patients [13].

HIV-associated Reiter's syndrome may precede symptomatic HIV infection by up to 12 months, although most patients develop it along with manifestations of immunodeficiency. It is unclear whether Reiter's syndrome is the result of an immune alteration secondary to HIV infection or the consequence of known risk factors, such as enteric or sexually transmitted pathogens. Two preliminary studies found that among homosexual men the prevalence of Reiter's syndrome is the same regardless of HIV serostatus [24, 25].

Psoriatic Arthritis

Arthritis occurs in approximately 7 percent of patients with psoriasis [26]. An asymmetric oligoarthritis is the most common finding on presentation; others include a symmetric polyarthritis similar to rheumatoid arthritis, classic distal interphalangeal joint (DIP) disease, arthritis mutilans, and spondyloarthropathy [26]. HLA-B27 is associated only with spondyloarthropathy [27].

A wide variety of psoriatic or psoriasiform skin lesions, including vulgaris, guttate, and erythrodermic varieties, have been described in HIV-infected patients [28]. Psoriatic arthritis has also been reported in a small number of individuals [1, 14, 29]. As in Reiter's syndrome, enthesopathy and dactylitis, especially of the foot, are common. Onychodystrophy is highly correlated with arthritis, particularly of the DIP joints [14]. HIV p24 antigen has been detected in synoviocytes and lymphocytes in synovial biopsy material from HIV-infected patients with psoriatic arthritis [30]. Since psoriatic fibroblasts in vitro have an increased response to growth factor stimulation (including epidermal growth factor, transforming growth factor beta, and platelet-derived growth factor), similar proteins could be encoded by HIV genes, inducing direct stimulation of keratinocytes, fibroblasts, and vascular cells, and resulting in dermal, synovial, and blood vessel proliferation [31].

Nonspecific Oligoarthritis

A few HIV-infected patients with arthritis cannot be classified as having either Reiter's syndrome or psoriatic arthritis [1, 16]. Typically, they have lower-extremity oligoarthritis with pain out of proportion to the degree of inflammation [2, 16]. No association with HLA-B27 or other autoantibodies has been found. Synovial biopsy demonstrates mild chronic synovitis, and synovial fluid is characteristically noninflammatory [16].

Septic Arthritis

Joint infection due to a variety of pathogens, including *Staphylococcus aureus*, *Campylobacter* species, *Cryptococcus neoformans*, and *Sporothrix schenckii*, has been described in patients with HIV disease [10, 32, 33]. Although no studies have addressed the prevalence of joint infection in this population, it appears to be less frequent than might be expected given the profound state of immunodeficiency that can occur [18]. Septic arthritis caused by *S. aureus* in patients with HIV infection presents much the same way as in seronegative persons. Injection drug use is a common risk factor, and, although the presentation most often seen is large-joint, lower-extremity monarthritis, unusual sites of articular infection, including the acromioclavicular joint, have been described [10]. Hemophiliacs with HIV infection may be particularly prone to joint sepsis due to the high frequency of hemarthrosis [34, 35]. The outcome of septic arthritis in HIV disease is dependent on the duration of symptoms before diagnosis and institution of antimicrobial therapy.

Myositis

A variety of myopathies have been described in patients with HIV infection, including polymyositis, zidovudine (ZDV)-associated mito-chondrial myopathy, and pyomyositis [8, 9, 36, 37]. Polymyositis in the setting of HIV infection presents with myalgias and proximal muscle weakness with increased serum creatine phosphokinase (CPK) levels. In one report, polymyositis was the only clinical manifestation of HIV infection [8]. Immunohistochemical studies of muscle biopsy specimens have shown that anti-HIV antibodies react with CD4 lymphocytes in the inflammatory infiltrate but not with muscle fibers, suggesting that HIV induces an autoimmune inflammatory response rather than a direct cytopathic effect [8]. Long-term ZDV therapy has been shown to pro-duce a mitochondrial myopathy that may be clinically indistinguish-able from that caused by HIV alone [37]. Muscle biopsy specimens in this condition show abundant "ragged red" fibers indicative of abnor-mal mitochondria with paracrystalline inclusions [37]. Interestingly, ZDV-associated myopathy, HIV-associated myopathy, and HIV-seronegative polymyositis all appear to be mediated by suppres-sor-cytotoxic (CD8) T cells and macrophages expressing class I major histocompatibility complex (MHC-I) antigens. This suggests the possi-bility of a common inflammatory mechanism [37].

Sjögren's-like Syndrome

Sjögren's syndrome is a chronic, inflammatory autoimmune disease characterized by diminished lacrimal and salivary secretions, resulting in the keratoconjunctivitis sicca symptom complex [38]. Rarely, associ-ated polymyositis, renal tubular acidosis, or vasculitis occurs. Ninety percent of patients with idiopathic Sjögren's syndrome are women. Salivary gland biopsy specimens typically show an inflammatory infil-trate consisting of predominantly CD4 cells, and there is a strong association with SSA/Ro and SSB/La autoantibodies [38, 39]. A secondary form of Sjögren's syndrome may be associated with rheumatoid arthritis, systemic lupus erythematosus, or scleroderma [38].

A Sjögren's-like syndrome, also known as diffuse lymphocytosis syndrome (DLS), has been reported in a number of patients with HIV infection [5, 6]. The majority have dry mouth but not dry eyes, and most have generalized lymphadenopathy [6]. Table 15-2 contrasts the features of DLS with those of primary or secondary forms of Sjögren's syndrome. Of particular note is the prominence of extraglandular features in the HIV syndrome, typically lymphoid interstitial pneumonitis (LIP), which was present in 10 of 17 patients in one series [6]. The severity of parotid involvement and LIP correlates directly with the peripheral CD8 count [6]. It is of interest that the rate of progression to AIDS may be slowed in patients with DLS, although the reason for this observation is unclear [6].

Vasculitis

A small number of cases of necrotizing vasculitis have been associated with HIV disease (Table 15-3). Underlying infection has been a prominent feature, although seven apparent cases of polyarteritis nodosa had negative hepatitis B serologies [12, 40]. All of these patients had a peripheral sensory or sensorimotor neuropathy, and many were found to have vasculitis on sural nerve biopsy [12, 40]. Of particular interest are six cases of angiocentric lymphoproliferative disorder, also known as lymphomatoid granulomatosis; three were associated with non-Hodgkin's lymphoma [11]. On biopsy, an angiocentric lesion without HIV antigen was found, suggesting that HIV-induced immune dysregulation led to uncontrolled T-cell proliferation, which eventu-

Table 15-2 *Comparison of Sjögren's syndrome and HIV diffuse lymphocytosis syndrome*

Feature	Sjögren's syndrome	Diffuse lymphocytosis syndrome
Extraglandular manifestations	Infrequent	Prominent
Infiltrative lymphocytic phenotype	CD4	CD8
Autoantibodies	High frequency of RF, ANA, anti-SSA/Ro, anti-SSB/La	Low frequency of RF, absent ANA, absent anti-SSA/Ro, SSB/La
HLA association	B8, DR2, DR3, DR4	DR5

RF = rheumatoid factor; ANA = antinuclear antibody.
Source: Adapted from S Itescu, L Brancato, J Buxbaum, et al. A diffuse infiltrative CD8 lymphocytosis in human immunodeficiency virus (HIV) infection: A host immune response associated with HLA-DR5. *Ann Intern Med* 112:3–10, 1990.

Table 15-3 *Necrotizing vasculitis associated with HIV infection*

Vasculitis type	Number (n = 47)	Associated condition
PAN	7	None
PA-CNS	2	1 disseminated varicella-zoster
LCV	7	1 CMV infection
		4 drug reactions
AIL	6	3 non-Hodgkin's lymphoma
		1 staphylococcal, cryptococcal infection
HSP	1	None
Overlap/unspecified	24	1 Kaposi's sarcoma

PAN = polyarteritis nodosa; PA-CNS = primary angiitis of central nervous system; LCV = leukocytoclastic vasculitis; AIL = angiocentric lymphoproliferative disorder; CMV = cytomegalovirus; HSP = Henoch-Schönlein purpura.
Source: Adapted from [12] and [40].

ally resulted in lymphoma [11]. Leukocytoclastic or hypersensitivity vasculitis has also been reported in association with HIV disease [12, 40]. Medications, including penicillin, trimethoprim-sulfamethoxazole, amitriptyline, and griseofulvin, have often been implicated as the precipitant [40].

Laboratory Data

Serologic Studies

A wide variety of autoantibodies have been described in association with HIV infection (Table 15-4). Their significance is unknown, although the majority likely represent epiphenomena of polyclonal B-cell activation [17]. Anticardiolipin antibodies, for example, are found in up to 40 percent of patients with HIV infection, but are not associated with clinical thrombosis as in systemic lupus erythematosus [41]. The presence of lupus anticoagulant antibody may mirror the activity of opportunistic infections [42]. Patients with systemic lupus erythematosus appear

Table 15-4 *Autoantibodies associated with HIV infection*

Anticardiolipin antibodies
Rheumatoid factor
Circulatory immune complexes
Antilymphocyte antibodies
Antisperm antibodies
Antimyelin antibodies
Antiplatelet antibodies
Anti–red blood cell antibodies

to have a higher than expected rate of HIV seropositivity by enzyme-linked immunosorbent assay. However, in one large series of 159 lupus patients, none met World Health Organization criteria (i.e., presence of bands reactive against at least two viral envelope antigens) for a positive result on the confirmatory Western blot test [43, 44].

Creatine phosphokinase is the most sensitive marker of inflammatory muscle disease, although it is similarly elevated in HIV-associated polymyositis and ZDV-associated myopathy and, therefore, cannot be used to distinguish between these two disorders [37].

Synovial Fluid and Synovial Biopsy

Synovial fluid white blood cell (WBC) count is elevated in Reiter's syndrome (approximately 11,000 WBC/mm^3) and psoriatic arthritis (approximately 15,000 WBC/mm^3), with a predominance of polymorphonuclear leukocytes [1]. Nonspecific HIV-associated oligoarthritis typically demonstrates noninflammatory synovial fluid, with the WBC count generally less than 2,000 cells/mm^3; HIV is rarely isolated [16, 45]. In one patient with HIV-associated oligoarthritis, in situ HIV DNA was found in small numbers of synovial fluid lymphocytes and dendritic cells [46]. Synovial fluid findings in HIV-infected patients with septic arthritis generally show WBC counts exceeding 50,000 cells/mm^3, low glucose levels, and organisms on Gram's stain and culture [10].

Synovial biopsy studies in patients with nonspecific oligoarthritis demonstrate only mild, chronic inflammatory changes [16]. Synovial biopsy may show noncaseating granulomas in patients with *S. schenckii* infection [33].

Muscle Studies

Electromyography

Electromyography (EMG) in patients with HIV-associated polymyositis shows nonspecific myopathic changes, such as low-amplitude EMG signals, increased insertional activity with fibrillation potentials, and F waves [8, 9].

Muscle Biopsy

Muscle biopsy specimens of both HIV-associated myopathy and ZDV-associated polymyositis show perivascular or endomysial inflammation, varying degrees of necrotic muscle fibers, rod (nemaline) bodies, and cytoplasmic bodies in many fibers [37]. Only ZDV-associated myopathy, however, demonstrates the presence of "ragged red" fibers, indicative of abnormal mitochondria, with paracrystalline inclusions by electron microscopy [37].

Roentgenographic Studies

Roentgenographic studies of patients with Reiter's syndrome, psoriatic arthritis, and septic arthritis may show evidence of joint destruction but are typically normal in patients with arthralgia, FMS, myositis, and vasculitis [47]. In patients with HIV-associated Sjögren's-like syndrome, chest x-ray may show interstitial changes characteristic of LIP [6].

HLA Testing

HLA-B27 is found in approximately 80 percent of patients with or without HIV infection who have Reiter's syndrome [13].

Clinical Evaluation

History and Physical Examination

Patients with rheumatic symptoms should undergo a careful history and physical examination. The history should focus on specific joint or muscle complaints, including the presence of joint swelling or muscle weakness. A detailed functional history is also critical; for example, eliciting a history of difficulty in combing the hair or rising from a seated position is suggestive of proximal myopathy. For patients with suspected Reiter's syndrome, a prior history of enteric or sexually transmitted infection and transient eye or urethral symptoms is important. Physical examination should focus on the joint and periarticular examination, including enthesopathy (Achilles tendonitis or plantar fasciitis) and nonarticular point tenderness. The presence of a joint effusion is almost always indicative of arthritis and should prompt further evaluation.

Laboratory Evaluation

Patients with FMS should have serum CPK level and thyroid function assessed to rule out polymyositis and hypothyroidism. Patients with muscle weakness should have CPK level measured and consideration of further evaluation, including EMG and muscle biopsy. Patients with arthritis and joint effusion(s) should generally undergo arthrocentesis; this is essential in the case of suspected joint infection. Roentgenographic studies of involved joints are helpful if a destructive arthropathy is part of the differential diagnosis, and HLA-B27 testing should be considered in patients with suspected Reiter's syndrome. For patients with possible vasculitis (e.g., palpable purpura, mononeuritis multiplex), biopsy of the involved organ should be considered before treatment is initiated.

Management

Arthralgia

Most arthralgias without arthritis can be managed with nonnarcotic analgesics, such as acetaminophen or nonsteroidal antiinflammatory drugs (NSAIDs). On occasion, short courses of narcotic analgesics may be required [1].

Fibromyalgia Syndrome

Most patients with FMS can be managed with the combination of low-dose tricyclic antidepressants and nonnarcotic analgesics. Severely depressed patients may require intensive antidepressant therapy and psychiatric referral.

Reiter's Syndrome, Psoriatic Arthritis, and Nonspecific Oligoarthritis

These disorders are generally treated with NSAIDs initially, although this therapy is not uniformly effective [13]. Sulfasalazine has been tried in several patients with Reiter's syndrome without substantial benefit [13]. Methotrexate should be used with caution, since rapid progression to AIDS was noted in two patients shortly after this agent was initiated in low doses for the treatment of Reiter's syndrome [13]. Zidovudine appears to improve psoriasis, but not psoriatic arthritis, in the setting of HIV infection [48].

Septic Arthritis

The management of septic arthritis in patients with HIV disease includes systemic antibiotic therapy and adequate joint drainage. Most authorities recommend a minimum of 4 weeks of treatment for bacterial arthritis.

Zidovudine-Associated Myopathy and HIV-Associated Polymyositis

It is not known whether ZDV-associated myopathy is dose related and whether the lower doses currently recommended will prove less myotoxic with long-term therapy. The management of these myopathies was reviewed by Dalakas and associates [37]. An NSAID should be tried first, with or without dose reduction of ZDV. If this is not effective, ZDV should be discontinued, and the patient's level of strength monitored (serum CPK level may normalize without improvement in muscle strength). If the patient's strength increases, another antiretroviral agent should be considered; if the patient's strength decreases or remains unchanged, ZDV can be resumed along with a course of prednisone therapy (40–60 mg daily).

Sjögren's-like Syndrome

In one study, early corticosteroid or chlorambucil therapy appeared to prevent progression to interstitial fibrosis [6].

Vasculitis

Once the possibility of infection as the underlying cause has been eliminated, a cautious trial of prednisone and a cytotoxic drug should be considered, particularly in the patient with more serious organ involvement.

References

1. Berman A, Espinoza LR, Diaz JD, et al. Rheumatic manifestations of human immunodeficiency virus infection. *Am J Med* 85:59–64, 1988.
2. Buskila D, Gladman DD, Langevitz P, et al. Fibromyalgia in human immunodeficiency virus infection. *J Rheumatol* 17:1202–1206, 1990.
3. Simms RW, Zerbini CAF, Ferrante N, et al. Fibromyalgia syndrome in patients infected with the human immunodeficiency virus. *Am J Med* 92:368–374, 1992.
4. De Clerck LS, Couttenye MM, de Broe ME, Stevens WJ. Acquired immunodeficiency syndrome mimicking Sjögren's syndrome and systemic lupus erythematosus. *Arthritis Rheum* 31:272–275, 1988.
5. Ulirsch RC, Jaffe ES. Sjögren's syndrome-like illness associated with the acquired immunodeficiency syndrome-related complex. *Hum Pathol* 18:1063–1068, 1987.
6. Itescu S, Brancato L, Buxbaum J, et al. A diffuse infiltrative CD8 lymphocytosis in human immunodeficiency virus (HIV) infection: A host immune response associated with HLA-DR5. *Ann Intern Med* 112:3–10, 1990.
7. Dalakas MC, Pezeshkpour GH, Gravell M, Sever JL. Polymyositis associated with AIDS retrovirus. *JAMA* 256:2381–2383, 1986.
8. Nordstrom DM, Petroposis AA, Giorno R, et al. Inflammatory myopathy and acquired immunodeficiency syndrome. *Arthritis Rheum* 32:475–479, 1989.
9. Glickstein SL, Strickland SR, Rusin LH. Acute myositis in a patient with acquired immunodeficiency syndrome. *Arthritis Rheum* 33:298, 1990.
10. Zimmerman B, Erickson AD, Milkolich DJ. Septic acromio-clavicular arthritis and osteomyelitis in a patient with acquired immunodeficiency syndrome. *Arthritis Rheum* 32:1175–1178, 1989.
11. Calabrese LH, Estes M, Yen-Lieberman B, et al. Systemic vasculitis in association with human immunodeficiency virus infection. *Arthritis Rheum* 32:569–576, 1989.
12. Marcef-Valeriano J, Ravichandran L, Kerr LD. HIV-associated systemic necrotizing vasculitis. *J Rheumatol* 17:1091–1093, 1990.
13. Winchester R, Bernstein H, Fischer H, et al. The co-occurrence of Reiter's

syndrome and acquired immunodeficiency. *Ann Intern Med* 106:19–26, 1987.

14. Duvic M, Johnson TM, Rapini RP, et al. Acquired immunodeficiency syndrome–associated psoriasis and Reiter's syndrome. *Arch Dermatol* 123:1622–1632, 1987.

15. Espinoza LR, Berman A, Vasey FB, et al. Psoriatic arthritis and acquired immunodeficiency syndrome. *Arthritis Rheum* 31:1034–1040, 1988.

16. Rynes RI, Goldenberg DL, di Giacomo R, et al. Acquired immunodeficiency syndrome–associated arthritis. *Am J Med* 84:810–816, 1988.

17. Calabrese LH. Autoimmune manifestations of human immunodeficiency virus (HIV) infection. *Clin Lab Med* 8:269–279, 1988.

18. Monteagndo I, Rivera J, Lopez-Lungo J, et al. AIDS and rheumatic manifestations in patients addicted to drugs. An analysis of 106 cases. *J Rheumatol* 18:1038–1041, 1991.

19. Wolfe F, Smythe HA, Yunus M, et al. The American College of Rheumatology 1990 criteria for the classification of fibromyalgia: Report of the multicenter criteria committee. *Arthritis Rheum* 33:160–172, 1990.

20. Hudson JI, Hudson MS, Pliner LF, et al. Fibromyalgia and psychopathology: Is fibromyalgia a form of "affective spectrum disorder" *J Rheumatol* 16 (suppl):15–22, 1989.

21. Goldenberg DL. Fibromyalgia and other chronic fatigue syndromes: Is there evidence for chronic viral disease? *Semin Arthritis Rheum* 18:111–120, 1988.

22. Calin A. Reiter's Syndrome. In WN Kelly, E Harris, S Ruddy, C Sledge (eds), *Textbook of Rheumatology* (3rd ed). Philadelphia: Saunders, 1989. Pp 1038–1049.

23. Calin A, Fries JF. An "experimental" epidemic of Reiter's syndrome revisited: Follow-up evidence on genetic and environmental factors. *Ann Intern Med* 84:564, 1976.

24. Clark M, Kinsolving M, Chernoff D. The prevalence of arthritis in two HIV-infected cohorts (abstract). *Arthritis Rheum* 32:S85, 1989.

25. Hochberg MC, Fox R, Nelson KR. Reiter's syndrome is not associated with HIV infection (abstract). *Arthritis Rheum* 33:17S, 1989.

26. Kammer GM, Soter NA, Gibson DJ, Schur PH. Psoriatic arthritis: A clinical immunologic and HLA study of 100 patients. *Semin Arthritis Rheum* 9:75–97, 1979.

27. Bennett RM. Psoriatic Arthritis. In DJ McCarty (ed), *Arthritis and Allied Conditions* (11th ed). Philadelphia: Lea & Febiger, 1989. Pp 954–971.

28. Kaplan MH, Sadick N, McNutt S, et al. Dermatologic findings and manifestations of acquired immunodeficiency syndrome (AIDS). *J Am Acad Dermatol* 16:485–506, 1987.

29. Reveille JD, Cewant MA, Dovic M. Human immunodeficiency virus–associated psoriasis, psoriatic arthritis, and Reiter's syndrome: A disease continuum? *Arthritis Rheum* 33:1574–1578, 1990.

30. Aguilar JL, Espinoza LR, Berman A, et al. HIV antigen demonstration in synovial membrane from patients with HIV-associated arthritis and HIV-associated psoriatic arthritis. *Arthritis Rheum* 32:587, 1989.

31. Aguilar JL, Espinoza LR. Psoriatic arthritis: A current perspective. *J Musculoskel Med* 6:11–28, 1989.

32. Ricciardi DD, Sepkowitz LB, Bienenstoch H, Maslow ML. Cryptococcal arthritis in a patient with acquired immune deficiency syndrome: A case report and review of the literature. *J Rheumatol* 13:455–458, 1986.

33. Lipstein-Kresch E, Isenberg HD, Singer C, et al. Disseminated *Sporothrix schenckii* infection with arthritis in a patient with acquired immunodeficiency syndrome. *J Rheumatol* 12:805–808, 1985.

34. Pappo AS, Buchanan GR, Johnson A. Septic arthritis in children with hemophilia. *Am J Dis Child* 143:1226–1228, 1989.

35. Rogni MV, Hanley EN. Septic arthritis in hemophiliac patients and infection with human immunodeficiency virus. *Ann Intern Med* 110:168–169, 1989.

36. Widrow CA, Kellie SM, Saltzman BR, Mathur-Wagh V. Pyomyositis in patients with the human immunodeficiency virus: An unusual form of disseminated bacterial infection. *Am J Med* 91:129–136, 1991.

37. Dalakas MC, Illa I, Pezeshkpour GH, et al. Mitochondrial myopathy caused by long-term zidovudine therapy. *N Engl J Med* 322:1098–1105, 1990.

38. Talal N. Sjögren's Syndrome and Connective Tissue Diseases Associated with Other Immunologic Disorders. In DJ McCarty (ed), *Arthritis and Allied Conditions* (11th ed). Philadelphia: Lea & Febiger, 1989. Pp 1197–1213.

39. Adamson TC, Fox RI, Frismen DM, et al. Immunohistochemical analysis of lymphoid filtrates in primary Sjögren's syndrome using monoclonal antibodies. *J Immunol* 130:203–208, 1983.

40. Gherardi R, Belec L, Mhiri C, et al. The spectrum of vasculitis in human immunodeficiency virus-infected patients: A clinicopathologic evaluation. *Arthritis Rheum* 36:1164–1174, 1993.

41. Canoso RT, Zow LI, Goopman JE. Anticardiolipin antibodies associated with HTLV-III infection. *Br J Haematol* 65:495–498, 1987.

42. Cohen A, Phillips TM, Kessler CM. Circulating coagulation inhibitors in the acquired immunodeficiency syndrome. *Ann Intern Med* 104:175–180, 1986.

43. Barthel HR, Wallace DJ. False-positive human immunodeficiency virus testing in patients with lupus erythematosus. *Semin Arthritis Rheum* 23:1–7, 1993.

44. Soriano V, Ordi J, Grau J. Tests for HIV in lupus. *N Engl J Med* 331:881, 1994.

45. Withrington RH, Cornes P, Harris JRW, et al. Isolation of human immunodeficiency virus from synovial fluid of a patient with reactive arthritis. *Br Med J* 294:484, 1987.

46. Espinoza LR, Aguilar JL, Espinoza CW, et al. HIV associated arthropathy: HIV antigen demonstration in the synovial membrane. *J Rheumatol* 17:1195–1201, 1990.

47. Rosenberg ZS, Norman A, Solomon G. Arthritis associated with HIV infection: Radiographic manifestations. *Radiology* 173:171–176, 1989.

48. Duvic M, Crane MM, Conant M, et al. Zidovudine improves psoriasis in human immunodeficiency virus–positive males. *Arch Dermatol* 130:447–451, 1994.

Endocrinologic Manifestations

16

Melanie J. Brunt, Stuart R. Chipkin

The endocrine manifestations of HIV infection are protean and incompletely understood. Infiltration and destruction of endocrine organs by opportunistic infection or neoplasm are common findings at autopsy in patients with HIV disease, although most do not have clinical evidence of endocrine dysfunction during life (Table 16-1). HIV-related endocrinopathy may also be mediated by antibodies against endocrine cells or by cytokines such as tumor necrosis factor, interleukin-1, and interferon. In addition, endocrine function may be adversely affected by therapeutic agents.

Adrenal Function

HIV-infected patients often have nonspecific symptoms similar to those of adrenal insufficiency. Autopsy studies have documented a high prevalence of infiltration of the adrenals by cytomegalovirus (CMV), other pathogens, and neoplasia. Despite these findings, most patients with HIV disease do not have measurable cortisol deficiency. Similar observations have been made in persons with extensive adrenal involvement by metastatic disease, tuberculosis, or hemorrhage [1–3]. While destruction of 80 to 90 percent of the adrenal gland is a prerequisite for cortisol deficiency, CMV is usually found to involve only 50 to 60 percent of the gland in HIV-infected patients at autopsy [4].

Clinical Manifestations

The clinical manifestations of adrenal insufficiency are nonspecific and cannot be readily distinguishable from wasting syndrome. Most often,

225

Table 16-1 *Mechanisms of endocrine dysfunction in HIV infection*

I. Destruction of endocrine tissue
    Cancer
    Infection
    Hemorrhage
    Nonspecific inflammation
II. Interference with endocrine function
    Acute illness
    Chronic illness
    Cytokines (tumor necrosis factor, interleukin-1, interferon)
    Antibodies
III. Action of therapeutic agents
    Ketoconazole—reduced adrenal and testicular steroidogenesis and 1,25-
        dihydroxyvitamin D formation
    Rifampin—increased cortisol metabolism
    Phenytoin—increased cortisol metabolism
    Opiates—increased cortisol metabolism
    Trimethoprim-sulfamethoxazole—pancreatic inflammation
    Pentamidine—inflammation and destruction of pancreatic beta cells
    Didanosine—pancreatic inflammation
    Foscarnet—decreased serum ionized calcium
    Megestrol acetate—pituitary suppression of LH, FSH, ACTH; transient
        diabetes mellitus due to glucocorticoid effects

LH = luteinizing hormone; FSH = follicle stimulating hormone; ACTH = adrenocorticotropin.
Source: Adapted from SK Grinspoon, JP Bilezikian. HIV disease and the endocrine
system. *N Engl J Med* 327:1360–1366, 1992.

the question of cortisol deficiency is raised in patients with advanced
HIV disease who are experiencing weight loss, fatigue, anorexia, nausea, diarrhea, and malaise (Table 16-2). Physical findings are few and
may be limited to postural hypotension and weight loss.

HIV-related adrenal insufficiency is usually a result of primary
hypofunction; secondary adrenal insufficiency is much less common.
Infiltration of the pituitary by tumor or infection has been reported, but
it usually occurs in conjunction with other endocrinopathies such as
hypothyroidism and hypogonadism. Additionally, hypotension and
electrolyte abnormalities may be less prominent in secondary adrenal
insufficiency because adrenal aldosterone production is maintained by
the renin-aldosterone axis, which is largely independent of pituitary
adrenocorticotropin (ACTH).

Laboratory Data

Ninety percent of patients with primary adrenal insufficiency have
hyponatremia, 66 percent have hyperkalemia, and 40 percent have
hypoglycemia (see Table 16-2). Other metabolic abnormalities including hypercalcemia may also occur.

Table 16-2 *Clinical presentation of primary adrenal insufficiency*

	Frequency (%)
Symptoms	
Weakness and fatigue	100
Anorexia	100
Nausea and diarrhea	56
Signs	
Weight loss	100
Hyperpigmentation	97
Hypotension	91
Vitiligo	Rare
Laboratory findings	
Hyponatremia	90
Hyperkalemia	66
Hypoglycemia	40
Hypercalcemia	6

Source: From MJ Brunt, JC Melby. Adrenal Gland Disorders. In J Noble (ed). *Textbook of Primary Care Medicine*. St. Louis: Mosby, 1995.

Hormonal studies have been conducted in HIV-infected patients without symptoms of adrenal insufficiency to determine the prevalence of subclinical adrenal dysfunction. Results vary, but the predominant findings have included increased basal levels of cortisol in asymptomatic patients or patients with early-stage disease, and subclinical adrenal dysfunction in those with advanced disease [5–8]. Aldosterone synthesis may also be abnormal in HIV-infected patients who do not have clinical evidence of mineralocorticoid deficiency [7].

Pathophysiology

The high cortisol production and low aldosterone and adrenal androgen levels found in HIV disease may represent a shift in adrenal production to cortisol related to the metabolic stress of a chronic systemic illness [9]. Alternatively, interference with the action of cortisol may be a factor. One group of investigators identified anti-corticosteroid antibodies in AIDS patients, and peripheral resistance to the action of cortisol has been postulated by others [10, 11]. In addition, cytokines have been found to affect adrenal function at all levels of the hypothalamic-pituitary-adrenal axis. Production of interleukin-1 and tumor necrosis factor by macrophages is increased in HIV disease, as is the production of interferon by monocytes [10]. Interleukin-1, in turn, appears to stimulate the release of corticotropin releasing factor from the hypothalamus, and has been reported to cause pituitary cells in vitro to secrete ACTH. Interferon may also increase ACTH secretion.

Differential Diagnosis

A summary of adrenal findings at autopsy in HIV-infected patients is presented in Table 16-3. Cytomegalovirus is found in 50 to 88 percent of patients; other pathogens described include mycobacteria, *Cryptococcus neoformans*, and *Toxoplasma gondii* [4, 12, 13]. Autopsy findings have also shown infiltration by lymphoma and Kaposi's sarcoma, hemorrhage, and cortical lipid depletion [4].

In HIV-infected patients with weight loss and constitutional symptoms who do not have an identifiable opportunistic disease, the differential diagnosis includes wasting syndrome and adrenal insufficiency. Although hyponatremia may result from cortisol deficiency in this setting, it is often caused by other conditions. Possibilities include severe volume depletion, the syndrome of inappropriate antidiuretic hormone secretion (SIADH) secondary to pulmonary or central nervous system infection, and renal sodium wasting from nephrotoxic drugs such as pentamidine and amphotericin B [14, 15].

Several medications commonly used in patients with HIV disease are associated with decreased cortisol levels. Ketoconazole interferes with adrenal steroidogenesis, and rifampin, phenytoin, and opiates accelerate cortisol degradation [4]. Megestrol acetate, a synthetic progestin used as an appetite stimulant in HIV-infected patients, interferes with cortisol production at the level of the pituitary by decreasing ACTH secretion [16].

Evaluation

Routine screening of HIV-infected patients for adrenal insufficiency is not recommended. Diagnostic evaluation should be considered in the following situations: (1) patients with wasting without an identifiable gastrointestinal cause, (2) patients with hyponatremia of uncertain etiology, (3) patients with disseminated CMV or other opportunistic

Table 16-3 *Adrenal pathologic findings in patients with AIDS*

Organism or process	Reported prevalence (%)
Cytomegalovirus	50–88
Lipid depletion	30–100
Hemorrhagic infarction	22
Fibrosis	24
Massive necrosis	8
Acid-fast bacilli	2–12
Kaposi's sarcoma	3–5
Cryptococcus neoformans	1–7
Toxoplasma gondii	1

Source: Adapted from DS Donovan, RG Dluhy. AIDS and its effect on the adrenal gland. *Endocrinologist* 1:228, 1991.

infections, and (4) for preoperative evaluation. The screening tests commonly employed are the morning serum cortisol level and rapid ACTH test. A morning cortisol level higher than 15 µg/dl indicates adequate endogenous adrenal function. If the serum cortisol level is below this value, a rapid ACTH test should be performed. This consists of a bolus intravenous injection of 250 µg of cosyntropin (synthetic 1,25-alpha-ACTH) with measurement of the serum cortisol just prior to injection and 60 minutes later. A serum cortisol level of 18 µg/dl or higher excludes adrenal insufficiency [17]. If the response indicates hypoadrenalism, serum endogenous ACTH levels should be measured between 8 and 10 AM to distinguish between primary and secondary adrenal dysfunction.

If cortisol deficiency is found in conjunction with an elevated ACTH level, the patient should be evaluated for causes of primary adrenal insufficiency and screened for appropriate opportunistic diseases. If cortisol deficiency is found in conjunction with a low or normal ACTH level, the patient is considered to have secondary adrenal insufficiency. Thyroid and reproductive hormone status should be investigated to rule out concurrent deficiency of other pituitary hormones, and magnetic resonance imaging (MRI) of the brain should be performed to exclude an intracerebral mass involving the pituitary gland.

Management

Empiric management of acute adrenal crisis should be initiated for all HIV-infected patients who develop hemodynamic collapse refractory to volume expansion or vasoconstricting agents (Table 16-4). Treatment can be instituted immediately after the rapid ACTH test is performed and discontinued if the results indicate that adrenal function is adequate.

Maintenance therapy for chronic hypoadrenalism consists of daily oral corticosteroid replacement, most commonly hydrocortisone or

Table 16-4 *Evaluation and management of acute adrenal insufficiency*

1. Draw blood for measurement of cortisol and ACTH.
2. Infuse sufficient normal saline with 5% dextrose to restore normotension.
3. Administer dexamethasone 2 mg IV stat (will not interfere with further testing).
4. Give 250 µg cosyntropin (ACTH) IV and measure 30-minute cortisol level.
5. Begin IV hydrocortisone as a continuous infusion to total of 200 mg in 24 hours; or dose can be given in bolus form of 50 mg every 6 hours.
6. Investigate underlying etiology of adrenal insufficiency as outlined in text.
7. Chronic replacement therapy can begin as soon as the patient is medically stable and able to take orally.

Source: From MJ Brunt, JC Melby. Adrenal Gland Disorders. In J Noble (ed), *Textbook of Primary Care Medicine*. St. Louis: Mosby, 1995.

prednisone. In patients with primary adrenal insufficiency, the mineralocorticoid fludrocortisone is added (Table 16-5). For a severe illness, such as a major acute infection requiring hospitalization, doses should be increased to "stress level" until the patient is stabilized. In patients with primary adrenal insufficiency, hydrocortisone may be a better choice than prednisone because of its higher mineralocorticoid activity.

Clinical symptoms are used to assess the adequacy of the glucocorticoid dose; 24-hour urine free cortisol levels can also be monitored [18]. Care should be taken to avoid excess replacement of glucocorticoids, which can result in osteoporosis or metabolic complications such as hyperglycemia. Mineralocorticoid therapy is monitored by serum electrolyte levels, postural blood pressure measurements, and plasma renin activity, which should be increased if the dose is insufficient. Excessive mineralocorticoid replacement may cause hypertension and hyperkalemia.

Thyroid Function

Clinical Manifestations

As with the adrenal gland, biochemical abnormalities of thyroid function are much more common in patients with HIV infection than is clinical thyroid disease. A small number of cases of thyroid involvement with opportunistic infections, especially with *Pneumocystis carinii*, have been reported [19, 20]. In most instances, thyroid function studies

Table 16-5 *Glucocorticoid characteristics*

Medication	T $^1/_2$	Dosages Replacement[a]	Stress[b]	Potencies GC[c]	MC[d]
Hydrocortisone (cortisol)	8–12 hr	20 mg	200 mg	1	1
Prednisone	12–36 hr	5 mg	50 mg	4	0.25
Methylprednisolone	12–36 hr	4 mg	40 mg	5	0.25
Dexamethasone	36–72 hr	0.75 mg	7.5 mg	25	0
Fluodrocortisone	12–20 hr	0.05–2.00 mg	Increase dietary sodium	10	125

T $^1/_2$ = drug half-life.
[a]Replacement refers to the dose required to replace the 24-hour cortisol production of nonstressed adrenal glands.
[b]Stress refers to the dose required to replace the 24-hour cortisol production of the adrenals in situations of severe metabolic stress.
[c]GC refers to the glucocorticoid potency of the medication as compared to cortisol.
[d]MC refers to the mineralocorticoid potency of the medication as compared to cortisol.
Source: From MJ Brunt, JC Melby. Adrenal Gland Disorders. In J Noble (ed), *Textbook of Primary Care Medicine*. St. Louis: Mosby, 1995.

are performed in HIV-infected patients for evaluation of weight loss, fatigue, and other constitutional symptoms.

Laboratory Data

The thyroid function test abnormalities reported in HIV disease are outlined in Table 16-6. In asymptomatic patients with HIV infection, thyroid function parameters are usually normal, with the exception of thyroid binding globulin (TBG), which may be increased, resulting in elevated total thyroxine (T_4) and triiodothyronine (T_3) concentrations with low resin uptake and normal thyroid stimulating hormone (TSH) levels [21–23]. Unlike other illnesses in which TBG is elevated, this finding does not appear to correlate with hepatic dysfunction. As HIV disease progresses, thyroid function abnormalities, including low total T_4, total T_3, and free T_4 levels, often develop, as in other types of chronic, nonthyroidal illness. Possible explanations of these findings include lower TBG levels resulting from decreased protein synthesis and decreased peripheral conversion of T_4 to T_3 [8, 10, 23, 24]. TSH levels in HIV disease are usually normal, and TSH response to thyrotropin releasing factor (TRH) was similar to normal control responses in one study of asymptomatic HIV-infected patients [5, 23]. Although total T_3 levels are generally reduced in HIV disease, they are not as low as in

Table 16-6 *Thyroid function test (TFT) abnormalities in HIV disease*

Stage	*TFT abnormality*	*Postulated mechanism*
Asymptomatic HIV positive	1. Usually none, or	
	2. High TBG, causing $\uparrow T_4$, $\uparrow T_3$, low resin uptake, normal TSH	Possibly nonspecific inflammatory response with diffuse increase in serum proteins or defective hepatic degradation
AIDS	1. $\downarrow$ total T_3 by 19%	$\downarrow T_4 {\rightarrow} T_3$ conversion (postulated adaptive response to conserve metabolic energy in acute or chronic illness)
	2. $\downarrow T_4$, $\downarrow$ free T_4	Unknown
	3. $\downarrow$ TSH	$\downarrow$ Pituitary secretion
	4. $\uparrow$ TSH	Unknown
	5. $\uparrow$ TBG	Nonspecific inflammatory response
	6. $\downarrow$ TBG	Malnutrition/starvation

TBG = thyroid binding globulin; TSH = thyroid stimulating hormone.

other types of chronic illness [24]. There has been some speculation that this may be maladaptive and contribute to the weight loss seen in AIDS patients [21].

Pathophysiology

The mechanisms of most thyroid function abnormalities in HIV disease are unknown [10]. Some authors have suggested that in other nonthyroidal illnesses, cytokines or other binding inhibitor proteins may block extrathyroidal conversion of T_4 to T_3 and interfere with pituitary TSH secretion [25].

Differential Diagnosis

If thyroid function test abnormalities are identified in the context of normal or low TSH levels, the differential diagnosis includes nonthyroidal illness and secondary or tertiary hypothyroidism. Hypothyroidism is much less common than nonthyroidal illness in HIV disease. True secondary or tertiary hypothyroidism should be accompanied by characteristic clinical findings, such as abnormal deep tendon reflexes or skin changes, and may be associated with other endocrinopathies, including hypogonadism and hypoadrenalism.

Nonthyroidal illness may also be confused with early subclinical primary hypothyroidism, particularly if the TSH level is slightly increased and clinical findings are nonspecific. Following resolution of an acute illness, TSH levels can rise during a "recovery phase," after which they return to normal. If thyroid function tests are performed during this period, the findings of an increased TSH level and low T_4 and free T_4 levels mimic primary hypothyroidism.

Evaluation

Initial laboratory evaluation of a patient with possible thyroid dysfunction should include measurements of TSH and T_4. Total T_3 measurement may occasionally help in establishing the presence of hyperthyroidism but should not be used to diagnose hypothyroidism. A T_3 resin uptake can be used to assess TBG level. Further laboratory evaluation is usually not required. Abnormalities found on thyroid function tests resulting from nonthyroidal illness typically resolve with the acute illness. If secondary or tertiary hypothyroidism is suspected, referral to an endocrine consultant is recommended.

Management

Treatment is not indicated in HIV-infected patients with thyroid function abnormalities that are consistent with nonthyroidal illness. Patients with TSH levels that are increased, but less than 15 mU/L, can be safely monitored for 1 to 2 months to determine whether clinical hypo-thyroidism develops.

Pituitary Function

Interference with hormone secretion and regulation in HIV disease has been found to occur at the level of the pituitary gland, affecting the thyroid, adrenals, and gonads. Cytokines such as interferon, interleukin-1, and tumor necrosis factor may mediate this dysfunction [10]. Additionally, autopsy studies have revealed pituitary involvement with opportunistic infections, tumor, infarction, or hemorrhage in many patients with HIV infection [9, 12, 26, 27]. None of these patients were known to have pituitary insufficiency during life, suggesting that massive destruction is required before clinical panhypopituitarism develops.

Megestrol acetate causes suppression of pituitary function, resulting in diminished secretion of follicle stimulating hormone (FSH), luteinizing hormone (LH), and ACTH [16]. This is probably related to the glucocorticoid-like effects of the drug.

Laboratory data, evaluation, differential diagnosis, and management for pituitary pathology typically relate to the specific end-organ involved. Differentiating pituitary from hypothalamic disease can be extremely challenging, and consultation with an endocrinologist often proves helpful in these situations.

Testicular Function

Clinical Manifestations

Symptoms of testosterone deficiency occur commonly in HIV disease. In one series, 67 percent of male patients with AIDS reported decreased libido, and 33 percent reported impotence [28]. Muscle wasting and loss of body hair have also been reported frequently in men with HIV infection, as has gynecomastia [29, 30].

Laboratory Data

When testosterone deficiency is present, its severity appears to depend on the stage of HIV disease. In one study, asymptomatic HIV-infected homosexual men had mean testosterone levels that were no different from levels in seronegative control subjects [29]. In men with AIDS, mean testosterone levels were significantly lower than control levels. Mean serum LH, FSH, and prolactin levels also rose progressively with advancing disease, although statistical significance was achieved only in the AIDS group. The mechanism of hypogonadism in the cohort of men with advanced HIV disease appears to be primary testicular failure, as indicated by low testosterone levels with compensatory increases in FSH and LH. Prolactin elevations were small and not in the range likely to cause sexual dysfunction. Other studies of heterosexual patients and injection drug users with HIV disease showed findings more consistent with endocrinologic dysfunction at the secondary or tertiary level (hypogonadotropic hypogonadism), which worsen with disease progression [8, 12].

Testosterone levels have also been reported to be increased in asymptomatic HIV-infected men [5]. Results of stimulation testing with gonadotropin releasing hormone were also abnormal, with an exaggerated LH response, consistent with hyperfunction at the pituitary-hypothalamic level. In asymptomatic HIV-infected men, semen analysis generally shows normal findings, indicating that fertility may not be impaired. In contrast, men with AIDS often have abnormal semen, with white blood cell infiltration [31].

Pathophysiology

The mechanism of hypothalamic or pituitary dysfunction in men with HIV disease and hypotestosteronemia or hypertestosteronemia is unknown. As with other endocrine organ dysfunction, cytokines are thought to play a role in influencing central secretion of reproductive hormone stimulating factors. Hypogonadotropic hypogonadism is a common finding in severe illness of any type and has been postulated to occur as a means of energy conservation when bodily resources are needed elsewhere [32]. In HIV disease, loss of function at the secondary or tertiary level may also result from partial pituitary destruction or infiltration by opportunistic infection or tumor, as suggested by autopsy findings.

Primary hypogonadism may also be caused by infiltration or destruction of testicular tissue. A variety of pathologic findings at autopsy have been reported, including hyalinization of seminiferous tubules, interstitial lymphocytic infiltration, azoospermia, impaired spermatogenesis, interstitial fibrosis, and opportunistic infections [33–36]. In one series, there was a 39 percent prevalence of opportunistic infections, including CMV, *T. gondii*, and *Mycobacterium avium* complex involving the testes [36]. In addition, medications may have hypogonadal effects. Ketoconazole is a potent inhibitor of testicular testosterone synthesis, resulting in the syndrome of primary hypogonadism and gynecomastia. Megestrol acetate may induce partial secondary hypogonadism related to pituitary suppression of gonadotropins [16].

Evaluation

HIV-infected men who complain of decreased libido or erectile dysfunction and are not taking medications associated with hypogonadism should be evaluated initially by physical examination for evidence of diminished secondary sex characteristics, including decreased beard growth, loss of male-pattern body hair, and gynecomastia. The testes should be examined for evidence of atrophy; testicular length should be at least 3.5 cm in normal adult men. Initial laboratory studies should include measurements of serum free testosterone, prolactin, and FSH.

Differential Diagnosis

Primary hypogonadism is suggested by an increased FSH level and a low free testosterone level, while in secondary or tertiary hypogonadism, values for both are low. If the hormonal results are consistent with secondary or tertiary hypofunction or if the prolactin level is increased, MRI of the brain may be needed to exclude a hypothalamic or pituitary mass lesion such as toxoplasmosis or lymphoma.

If results of the above-mentioned laboratory studies are normal, sexual dysfunction is not related to hormonal deficiency. Differential diagnosis in men with normal hormone levels includes vascular insufficiency, neurologic dysfunction, and depression. Evidence of vascular or neurologic impairment is usually suggested by findings on physical examination.

Management

HIV-infected men who have testosterone deficiency related to endocrine dysfunction at any level can be treated with testosterone injections or a testosterone patch, unless contraindicated by the presence of severe liver disease, prostatic hyperplasia, or cancer. Testosterone injections are generally administered intramuscularly in a dose of 150 to 250 mg every 2 to 3 weeks. Efficacy is monitored by clinical response and trough serum testosterone levels. Trough levels are measured after several cycles, just prior to the next injection, and should be low-normal. Testosterone skin patches, which are applied daily to a shaved area of the scrotum, are more expensive but provide a more continuous clinical effect and serum levels.

Ovarian Function

Ovarian function has not been evaluated directly in women with HIV disease, but limited epidemiologic data suggest a relationship between female infertility and HIV infection in some populations. In Gabon, women with primary infertility had higher HIV seroprevalence rates than did the fertile population [37]. Among Tanzanian women working as prostitutes in Kenya, HIV seropositivity was associated with reduced fecundity, independent of the presence of other sexually transmitted diseases and oral contraceptive use [38]. However, among Zairian women followed prospectively after their most recent childbirth, rates of term pregnancy were no different in HIV-positive women than in seronegative control subjects [39]. Similar findings were noted in a study of New York State female prison inmates in 1988 [40]. Data are unavailable regarding other parameters of ovarian function in HIV-infected women, including menstrual cycle behavior, libido, and estrogen sufficiency.

Pancreatic Endocrine Function

Clinical Manifestations

Pancreatic dysfunction is uncommon in HIV disease, despite a more than 50 percent prevalence of abnormalities at autopsy [41]. Clinical evidence of pancreatic endocrine dysfunction does occur in association with intravenous pentamidine therapy. Pentamidine is directly toxic to pancreatic beta cells, initially causing excess release of insulin through their destruction, and eventually resulting in insulin deficiency as synthetic capacity is destroyed. Clinically, this effect is manifested first by hypoglycemia, which occurs within a few days to weeks of therapy, followed by clinical diabetes mellitus in some patients [42]. Depending on the degree of insulin deficiency, patients may present with frank diabetic ketoacidosis or with milder disease with nonketotic hyperglycemia [43]. Acute pancreatitis has been reported to precede the development of diabetes mellitus on occasion [42]. Pentamidine-induced diabetes mellitus is usually, but not always, permanent [44]. Aerosol pentamidine does not appear to cause diabetes mellitus, but cases of acute pancreatitis have been reported [42].

Megestrol acetate has also been associated with diabetes mellitus in AIDS patients [43, 45]. The mechanism is thought to be related to insulin resistance from the mild glucocorticoid action of this drug in conjunction with the increased caloric intake and weight gain that may result from its use [46]. The effect is transient and resolves when the medication is discontinued.

Laboratory Data

Hyperamylasemia is common in patients with acute pentamidine-associated pancreatic damage [41]. Endogenous insulin levels, as assessed by C-peptide measurement, are reduced later in the course, indicating beta-cell destruction [47].

Evaluation and Differential Diagnosis

Classic symptoms of diabetes mellitus in the context of prior pentamidine or megestrol acetate therapy generally indicate the etiology of pancreatic endocrine dysfunction.

Management

Treatment consists of discontinuation of the offending medication and conventional diabetic management with either insulin or oral hypoglycemic agents. Oral sulfonylureas are usually less effective in treating patients with pentamidine-associated beta-cell destruction.

Calcium Metabolism

Both hypocalcemia and hypercalcemia have been reported in HIV disease. In one retrospective study of HIV-infected patients, most of whom were injection drug users, 17.9 percent had hypocalcemia and 2.9 percent had hypercalcemia [48]. In acutely ill patients with HIV disease, hypocalcemia can occur from the same mechanisms that have been reported in other types of severe illness, including hypoalbuminemia, increased calcium binding to albumin, and parathyroid hormone resistance [10]. Medications may also result in hypocalcemia. Foscarnet, used in the treatment of CMV infection, forms a complex with ionized calcium, resulting in carpopedal spasm and neuromuscular irritability [49]. Ketoconazole can interfere with the formation of 1,25-dihydroxyvitamin D, causing decreased calcium absorption [10]. Malabsorption of any etiology can also result in vitamin D deficiency. Hypercalcemia is uncommon in HIV-infected patients and is usually caused by a coexistent illness such as lymphoma or human T-cell lymphotropic virus, type I, infection [10].

References

1. Ihde JK, Turnbull AD, Bajorunas DR. Adrenal insufficiency in the cancer patient: Implications for the surgeon. *Br J Surg* 77:1335–1337, 1990.
2. Siu SCB, Kitzman DW, Sheedy PF, Northcutt RC. Adrenal insufficiency from bilateral hemorrhage. *Mayo Clin Proc* 65:664–670, 1990.
3. Gamelin E, Beldent V, Rousselet MC, et al. Non-Hodgkin's lymphoma presenting with primary adrenal insufficiency. *Cancer* 69:2333–2336, 1992.
4. Donovan DS, Dluhy RG. AIDS and its effect on the adrenal gland. *Endocrinologist* 1:227–232, 1991.
5. Merenich JA, McDermott MT, Asp AA. Evidence of endocrine involvement early in the course of human HIV infection. *J Clin Endocrinol Metab* 70:566–571, 1990.

6. Villette JM, Bourin P, Doinel C, et al. Circadian variations in plasma levels of hypophyseal, adrenocortical and testicular hormones in men infected with human immunodeficiency virus. *J Clin Endocrinol Metab* 70:572–577, 1990.
7. Membreno L, Irony J, Dere W, et al. Adrenocortical function in AIDS. *J Clin Endocrinol Metab* 65:482–487, 1987.
8. Rain F, Brisseau JM, Planchon B, et al. Endocrine function in 98 HIV-infected patients. A prospective study. *AIDS* 5:729–733, 1991.
9. Dluhy RG. The growing spectrum of HIV-related endocrine abnormalities. *J Clin Endocrinol Metab* 90:563–564, 1990.
10. Grinspoon SK, Bilezikian JP. HIV disease and the endocrine system. *N Engl J Med* 327:1360–1365, 1992.
11. Norbiato G, Berilaqua M, Vago T, et al. Cortisol resistance in acquired immunodeficiency syndrome. *J Clin Endocrinol Metab* 74:608–613, 1992.
12. Groll A, Schneider M, Althoff PH, et al. The morphology and clinical significance of pathologic changes of the adrenals and hypophysis in AIDS [German]. *Dtsche Med Wochenschr* 115:483–488, 1990.
13. Jautzke G, Sell M, Thalman U, et al. Extracerebral toxoplasmosis in AIDS—histological and immunohistological findings based on 80 autopsy cases. *Pathol Res Pract* 189:428–436, 1993.
14. Tang WW, Kaptein EM, Feinstein EL, Massey SG. Hyponatremia in hospitalized patients with AIDS and the AIDS-related complex. *Am J Med* 94:169–174, 1993.
15. Faber M, Flachs H, Frimodt-Moller N, Lindholm J. Hyponatremia and adrenocortical function in patients with severe bacterial infections. *Scand J Infect Dis* 25:101–105, 1993.
16. Loprinzi CL, Jensen MD, Jiang NS, Schaid DJ. Effect of megestrol acetate on the human pituitary axis. *Mayo Cln Proc* 67:1160–1162, 1992.
17. Oelkers W, Diederich S, Bahr V. Diagnosis and therapy surveillance in Addison's disease—rapid ACTH test and measurement of plasma ACTH, renin activity, and aldosterone. *J Clin Endocrinol Metab* 75:259–264, 1992.
18. Trainer PJ, McHardy KC, Harvey RD, Reid LW. Urinary free cortisol in the assessment of hydrocortisone replacement therapy. *Horm Metab Res* 25:117–120, 1993.
19. Battan R, Mariuz P, Raviglione MC, et al. *Pneumocystis carinii* infection of the thyroid in a hypothyroid patient with AIDS: Diagnosis by fine needle aspiration. *J Clin Endocrinol Metab* 72:724–726, 1991.
20. Drucker DJ, Bailey D, Rotstein L. Thyroiditis as the presenting manifestation of disseminated extrapulmonary *Pneumocystis carinii* infection. *J Clin Endocrinol Metab* 71:1663–1665, 1990.
21. Lopresti JS, Fried JC, Spencer CA, Nicoloff JT. Unique alterations of thyroid hormone indices in AIDS. *Ann Intern Med* 110:970–975, 1989.
22. Lambert M, Zech F, DeNayer P, et al. Elevation of TBG in association with progression of HIV infection. *Am J Med* 89:748–751, 1990.
23. Feldt-Rasmussen U, Sestoft L, Berg H. Thyroid function tests in patients with AIDS and healthy HIV1-positive outpatients. *Eur J Clin Invest* 21:59–63, 1991.
24. Grumfeld C, Pang M, Doerrler W, et al. Indices of thyroid function and weight loss in HIV infections and AIDS. *Meta Clin Exp* 42:1270–1276, 1993.

25. Docter R, Krenning EP, de Jong M, Hennemann G. The sick euthyroid syndrome: Changes in thyroid hormone serum parameters and hormone metabolism (review). *Clin Endocrinol (Oxf)* 39:499–518, 1993.
26. Grampolmo A, Buiffa P, Quajlia AC. AIDS pathology: Various critical considerations [Italian]. *Pathologica* 82:663–677, 1992.
27. Mosca L, Costanzi G, Antonacci C, et al. Hypophyseal pathology in AIDS. *Histol Histopathol* 7:291–300, 1992.
28. Dobs AE, Dempsey MA, Ladenso PW, et al. Endocrine disorders in men infected with HIV. *Am J Med* 84:611–616, 1988.
29. Croxson TS, Chapman WE, Miller LK, et al. Changes in the HPA axis in HIV-infected homosexual men. *J Clin Endocrinol Metab* 68:317–321, 1989.
30. Couderc LJ, Clauvel JP. HIV-induced gynecomastia. *Ann Intern Med* 107:257, 1987.
31. Krieger JN, Coombs RW, Collier AC, et al. Fertility parameters in men infected with HIV. *J Infect Dis* 164:464–469, 1991.
32. Woolf PD, Hamill RW, McDonald JV, et al. Transient hypogonadotrophic hypogonadism caused by severe illness. *J Clin Endocrinol Metab* 60:444–450, 1985.
33. Pudney J, Anderson D. Orchitis and HIV type 1 infected cells in reproductive tissues from men with AIDS. *Am J Pathol* 139:149–160, 1991.
34. Dalton AD, Harcourt-Webster JN. The histopathology of the testes and epididymis in AIDS—a post-mortem study. *J Pathol* 163:47–52, 1991.
35. da Silva M, Shevchuk MM, Cronin WJ, et al. Detection of HIV-related protein in testes and prostates of patients with AIDS. *Am J Clin Pathol* 93:196–201, 1990.
36. DePaepe ME, Guerrieri C, Waxman M. Opportunistic infections of the testis in AIDS. *Mt Sinai J Med* 57:25–29, 1990.
37. Schrijvers D, Delaport E, Peeters M, et al. Sero-prevalence of retroviral infection in women with different fertility statuses in Gabon. *J Acquir Immune Defic Syndr* 4:468–470, 1991.
38. Simonsen JN, Plummer FA, Ngugi EN, et al. HIV infection among lower SES prostitutes in Nairobi. *AIDS* 4:139–144, 1990.
39. Ryder RW, Baiter VL, Nsuami M, et al. Fertility rates in 238 HIV-1 seropositive women in Zaire followed for 3 years postpartum. *AIDS* 5:1521–1527, 1991.
40. Smith PF, Mikl J, Truman BI, et al. HIV infection entering the New York State Correctional System. *Am J Public Health* 81 (suppl):35–40, 1991.
41. Schwartz MS, Brandt LJ. The spectrum of pancreatic disorders in patients with AIDS. *Am J Gastroenterol* 84:459–462, 1989.
42. Wood G, Metzig N, Hogan P, Whitby M. Survival from pentamidine-induced pancreatitis and diabetes mellitus. *Aust N Z J Med* 21:341–342, 1991.
43. Abourizk NN, Lyons RW, Madden GM. Transient state of NIDDM in a patient with AIDS. *Diabetes Care* 16:931–933, 1993.
44. Herchline TE, Plouffe JF, Para MF. Diabetes mellitus presenting as ketoacidosis following pentamidine therapy in patients with AIDS. *J Infect* 22:41–44, 1991.
45. Salinas L, Lucas A, Clotet B. Secondary diabetes induced by megestrol acetate therapy in a patient with AIDS-associated cachexia (letter). *AIDS* 7:894, 1993.

46. Henry K, Rathgaber S, Sullivan C, McCabe K. Diabetes mellitus induced by megestrol acetate in a patient with AIDS and cachexia. *Ann Intern Med* 116:53, 1992.
47. Perronne C, Bricaire F, Leport C, et al. Hypoglycemia and diabetes mellitus following parenteral pentamidine mesylate treatment in AIDS patients. *Diabetic Med* 7:585–589, 1990.
48. Peter SA. Disorders of serum calcium in AIDS. J *Natl Med Assoc* 84:626–828, 1992.
49. Jacobson MA, Gambertoglio JG, Aweeka FL, et al. Foscarnet-induced hypocalcemia and effects on calcium metabolism. *J Clin Endocrinol Metab* 72:1130, 1991.

Neurologic Manifestations   *17*

Nagagopal Venna

Manifestations of HIV disease involving the central, peripheral, and autonomic nervous systems are protean [1, 2] (Table 17-1). Disorders characteristic of primary HIV infection include acute aseptic meningitis and encephalitis, demyelinating polyneuropathy, and acute mononeuropathy; HIV encephalopathy, vacuolar myelopathy, distal symmetric polyneuropathy, and opportunistic infections and neoplasms generally occur with advanced HIV disease. Many neurologic disturbances in HIV-infected patients improve in response to therapeutic intervention. As patients live longer with lower CD4 lymphocyte counts, the rate of neurologic complications appears to be rising [3].

HIV Meningoencephalitides

See Table 17-2 for a list of brain and meningeal disorders associated with HIV disease.

Chronic Asymptomatic Meningitis

Human immunodeficiency virus penetrates the blood-brain barrier early in the course of infection, as demonstrated by the presence of increased cerebrospinal fluid (CSF) mononuclear cells and protein, oligoclonal immunoglobulins, and positive HIV culture. While meningeal inflammation persists throughout the course of the disease, the factors affecting neurologic progression are unknown.

Acute Meningitis

Acute meningitis may appear during HIV seroconversion, presenting as fever, myalgias, headache, neck stiffness, and rarely, transient Bell's

241

Table 17-1 *Neurologic manifestations of HIV disease*

Brain and meninges
  HIV-related meningoencephalitides
  Opportunistic infections
  Neoplasms
  Stroke syndrome
  Seizure disorder
Spinal cord
  HIV-related vacuolar myelopathy
  Acute myelopathy due to opportunistic infections
Peripheral nerves
  Distal symmetric polyneuropathy
  Drug-induced symmetric neuropathy
  Bell's palsy
  Neuralgic amyotrophy
  Mononeuritis multiplex
  Lumbosacral polyradiculopathy
  Demyelinating polyneuropathies
  Autonomic neuropathy

Table 17-2 *Brain and meningeal disorders in HIV disease*

HIV infection
  Chronic asymptomatic meningitis*
  Acute meningitis
  Acute encephalitis
  HIV encephalopathy*

Opportunistic infections
  Viral infections
    Cytomegalovirus encephalitis
    Varicella-zoster virus meningoencephalitis
    Herpes simplex virus encephalitis
    Progressive multifocal leukoencephalopathy*
  Protozoal infections
    Toxoplasmic encephalitis*
    Chagas' disease
    Amebic encephalitis
  Fungal infections
    Cryptococcosis*
    Mucormycosis
    Aspergillosis
    Candidiasis
  Bacterial infections
    Nocardiosis
    Tuberculosis*
    Syphilis*
    Bacillary angiomatosis

Neoplastic diseases
  Lymphoma, primary and metastatic*
  Kaposi's sarcoma

*Most common disorders.

palsy [4]. Cerebrospinal fluid analysis shows lymphocytosis, moderately increased protein level, normal glucose concentration, and positive HIV culture. Clinical recovery generally occurs within 2 weeks, but the syndrome may recrudesce periodically.

Acute Encephalitis

Acute encephalitis is rarely associated with HIV seroconversion and manifests as fever, malaise, confusion, lethargy, seizures, and focal neurologic signs evolving over a few days [5]. Cerebrospinal fluid analysis shows mild lymphocytosis, increased protein level, and normal glucose concentration; radiologic imaging of the brain is not revealing. Patients recover spontaneously.

HIV Encephalopathy

This common and progressive complication of HIV infection usually becomes evident in patients with advanced disease but may present earlier [6, 7]. Pathologic abnormalities, identified in approximately 90 percent of patients dying from AIDS, include demyelination, accumulation of mononuclear cells, microglial nodules, and multinucleated cells in the subcortical gray and white matter. HIV antigens are demonstrable in macrophages, monocytes, microglia, oligodendrocytes, astrocytes, and capillary endothelial cells but not in neurons. Specifically how HIV infection produces neurologic derangement remains unknown. Cytokines released by HIV-infected macrophages, the HIV gp120 viral envelope protein, and breakdown of the blood-brain barrier probably all contribute to this process. Characteristic pathologic changes are not found in asymptomatic individuals with HIV infection who die from unrelated causes [8].

The syndrome begins with insidious alteration of behavior, intellect, and motor control. Behavioral changes are usually noted by family and friends as a decline in spontaneity and drive resembling depression. Cognitive changes lead to difficulty in tasks that demand sustained concentration and complex sequential steps. Later, memory becomes increasingly impaired. These changes are punctuated or sometimes brought to light by dramatic psychosis [9]. Mania, acute schizophreniform illness with bizarre behavior, suicidal ideation, and labile affect have all been described. The patient experiences gradual disintegration of motor skills: Hands become clumsy, gait is slowed and unsteady, and eye movements lose normal smoothness in pursuit.

In the early stages of HIV encephalopathy, neuropsychological tests may help detect subtle changes of memory, concentration, and frontal system function, such as speed of processing information and sequential complex tasks. The impairment of ocular pursuit, decrease in rapid fine finger movements, and other early signs of upper motor neuron system dysfunction provide supportive evidence for the diagnosis. Computed tomographic (CT) and magnetic resonance imaging (MRI) scans show diffuse and progressive cerebral gyral atrophy, dilatation of ventricles, and patchy abnormal signals in subcortical white and gray matter (Fig. 17-1). Electroencephalography (EEG) shows nonspecific slowing over the hemispheres, and positron emission tomographic (PET) and single-photon emission computed tomographic (SPECT) scans may indicate subcortical hypometabolism. Cerebrospinal fluid analysis reveals mononuclear pleocytosis, modestly increased protein level, and sometimes oligoclonal bands.

Although nonspecific, the clinical picture of dementia without decreased alertness is characteristic of HIV encephalopathy. Differential diagnosis includes depression, infectious and neoplastic diseases of the central nervous system (CNS), and toxic and drug-induced encephalopathies. Zidovudine (ZDV) has produced modest clinical improvement in some patients as documented by brain metabolic mapping studies [10]. The efficacy of other antiretroviral agents is unknown. Careful use of tricyclic antidepressant drugs, methylphenidate (to treat apathy), and neuroleptics may be helpful in ameliorating symptoms.

Figure 17-1. Computed tomographic scan of cerebral atrophy associated with HIV encephalopathy. (From DM Barnes. AIDS-related brain damage unexplained. *Science* 232:1091–1093. Copyright 1986 by the American Association for the Advancement of Science.)

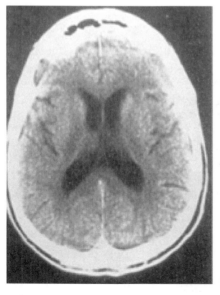
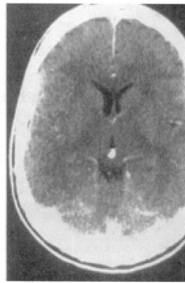

Meningoencephalitides Caused by Opportunistic Infections

Cytomegalovirus Encephalitis

Cytomegalovirus (CMV) encephalitis is a common pathologic finding in patients who died from AIDS [11]. Microglial nodules, some of which contain CMV, are scattered in the subcortical gray and white matter, accompanied by multifocal parenchymal necrosis without inflammation. This syndrome is more commonly associated with advanced HIV disease, often in the context of CMV retinitis [12]. It evolves subacutely over a few weeks, with fever and encephalopathy characterized by confusion, disorientation, and forgetfulness. Cranial neuropathies of the third, fifth, sixth, seventh, and eighth nerves may accompany the dementia, a feature that is rare in HIV encephalopathy. Brain CT and MRI scans are generally nonfocal, but may show periventricular and meningeal enhancement due to ventriculitis and small multifocal subcortical lesions. The CSF reveals lymphocytosis, increased CMV antibody titers, and occasionally, a positive CMV culture. In a third of patients, CMV can be identified by polymerase chain reaction (PCR) testing of the CSF, and the CSF glucose level may be low. While the antiviral agent ganciclovir, used in the treatment of CMV retinitis, penetrates the brain well, its role in the management of encephalitis has not been established. The therapeutic efficacy of foscarnet is also unknown.

Varicella-Zoster Virus Meningoencephalitis

Varicella-zoster virus (VZV) encephalitis is characterized pathologically by multifocal demyelination, necrosis, and thrombosis with viral antigens and inclusions in neurons and glia [13]. This rare illness manifests as the subacute onset of confusion, lethargy, memory impairment, upper motor neuron paresis, and ataxia [14]. Brain CT and MRI scans may be normal or show multifocal white and gray matter lesions. Cerebrospinal fluid abnormalities are nonspecific, and VZV antibodies are rarely present. Brain biopsy and culture are necessary for definitive diagnosis. Therapy with acyclovir may be beneficial but has not been demonstrated to be effective.

Herpes Simplex Virus Encephalitis

Herpes simplex virus (HSV) may coinfect the CNS with CMV in patients with advanced HIV disease, but the focal, frontotemporal encephalitis characteristic of HSV infection in immunocompetent patients has not been documented.

Progressive Multifocal Leukoencephalopathy

Progressive multifocal leukoencephalopathy (PML) is caused by JC virus infection of oligodendroglia. This previously rare condition affects approximately 3 percent of AIDS patients, resulting in large patches of demyelination without inflammation in the cerebral, brainstem, and cerebellar white matter [15, 16]. Patients have hemiparesis, dysarthria, hemianopsia, cortical blindness, cerebellar ataxia, evidence of brainstem dysfunction, and dementia, but remain alert and without seizures. Computed tomographic scan shows hypodense, nonenhancing white matter lesions. Magnetic resonance imaging demonstrates distinctive abnormalities in the subcortical region, including sparing of the cortex, lack of mass effect, predilection to periventricular areas, and lack of contrast enhancement (Fig. 17-2). Cerebrospinal fluid analysis is typically normal, and EEG often reveals delta wave slowing. Brain biopsy, necessary for definitive diagnosis, shows demyelination, axonal sparing with bizarre astrocytes, and viral particles in the oligodendrocytes. No treatment has been demonstrated effective, although anecdotal reports of improvement with alpha-interferon, acyclovir, and adenine arabinoside have been described. Patients generally experience a progressive downhill course over months, but extended survival and spon-

Figure 17-2. Progressive multifocal leukoencephalopathy on T2-weighted MRI of the brain. The image on the left shows an extensive area of abnormal high signal in the cerebellar peduncles; the image on the right shows high signal in the white matter of the pons.

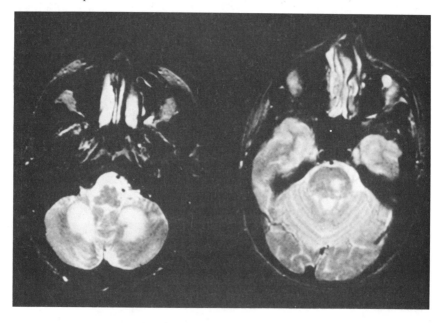

taneous clinical improvement have been reported in some cases [17, 18].

Toxoplasmic Encephalitis

Toxoplasmosis, which causes a multifocal necrotizing encephalitis, is the most common opportunistic infection of the brain in AIDS, affecting approximately 10 percent of patients [19]. Clinical manifestations include headache, confusion, lethargy, and less commonly, focal abnormalities, such as seizures, hemiparesis, gait ataxia, hemiballismus, and evidence of brainstem dysfunction. Brain CT scan shows single or multiple, noncalcified mass lesions with contrast enhancement (Fig. 17-3); gadolinium-enhanced MRI appears to be even more sensitive. Most patients with cerebral toxoplasmosis have detectable serum *Toxoplasma* antibodies; the role of CSF antibodies is uncertain. Brain biopsy, although necessary for definitive diagnosis, is generally performed only in patients who fail to respond to therapy.

Empiric treatment with pyrimethamine/sulfadiazine is indicated when toxoplasmic encephalitis is suggested by clinical and radiologic findings (see Chap. 22). Improvement usually occurs within days to a couple of weeks of initiation of therapy. Dexamethasone should be administered if clinically significant cerebral edema is present, although its indiscriminate use may obscure the diagnostic value of empiric antimicrobial therapy. Chronic maintenance therapy with reduced doses of the antimicrobial drugs used for initial management is necessary to prevent relapse.

Cryptococcal Meningitis

Cryptococcus neoformans causes a subacute or chronic basal meningitis, with occasional involvement of the lumbosacral, cervical, or thoracic meninges and nerve roots [20]. The basal meningitis may lead to hydrocephalus, intracranial hypertension, and cranial nerve palsies.

Cryptococcal meningitis is manifested by headache, lethargy, confusion, and numbness and weakness in the extremities; neck stiffness is frequently absent. Papilledema, blindness, and deafness may occur. Cerebral granulomas or cysts may cause progressive hemiparesis or other focal signs. Brain CT and MRI scans are generally normal, but granulomas are occasionally seen. Diagnosis is made by lumbar puncture with CSF analysis, which shows variable pleocytosis, increased protein level, and/or decreased glucose concentration. Cerebrospinal fluid cryptococcal antigen and India ink preparation findings are usually positive, and organisms can be readily cultured. In some patients, very high CSF pressure develops without hydrocephalus by an unknown mechanism.

Amphotericin B or fluconazole is used for primary treatment; fluconazole is the drug of choice for maintenance therapy (see Chap.

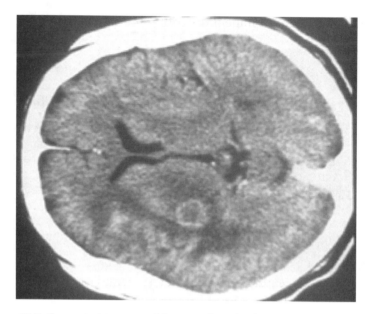

Figure 17-3. Computed tomographic scan of cerebral toxoplasmosis.

21). In patients with progressive obtundation and visual failure associated with high CSF pressure without hydrocephalus, large-volume spinal taps or lumboperitoneal shunt should be attempted [21]. Obstructive hydrocephalus is managed by ventricular drainage with a CSF reservoir or ventriculoperitoneal shunt.

Cerebral Mucormycosis

Cerebral mucormycosis is a rare cause of focal necrotizing encephalitis that should be considered in HIV-infected patients who inject drugs [22]. The clinical presentation is nonspecific. Brain scans show focal mass lesions, and organisms cannot generally be recovered from the CSF. Unlike mucormycosis associated with diabetic ketoacidosis, paranasal sinusitis and orbital cellulitis are typically absent in HIV-infected patients. Diagnosis is by brain biopsy with methenamine silver stain, which shows nonseptate hyphae with right-angled branches. Treatment consists of amphotericin B.

Cerebral Aspergillosis

Cerebral aspergillosis is a focal encephalitis that is uncommon in AIDS, developing in the context of severe systemic illness and broad-spectrum antibiotic therapy [23]. Fulminant hemorrhagic infarction of the brain with prominent invasion of blood vessels by the fungus is characteristic. Diagnosis is generally by brain biopsy, although repeated CSF examinations, especially by cisternal tap, may sometimes reveal the pathogen. Therapy is with amphotericin B, but the prognosis is poor.

Candidal Encephalitis

Only a few cases of candidal abscesses of the CNS have been described in AIDS patients despite the high prevalence of mucocutaneous candidiasis in HIV infection. The clinical picture is nonspecific, with brain imaging studies showing multiple small abscesses. *Candida albicans* is often cultured from the blood and CSF. Amphotericin B is the drug of choice.

Nocardial Encephalitis

Nocardial abscesses have been documented in AIDS but are unusual [24]. Clinical features and CSF analysis are nonspecific, and brain scans show focal ring-like abscesses. Diagnosis is made by biopsy of the brain or other involved sites. Antibiotic therapy with trimethoprim-sulfamethoxazole or sulfonamides is effective, but surgical excision may be necessary for large multiloculated lesions.

Mycobacterial Infection

Extrapulmonary infection with *Mycobacterium tuberculosis* is commonly associated with HIV infection [25]. Neurologic involvement is characterized by subacute basal meningitis complicated by cranial nerve palsies, hydrocephalus, and infectious arteritis leading to brain infarction. Brain tuberculomas and abscesses may occur with or without meningitis. Pulmonary disease may not be evident, and the response to the tuberculosis skin test (purified protein derivative) and controls may be negative with advanced immunodeficiency.

Fever, headache, confusion, lethargy, and cranial nerve palsies steadily progress over days. Sudden stroke syndrome may be the presenting feature or punctuate the illness, and seizures are common with intra-cerebral tuberculomas. Brain CT and MRI scans often reveal basal meningeal enhancement, obstructive hydrocephalus, focal hypo-densities due to brain infarction, granulomas with or without calcification, and rarely, abscesses. Cerebrospinal fluid analysis shows progressive lymphocytic pleocytosis, increased protein level, and decreased glucose concentration. Acid-fast stains rarely reveal the organism, but CSF culture is generally positive. Occasionally, brain biopsy may be necessary for diagnosis.

Treatment should be started promptly based on the clinical presentation and CSF analysis pending definitive diagnosis (see Chap. 20).

Combination antituberculous drug therapy with isoniazid, rifampin, ethambutol, and pyrazinamide is indicated pending culture and drug sensitivity testing results. Corticosteroids may have a role in the management of severe meningitis. Clinical and radiologic improvement generally occurs within a few weeks of initiation of therapy.

Syphilitic Meningoencephalitis

Central nervous system infection with *Treponema pallidum* in HIV-infected patients may be asymptomatic or present with acute meningitis, meningitis with cerebral vasculitis, or encephalitis [25]. In the meningovascular form, obliterative vasculitis of the small and the penetrating arteries causes small lacunar infarctions. In the rare encephalitic form, characterized by dementia, seizures, and myoclonus, there is diffuse infection of the brain. Some HIV-infected patients with syphilis may have atypical clinical manifestations, accelerated disease progression, false-negative results on serologic studies, and inadequate therapeutic responses to conventional antibiotic regimens [26, 27].

Acute syphilitic meningitis causes fever, headache, neck stiffness, and sometimes, cranial nerve palsies, especially of the second and eighth nerves; conjunctivitis, uveitis, and retinitis may accompany the neurologic syndrome. Cerebrospinal fluid examination shows lymphocytosis, increased protein level, and decreased glucose level, and the CSF VDRL test result is generally positive. Meningovascular syphilis is most often characterized by the abrupt onset of hemiplegia, but a variety of cerebral and brainstem syndromes have also been noted. Brain CT and MRI scans show focal infarctions, especially of the basis pontis and internal capsule.

Syphilis should be considered in the differential diagnosis of any HIV-related neurologic problem, and serum and CSF serologies should always be obtained (see Chap. 23). Nervous system involvement may be associated with other manifestations of syphilis or occur in isolation. Conventional treatment of neurosyphilis consists of parenteral penicillin G, 12 to 24 million units per day for 10 to 14 days, followed by benzathine penicillin, 2.4 million units given intramuscularly for 3 consecutive weeks. Persons who are allergic to penicillin should be desensitized. Patients diagnosed with syphilis should be monitored clinically and serologically following completion of their treatment regimen.

Miscellaneous Infections

A case of focal encephalitis caused by the protozoan *Trypanosoma cruzi* was described in an AIDS patient who came from an endemic area [28]. Temporal lobe bacillary angiomatosis was reported in a patient who had a characteristic skin lesion [29]. Biopsy of skin and brain lesions confirmed the presence of microvascular proliferation of pleomorphic bacilli, and the condition responded to erythromycin therapy. Focal hemorrhagic encephalitis caused by ameba also has been described in association with HIV infection [30].

Neoplastic Meningoencephalopathies

Primary CNS Lymphoma

Primary B-cell brain lymphoma occurs in approximately 5 to 10 percent of patients with AIDS but is an otherwise rare tumor [31]. Highly malignant and multicentric, it has a predilection for the basal ganglia, thalami, and periventricular regions. The tumor presents with headache, lethargy, and confusion, sometimes accompanied by hemiparesis and cerebellar or brainstem dysfunction. The patient experiences steady clinical deterioration over a few weeks, with increasing obtundation secondary to infiltrating tumor or hydrocephalus, or both. Brain CT and MRI scans show single or multiple lesions with minimal mass effect (Fig. 17-4). Following administration of contrast material, there is diffuse irregular enhancement of the mass and sometimes, ventricular lining. In approximately 25 percent of patients, immunocytology of the CSF reveals monoclonal malignant cells. Definitive diagnosis requires

Figure 17-4. Primary central nervous system lymphoma on an MRI of the brain. The image on the left shows a large gadolinium-enhanced lesion of the frontal lobe with surrounding edema; the image on the right is without enhancement.

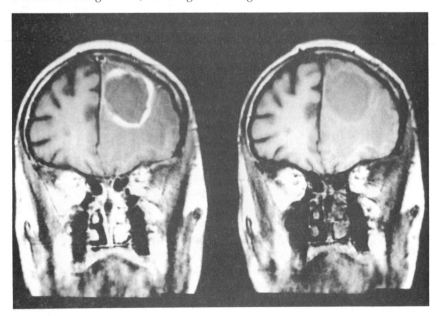

brain biopsy, although diagnosis is sometimes made presumptively on the basis of clinical and radiologic features. Dexamethasone combined with radiation treatment is used for palliation, but the survival time rarely exceeds 3 months.

Metastatic Lymphoma

Systemic lymphoma may spread to the brain and meninges. Meningeal lymphomatosis presents with multiple cranial and extremity nerve palsies and may be complicated by obstructive hydrocephalus. Cytologic examination of CSF reveals malignant cells. Intrathecal methotrexate and cytosine arabinoside have been used therapeutically.

Kaposi's Sarcoma

Central nervous system involvement with Kaposi's sarcoma is very rare and is manifested by the rapid onset of focal neurologic signs [32]. Brain CT scan shows multiple, hemorrhagic nodules with mass effect, but definitive diagnosis requires brain biopsy. There are no data available regarding the efficacy of therapy.

Stroke Syndrome

HIV-infected patients have a markedly increased incidence of stroke. Cerebral infarctions may be sequelae to infectious vasculitis of mycobacterial, treponemal, viral, or cryptococcal origin, or to embolism from endocarditis [33]. Thrombocytopenia, commonly seen in HIV disease, may predispose to intracerebral hemorrhage. In some patients, cerebral infarction occurs without a specific identifiable etiology and is ascribed to an "HIV arteriopathy." The CSF should be examined for evidence of infection in all HIV-infected patients who present with stroke.

Seizure Disorder

Seizure activity occurs frequently in HIV infection and may be a presenting symptom of neurologic disease [34]. In approximately 50 percent of patients, it indicates the presence of a focal meningoencephalitis. In about 25 percent, it is a manifestation of HIV encephalopathy, and in the remaining patients, no specific cause can be found. Although seizure activity generally responds well to conventional anticonvulsive agents, HIV-infected patients seem to have an unusually high incidence of hypersensitivity reactions to phenytoin. Carbamazepine and valproic acid should be used with caution in this population because of the frequent coexistence of bone marrow and liver dysfunction. Newer anticonvulsant drugs with less overall toxicity, such as gabapentin, may be preferable.

Diagnostic Approach to Meningoencephalitis

Because clinical manifestations are often nonspecific, all HIV-infected patients with evidence of significant CNS dysfunction should undergo brain CT with contrast or MRI with gadolinium, followed by lumbar puncture with CSF analysis (Table 17-3). Syphilis and *Toxoplasma* serologies should be performed, and a PPD with appropriate controls placed. Psychiatric examination or neuropsychological testing, or both, are also indicated if depression is part of the differential diagnosis. Injection drug and alcohol abuse histories should be reviewed, as both intoxication and withdrawal syndromes may result in altered mental states. Toxicity from prescription medications should also be considered.

Table 17-3 *Evaluation of HIV-related meningoencephalitis*

History
    History of syphilis, tuberculosis
    Vegetative symptoms of depression
    Injection drug use
    Alcoholism
    Medication toxicity

Physical examination
    Alteration in mental status
    Focal neurologic findings

Laboratory evaluation
    CD4 cell count
    Syphilis serologies
    Toxoplasma serology
    PPD and controls
    Neuropsychological testing
    Brain CT with contrast or MRI with gadolinium
    Lumbar puncture with CSF analysis
        Cell count
        Glucose, protein
        Gram's, acid-fast, India ink stains
        Bacterial, mycobacterial, fungal cultures
        Cryptococcal antigen
        VDRL
    Brain biopsy*

*Indicated only if the diagnosis is uncertain based on less invasive tests or if clinical progression occurs despite empiric therapy.

Opportunistic infections of the CNS are more common with advanced immunodeficiency (CD4 cell count < 200/mm^3), and patients with suspected toxoplasmosis or tuberculosis should be treated empirically. Brain biopsy is indicated if the diagnosis remains uncertain or if clinical progression occurs despite empiric therapy. Stereotactic technique permits biopsy of even deep brain lesions with little morbidity and is quite safe in the absence of a bleeding diathesis. Specimens should be examined with fungal, acid-fast, and immunoperoxidase stains, by dark-field microscopy for spirochetes, and by electron microscopy for viral inclusions.

Spinal Cord Syndromes

The most common spinal cord syndrome associated with HIV infection is subacute vacuolar myelopathy. Rare cases of acute myelitis are caused by VZV, HSV, CMV, and *Toxoplasma gondii,* and as a complication of tuberculous and syphilitic meningitides.

Vacuolar Myelopathy

The striking pathologic picture seen with vacuolar myelopathy resembles subacute combined degeneration of the spinal cord related to vitamin B$_{12}$ deficiency, with vacuolation of the lateral and posterior columns, minimal inflammation, and no vascular changes [35]. HIV antigen has been identified in macrophages.

Vascuolar myelopathy may be overshadowed clinically by HIV encephalopathy and peripheral neuropathy, but presents as a subacute spastic, ataxic paraparesis associated with upper motor neuron signs and impaired proprioception in the limbs. A mass lesion should be ruled out by MRI with gadolinium, and CSF analysis should be performed to exclude syphilis and tuberculosis. The role of antiretroviral therapy has not been examined in a controlled fashion, although one case report suggested improvement with ZDV [36].

Acute Myelopathies

Although rare, acute myelopathies are important because some are potentially treatable [37–40]. Patients have rapidly developing paraparesis, bladder and bowel incontinence, and a transverse sensory level. VZV myelitis is suggested by its association with shingles. MRI of the spinal cord with gadolinium may reveal epidural abscess in the drug-using patient or focal swelling suggesting *Toxoplasma* or tuberculous myelitis. Cerebrospinal fluid examination should be performed to rule out syphilis, tuberculosis, or CMV infection as the cause.

Peripheral Neuropathies

A variety of peripheral nerve disorders have been reported in HIV infection [41].

Distal Symmetric Polyneuropathy

Distal symmetric polyneuropathy is a common neuropathy of unknown etiology that is characterized pathologically by diffuse axonal loss with variable lymphocytic infiltration and HIV antigen in the axoplasm and mononuclear cells. It presents insidiously with prominent paresthesias and shooting pains in the lower extremities accompanied by contact hypersensitivity. Physical findings may be minimal early in the disorder, with reduction in proprioception and diminished ankle reflexes, but later sensory impairment occurs in a stocking and glove distribution. Motor abnormalities are unusual. Nerve conduction velocity tests and electromyography (EMG) demonstrate a symmetric, predominantly axonal neuropathy with decreased sensory action potentials. Cerebrospinal fluid analysis may show mild pleocytosis and increased protein level, and sural nerve biopsy reveals nonspecific axonal degeneration. Other causes of neuropathy, such as alcoholism and neurotoxic drugs, should be considered in the differential diagnosis.

The neuropathy has an indolent course and may stabilize spontaneously. One report suggested that ZDV therapy may be beneficial [42]. Treatment of pain and dysesthesia is challenging. Tricyclic antidepressant drugs, such as amitriptyline, doxepin, and desipramine, given in modest doses are often helpful. Carbamazepine, clonazepam, baclofen, phenytoin, mexiletine, and acupuncture have been used alternatively. In severe cases, narcotic analgesics may be necessary.

Drug-Induced Symmetric Polyneuropathy

This predominantly sensory polyneuropathy is a common toxicity of the antiretroviral agents ddI, zalcitabine (formerly dideoxycytidine or ddC), stavudine (d4T), and lamivudine (3TC) [43]. Significant symptoms may necessitate discontinuation of the drug but take weeks to months to abate. Vincristine, used in the treatment of Kaposi's sarcoma, is associated with a similar dose-dependent, reversible polyneuropathy. Isoniazid, lithium carbonate, and dapsone are other potential causes of polyneuropathy.

Bell's Palsy

Self-limited unilateral or bilateral Bell's palsy may develop with primary HIV infection, sometimes in association with aseptic meningitis.

Neuralgic Amyotrophy

A syndrome of self-limited unilateral or bilateral shoulder girdle neuropathy may also develop during HIV seroconversion. Intense pain in the shoulders is followed by rapid development of weakness and atrophy of the girdle muscles. Weakness of the serratus anterior, associated with winging of the scapula, is particularly characteristic.

Mononeuritis Multiplex

In mononeuritis multiplex, an unusual variant of peripheral neuropathy, multiple cranial, limb, and truncal nerves are affected serially over days to weeks in a patchy, scattered pattern. Cerebrospinal fluid analysis is nonspecific; sural nerve biopsy may show mononuclear cell infiltration and occasionally, necrotizing vasculitis. The condition may evolve into a symmetric, diffuse demyelinating polyneuropathy; stabilize; or improve spontaneously. Patients with progressive disease may respond to plasmapheresis, corticosteroids, and intravenous immunoglobulin therapy.

Lumbosacral Polyradiculopathy: Cauda Equina Syndrome

In lumbosacral polyradiculopathy, an unusual and potentially treatable neuropathy, the nerve roots of the cauda equina are affected by a necrotizing vasculitis resulting from CMV infection [44]. Rapidly progressive weakness and numbness of the legs and the perianal area lead to sphincter paralysis. Physical examination shows bilateral asymmetric, areflexic paraparesis and anesthesia over the buttocks. Cerebrospinal fluid analysis is remarkable for polymorphonuclear pleocytosis, increased protein level, decreased glucose concentration, and the presence of CMV antibodies. Cytomegalovirus can be cultured from the CSF, and sural nerve biopsy may reveal CMV inclusions in giant cells. The PCR technique is helpful in detecting CMV in the CSF. Lumbar spine CT scan after intrathecal administration of contrast material and gadolinium-enhanced MRI show thickened lumbosacral nerve roots and enhancement of the lumbar thecal sac. Differential diagnosis includes syphilitic, tuberculous, cryptococcal, and lymphomatous meningoradiculopathies, and toxoplasmosis of the conus medullaris [45]. Empiric treatment with ganciclovir or foscarnet should be initiated based on characteristic clinical and CSF findings, and may prevent progressive neurologic deterioration.

Acute and Chronic Inflammatory Demyelinating Polyneuropathies

These conditions characteristically occur with primary HIV infection. The ascending quadriparesis usually begins in the lower limbs and spreads to the upper extremities, bulbar and facial muscles, and in severe cases, the respiratory muscles. The acute form (Guillain-Barré syndrome) evolves over 2 to 4 weeks, whereas the chronic variety develops over months and has a tendency to relapse. Cerebrospinal fluid analysis shows mononuclear pleocytosis. Nerve conduction velocity testing reveals marked slowing in multiple peripheral nerves. Plasmapheresis accelerates neurologic recovery, and intravenous immunoglobulin therapy has been reported to ameliorate symptoms [46].

Autonomic Neuropathy

Evidence of autonomic dysfunction is being increasingly recognized in HIV-infected patients. Although usually asymptomatic, it may cause orthostatic hypotension, gastrointestinal dysfunction, urinary incontinence, impotence, and rarely, cardiopulmonary arrest [47].

References

1. Snider WD, Simpson DM, Nielsen J. Neurological complications of acquired immunodeficiency syndrome: Analysis of 50 patients. *Ann Neurol* 14:403–418, 1983.
2. McArthur JC. Neurological manifestation of AIDS. *Medicine (Baltimore)* 66:407–437, 1987.
3. Bacellar HB, et al. Temporal trends in the incidence of HIV-1-related neurologic diseases: Multicenter AIDS Cohort Study, 1985–1992. *Neurology* 44:1892–1900, 1994.
4. Hollander H, Stringari S. Human immunodeficiency virus associated meningitis: Clinical course and correlations. *Am J Med* 83:813–815, 1987.
5. Carne CA, Smith A, Elkington SG, et al. Acute encephalopathy coincident with seroconversion for HTLV-III. *Lancet* 2:1206–1208, 1985.
6. Navia BA, Jordan BD, Price RW. The AIDS dementia complex: I. Clinical features. *Ann Neurol* 19:517–524, 1986.
7. Navia BA, Cho ES, Petito CK, et al. AIDS dementia complex: II. Neuropathology. *Ann Neurol* 19:525–535, 1986.
8. Bell JE, et al. Human immunodeficiency virus and the brain: Investigation of virus load (?) and neuropathologic changes in pre-AIDS subjects. *J Infect Dis* 168:818–824, 1993.
9. Perry SW. Organic mental disorders caused by human immunodeficiency virus: Update on early diagnosis and treatment. *Am J Psychiatry* 147:696–710, 1990.
10. Schmitt FA, Bigley JW, McKinnis R, et al. Neuropsychological outcome of zidovudine (AZT) in the treatment of patients with AIDS and AIDS-related complex. *N Engl J Med* 319:1573–1578, 1987.
11. Morgello S, Cho ES, Nielsen S, et al. Cytomegalovirus encephalitis in patients with acquired immunodeficiency syndrome: An autopsy study of 30 cases and a review of the literature. *Hum Pathol* 18:289–297, 1987.

12. Holland NR, Power C, Matthews VP, et al. Cytomegalovirus encephalitis in acquired immunodeficiency syndrome (AIDS). *Neurology* 44:507–514, 1994.
13. Morgello S, Block GA, Price RW, et al. Varicella-zoster leukoencephalitis and cerebral vasculopathy. *Arch Pathol Lab Med* 112:173–177, 1988.
14. Gilden DH, Murray RS, Wellish M, et al. Chronic progressive varicella-zoster encephalitis in an AIDS patient. *Neurology* 38:1150–1153, 1988.
15. Berger JR, Kaszovitz B, Donovan MJ, et al. Progressive multifocal leukoencephalopathy associated with human immunodeficiency virus infection: A review of the literature with a report of sixteen cases. *Ann Intern Med* 107:78–87, 1987.
16. Gillespie SM, et al. Progressive multifocal leukoencephalopathy in persons infected with human immunodeficiency virus, San Francisco, 1981–89. *Ann Neurol* 30:597–604, 1991.
17. Karahalios D, et al. Progressive multifocal leukoencephalopathy in patients with HIV infection: Lack of impact of early diagnosis of stereotactic brain biopsy. *J Acquir Immune Defic Syndr* 5:1030–1038, 1992.
18. Berger JR, Mucke L. Prolonged survival and partial recovery in AIDS associated progressive multifocal leukoencephalopathy. *Neurology* 38:1060–1065, 1988.
19. Luft BJ, Hafner R, Korzum AH, et al. Toxoplasmic encephalitis in patients with acquired immunodeficiency syndrome. *N Engl J Med* 329:995–1000, 1993.
20. Dismukes WE. Cryptococcal meningitis in patients with AIDS: AIDS commentary. *J Infect Dis* 157:624–628, 1988.
21. Denning D, Armstrong RW, Steven DA. Elevated cerebrospinal fluid pressure in patients with cryptococcal meningitis and acquired immunodeficiency syndrome. *Am J Med* 91:267–272, 1991.
22. Cuadrado LM, Guerrero A, Asenjo LG, et al. Cerebral mucormycosis in two cases of acquired immunodeficiency syndrome. *Arch Neurol* 45:109–111, 1988.
23. Woods GL, Goldsmith JC. Aspergillus infection of the central nervous system in patients with acquired immunodeficiency syndrome. *Arch Neurol* 47:181–184, 1990.
24. Adair JC, Beck AC, Apfelbaum RI, et al. Nocardial brain abscess in the acquired immunodeficiency syndrome. *Arch Neurol* 44:548–550, 1987.
25. Berenguer J, Moreno S, Laguna F, et al. Tuberculous meningitis in patients infected with the human immunodeficiency virus. *N Engl J Med* 326:668–672, 1992.
26. Katz DA, Berger JR. Neurosyphilis in acquired immunodeficiency syndrome. *Arch Neurol* 46:895–898, 1989.
27. Musher DM, Hanill RJ, Baughn RE. Effect of human immunodeficiency virus infection on the course of syphilis and on the response to treatment. *Ann Intern Med* 113:872–881, 1990.
28. Gluckstein D, Ciferri F, Ruskin J. Chagas' disease: Another cause of cerebral mass in the acquired immunodeficiency syndrome. *Am J Med* 92:429–432, 1992.
29. Spach DH, Panther LA, Thorning DR, et al. Intracerebral bacillary

angiomatosis in a patient infected with human immunodeficiency virus. *Ann Intern Med* 116:740–742, 1992.

30. Gordner HAR, Martinez AJ, Visvesvara GS, et al. Granulomatous amebic encephalitis in an AIDS patient. *Neurology* 41:1993–1995, 1991.
31. Remick SC, Diamond C, Migliozzi JA, et al. Primary central nervous system lymphoma in patients with and without the acquired immunodeficiency syndrome. *Medicine (Baltimore)* 69:345–360, 1990.
32. Gorin FA, Bale TF, Halks-Miller M, et al. Kaposi sarcoma metastatic to the CNS. *Arch Neurol* 42:162–165, 1985.
33. Engstrom JW, Lowenstein DH, Bredesen DE. Cerebral infarction and transient neurological deficits associated with acquired immunodeficiency syndrome. *Am J Med* 86:528–532, 1989.
34. Wong MC, Suite NDA, Labar DR. Seizures in human immunodeficiency virus infection. *Arch Neurol* 47:640–642, 1990.
35. Petito CK, Mavia BA, Cho ES, et al. Vacuolar myelopathy pathologically resembling subacute combined degeneration in patients with acquired immunodeficiency syndrome. *N Engl J Med* 312:874–879, 1985.
36. Oksenhendler E, Ferchal F, Cadranel J, et al. Zidovudine for HIV-related myelopathy. *Am J Med* 88:65N–66N, 1990.
37. Britton CB, Mesa-Tejada R, Fenoglio CM, et al. A new complication of AIDS: Thoracic myelitis caused by herpes simplex. *Neurology* 35:1071–1074, 1985.
38. Woolsey RM, Chambers TJ, Chung HD, et al. Mycobacterial meningomyelitis associated with human immunodeficiency virus infection. *Arch Neurol* 45:691–693, 1988.
39. Berger JR. Spinal cord syphilis associated with human immunodeficiency virus infection: A treatable myelopathy. *Am J Med* 922:101–103, 1992.
40. Herskovitz S, Siegel SE, Schneider AT, et al. Spinal cord toxoplasmosis in AIDS. *Neurology* 39:1552–1553, 1989.
41. Dalakas MC, Perzeshkpour GH. Neuromuscular disease associated with human immunodeficiency virus infection. *Ann Neurol* 23 (suppl):38–48, 1988.
42. Dalakas MC, Harchoan MD, Spitzer R, et al. Treatment of human immunodeficiency virus-related polyneuropathy with 3-azido-2-3-dideoxythymidine. *Ann Neurol* 23 (suppl):92–94, 1988.
43. Berger AR, Arezzo JC, Achumburg HH, et al. 2',3'-Dideoxycytidine (ddC) toxic neuropathy: A study of fifty-two patients. *Neurology* 43:358–362, 1993.
44. Miller RG, Storey JR, Greco CM. Gancyclovir in the treatment of progressive AIDS-related polyradiculopathy. *Neurology* 40:569–574, 1990.
45. Lanska MJ, Lanska J, Schmidley JW. Syphilitic polyradiculopathy in an HIV-positive man. *Neurology* 38:1277–1301, 1988.
46. Malamut RI, Leopold N, Chester PA, et al. The treatment of HIV associated chronic inflammatory demyelinating polyneuropathy with intravenous immunoglobulin. *Neurology* 42 (suppl 3):355, 1992.
47. Cohen JA, Miller L, Polish L. Orthostatic hypotension in human immunodeficiency virus infection may be the result of generalized autonomic nervous system dysfunction. *J Acquir Immune Defic Syndr* 4:32, 1991.

Neuropsychiatric Manifestations

18

Alexandra Beckett, Marshall Forstein

Altered Mental Status in HIV Infection

HIV-infected patients with neuropsychiatric symptoms require careful clinical assessment. Although psychological problems are common in this population, the assumption should always be that the etiology of mental status abnormalities is central nervous system (CNS) dysfunction. Primary causes ensue directly from HIV infection, while secondary causes derive from opportunistic infections and malignancies, systemic derangements, and treatment complications (Table 18-1). Primary CNS dysfunction is often insidious in onset; a rapid or sudden change in mental state is more likely to represent a secondary disorder. Many causes of neuropsychologic symptoms are treatable or even reversible. These include anemia, hypoxia, electrolyte imbalance, drug toxicities (Table 18-2), and opportunistic infections and malignancies. Individuals with preexisting HIV encephalopathy, even of relatively minor clinical significance, may be particularly vulnerable to the superimposed psychological and neurologic challenges of acute medical illness. The evaluation of altered mental status in the HIV-infected patient is guided by clinical presentation and will often include head computed tomographic (CT) or magnetic resonance imaging (MRI) scan, lumbar puncture, electroencephalography (EEG), and neuropsychological testing.

HIV-Related Neurocognitive Disease

By 1982, clinicians noted a syndrome of depression, apathy, and social withdrawal that was often associated with AIDS. It was suspected that

Table 18-1 *Causes of altered mental status in the HIV-infected patient*

HIV-related syndromes
   Primary infection
   HIV encephalopathy
Infections
   Bacterial (tuberculosis, syphilis)
   Fungal (cryptococcosis, candidiasis)
   Parasitic (toxoplasmosis)
   Viral (herpes simplex, cytomegalovirus)
Neoplasms
   Primary or metastatic lymphoma
   Kaposi's sarcoma (rarely)
Cerebrovascular disease
Toxic/metabolic disorders
   Drug-related neurotoxicities
   Anemia
   Nutritional deficiencies
   Dehydration
   Hypoxia secondary to pulmonary disease
   Adrenal insufficiency
   Renal disease
   Hepatic encephalopathy
Psychiatric disorders
   Adjustment disorder
   Major depression/bipolar disorder
   Psychosis
   Anxiety disorders
   Substance abuse disorders

Table 18-2 *Neuropsychiatric side effects of medications*

Drug	Neuropsychiatric effects
Acyclovir	Visual hallucinations, depersonalization, tearfulness, confusion, hyperesthesia, hyperacusia, thought insertion, insomnia, agitation
Amphotericin B	Delirium, peripheral neuropathy, diplopia, weight loss, loss of appetite
Corticosteroids	Depression, euphoria, psychosis
Ganciclovir	Manic psychosis, agitation, delirium, irritability
Alpha-interferon	Depression, weakness
Isoniazid	Depression, agitation, hallucinations, paranoia, impaired memory
Methotrexate	Encephalopathy (high dose)
Pentamidine	Hypoglycemia, hypotension (leading to CNS dysfunction)
Procarbazine	Mania, loss of appetite, insomnia, nightmares, confusion, malaise
Trimethoprim-sulfamethoxazole	Depression, loss of appetite, insomnia, apathy, headache
Vinblastine	Depression, loss of appetite, headache
Vincristine	Hallucinations, headache, ataxia, sensory loss, depression, agitation
Zidovudine	Headache, restlessness, severe agitation, insomnia, mania, depression, irritability

this syndrome, which was termed *subacute encephalitis* or *AIDS encephalopathy*, had an organic etiology. Evidence rapidly accumulated that CNS involvement with HIV led to the development of encephalopathy [1]. In 1987, recognizing the prevalence and severity of HIV-related neurologic dysfunction, the Centers for Disease Control added dementia to its roster of AIDS-defining disorders [2]. In 1991, the American Academy of Neurology (AAN) published detailed criteria for what is now called HIV-associated dementia complex (HAD) [3]. In addition, the AAN proposed a separate classification, HIV-associated minor cognitive-motor complex (HAMCM), to describe cognitive abnormalities that do not significantly impair work performance or activities of daily living. HIV-related disease has been described at all levels of the CNS and represents an important source of morbidity.

Pathogenesis

Evidence suggests that HIV gains access to the CNS early in the course of infection [4]. Neuroimmunologic research indicates that HIV-infected monocytes enter the circulation and then pass into the brain parenchyma through ruptured capillary endothelium [1]. When activated, HIV replicates within macrophages, with release of chemotactic factors, cytokines, and proteolytic enzymes. It also appears that HIV replicates in the cerebrospinal fluid (CSF) and sometimes in the brain itself. HIV has been recovered from brain tissue, CSF, spinal cord, and peripheral nerves of patients with neurologic dysfunction [5]. In a few cases, HIV has been isolated from the nervous system of patients in whom no virus was detected in peripheral blood [6]. Eighty to 90 percent of autopsied AIDS cases manifest histopathologic changes in the brain, the most severe residing in the central and periventricular white matter with variable extension to the subcortical gray matter [7]. There may be small areas of active demyelination, usually in a perivascular distribution, as well as reactive astrocytosis. Focal and diffuse vacuolation, from which atrophy derives, is seen in white matter.

Clinical Manifestations

HIV-associated neurocognitive disorders are comprised of cognitive, affective, behavioral, and motor abnormalities (Table 18-3). The clinical findings are often subtle and insidious in onset. Forgetfulness and loss of concentration are the most frequent early symptoms [8]. Patients may complain of difficulty with attention, confusion, and mental slowing. Attentional lapses may appear as an inability to read a book, follow a television program, or sustain a conversation. Patients may have trouble accomplishing complex tasks that were formerly automatic, and vegetative signs of depression, including loss of energy and appetite, sexual dysfunction, and sleep disturbance, are common. Some patients may become apathetic, socially withdrawn, or irritable. Persons familiar with

Table 18-3 *Stages of HIV encephalopathy*

Early
   Cognitive: Short-term memory loss, impaired attention and concentration, comprehension difficulties, slowed information processing, mild frontal lobe dysfunction
   Behavioral: Apathy, withdrawal, irritability
   Motor: Slowing, unsteady gait, dysgraphia, dysarthria, hyperreflexia, weakness
   Affective: Depression, psychotic features, hypomania

Late
   Cognitive: Severe memory impairment, severe attention difficulties, marked frontal lobe dysfunction
   Behavioral: Disinhibition, withdrawal
   Motor: Slowing, spasticity, incontinence, ataxia
   Affective: Depression, psychosis, hypomania/mania

End stage
   Mutism, aphasia, incontinence, myoclonus, seizures

the patient may notice a "change in personality" characterized by heightened anxiety in response to change and the development of a rigid, inflexible lifestyle [7]. The presentation of HAD is occasionally much more dramatic, with acute agitated psychosis, hallucinations, paranoid ideation, or frank mania [9, 10]. In this setting, there is often evidence of cognitive dysfunction or focal neurologic deficits supporting the diagnosis of an organic mental disorder.

Nearly 50 percent of patients with HAD complain of motor dysfunction [11]. Motor impairments may include weakness, particularly of the lower extremities, and difficulty with fine motor coordination. There is often dysarthria, tremor, and physical slowing [4]. Patients may notice difficulty when walking or climbing stairs, deterioration in handwriting, or a slight slurring of speech. Some of these motor deficits may result from concomitant spinal cord disease (vacuolar myelopathy) and not solely from cerebral involvement.

The course of HAD is highly variable. There may be little or no progression of deficits, and affected individuals can often compensate for cognitive problems by keeping written records, using a pocket calendar, or preparing a daily medication sheet. For some patients, the cognitive problems progress, rendering them dependent on others for help with daily tasks. Occasionally the syndrome is characterized by a dramatic and catastrophic decline in mental function, resulting in severe dementia within weeks.

Diagnostic Evaluation

Both HAMCM and HAD are diagnoses of exclusion. The clinical evaluation for HIV-associated neurocognitive disorders should include (1) a general medical assessment to identify potentially treatable causes such as drug toxicity, metabolic abnormalities, and opportunistic infections and malignancies; (2) a psychiatric evaluation; (3) a screening cognitive examination; and (4) a functional status assessment.

Neuroradiologic Imaging

The head CT scan in HAD may be normal or demonstrate diffuse cerebral atrophy (see Fig. 17-1). In advanced cases, the scan often shows a widening of the frontal horns or bilateral low density of the adjacent white matter [1]. Magnetic resonance imaging is more sensitive than CT because of its superior capacity to distinguish white matter disease [12]. MRI findings in HAD include cerebral atrophy and ventricular enlargement. In addition, MRI may demonstrate hemispheric white matter abnormalities such as patchy or diffusely increased signal on the T2-weighted image. Single-photon emission computed tomography (SPECT) is a technique that visualizes blood perfusion in the brain. The imaging of individuals with HAD using 123-I-N-isopropyl-p-iodoamphetamine (123-I-IMP) has identified focal uptake deficits, although correlation with clinical findings has not been established [13].

Cerebrospinal Fluid Abnormalities

Cerebrospinal fluid abnormalities may occur in individuals without clinical findings of neurocognitive disorder, although the incidence of abnormal findings is greater in those who are symptomatic. The absence of abnormal CSF findings does not rule out an HIV-related neurocognitive disorder. In two-thirds of patients with HAD [8], CSF abnormalities include mononuclear pleocytosis (4–50 cells/mm^3) and mildly increased protein levels (42–189 mg/dl). HIV-specific immunoglobulin G (IgG), p24 antigen, and positive viral culture, while corroborating the presence of HIV in the CNS, do not correlate with neuropsychiatric impairment. The most important purpose of CSF examination in this setting is to rule out secondary causes for neurocognitive dysfunction. Cerebrospinal fluid analysis should include India ink preparation and cryptococcal antigen assay, fungal culture, VDRL, acid-fast bacilli stain and culture, and viral cultures.

Neuropsychological Testing

There is a consensus among investigators that clinically significant cognitive impairment occurs in persons diagnosed with AIDS, although its prevalence is uncertain. Disagreement exists as to whether subtle neuropsychological impairment occurs in asymptomatic seropositive individuals [14]. Among large numbers of patients followed neuropsychologically in the Multicenter AIDS Cohort Study, no difference was detected between asymptomatic seropositive individuals and seronegative control subjects [15–17].

Neuropsychological testing has been found to be useful in assessing the HIV-infected population. These include measures of attention and concentration, psychomotor speed, motor performance, short-term memory, abstraction, information processing, and complex tasks involving sequencing. Brief clinical instruments to screen for cognitive impairment have also been described [18].

Psychiatric Disorders

The most common psychiatric diagnoses in patients with HIV disease are adjustment disorder, major depression, anxiety disorder, and substance abuse [19, 20]. Because of the high incidence of organic brain disease in this population, a syndrome that manifests itself primarily as a psychiatric disorder merits careful evaluation [21, 22]. Psychological symptoms may be part of an organic syndrome warranting medical intervention. For example, mania in a patient with HIV infection may signal an intracranial process, such as infection or tumor, or may represent an adverse drug effect (e.g., zidovudine [ZDV] or ganciclovir).

Symptoms of anxiety and depression are the most common findings in patients without clear organic pathology. Adjustment disorder with depressed or anxious mood, considered to be a reaction to the illness, is common and may be severe enough to warrant psychotherapeutic or pharmacologic treatment. A clinical distinction can be made between the withdrawal, apathy, avoidance of complex tasks, and mental slowing associated with early HIV-associated neurocognitive disorder and the low self-esteem, irrational guilt, and other signs of psychological depression. However, studies that suggest unusually high rates of mood disturbance in people with and at risk for HIV infection sometimes make the distinction between organic disorders and psychological depression problematic [23, 24].

In addition to the CNS effects of HIV itself, the complications of HIV disease and its treatment may alter brain function. More difficult to assess completely are the external (societal) and internal (intrapsychic) stressors associated with HIV infection. These stressors, which make the accommodation to neuropsychiatric disturbances more difficult, include (1) all of the psychological issues associated with a life-threatening illness, (2) the stigmatization that threatens the patient's premorbid status in society, (3) uncertainty about the course of illness, (4) difficulty in obtaining adequate health care or financial resources, and (5) loss of significant numbers of one's social support network to AIDS [25].

Suicidality

Assessment of suicidal risk in the HIV-infected population is important [26]. The use of suicidal ideation as a means of coping with difficult and intractable life circumstances is common. Neuropsychiatric disorders, such as delirium, dementia, or depression, may be contributing factors. Psychodynamically, suicidal ideation may be used to cope with the fear of pain, death, or disfigurement. It may represent a wish to have ultimate control over one's fate when all else seems to be slipping away. The onset of a new medical illness, a relapse of substance abuse, a precipitous drop in CD4 lymphocyte count, a loss of someone important, financial devastation, loss of living quarters, or rejection by others may engender suicidal thinking or behavior.

Assurance from the clinician that pain, depression, and cognitive impairment will be aggressively treated is comforting to patients and reduces the intrusive nature of self-destructive thoughts. Suicidal ideation may be the way that patients begin to talk about the fears and anxieties associated with dying and death. As patients become more impaired and face the inevitability of death, they may begin to withdraw emotionally from others, focusing more on themselves and the approaching end of life. Patients who perceive their clinician as one willing to speak openly about suicide, decisions concerning the rational termination of treatment, and anxiety about dying will be more likely to seek help before acting impulsively. The use of disinhibiting substances may contribute to self-destructive behavior.

Clinicians must recognize that, in the presence of treatable organic illness or depression, suicide is not a rational choice. A newly diagnosed asymptomatic patient with early HIV disease who believes he or she is going to die soon cannot be considered to be acting reasonably. Conversely, an end-stage patient's decision to forgo further treatment when there is little to be accomplished medically, as opposed to reversing an acute condition, must be differentiated from suicide.

Pain

HIV-infected patients often experience pain during the course of their illness [27]. Since the severity of pain is impossible to measure objectively, clinicians are often faced with difficult management issues in affected patients, especially those with a history of drug abuse. Chronic, severe pain should be treated with a sufficient standing dose of a long-acting narcotic. Pain or the fear of pain may be a precipitant to suicidal ideation and behavior.

Sleep Disorders

Most patients with HIV infection complain of sleep disturbance at some time during the course of illness. Sleep may be disturbed as a consequence of acute anxiety or depression, or as a result of drug toxicity or the direct effect of HIV on the CNS [28]. Sleep deprivation may cause significant psychiatric morbidity and requires careful evaluation and treatment.

Management

HIV-Related Neurocognitive Disease

High-dose ZDV therapy (200 mg PO 5 times/day) may be beneficial in some patients with HAD. Yarchoan and associates [29] reported improvement in clinical status, motor function, nerve conduction velocities, memory, general cognitive ability, and findings on neuroradiologic imaging. Schmitt and colleagues [30] noted a significant improvement in neuropsychological performance in a double-blind, placebo-controlled trial of ZDV for persons with neurocognitive dysfunction and AIDS. Measures of subjective distress were also lower in ZDV recipients.

Psychostimulants provide significant relief of symptoms for a number of patients. Fernandez and associates [31] and Holmes and colleagues [32] found improvement in most neuropsychological tests in cognitively impaired AIDS-related complex (ARC) and AIDS patients treated with psychostimulants. Pharmacotherapy with either methylphenidate or dextroamphetamine was "clinically effective" in 91 percent and moderately to markedly effective in 82 percent. Therapy was helpful in bringing about qualitative and quantitative improvement in higher cortical functions, self-esteem, and self-sufficiency; few side effects were seen.

Psychiatric Disorders

Recommendations on the use of antidepressants, antipsychotics, and benzodiazepines in HIV-infected patients are outlined in this section. General recommendations for prescribing psychoactive medications include the following:

1. Start with a low drug dose and increase it slowly; HIV-infected patients generally respond more quickly and at lower doses than do seronegative individuals.
2. Monitor the patient closely for side effects, particularly when using drugs with high anticholinergic affinity.
3. Prescribe limited supplies in potentially suicidal patients.

Depression

For depression with marked slowing, apathy, and hypersomnia, treatment with desipramine or an activating selective serotonin reuptake inhibitor such as fluoxetine should be considered. Desipramine therapy should begin with a daily oral dose of 10 mg and be increased by 10 mg every 3 days; response is usually achieved at well below the maximum daily dose of 200 to 250 mg. Fluoxetine can be started at 5 to 10 mg per day, with dose increases no more often than every 2 weeks; most patients respond at 10 to 20 mg each day, although some may require higher doses.

For depression with difficulty in falling asleep or early-morning awakening, trazodone or doxepin should be considered. Trazodone dosing should begin at 25 mg at bedtime, with 25-mg increases every 3 days to achieve antidepressant effect, generally noted daily at 100 to 200 mg. Doxepin therapy should be initiated at 10 mg and increased by 10 mg every 3 days to a maximum daily dose of 150 mg.

Other useful antidepressants include nortriptyline, bupropion, sertraline, paroxetine, and venlafaxine.

Psychosis

Antipsychotics are indicated for the treatment of psychosis, mania, delirium, and agitation. Caution is warranted with respect to anticholinergic side effects and extrapyramidal symptoms. Haloperidol, perphenazine, molindone, and risperidone have been effective and well tolerated in this population. Haloperidol, 0.5 to 1.0 mg once to twice a day orally or intramuscularly, can be used initially; agitated patients may require significantly higher doses. Adjunctive treatment with lorazepam may be helpful and often reduces the neuroleptic dose requirement for agitated patients.

Carbamazepine, valproic acid, and lithium have all been used successfully for prophylaxis against recurrent manic episodes.

Anxiety

Benzodiazepines may exacerbate underlying cognitive problems. In general, they should be used sparingly, and, when possible, nonpharmacologic interventions should be attempted. Benzodiazepines are generally considered the drugs of first choice when a time-limited cause of anxiety can be identified. Lorazepam and oxazepam are primarily conjugated and therefore less likely to accumulate and cause sedation or other untoward effects. Buspirone may be effective for management of chronic anxiety.

Chronic Pain

When pain is neuropathic in origin, carbamazepine, valproic acid, or amitriptyline in low doses should be considered, increasing the dose as tolerated. Opiates should be used where necessary in doses sufficient to completely relieve rather than ameliorate severe pain. Acupuncture should be considered as adjunctive therapy for chronic pain.

CNS Drug Toxicities

Anticholinergic side effects of tricyclic antidepressants, antipsychotic agents, antihistamines, and antiemetics may cause CNS symptoms, including confusion, delirium with disorientation, agitation, visual and auditory hallucinations, anxiety, and motor restlessness; they may also cause peripheral nervous system manifestations, including constipation, urinary retention, anhidrosis, mydriasis, dry mouth, flushing, and tachycardia. Extrapyramidal syndromes characteristic of antipsychotic agents include acute dystonic reactions (involuntary movements or oculogyric crisis), motor restlessness, Parkinson's syndrome (tremor, rigidity, akinesia, or bradykinesia), and tardive dyskinesia (abnormal, involuntary choreoathetotic movements involving tongue, lips, jaw, face, and extremities).

Psychotherapy

The physician may be the most constant, stabilizing influence on the HIV-infected patient. It is important that the clinician conceptualize his or her role as having psychotherapeutic power but not feel as if he or she has to carry that burden alone; the emotional needs of someone with AIDS can be exhausting to both provider and patient. Thus, making use of other available resources such as individual and group psychotherapy and peer-run support and psychoeducational groups is essential. Many patients resist seeing a psychotherapist based on previous experience or cultural biases, or out of fear of losing control over their lives to someone else. Additionally, an unspoken fear may be that the therapist will identify cognitive impairment. Primary care providers can facilitate psychotherapy referral by talking with the patient about his or her fears and considering the need for further evaluation and treatment.

References

1. Levy, JA. The Biology of the Human Immunodeficiency Virus and its role in Neurological Disease. In Rosenblum, RM Levy, DE Bredesen (eds), *AIDS and the Nervous System*, New York: Raven, 1988. Chap. 16.
2. Centers for Disease Control. Revision of the CDC surveillance case definition for acquired immunodeficiency syndrome. *MMWR* 36 (suppl):1–16, 1987.
3. Janssen R, Cornblath DR, Epstein LG, et al. Nomenclature and research case definitions for neurological manifestations of human immunodeficiency virus type-1 (HIV-1) infection: Report of a working group of the American Academy of Neurology Task Force. *Neurology* 5:41, 1991.
4. Brew BJ, Sidtis JJ, Rosenblum M, et al. AIDS dementia complex. *J Royal College of Physicians of London* 3(5):140–144, 1988.

5. Ho DD, Sarngadharan MG, Resnick L, et al. Primary human T-lymphotropic virus type III infection. *Ann Intern Med* 103:880–883, 1985.
6. Hollander H, Levy J. Neurological abnormalities and human immunodeficiency virus recovery from cerebrospinal fluid. *Ann Intern Med* 106:692–695, 1987.
7. Navia BA, Cho ES, Rosenblum ML. The AIDS dementia complex: II. Neuropathology. *Ann Neurol* 19:525–535, 1986.
8. Navia BA, Jordan BD, Price RW. The AIDS dementia complex: I. Clinical features. *Ann Neurol* 19:517–524, 1986.
9. Beckett A, Summergrad P, Manschreck T, et al. Symptomatic HIV infection of the CNS in a patient without clinical evidence of immune deficiency. *Am J Psychiatry* 144:1342–1344, 1987.
10. Harris MJ, Jeste DV, Gleghorn A, Sewell DD. New-onset psychosis in HIV-infected patients. *J Clin Psychiatry* 52:369–376, 1991.
11. Gabuzda DH, Hirsch MS. Neurologic manifestations of infection with human immunodeficiency virus: Clinical features and pathogenesis. *Ann Intern Med* 107:383–391, 1987.
12. Post MJD, Sheldon JJ, Hensley GT, et al. Central nervous system disease in acquired immunodeficiency syndrome. Prospective correlation using CT, MR imaging, and pathologic studies. *Radiology* 158:141–148, 1986.
13. Pohl P, Vogle G, Heiko F, et al. Single photon emission computed tomography in AIDS dementia complex. *J Nucl Med* 29:1382–1386, 1988.
14. Perry SW. Organic mental disorders caused by HIV: Update on early diagnosis and treatment. *Am J Psychiatry* 147:696–710, 1990.
15. Neel JR. Predict no epidemic of dementing illness in HIV seropositives. *Clin Psychiatry News* Vol 6, 1988.
16. McArthur JC, Cohen BA, Selnes OA. Low prevalence of neurological and neuropsychiatric abnormalities in healthy HIV-1 infected individuals: Results from the Multicenter AIDS Cohort Study. *Ann Neurol* 26:5, 1989.
17. Goethke KE, Mitchell JE, Marshall DW, et al. Neuropsychological and neurological function of human immunodeficiency virus seropositive asymptomatic individuals. *Arch Neurol* 46:129–133, 1989.
18. Jones BN, et al. A new bedside test of cognition for patients with HIV infection. *Ann Intern Med* 119:1001–1204, 1993.
19. Holland JC, Tross S. The psychosocial and neuropsychiatric sequelae of the acquired immunodeficiency syndrome. *Ann Intern Med* 103:760–764, 1985.
20. Perry SW, Jacobsen P. Neuropsychiatric manifestations of AIDS spectrum disorders. *Hosp Community Psychiatry* 37:135–142, 1986.
21. Forstein M, Baer J. HIV Infection. In Sederer (ed), *Inpatient Psychiatry: Diagnosis and Treatment*. Baltimore: Williams & Wilkins, 1991. P. 189–211.
22. Beckett A. Neurobiology of HIV Infection. In A Tasman, SM Goldfinger, C Kaufmann (eds), *Review of Psychiatry*. Washington, DC: American Psychiatric Press, 1990.
23. Atkinson JH, Grant I, Kennedy J, et al. Prevalence of psychiatric disorders among men infected with human immunodeficiency virus. *Am J Psychiatry* 145:859–864, 1988.
24. Perry SW, Jacobsen LB, Fishman B, et al. Psychiatric diagnosis before

serologic testing for the human immunodeficiency virus. *Am J Psychiatry* 147:89–93, 1990.

25. Dilley JW, Forstein M. Psychosocial Aspects of the Human Immunodeficiency Virus Epidemic. In A Tasman, SM Goldfinger, CA Kaufmann (eds), *Review of Psychiatry*. Washington, DC: American Psychiatric Press, 1990.

26. Beckett A, Shenson D. Suicide risk in HIV infection and AIDS. *Harvard Rev Psychiatry* 1:27–35, 1993.

27. O'Neill WM, Sherrard JS. Pain in human immunodeficiency virus disease: A review. *Pain* 54:3–14, 1993.

28. Wiegand M, Moller AA, Schreiber W, et al. Alterations of nocturnal sleep in patients with HIV infection. *Acta Neurol Scand* 83:141–142, 1991.

29. Yarchoan R, Berg G, Brouwers P, et al. Response of human-immunodeficiency-virus–associated neurological disease to 3'-azido-3'-deoxythymidine. *Lancet* 1:132–135, 1987.

30. Schmitt FA, Bigley JW, McKinnis R, et al. Neuropsychological outcome of zidovudine (AZT) treatment of patients with AIDS and AIDS-related complex. *N Engl J Med* 319:1573–1578, 1988.

31. Fernandez F, Adams F, Levy JK, et al. Cognitive impairment due to AIDS-related complex and its response to psychostimulants. *Psychosomatics* 1:38–46, 1988.

32. Holmes VF, Fernandez F, Levy JK. Psychostimulant response in AIDS-related complex (ARC) patients. *J Clin Psychiatry* 50:5–8, 1989.

Opportunistic
Diseases

Pneumocystis Pneumonia 19

Brant L. Viner

Epidemiology

Despite ultrastructural and genomic sequence data suggesting that *Pneumocystis carinii* may be a fungus, it has traditionally been classified as a protozoan [1, 2]. *Pneumocystis carinii* is a unicellular organism of global distribution that has been recovered from the lungs of many mammals including humans. Serologic evidence of infection with *P. carinii* develops in virtually all children before 4 years of age [3, 4]. Autopsy series of adults have demonstrated the organism in 4 to 8 percent of lung specimens, often without evidence of pneumonia [3, 5].

The first association of *P. carinii* with human disease was made after World War II, when outbreaks of interstitial plasma cell pneumonitis occurred in foundling homes that sheltered premature and debilitated infants. This epidemic form of disease has been seen subsequently in Korea, Iran, and Vietnam, and appears to represent primary infection in immunosuppressed hosts. Although evidence in humans is lacking, animal studies suggest the possibility of person-to-person respiratory transmission of the organism.

A totally distinct form of pneumocystosis emerged in the mid-1950s, manifesting as a diffuse alveolar pneumonitis that affected children and adults suffering from drug-induced, neoplastic, or congenital immune deficiency. Although sporadic in distribution, this reactivation type of pneumocystosis was the most common variety seen in developed countries before the AIDS epidemic. Extrapulmonary and disseminated disease was rare, almost always appearing in conjunction with pneumonitis [6, 7].

Pneumocystis carinii pneumonia (PCP) was one of the first opportunistic diseases described in association with AIDS. Initial reports identified PCP as the AIDS-defining diagnosis in approximately 60 percent of HIV-infected patients [8–12]. Although recent data suggest that the widespread use of chemoprophylaxis has decreased the incidence of PCP [13–15] and that the disease may not be as prevalent in underdeveloped countries [16], it remains one of the most important HIV-related infections.

Clinical Manifestations

HIV-related PCP is etiologically and pathologically similar to the sporadic form of the disease previously described. However, its clinical features are unique [17]. Patients with non–HIV-related PCP experience the sudden onset of severe respiratory compromise. Although AIDS patients may present in a similar fashion, they typically describe a subacute process that lasts for weeks to months. The indolent nature of this illness frequently permits a remarkable degree of physiologic compensation. Constitutional symptoms, such as fever, anorexia, and lethargy, may overshadow localized pulmonary complaints (Table 19-1). Although cough occurs, it is seldom productive. Dyspnea is common but may go unnoticed in a sedentary patient, and chest pain is rare. The patient may have a low-grade fever, and the lungs are either clear or reveal dry bibasilar rales on auscultation.

Routine laboratory studies may not be helpful. Serum lactate dehy-

Table 19-1 *Clinical and laboratory features of Pneumocystis pneumonia*

History
CD4 cell count < 200/mm^3 or prior history of PCP
Subacute or chronic onset
Constitutional and/or respiratory symptoms

Physical examination
Fever
Lungs are clear or show nonspecific findings

Laboratory evaluation
Nonspecific findings
Increased serum lactic dehydrogenase (LDH) level
Increased alveolar-arterial oxygen gradient
Diffuse interstitial pattern on chest x-ray[a]
Abnormal postexercise diffusing capacity (DLCO)
Positive gallium scan
Specific findings
Positive induced sputum
Positive bronchoalveolar lavage
Positive transbronchial or open lung biopsy[b]

[a]Normal chest x-ray in up to 39% of patients; atypical radiologic presentations are more common in patients receiving aerosol pentamidine prophylaxis.
[b]Rarely necessary for diagnosis.

drogenase (LDH) levels are usually increased but nonspecific, and normal values do not rule out PCP. Resting arterial blood gases generally show an increased alveolar-arterial oxygen gradient. Chest radiography is often remarkable for a diffuse interstitial infiltrate but may be normal in early disease.

AIDS-related extrapulmonary *P. carinii* infection has proved both more common and varied than that seen in other populations [6, 7, 18–20]. Over 70 cases have been reported, approximately one-third of which have presented as fulminant, disseminated disease in patients previously diagnosed with AIDS. The vast majority of cases were fatal, and 50 percent were associated with pneumonia. Other cases took the form of more indolent, focal disease without pneumonia. While extrapulmonary pneumocystosis usually presents nonspecifically, symptomatic infiltration of lymph nodes, liver, spleen, pleura, bone marrow, gastrointestinal tract, thyroid, ears/mastoid, eyes, and skin has also been described. Patients receiving aerosol pentamidine (AP) prophylaxis appear to be at greatest risk for the development of extrapulmonary disease.

Diagnosis

Chest radiography is an imprecise tool for the diagnosis of PCP. A nonspecific diffuse interstitial pattern is described in the majority of cases, but up to 39 percent are associated with a normal study [21–23] (see Table 19-1, Fig. 19-1). Typically, infiltrates are bilateral (95%) and involve both central and peripheral fields (84%); localized infiltrates generally affect the lower lobes. Thin-walled cystic lesions and infiltrates with spontaneous pneumothorax, although infrequent, are highly suggestive of PCP. While unilobar or unilateral disease, cavitation, nodularity, pleural effusion, and intrathoracic adenopathy should raise suspicion for a different disease process, all have been described with PCP. Conversely, radiographic patterns that are "classic" for PCP may be seen with cytomegalovirus pneumonia, pulmonary Kaposi's sarcoma, nonspecific interstitial pneumonitis, tuberculosis, and cryptococcosis. Up to 15 percent of AIDS patients with a diffuse interstitial pattern on chest x-ray do not have PCP [23].

The use of AP prophylaxis appears to alter the radiographic presentation of PCP, resulting in an increased incidence of cystic disease and spontaneous pneumothorax [24, 25]. It also appears to be highly associated with pleural effusion [26]. Only 26 to 52 percent of those receiving AP present with a diffuse interstitial pattern on chest x-ray [24, 27–32]. Infiltrates are often limited to, or predominate in, the upper lung fields.

Pulmonary function tests (PFTs) are not useful in establishing the diagnosis of PCP but may be helpful in excluding it. Postexertional

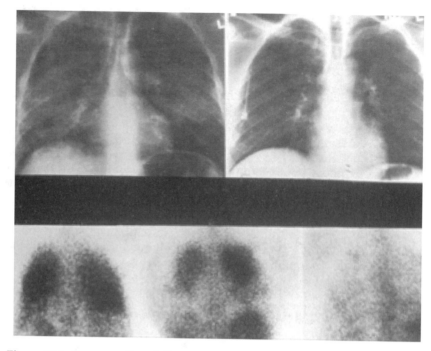

Figure 19-1. *Pneumocystis carinii* pneumonia on chest x-ray (*top*) and gallium scan (*bottom*): at time of diagnosis (*left*), following treatment (*right*). (Reprinted with permission of JA Golden et al. *Pneumocystis carinii* pneumonia treated with α-difluoromethylornithine: A prospective study among patients with acquired immunodeficiency syndrome. *West J Med* 141:613–622, 1984.)

arterial blood gases and diffusing capacity (DLCO) are extremely sensitive (90–100%) but not specific [33–35]. Thus, the finding of normal PFTs makes the diagnosis of PCP very unlikely.

Nuclear lung scans suffer from the same limitations as PFTs. Gallium scans demonstrate high sensitivity (94–100%) but low specificity (20–74%) for PCP [36–39] (see Fig. 19-1). High-grade, diffuse gallium uptake in the lungs, classic for AIDS-related PCP, may be associated with other pulmonary processes, and atypical patterns have been reported in PCP patients receiving therapy [39]. Cases that "break through" AP prophylaxis may present with focal and/or decreased tracer uptake [24]. Thus, a negative gallium scan only excludes PCP when clinical suspicion is low.

The definitive diagnosis of PCP requires direct visualization of *P. carinii* on sputum or tissue stains (Fig. 19-2). Experienced observers can readily identify sporozoites, trophozoites, and cysts with Giemsa, Wright, or methylene blue stains, but cysts are more easily seen with toluidine blue or methenamine silver stains [40]. Immunofluorescent techniques employing monoclonal antibodies specific for *P. carinii* have now replaced traditional staining methods in many institutions.

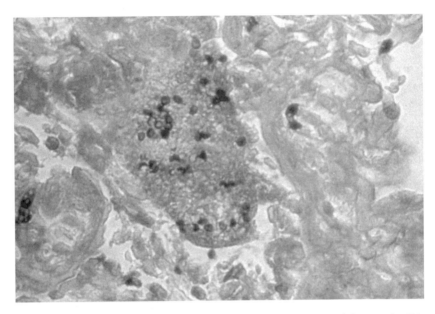

Figure 19-2. *Pneumocystis carinii* cysts in lung tissue. (Courtesy of Centers for Disease Control, Atlanta, GA.)

In contrast to other immunocompromised hosts in whom open lung biopsy is frequently required to demonstrate pneumocysts, fiberoptic bronchoscopy has proven a sensitive and reliable method of obtaining diagnostic specimens in HIV-infected patients. Transbronchial biopsy (TBB) provides the highest yield, with pneumocysts detected in 88 to 97 percent of PCP cases [11, 41–43]. However, pneumothorax occurs in 9 to 16 percent of patients who undergo this procedure, and, in those with a tenuous pulmonary and/or hematologic status, such risk may be prohibitive [41, 42, 44].

In most cases, bronchoalveolar lavage (BAL) is only slightly less sensitive for the diagnosis of PCP than TBB [41, 42, 45]. It is a relatively benign procedure that is well tolerated by all except the most fragile patients. Because of its high sensitivity and low morbidity, BAL alone is generally satisfactory for the initial assessment of diffuse lung disease in the HIV-infected patient. Although some investigators have found that BAL is less sensitive in persons receiving AP prophylaxis [24], others have found this not to be the case [32, 46–48]. Multiple lobe lavage, with or without sampling of an upper lobe, appears to compensate for whatever decreased sensitivity AP prophylaxis may confer [47, 49]. If BAL is negative or if there is accessible focal lung disease, repeat bronchoscopy with TBB may be useful. When TBB is combined with BAL, the sensitivity of flexible bronchoscopy approaches 100 percent, even in patients receiving AP [24, 41, 43]. Negative studies argue strongly against the diagnosis of PCP [50].

At many institutions, examination of induced sputum is the diagnostic modality of choice, with bronchoscopy reserved for cases in which it is unrevealing. In experienced hands, traditional stains of concentrated sputum obtained by induction with an ultrasonic saline nebulizer have achieved a sensitivity of 55 to 80 percent compared to fiberoptic bronchoscopy [51–55]. Direct or indirect fluorescent antibody stains increase the sensitivity to 85 to 92 percent [29, 52, 56, 57]. Preliminary reports suggest that polymerase chain reaction (PCR) tests may be useful in the evaluation of induced or expectorated sputum or the blood of patients with disseminated infection [58].

Clinical Course

In non–HIV-infected populations, PCP typically responds rapidly to appropriate therapy, with clinical and radiologic improvement within several days; 2 weeks of treatment are sufficient for all but the exceptional case [17, 59]. In contrast, many AIDS patients demonstrate few, if any, objective signs of resolution during the first week of therapy. Improved oxygenation on arterial blood gases may be seen as soon as 2 or 3 days into treatment, but should not be expected for at least a week to 10 days. Patients may defervesce within a day or two but frequently this does not occur until the second week of therapy [9, 60].

Chest x-rays are also unreliable for evaluating clinical response. As many as 50 percent of patients who eventually improve have worsening radiographic studies early in therapy [12, 21]. Resolution of infiltrates may take as long as 2 weeks, and some patients never clear them entirely [9, 17, 21, 60]. Extreme increases in serum LDH and failure of serum LDH to fall with therapy have been associated with poor outcome [61–63]. Sequential PFTs have been shown to be of little value in the management of PCP [64].

Unless a patient is clearly deteriorating and the question of a second pulmonary process has been raised, follow-up bronchoscopy is seldom useful. In contrast to other immunocompromised hosts, AIDS patients will continue to show *P. carinii* cysts in 38 to 90 percent of bronchoscopy specimens obtained after 2 to 3 weeks of therapy and in up to 25 percent of specimens obtained after more than 5 weeks of therapy [65–67]. Although one report suggested that the failure to decrease *P. carinii* burden by at least 50 percent on BAL performed 21 days into therapy is predictive of early relapse, other investigators found that neither the persistence nor the quantity of organisms recovered on follow-up bronchoscopy correlates with clinical status, outcome, or tendency to relapse [65, 68, 69].

Although the rate of clinical improvement is slower, AIDS patients with a first episode of PCP otherwise respond much the same as other immunocompromised hosts [9, 17, 59, 70–72]. Ninety percent of patients in good clinical condition can be expected to improve on therapy, although, without prophylaxis, many would suffer recurrent PCP within months of the initial episode. Annual relapse rates of 25 to 85 percent have been reported in patients not receiving prophylactic therapy, with a median time of 6 to 10 months [70, 73, 74]. The overall survival rate of recurrent AIDS-related PCP is approximately 60 percent, significantly lower than that of the first episode [9, 17, 70, 72]. However, patients with mild recurrent disease generally do well [75]. Mortality from individual PCP episodes can be estimated using an algorithm which includes alveolar-arterial oxygen gradient, body mass index, and total lymphocyte count [76].

Early reports documented a survival rate of 0 to 15 percent among AIDS patients who required intubation for respiratory distress [10, 17, 77]. Many died in the intensive care unit, and those who were successfully extubated often succumbed to other processes before they could leave the hospital. The grim prognosis of severe AIDS-related PCP has led some authors to question the value of intubation in this setting [10, 77]. However, using current standard management techniques, more recent studies describe a 40 to 53 percent immediate survival and 30 to 38 percent survival at 9 months in PCP patients who required intubation [61, 78].

Treatment

Despite scant scientific evidence, many clinicians believe that AIDS patients require a longer treatment course than other hosts with PCP. Three weeks of therapy is standard for uncomplicated cases. There are two widely accepted regimens for the treatment of PCP: pentamidine and trimethoprim-sulfamethoxazole (TMP-SMX). Neither is fully satisfactory with respect to clinical outcome and toxicity.

Pentamidine

Pentamidine is one of a family of guanidine analogues that were discovered to have antiprotozoal activity in the late 1930s. While its mechanism of action is not firmly established, it appears to function by inhibition of dihydrofolate reductase and interference with nucleic acid synthesis [79]. Pentamidine was first employed in the treatment of PCP in the late 1950s. When used early in the course of disease, pentamidine reduced the mortality of infantile plasma cell pneumo-nitis from 50 percent to as low as 3 percent, and of alveolar disease in immunocompromised hosts from 100 percent to 25–32 percent [80].

Pentamidine must be administered parenterally. In the past, because of reports of severe hypotension following rapid intravenous administration, the intramuscular route was advised. Experience with AIDS patients suggest that this problem was rate-related rather than route-related. The Centers for Disease Control (CDC) reviewed the first 108 AIDS cases in which pentamidine was employed; severe hypotension was documented only in patients treated intramuscularly [81]. When administered slowly over the course of at least one hour, intravenous pentamidine appears to be well tolerated. The recommended dosage of pentamidine isethionate is 4 mg/kg/day regardless of the route chosen.

The pharmacokinetics of pentamidine have not been fully defined. However, since it is in part cleared by the kidneys, dosage adjustment is required in the presence of renal failure. For a glomerular filtration rate (GFR) of 10 to 50 ml per minute, doses should be administered every 24 to 36 hours; if the rate is less than 10 ml per minute, doses should be given every 48 hours [82].

Toxicity

The major limitation of pentamidine is its toxicity. Although small series in patients with mild to moderate PCP suggest that a dose reduction to 3 mg/kg/day reduces the frequency and severity of side effects without lessening efficacy, most reports using the conventional dose confirm the pre-AIDS experience of a 40 to 50 percent risk of major adverse reactions [73, 79, 80, 83–86]. The more important toxicities of pentamidine include renal failure, hypotension, hematologic disturbances, hypoglycemia, and hepatic dysfunction. Less common adverse reactions include sterile abscess formation at intramuscular injection sites, rash (including Stevens-Johnson syndrome), hyperkalemia, hypocalcemia, acute pancreatitis, ventricular tachycardia, Jarisch-Herxheimer reaction, fever, anorexia, nausea, and acute confusional states [79, 80, 84, 86].

Renal Failure (Approximately 25%).   Although pentamidine-induced nephrotoxicity usually presents with isolated increased serum creatinine, a clinical syndrome indistinguishable from type IV renal tubular acidosis has also been reported [87]. Occasional severe cases have required dialysis and/or treatment of hyperkalemia. Far more commonly, renal dysfunction has been mild and reversible with discontinuation of the agent. Preexisting renal failure is a relative contraindication to the use of pentamidine.

Hypotension (Approximately 10%).   This appears to be less common when pentamidine is given by slow intravenous infusion. If hypotension occurs during intravenous administration, the infusion should be stopped, and crystalloids and pressors should be used as needed. Once the patient's blood pressure has returned to baseline, there is no contraindication to restarting pentamidine at a slower infusion rate under close observation.

Hematologic Disturbances (Approximately 15%). Leukopenia is the most common problem but is usually mild. Severe neutropenia may require discontinuation of pentamidine in up to 7 percent of AIDS patients [88]. Thrombocytopenia has been described more rarely. Hematologic problems are almost always reversible.

Hypoglycemia (6–35%). Most pentamidine-induced hypoglycemia is subclinical, but severe hypoglycemia can occur within hours of the first dose and is seen more commonly late in the first week of therapy. Hypoglycemia can usually be controlled with glucose infusion and discontinuation of the drug, but diazoxide therapy may occasionally be required. Some patients who have suffered pentamidine-induced hypoglycemia have developed irreversible insulin-dependent diabetes mellitus within 6 to 150 days of initiation of the drug. Derangements of glucose metabolism are believed to be secondary to a streptozocin-like action of pentamidine on pancreatic beta cells [89].

Hepatic Dysfunction (Approximately 10%). Increased serum transaminase values is generally mild and reversible.

Trimethoprim-Sulfamethoxazole

Trimethoprim-sulfamethoxazole was first used for the treatment of pneumocystosis in the mid-1970s. Studies of immunocompromised children with alveolar PCP demonstrated equal efficacy for the pentamidine, 4 mg/kg/day parenterally, and TMP, 20 mg/kg/day, plus SMX, 100 mg/kg/day orally. Adverse effects were seen far less often in patients with TMP-SMX, and, for this reason, it came to be regarded as the drug of choice for PCP [71, 80].

Trimethoprim-sulfamethoxazole seems to derive its antiprotozoal activity from interference with folate metabolism. The drug is available in oral and parenteral preparations, and both have proved effective in the treatment of PCP. In patients who are severely ill or who might not absorb a drug well from the gastrointestinal tract, parenteral therapy is indicated; for all others, there is no evidence to suggest it is superior to oral treatment.

Trimethoprim-sulfamethoxazole should be avoided in patients with sulfa allergy or glucose 6-phosphate dehydrogenase (G6PD) deficiency. Because TMP-SMX must be given as a very dilute solution, it should be administered carefully in individuals with a low cardiac ejection fraction. Because TMP-SMX is excreted primarily by the kidneys, dosage adjustment is required in the presence of renal failure. For a GFR greater than 50 ml per minute, TMP-SMX should be given as 5 mg/kg TMP every 6 hours. For a GFR of 10 to 50 ml per minute, the same dose should be given every 8 hours, and, if the GFR is less than 10 ml per minute, every 12 hours [82.]

The side effects of TMP-SMX include drug fever, rash (including

Stevens-Johnson syndrome), hepatitis, hepatic necrosis, serum sickness, hyperkalemia, acute hemolytic anemia, agranulocytosis, thrombocytopenia, and aplastic anemia. The concurrent administration of folate or folinic acid does not ameliorate the hematologic effects of the drug. AIDS patients experience a high rate of toxicity to TMP-SMX, with a 38 to 65 percent incidence of major adverse reactions [9, 17, 70, 86, 90]. As many as 18 to 54 percent of patients require alteration of therapy, usually for drug fever, rash, leukopenia, thrombocytopenia, or increased serum transaminases. Classically, TMP-SMX reactions occur 7 to 14 days into therapy and are almost always reversible with discontinuation of the drug. They may be less common in patients with very low CD4 counts and in those receiving concurrent corticosteroid therapy [91, 92]. The use of diphenhydramine or epinephrine, or both, may permit continued treatment with TMP-SMX in the setting of drug toxicity [93]. Oral desensitization techniques have also been used successfully in the majority of patients with a history of mild to moderate hypersensitivity reactions [94, 95].

There is tenuous evidence in the pre-AIDS literature to suggest that successful clinical outcome correlates with achieving a peak TMP level of 3 to 8 μg/ml and a peak SMX level of 100 to 150 μg/ml between 60 and 90 minutes after dosing [71, 96]. More recent data suggest that the frequency and severity of TMP-SMX reactions can be reduced by maintaining serum levels in this same range [97]. Nevertheless, in most institutions, serum TMP-SMX levels are not routinely monitored.

Initial Drug Therapy

There has been considerable debate about whether to use pentamidine or TMP-SMX as the first-line agent in the treatment of AIDS-related PCP (Table 19-2). This question is impossible to answer with certainty because available data are derived largely from retrospective analysis of small samples of patients who were switched from one drug to the other according to variable definitions of "adverse drug reaction" and "therapeutic failure."

Trimethoprim-sulfamethoxazole has been studied far more extensively than pentamidine in AIDS patients. Of all patients with PCP, 58 to 86 percent responded to TMP-SMX therapy, with patients treated for an initial episode doing better than those with recurrent disease [17, 60, 80, 97]. Of patients started on TMP-SMX, 42 to 85 percent were switched to pentamidine because of therapeutic failure or adverse reactions [11, 17, 60, 80, 86, 90]. In general, survival rates were much higher for patients switched to pentamidine because of TMP-SMX reactions (69–100%) than in those switched because of TMP-SMX failure (11–46%) [11, 17, 60, 70, 90, 98].

Investigators have reported a response rate of 44 to 100 percent in PCP patients treated with pentamidine; there are no good data com-

Table 19-2 *Treatment of Pneumocystis pneumonia**

Drug therapy of choice
  Trimethoprim-sulfamethoxazole: TMP, 20 mg/kg/day, and SMX, 100 mg/
    kg/day, in four divided doses orally or intravenously, *or*
  Pentamidine isethionate, 4 mg/kg/day intravenously, *and* if $PaO_2 < 70$ or
    alveolar-arterial gradient > 35, *add*
  Prednisone, 40 mg orally bid × 5 days, followed by 40 mg qd orally × 5 days,
    followed by 20 mg qd orally × 11 days
Alternative agents
  Trimethoprim-dapsone
  Primaquine-clindamycin
  Atovaquone
  Trimetrexate

*See text for drug toxicities and additional information.

paring response rates of initial compared to recurrent disease [17, 60, 70, 83, 85, 86, 97, 98]. Of patients started on pentamidine, 22 to 92 percent were switched to TMP-SMX because of therapeutic failure or adverse reactions [17, 86, 98]. Few data are available concerning the prognostic significance of a change in regimen. Survival rates among patients switched to TMP-SMX because of pentamidine reactions have ranged from 11 to 94 percent, and rates in those switched for pentamidine failure have ranged from 33 to 56 percent [17, 98].

There have been three prospective, randomized studies comparing TMP-SMX to pentamidine in the treatment of AIDS-related PCP. Both Wharton and colleagues [86] and Klein and colleagues [98] found that patients started on pentamidine had higher overall survival rates than those begun on TMP-SMX. However, the difference was not statistically significant, and 60 to 80 percent of each study group crossed over to the other agent because of therapeutic failure or adverse drug reaction. In a non-crossover study, Sattler and colleagues [97] found a significant difference in survival between patients treated with TMP-SMX and those given pentamidine (86 vs. 61%).

Alternative and Adjunctive Therapies

TMP-SMX and Pentamidine
Data on the simultaneous use of TMP-SMX and pentamidine are scarce. Work with a rat model of PCP failed to demonstrate clinical benefit with this regimen, but human experience has been limited by concerns about combined toxicity [99]. In one study, 21 AIDS patients were incidentally discovered to have received 3 or more days of combination therapy after TMP-SMX failure [70]. These patients fared slightly worse than others given pentamidine alone, but the difference was not significant.

TMP-Dapsone

In the rat model, dapsone and TMP-dapsone seem to be as effective as TMP-SMX. Although dapsone monotherapy has not proved very successful in HIV-related PCP, TMP-dapsone appears more promising [100]. In an uncontrolled, nonblinded study, Leoung and associates [101] treated 15 AIDS patients suffering their first episode of mild to moderate PCP with TMP, 20 mg/kg/day in four divided doses, plus dapsone, 100 mg per day, for 3 weeks. All patients survived, and only two were switched to alternative therapy because of adverse reactions. Medina and colleagues [102] randomized 60 AIDS patients with similar characteristics to receive either TMP-dapsone or a standard course of oral TMP-SMX. Both groups had over a 90 percent survival rate, but significantly fewer of those treated with TMP-dapsone required a change in therapy because of adverse reactions (30 vs. 57%). Common side effects included rash, nausea and vomiting, methemoglobinemia, hematologic derangements, and hepatitis. Patients being considered for dapsone therapy should be screened for G6PD deficiency.

Primaquine-Clindamycin

In the rat model, primaquine-clindamycin has demonstrated efficacy in the treatment and prophylaxis of PCP, and a growing body of evidence suggests that this combination may be useful in the treatment of HIV-related disease. In an ongoing study, Toma [103] has given primaquine, 15 mg orally once a day, and clindamycin, 300 to 450 mg every 6 hours orally, or 450 to 600 mg every 6 hours intravenously, for 3 weeks to a group of 109 patients, 36 percent of whom did not have firmly diagnosed PCP and 73 percent of whom had received prior treatment with standard agents; 73 percent were "cured" and another 19 percent "improved" with therapy. Black and associates [104] conducted a multicenter, nonrandomized, open-label, pilot study for mild to moderate AIDS-related PCP. Patients were treated with primaquine, 30 mg orally once a day, and clindamycin, 1,800 to 2,700 mg per day in divided doses every 6 to 8 hours, for 21 days. The clinical response rate was 92 percent, with treatment-limiting toxicity seen in only 4 of 36 subjects. Ruf and colleagues [105] treated a study group of 19 patients with a first episode of mild to moderate PCP with primaquine, 30 mg orally each day, and clindamycin, 900 mg orally or intravenously four times a day, for 3 weeks. Comparing these patients to matched historical control subjects who had been treated with TMP-SMX, no difference was found in response rate and no treatment-limiting toxicity was noted. Finally, Noskin and colleagues [106] achieved an 86 percent cure rate using the oral regimen of primaquine, 30 mg per day, and clindamycin, 900 mg every 8 hours, in patients who had failed or suffered adverse reactions on conventional regimens.

Side effects described in AIDS patients given primaquine-clindamycin, appear to be milder than those caused by TMP-SMX or pentamidine and rarely require alteration of treatment [103–105]. Rash occurs in about 50 percent of cases but usually resolves in 3 to 5 days. Methemoglobinemia is common, but seldom causes symptoms that require intervention. Diarrhea, hepatitis, and leukopenia are seen infrequently.

Aerosol Pentamidine

With appropriate equipment and technique, pentamidine can be nebulized and delivered directly to the lung, with minimal systemic absorption [107]. Small, uncontrolled pilot studies suggested that AP is effective, nontoxic therapy for mild to moderate AIDS-related PCP, but subsequent trials have not confirmed these results. Soo Hoo and associates [85] randomized 30 patients with mild to moderate PCP to receive either pentamidine aerosol, 8 mg/kg/day, or intravenous pentamidine, 4 mg/kg/day, for 3 weeks. Although much less drug toxicity was seen in the group receiving AP, the clinical outcome was significantly worse (55% response rate vs. 100%). Conte and colleagues [83] obtained similar results when they randomized 45 patients with mild to moderate PCP to receive either pentamidine aerosol, 600 mg per day nebulized, or intravenous pentamidine, 3 mg/kg/day, for 2 to 3 weeks. Subjects who received intravenous treatment had a response rate of 81 percent with no deaths or relapses, compared to a 53 percent response rate and 12 percent mortality in those receiving AP. Furthermore, 35 percent of the AP group recrudesced within 28 days of treatment and another 24 percent relapsed during a 3-month follow-up period. Given current regimens and delivery systems, AP does not appear particularly effective for the treatment of AIDS-related PCP.

Atovaquone

Atovaquone, a hydroxynaphthoquinone, has been shown to be a potent and selective inhibitor of de novo pyrimidine synthesis in a number of protozoa. In an early, open-label, dose-escalation phase I–II trial, Falloon and colleagues [108] studied atovaquone in 34 HIV-infected patients with mild to moderate PCP. Seventy-nine percent were treated successfully, and drug toxicity was minimal. Despite the fact that all patients successfully completing therapy were given PCP prophylaxis, recurrent infection developed in 26 percent within 6 months. Hughes and colleagues [109] subsequently performed a prospective, randomized, double-blind study comparing the oral regimen of atovaquone, 750 mg three times per day, to a fixed dose of TMP, 320 mg, plus SMX, 1,600 mg three times per day for 21 days in 322 AIDS patients with mild to moderate PCP. A significantly greater number of those receiving TMP-SMX responded to therapy (93 vs. 80%) and survived (98 vs. 93%). However, treatment-limiting side effects were also more common in this group (20 vs. 7%). Diarrhea on entry to the study was highly associated with low plasma drug concentrations, therapeutic failure, and death in patients receiving atovaquone. Dohn and colleagues [110] studied 109 HIV-infected patients with mild to moderate PCP, randomizing them to atovaquone, 750 mg orally three times per day, or to pentamidine, 3 to 4 mg/kg intravenously once a day for 21 days. More patients in the atovaquone group were successfully treated (57 vs. 40%), but more also failed to respond to therapy (29 vs. 17%). Only toxicity data achieved statistical significance, with treatment-limiting adverse events seen far less often in patients receiving atovaquone (4 vs. 36%).

Atovaquone is not as effective as TMP-SMX, absorption is variable, and a high PCP relapse rate has been described in early studies. It is currently reserved for patients with inadequate response or proven intolerance to standard therapies, with the recommended dosage of 750 mg three times a day. Side effects include fever, rash, hepatitis, neutropenia, and anemia. The drug is not well absorbed in patients with diarrhea or when administered on an empty stomach.

Trimetrexate

Trimetrexate, an antineoplastic agent related to methotrexate, was recently approved by the Food and Drug Administration for the treatment of PCP. It is a potent inhibitor of dihydrofolate reductase and, thus, highly myelosuppressive. The simultaneous administration of folinic acid ameliorates its hematologic toxicity. In an uncontrolled pilot study performed by Allegra and associates [111], subjects with PCP, including severely ill patients and individuals with recurrent disease, were given trimetrexate, 30 mg/m^2/day intravenously, and folinic acid, 20 mg/m^2 every 6 hours, for 21 days. Cure rates appeared comparable to those seen with standard agents, and the drug was well tolerated. In a subsequent phase I–II dose-escalation study, 54 patients with mild to moderate PCP were treated for 3 weeks, with an 85 percent survival rate [112]. Sattler and associates [113] reported the results of a randomized, prospective, double-blind study comparing trimetrexate, 45 mg/m^2 intravenously daily, plus folinic acid, 20 mg/m^2, with TMP-SMX at a dosage of 5 mg/kg TMP every 6 hours for 21 days in 215 AIDS patients with moderate to severe PCP. TMP-SMX was shown to be more effective than trimetrexate, producing significantly fewer treatment failures (20 vs. 38%) at day 21 and lower mortality at day 49 (16 vs. 31%). However, serious adverse events were much more common in patients randomized to TMP-SMX (28 vs. 8% by day 21).

Trimetrexate with folinic acid is well tolerated and will undoubtedly prove useful as a parenteral regimen for the treatment of PCP. However, it does not appear to be as effective as TMP-SMX and should therefore be reserved for patients who have either failed or been unable to tolerate standard therapy. Common side effects include neutropenia, hepatitis, fever, and rash; anemia, thrombocytopenia, and central nervous system dysfunction have also been reported. The recommended dosage is trimetrexate, 45 mg/m^2 intravenously daily, with folinic acid, 20 mg/m^2 every 6 hours. Both doses must be adjusted for hematologic toxicity.

Corticosteroids

Data from prospective, randomized trials have demonstrated corticosteroid therapy to be useful adjunctively in the treatment of moderate to severe PCP. Although a study by Clement and associates [114] failed to show a clinical benefit of methylprednisolone for AIDS patients with PCP and room air PaO_2 of 50 mm Hg or less, most had not received the agent until after at least 2 days of antimicrobial therapy. In contrast, three groups have been able to demonstrate clinical benefit from early administration of corticosteroids.

Montaner and associates [115] studied patients with first-episode PCP and a room air oxygen saturation of 85% or greater. Although no difference in survival was noted, subjects given adjunctive prednisone within 48 hours were significantly less likely to suffer early clinical deterioration than those given placebo (6 vs. 42%). Gagnon and colleagues [116] studied nonintubated patients with PCP who had a resting respiratory rate of greater than 30 per minute, an alveolar-arterial oxygen gradient of greater than 30 mm Hg on room air, and a PaO_2 of less than 75 mm Hg on 35% oxygen but greater than 60 mm Hg on 100% oxygen. Subjects given adjunctive methylprednisolone within 72 hours were significantly less likely to suffer respiratory failure (25 vs. 82%) and more likely to survive until discharge (75 vs. 18%) than those given placebo. Bozzette and coworkers [117] studied patients with presumed or confirmed PCP who were not intubated and had a hypoxemia ratio (PaO_2:FIO_2) of 75 or greater. Subjects who received adjunctive prednisone or methylprednisolone within 36 hours were significantly less likely to develop respiratory failure (14 vs. 30%) and more likely to survive (86 vs. 70%) than those who did not. In subgroup analysis, clinical benefit could only be demonstrated for patients with moderate to severe disease.

Although there have been case reports of new and accelerated Kaposi's sarcoma in AIDS patients receiving corticosteroid therapy, relatively few complications have been noted with the use of adjunctive steroids for PCP [118, 119]. An increased incidence of thrush and reactivation mucocutaneous herpes simplex infection has been described [92, 117]. There is no evidence that corticosteroid therapy is associated with an increased risk of serious opportunistic infection or PCP relapse [120, 121].

Despite considerable variation in study design, population examined, and steroid regimen employed, the aforementioned studies persuaded the National Institutes of Health (NIH) to issue a consensus statement on the use of corticosteroids as adjunctive therapy for AIDS-related PCP [122]. It recommends that steroids be given to all patients 13 years of age or older with HIV infection and documented or suspected PCP of at least moderate severity (defined as PaO_2 < 70 mm Hg or an alveolar arterial gradient of > 35 mm Hg). It advises that adjunctive steroid therapy be initiated at the same time that antimicrobial agents are started, with a regimen of prednisone, 40 mg orally twice a day for 5 days, followed by 40 mg orally once a day for 5 days, followed by 20 mg orally once a day for 11 days. Intravenous methylprednisolone at 75 percent of the above dosages can be used instead if parenteral treatment is necessary. In the opinion of the NIH, insufficient data exist to allow useful conclusions about the benefit of corticosteroid therapy for patients in whom standard regimens fail or for patients with mild PCP.

Prophylaxis

The issue of PCP prophylaxis was first addressed in the pediatric literature. Success in the animal model of PCP led to large-scale trials of TMP-SMX in children suffering from hematologic malignancies. In 1977, Hughes and colleagues [123] showed that an oral formulation of TMP, 150 mg/m^2/day, and SMX, 750 mg/m^2/day, given as two divided doses provided virtually complete protection in a population known to have an attack rate of 20 percent. Ten years later, Hughes and associates [124] examined a similar group and showed that the same dose of TMP-SMX given 3 consecutive days per week was just as effective for the prevention of PCP.

The high incidence of PCP in the HIV-infected population argues strongly for attempts at prophylaxis. Asymptomatic patients with an absolute CD4 lymphocyte count of less than 200 cells/mm^3 or a CD4–total lymphocyte ratio of less than 20 percent are at significant risk for PCP, as are individuals with a prior history of PCP [125, 126]. Patients with thrush or prolonged, unexplained fever may also be at increased risk for PCP despite a CD4 count of greater than 200 cells/mm^3 [126]. Several PCP prophylaxis regimens, including TMP-SMX, AP, dapsone, pyrimethamine-sulfadoxine, pyrimethamine-sulfadiazine, and zidovudine (ZDV), have been evaluated in HIV-infected patients. Studies examining the use of atovaquone for PCP prophylaxis are in progress.

Trimethoprim-Sulfamethoxazole

Fischl and associates [127] examined a group of 60 HIV-infected patients with biopsy-proven Kaposi's sarcoma and no history or evidence of opportunistic infection. Subjects were randomly assigned to receive either no therapy or an oral dose of 160 mg TMP and 800 mg SMX twice a day, and were followed for up to 3 years. No patients receiving TMP-SMX developed PCP, compared to 53 percent of the control group. Sixty percent of the patients randomized to TMP-SMX died during the course of the study, compared to 93 percent of the control group.

Data concerning low-dose, intermittent TMP-SMX prophylaxis of HIV-infected patients are beginning to become available. Wormser and associates [128] gave 160 mg TMP and 800 mg SMX orally every other day to 67 HIV-seropositive patients with either a CD4 count of less than 200 cells/mm^3 or a history of proven or probable PCP. No episodes of

PCP occurred among 32 subjects receiving primary prophylaxis over a mean of 7 months, and one case of recurrent PCP developed among 35 subjects receiving secondary prophylaxis over a mean of 11 months. Adverse reactions occurred in 40 percent of patients, usually leading to discontinuation of the drug. Ruskin and LaRiviere [129] evaluated the prophylactic use of TMP-SMX, 160 mg/800 mg orally three times a week, in 116 HIV-infected patients. No cases of PCP were seen in primary prophylaxis patients over a mean of 24 months or in secondary prophylaxis patients over a mean of 19 months. Although adverse reactions occurred in 28 percent of individuals, they rarely necessitated discontinuation of the drug. Of note, none of the study subjects developed toxoplasmosis.

Aerosol Pentamidine

Although AP has been disappointing for the treatment of AIDS-related PCP, there is considerable evidence of its efficacy in both primary and secondary prophylaxis. In a prospective, randomized, double-blind, placebo-controlled trial evaluating primary prophylaxis, Hirschel and associates [130] studied 223 HIV-infected patients with CD4 counts of less than $200/mm^3$, advanced AIDS-related complex (ARC), or AIDS without prior PCP. Within a year, 23 cases of PCP had occurred in the placebo group compared to only 8 in the group receiving 300 mg pentamidine isethionate by Respirgard II nebulizer every 28 days. Only 4 percent of those given AP discontinued treatment because of drug toxicity. Montaner and colleagues [131] achieved equally impressive results in a similar trial of secondary prophylaxis. They studied 164 HIV-infected patients who had suffered one prior episode of PCP and no other AIDS-defining opportunistic infection. Over a mean follow-up period of 15.5 weeks, 27 of 32 (84%) PCP recurrences had occurred in the placebo group. Only one subject receiving pentamidine reported clinically significant side effects. Large dose-ranging studies by Leoung and coworkers [132] and Murphy and associates [31] confirm the efficacy and safety of both the Respirgard and Fisoneb AP prophylactic regimens. A recent study suggests that high-dose AP (300 mg every 2 weeks or 600 mg once per month) may be more effective in preventing PCP than the traditional regimen [133].

Many patients treated with AP complain of metallic taste, but it usually resolves once treatment is completed and fluids are given. Drug-induced bronchospasm and coughing spells are common, especially in smokers and asthmatics. Inhaled bronchodilators given as needed or before treatment and cessation of smoking greatly ameliorate symptoms in most cases. Every effort must be made to rule out transmissible respiratory diseases such as tuberculosis before initiation of therapy. Since very little AP is absorbed from the lungs, systemic side effects are unusual. However, hypoglycemia and pancreatitis have been reported.

The failure of AP to achieve significant blood levels may not be altogether fortunate. Distribution of an aerosol drug is determined by ventilatory dynamics and the size of the particles generated by whatever delivery system is employed. Not all nebulizer systems are equally effective in delivering AP to the pulmonary alveoli [107]. Even under ideal circumstances, the upper lobes receive less drug than other regions. In patients who have preexisting lung damage or who are too debilitated to generate maximum inspiratory effort, drug distribution can be even more problematic. Breakthrough pneumocystosis may present atypically in patients receiving AP, displaying focal radiographic or gallium abnormalities predominantly in the upper lung fields [24, 27–31]. Furthermore, approximately 50 percent of the cases of HIV-related extrapulmonary pneumocystosis reported to date have occurred in patients receiving AP prophylaxis [6, 7, 18–20]. If AP cannot be tolerated or if there is concern about systemic pneumocystosis, monthly intramuscular pentamidine may be a reasonable alternative [134].

Dapsone

Dapsone provides highly effective PCP prophylaxis in the rat model. Early studies by Metroka and coworkers [135, 136] suggested that patients given dapsone, 25 mg orally four times a day, received effective primary and secondary prophylaxis compared to untreated historical controls and to patients given oral TMP-SMX, one double-strength tablet twice a day. Hughes and associates [137] gave dapsone—100, 200, or 300 mg weekly—to 61 AIDS patients as primary and secondary prophylaxis. Only one case of PCP developed over a time course in which 14 were expected based on historical controls. Lavelle and colleagues [138] are conducting a trial of dapsone, 200 mg once a week, with or without pyrimethamine, 25 mg once a week, for primary and secondary prophylaxis. Preliminary analysis of 45 patients over a median follow-up period of 40 weeks has documented only two cases of PCP, one in each group.

Studies suggest that 10 to 25 percent of patients treated with dapsone will experience side effects (described above), but they are seldom severe and almost always reversible with cessation of the drug. Dapsone can usually be employed safely in HIV-infected patients with a history of TMP-SMX intolerance, including those with severe reactions [139–141].

Pyrimethamine-Sulfadoxine

Fansidar contains 25 mg pyrimethamine and 500 mg sulfadoxine. Two open, uncontrolled studies documented the efficacy of one tablet per week for the prophylaxis of AIDS-related PCP [142, 143]. However, Fischl and Dickinson [144] found pyrimethamine-sulfadoxine to be ineffective primary prophylaxis in a group of 30 HIV-seropositive patients with newly diagnosed Kaposi's sarcoma and no history of opportunistic infection.

Pyrimethamine-sulfadoxine possesses the same toxicity profile as other sulfa-containing compounds, but severe mucocutaneous reactions may be more common than with shorter-acting agents. One fatal and several nonfatal cases of Stevens-Johnson syndrome have been reported [145]. Thus, despite the obvious appeal of a simple, inexpensive, oral regimen, many clinicians are reluctant to use this agent.

Pyrimethamine-Sulfadiazine

Pyrimethamine-sulfadiazine is commonly used in the treatment and prophylaxis of cerebral toxoplasmosis. In a large cohort study, Heald and associates [146] found that the incidence of PCP was substantially lower in patients receiving treatment for cerebral toxoplasmosis than in patients with other severe opportunistic infections and similar to that seen in individuals receiving AP prophylaxis. The most frequently used prophylactic regimens were 25 mg pyrimethamine with 3,000 mg sulfadiazine or 2,400 mg clindamycin daily. Only one of the six prophylaxis failures occurred in patients receiving pyrimethamine-sulfadiazine. There have been no prospective studies of pyrimethamine-sulfadiazine for PCP prophylaxis.

Zidovudine

Although ZDV has no intrinsic activity against *P. carinii*, it seems reasonable that an antiretroviral agent might have prophylactic value to the extent that it improves host immune function. In fact, several large, prospective, randomized trials found decreased PCP incidence and increased survival in ARC and AIDS patients receiving ZDV [132, 147, 148]. However, other studies have been less convincing. Recurrence rates equivalent to historical and untreated controls have been described in AIDS patients given ZDV after the first episode of PCP [148–151]. ARC and AIDS patients receiving ZDV alone suffer a significantly higher incidence of PCP than those also receiving specific prophylactic therapy [151–152]. Furthermore, in patients receiving AP who have been followed prospectively, it has not been possible to demonstrate additional prophylactic benefit from ZDV therapy [27, 131].

Comparison of Regimens

In controlled trials, TMP-SMX has been shown to be effective for primary PCP prophylaxis and AP effective for both primary and secondary prophylaxis [127, 130, 131]. However, it is only recently that data comparing these regimens have become available.

A study performed by the AIDS Clinical Trials Group has convincingly demonstrated the superiority of TMP-SMX over AP in secondary PCP prophylaxis [153]. In this trial, 310 participants were randomized to receive either TMP-SMX, one double-strength tablet daily, or AP, 300 mg every 4 weeks by means of a Respirgard II nebulizer, for secondary prophylaxis. Analysis showed that in 11.4 percent of subjects receiving TMP-SMX recurrent PCP developed within 18 months, compared to 27.6 percent of those receiving AP. Although side effect profiles were remarkably similar in the two groups, subjects initially treated with TMP-SMX had to be crossed over more frequently than those who received AP (27 vs. 4%).

Another prospective study has shown TMP-SMX to be superior to AP for primary PCP prophylaxis [154]. Subjects were randomized to receive AP, 300 mg once a month; TMP-SMX, one single-strength tablet daily; or TMP-SMX, one double-strength tablet daily. At a mean of 8.5 months follow-up, 8 percent of subjects receiving AP had a documented case of PCP, compared to none in both of the two TMP-SMX groups. Of subjects who received TMP-SMX, 25 percent experienced drug toxicity compared to 3 percent of those who received AP. An additional study demonstrated that TMP-SMX, AP, and dapsone were of comparable effectiveness in primary prevention of PCP in HIV-infected patients with CD4 counts of $100/mm^3$ or above [155]. However, for individuals with counts below $100/mm^3$, the risk for PCP was significantly lower in those receiving TMP-SMX compared to AP (19 vs. 33%).

Reports comparing dapsone to TMP-SMX or AP prophylaxis are more difficult to interpret since no dapsone regimen has been accepted as standard. However, preliminary data suggest that dapsone, with or without pyrimethamine, is somewhat less effective than TMP-SMX [156–158] and similar to AP [157, 159–161] for primary and secondary PCP prophylaxis. Dapsone is generally less toxic than TMP-SMX, but it may not be as well tolerated as AP.

Management Recommendations

Prophylaxis with TMP-SMX, AP, or dapsone reduces the incidence of PCP in patients with advanced HIV disease. Recent data indicate that the use of PCP prophylaxis is also associated not only with decreased incidence of PCP [13, 14] but also with delayed progression to AIDS [13] and prolonged survival [162]. Table 19-3 compares key features of available PCP prophylaxis regimens. In general, TMP-SMX appears to be the most effective agent but has the greatest toxicity. Aerosol pentamidine and dapsone have been associated with breakthrough PCP infection, and extrapulmonary disease seems to be a significant problem with AP because it is not systemically absorbed. TMP-SMX may be difficult to give to patients who are receiving other marrow suppressants such as ZDV; didanosine (ddI) may interfere with the absorption of dapsone if dosed at the same time. A potential benefit of AP therapy is the ability to monitor compliance. However, AP costs considerably

Table 19-3 *Comparison of PCP prophylaxis regimens*

Issue	TMP-SMX	Dapsone	AP
Efficacy	High	Moderate	Moderate
Toxicity	Moderate	Low	Lowest
Drug interaction	Zidovudine	Didanosine	None
Cost	Low	Low	High
Toxoplasmosis protection	Yes	Yes	No

more than either TMP-SMX or dapsone. TMP-SMX appears to afford additional protection against common bacterial infections [153] and toxoplasmosis [158, 160, 163, 164]. Dapsone also seems to have preventive activity against toxoplasmosis [158, 160, 161].

On the basis of available data, the United States Public Health Service has published guidelines for PCP prophylaxis [165, 166] (Fig. 19-3). Current recommendations are that, unless contraindicated, lifetime PCP prophylaxis be initiated in HIV-infected adults who have a prior history of PCP, a CD4 count of less than 200 cells/mm³, or constitu-

Figure 19-3. Algorithm for prophylaxis of *Pneumocystis carinii* pneumonia. (Adapted from Centers for Disease Control, Recommendations for prophylaxis against *Pneumocystis carinii* pneumonia for adults and adolescents infected with human immunodeficiency virus. *MMWR* 41[RR-4]:1–11, 1992.)

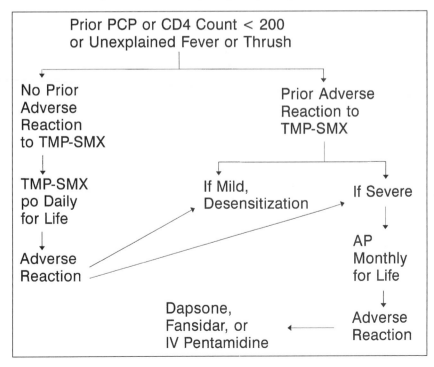

tional symptoms such as thrush or unexplained fever greater than 100°F for 2 weeks or longer. Several prophylaxis regimens have been endorsed, including: (1) 160 mg TMP and 800 mg SMX orally once a day; (2) 300 mg AP once a month by means of a Respirgard II jet nebulizer; and (3) 100 mg dapsone orally once a day. TMP-SMX should be used initially. In patients who experience a mild reaction to TMP-SMX, rechallenge using an oral desensitization technique is appropriate (Table 19-4). In individuals with a history of significant toxicity, AP or dapsone should be given as alternative therapy. In patients who experience breakthrough PCP or toxicity on AP or dapsone, the other agent should be administered.

Table 19-4 *TMP-SMX oral desensitization protocol**

	Regimen	*Dose concentrations**
Day 1	1 : 1,000,000 dilution Serial doses of 1 ml, 2 ml, 3 ml, 4 ml, 8 ml	0.00002 mg SMX in 1 ml 0.000004 mg TMP in 1 ml
Day 2	1 : 100,000 dilution Serial doses of 1 ml, 2 ml, 4 ml, 8 ml	0.0002 mg SMX in 1 ml 0.00004 mg TMP in 1 ml
Day 3	1 : 10,000 dilution Serial doses of 1 ml, 2 ml, 4 ml, 8 ml	0.002 mg SMX in 1 ml 0.0004 mg TMP in 1 ml
Day 4	1 : 1,000 dilution Serial doses of 1 ml, 2 ml, 4 ml, 8 ml	0.02 mg SMX in 1 ml 0.004 mg TMP in 1 ml
Day 5	1 : 100 dilution Serial doses of 1 ml, 2 ml, 4 ml, 8 ml	0.2 mg SMX in 1 ml 0.04 mg TMP in 1 ml
Day 6	1 : 10 dilution Serial doses of 1 ml, 2 ml, 4 ml, 8 ml	2.0 mg SMX in 1 ml 0.4 mg TMP in 1 ml
Day 7	50% standard oral suspension Serial doses of 1 ml, 2 ml, 4 ml, 8 ml	20.0 mg SMX in 1 ml 4.0 mg TMP in 1 ml
Day 8	Standard oral suspension Serial doses of 5 ml, 10 ml, 20 ml	40.0 mg SMX in 1 ml 8.0 mg TMP in 1 ml

On the last dose for day 8, give one double-strength tablet of TMP-SMX; following day 8, give one double-strength tablet every day.

*The protocol is administered over 8 days with doses of TMP-SMX given every 6 hours. Solutions are made from a standard oral suspension of TMP-SMX, which consists of 40 mg TMP and 200 mg SMX per 5 ml. The dilutions for TMP-SMX are based on 50% standard oral suspension.

Table 19-4 *(Continued)*

General management recommendations

1. The first dose of TMP-SMX should be administered in the office, and the patient should be observed for anaphylaxis for 1 hour.
2. Instruct patient to drink 3,000 ml of fluid daily.
3. Patient should use a no. 15 or higher sunscreen during exposure to sun.
4. Instruct patient not to interrupt therapy, even for 1 or 2 days, because allergic reaction may occur.
5. Regular telephone contact with patient and office visits are important to provide supervision and encouragement.

Management of drug reactions

Symptoms	Treatment
Low-grade fever, malaise, myalgia	Acetaminophen, 650 mg PO q4h as needed
Mild morbilliform eruption	Diphenhydramine hydrochloride, 25–50 mg PO q6–8h as needed
Significant fever and/or florid morbilliform eruption	Prednisone: 20 mg PO tid for 3 days
	15 mg PO tid for 3 days
	10 mg PO tid for 3 days
	10 mg PO qd for 3 days

Source: From MA Conant et al. Oral desensitization to trimethoprim/sulfamethoxazole. Eighth International Conference on AIDS, Amsterdam, July 1992.

References

1. Edman JC, Kovacs JA, Masur H, et al. Ribosomal RNA sequence shows *Pneumocystis carinii* to be a member of the fungi. *Nature* 334:519–522, 1988.
2. ul Haque A, Plattner SB, Cook RT, Hart MN. *Pneumocystis carinii*. Taxonomy as viewed by electron microscopy. *Am J Clin Pathol* 87:504–510, 1987.
3. Meuwissen JH, Tauber I, Leeuwenberg PJ, et al. Parasitologic and serologic observations of infection with pneumocystis in humans. *J Infect Dis* 136:43–49, 1977.
4. Pifer LL, Hughes WT, Stagno S, Woods D. *Pneumocystis carinii* infection: Evidence for high prevalence in normal and immuno-suppressed children. *Pediatrics* 61:35–41, 1978.
5. Esterly JA. *Pneumocystis carinii* in lungs of adults at autopsy. *Am Rev Respir Dis* 97:935–937, 1968.
6. Raviglione MC. Extrapulmonary pneumocystosis: The first fifty cases. *Rev Infect Dis* 12:1127–1138, 1990.
7. Nortfelt DW, Clement MJ, Safrin S. Extrapulmonary pneumo-cystosis: Clinical features in human immunodeficiency virus infection. *Medicine (Baltimore)* 69:392–398, 1990.

8. Catterall JR, Potasman I, Remington JS. *Pneumocystis carinii* pneumonia in the patient with AIDS. *Chest* 88:758–762, 1985.
9. Engelberg LA, Lerner CW, Tapper ML. Clinical features of *Pneumocystis* pneumonia in the acquired immune deficiency syndrome. *Am Rev Respir Dis* 130:689–694, 1984.
10. Mills J. *Pneumocystis carinii* and *Toxoplasma gondii* infections in patients with AIDS. *Rev Infect Dis* 8:1001–1010, 1986.
11. Murray JF, Felton CP, Garay SM et al. Pulmonary complications of the acquired immunodeficiency syndrome: Report of National Heart, Lung, and Blood Institute Workshop. *N Engl J Med* 310:1682–1688, 1984.
12. Stover DE, White DA, Romano PA et al. Spectrum of pulmonary diseases associated with the acquired immune deficiency syndrome. *Am J Med* 78:429–437, 1985.
13. Hoover DR, et al. Clinical manifestations of AIDS in the era of *Pneumocystis* prophylaxis. Multicenter AIDS Cohort Study. *N Engl J Med* 329:1922–1926, 1993.
14. Munoz A, et al. Trends in the incidence of outcomes defining acquired immunodeficiency syndrome (AIDS) in the Multicenter AIDS Cohort Study: 1985–1991. *Am J Epidemiol* 137:423–438, 1993.
15. Chien SM, et al. Changes in hospital admissions pattern in patients with human immunodeficiency virus infection in the era of *Pneumocystis carinii*. *Chest* 102:1035–1039, 1992.
16. Abouya YL, et al. *Pneumocystis carinii* pneumonia. An uncommon cause of death in African patients with acquired immunodeficiency syndrome. *Am Rev Respir Dis* 145:617–620, 1992.
17. Kovacs JA, Hiemenz JW, Macher AM, et al. *Pneumocystis carinii* pneumonia: A comparison between patients with the acquired immunodeficiency syndrome and patients with other immunodeficiencies. *Ann Intern Med* 100:663–671, 1984.
18. Cohen OJ, Stoeckle MY. Extrapulmonary *Pneumocystis carinii* infections in the acquired immunodeficiency syndrome. *Arch Intern Med* 151:1205–1214, 1991.
19. Sha BE, et al. *Pneumocystis carinii* choroiditis in patients with AIDS: Clinical features, response to therapy, and outcome. *J Acquir Immune Defic Syndr* 5:1051–1058, 1992.
20. Dieterich DT, et al. Gastrointestinal pneumocystosis in HIV-infected patients on aerosolized pentamidine: Report of five cases and literature review. *Am J Gastroenterol* 87:1763–1770, 1992.
21. DeLorenzo LJ, Huang CT, Maguire GP, Stone DJ. Roentgenographic patterns of *Pneumocystis carinii* pneumonia in 104 patients with AIDS. *Chest* 91:323–327, 1987.
22. Opravil M, et al. Shortcomings of chest radiography in detecting *Pneumocystis carinii* pneumonia. *J Acquir Immune Defic Syndr* 7:39–45, 1994.
23. Suster B, Akerman M, Orenstein M, Wax M. Pulmonary manifestations of AIDS: Review of 106 episodes. *Radiology* 161:87–93, 1986.
24. Jules-Elysee KM, Stover DE, Zaman MB, et al. Aerosolized pentamidine: Effect on diagnosis and presentation of *Pneumocystis carinii* pneumonia. *Ann Intern Med* 112:750–757, 1990.

25. Tietjen PA, Jules-Elysee KM, Stover DE. Increased incidence of pneumothoraces with aerosolized pentamidine. *Chest* 96:187S, 1989.
26. Horowitz ML, et al. *Pneumocystis carinii* pleural effusion. Pathogenesis and pleural fluid analysis. *Am Rev Respir Dis* 148;232–234, 1993.
27. Golden JA, Chernoff D, Hollander H, et al. Prevention of *Pneumocystis carinii* pneumonia by inhaled pentamidine. *Lancet* 1:654–757, 1989.
28. Lowery S, Fallat R, Feigal DW, et al. Changing patterns of *Pneumocystis carinii* pneumonia (PCP) on pentamidine aerosol prophylaxis. Fourth International Conference on AIDS, Stockholm, June 1988.
29. Levine SJ, Masur H, Gill VJ, et al. Effect of aerosolized pentamidine prophylaxis on the diagnosis of *Pneumocystis carinii* pneumonia by induced sputum examination in patients infected with the human immunodeficiency virus. *Am Rev Respir Dis* 144:760–764, 1991.
30. Chaffey MH, Klein JS, Gamsu G, et al. Radiographic distribution of *Pneumocystis carinii* pneumonia in patients with AIDS treated with prophylactic inhaled pentamidine. *Radiology* 175:715–719, 1990.
31. Murphy RL, Lavelle JP, Allan JD, et al. Aerosol pentamidine prophylaxis following *Pneumocystis carinii* pneumonia in AIDS patients: Results of a blinded dose-comparison study using an ultrasonic nebulizer. *Am J Med* 90:418–426, 1991.
32. Fahy JV, et al. Effect of aerosolized pentamidine prophylaxis on the clinical severity and diagnosis of *Pneumocystis carinii* pneumonia. *Am Rev Respir Dis* 146:844–848, 1992.
33. Curtis J, Goodman P, Hopewell P. Noninvasive tests in the diagnostic evaluation for *P. carinii* pneumonia in patients with or suspected of having AIDS. *Am Rev Respir Dis* 133:A182, 1986.
34. Smith DE, McLuckie A, Wyatt J, et al. Severe exercise hypoxemia with normal or near normal x-rays: A feature of *Pneumocystis carinii* infection. *Lancet* 2:1049–1051, 1988.
35. Stover DE, Greeno RA, Gagliardi AJ. The use of a simple exercise test for the diagnosis of *Pneumocystis carinii* pneumonia in patients with AIDS. *Am Rev Respir Dis* 139:1343–1346, 1989.
36. Barron TF, Birnbaum NS, Shane LB, et al. *Pneumocystis carinii* pneumonia studied by gallium-67 scanning. *Radiology* 154:791–793, 1985.
37. Coleman DL, Hattner RS, Luce JM, et al. Correlation between gallium lung scans and fiberoptic bronchoscopy in patients with suspected *Pneumocystis carinii* pneumonia and the acquired immune deficiency syndrome. *Am Rev Respir Dis* 130:1166–1169, 1984.
38. Kramer EL, Sanger JJ, Garay SM, et al. Gallium-67 scans of the chest in patients with acquired immunodeficiency syndrome. *J Nucl Med* 28:1107–1114, 1987.
39. Woolfenden JM, Carrasquillo JA, Larson SM, et al. Acquired immunodeficiency syndrome: Ga-67 citrate imaging. *Radiology* 162:383–387, 1987.
40. Kim HK, Hughes WT. Comparison of methods for identification of *Pneumocystis carinii* in pulmonary aspirates. *Am J Clin Pathol* 60:464–466, 1973.
41. Broaddus C, Dake MD, Stulbarg MS, et al. Bronchoalveolar lavage and transbronchial biopsy for the diagnosis of pulmonary infections in

the acquired immunodeficiency syndrome. *Ann Intern Med* 102:747–752, 1985.

42. Milligan SA, Luce JM, Golden J, et al. Transbronchial biopsy without fluoroscopy in patients with diffuse roentgenographic infiltrates and the acquired immunodeficiency syndrome. *Am Rev Respir Dis* 137:486–488, 1988.

43. Stover DE, White DA, Romano PA, Gellene RA. Diagnosis of pulmonary disease in acquired immune deficiency syndrome (AIDS). *Am Rev Respir Dis* 130:659–662, 1984.

44. Miller RF, Millar AB, Semple SJG. Complications of fiberoptic bronchoscopy in HIV-1 antibody positive patients undergoing investigations for pulmonary disease. *Thorax* 43:847A, 1988.

45. Golden JA, Hollander H, Stulbarg MS, et al. Bronchoalveolar lavage as the exclusive diagnostic modality for *Pneumocystis carinii* pneumonia: A prospective study among patients with acquired immunodeficiency syndrome. *Chest* 90:18–22, 1986.

46. Ng VL, et al. Lack of effect of prophylactic aerosolized pentamidine on the detection of *Pneumocystis carinii* in induced sputum or bronchoalveolar lavage specimens. *Arch Pathol Lab Med* 117:493–496, 1993.

47. Levine SJ, et al. Diagnosis of *Pneumocystis carinii* by multiple lobe, site-directed bronchoalveolar lavage with immunofluorescent monoclonal antibody staining in human immunodeficiency virus–infected patients receiving aerosolized pentamidine chemoprophylaxis. *Am Rev Respir Dis* 146:838–843, 1992.

48. Teuscher AU, et al. Predicted value of bronchoalveolar lavage in excluding a diagnosis of *Pneumocystis carinii* pneumonia during prophylaxis with aerosolized pentamidine. *Clin Infect Dis* 16:519–522, 1993.

49. Yung RC et al. Upper and middle lobe bronchoalveolar lavage to diagnose *Pneumoystis carinii* pneumonia. *Am Rev Respir Dis* 148:1563–1566, 1993.

50. Barrio JL, Harcup C, Baier JH, et al. Value of repeat fiberoptic bronchoscopies and significance of nondiagnostic bronchoscopic results in patients with the acquired immunodeficiency syndrome. *Am Rev Respir Dis* 135:422–425, 1987.

51. Bigby TD, Margolskee D, Curtis JL, et al. The usefulness of induced sputum in the diagnosis of *Pneumocystis carinii* pneumonia in patients with the acquired immunodeficiency syndrome. *Am Rev Respir Dis* 133:515–518, 1986.

52. Kovacs JA, Ng VL, Masur H, et al. Diagnosis of *Pneumocystis carinii* pneumonia: Improved detection in sputum with use of monoclonal antibodies. *N Engl J Med* 318:589–593, 1988.

53. Ng VL, Gartner I, Weymouth LA, et al. The use of mucolysed induced sputum for the identification of pulmonary pathogens associated with human immunodeficiency virus infection. *Arch Pathol Lab Med* 113:488–493, 1989.

54. Pitchenik AE, Ganjei P, Torres A, et al. Sputum examination for the diagnosis of *Pneumocystis carinii* pneumonia in the acquired immunodeficiency syndrome. *Am Rev Respir Dis* 133:226–229, 1986.

55. Zaman MK, Wooten OJ, Suprahmanya B, et al. Rapid noninvasive diag-

nosis of *Pneumocystis carinii* from induced liquified sputum. *Ann Intern Med* 109:7–10, 1988.

56. Ng VL, Yajko DM, McPhaul LW, et al. Evaluation of an indirect fluorescent-antibody stain for detection of *Pneumocystis carinii* in respiratory specimens. *J Clin Microbiol* 28:975–979, 1990.

57. Virani N, Ng VL, Chaisson RE, et al. Rapid diagnosis of *Pneumocystis carinii* pneumonia (PCP) in patients with AIDS using a direct fluorescent monoclonal antibody (DFA) assay. Fifth International Conference on AIDS, Montreal, June 1989.

58. Lipschick GY, et al. Improved diagnosis of *Pneumocystis carinii* infection by polymerase chain reaction on induced sputum and blood. *Lancet* 340:203–206, 1992.

59. Winston DJ, Lau WK, Gale RP, Young LS. Trimethoprim-sulfamethoxazole for the treatment of *Pneumocystis carinii* pneumonia. *Ann Intern Med* 92:762–769, 1980.

60. Small CB, Harris CA, Friedland GH, Klein RS. The treatment of *Pneumocystis carinii* pneumonia in the acquired immunodeficiency syndrome. *Arch Intern Med* 145:837–840, 1985.

61. Efferen LS, Nadarajah D, Palat DS. Survival following mechanical ventilation for *Pneumocystis carinii* pneumonia in patients with the acquired immunodeficiency syndrome: A different perspective. *Am J Med* 87:401–404, 1989.

62. Silverman BA, Rubinstein A. Serum lactate dehydrogenase levels in adults and children with acquired immune deficiency syndrome (AIDS) and AIDS-related complex: Possible indicator of B cell lymphoproliferation and disease activity. *Am J Med* 78:728–736, 1985.

63. Zaman MK, White DA. Serum lactate dehydrogenase levels and *Pneumocystis carinii* pneumonia. *Am Rev Respir Dis* 137:796–800, 1988.

64. Coleman DL, Dodek PM, Golden JA, et al. Correlation between serial pulmonary function tests and fiberoptic bronchoscopy in patients with *Pneumocystis carinii* pneumonia and the acquired immune deficiency syndrome. *Am Rev Respir Dis* 129:491–493, 1984.

65. DeLorenzo LJ, Maguire GP, Wormser GP, et al. Persistence of *Pneumocystis carinii* pneumonia in the acquired immunodeficiency syndrome: Evaluation of therapy by follow-up transbronchial lung biopsy. *Chest* 88:79–83, 1985.

66. Hartmann B, Koss M, Hui A, et al. *Pneumocystis carinii* pneumonia in the acquired immunodeficiency syndrome. (AIDS): Diagnosis with bronchial brushings, biopsy, and bronchoalveolar lavage. *Chest* 87:603–607, 1985.

67. Shelhamer JH, Ognibene FP, Macher AM, et al. Persistence of *Pneumocystis carinii* in lung tissue of acquired immunodeficiency syndrome patients treated for pneumocystis pneumonia. *Am Rev Respir Dis* 130:1161–1165, 1984.

68. Colangelo G, Baughman RP, Dohn MN, Frame PT. Follow-up bronchoalveolar lavage in AIDS patients with *Pneumocystis carinii* pneumonia: *Pneumocystis carinii* burden predicts early relapse. *Am Rev Respir Dis* 143:1067–1071, 1991.

69. Brenner M, Ognibene FP, Lack EE, et al. Prognostic factors and life ex-

pectancy of patients with acquired immunodeficiency syndrome and *Pneumocystis carinii* pneumonia. *Am Rev Respir Dis* 136:1199–1206, 1987.

70. Haverkos HW. Assessment of therapy for *Pneumocystis carinii* pneumonia: PCP therapy project group. *Am J Med* 76:501–508, 1984.
71. Hughes WT, Feldman S, Chaudhary SC, et al. Comparison of pentamidine isethionate and trimethoprim-sulfamethoxazole in the treatment of *Pneumocystis carinii* pneumonia. *J Pediatr* 92:285–291, 1978.
72. Kales CP, Murren JR, Torre RA, et al. Early predictors of in-hospital mortality for *Pneumocystis carinii* pneumonia in the acquired immunodeficiency syndrome. *Arch Intern Med* 147:1413–1417, 1987.
73. Conte JE, Hollander H, Golden JA. Inhaled or reduced-dose pentamidine for *Pneumocystis carinii* pneumonia: A pilot study. *Ann Intern Med* 107:495–498, 1987.
74. Feigal DW, Edison R, Leoung GS, et al. Recurrent *Pneumocystis carinii* pneumonia (PCP) in 201 patients before AZT or prophylaxis: Implications for clinical trials. Fourth International Conference on AIDS, Stockholm, June 1988.
75. Dohn MN, et al. Equal survival rates for first, second, and third episodes of *Pneumocystis carinii* pneumonia in patients with acquired immunodeficiency syndrome. *Arch Intern Med* 152:2465–2470, 1992.
76. Bennett CL, et al. A rapid preadmission method for predicting inpatient course of disease for patients with HIV-related *Pneumocystis carinii* pneumonia. *Am J Respir Crit Care Med* 150:1503–1507, 1994.
77. Wachter RM, Luce JM, Turner J, et al. Intensive care of patients with the acquired immunodeficiency syndrome: Outcome and changing patterns of utilization. *Am Rev Respir Dis* 134:891–896, 1986.
78. Wachter RM, Russi MB, Bloch DA, et al. *Pneumocystis carinii* pneumonia and respiratory failure in AIDS: Improved outcomes and increased use of intensive care units. *Am Rev Respir Dis* 143:251–256, 1991.
79. Drake S, Lampasona V, Nicks HL, Schwarzmann SW. Pentamidine isethionate in the treatment of *Pneumocystis carinii* pneumonia. *Clin Pharmacol* 4:507–516, 1985.
80. Hughes WT. *Pneumocystis carinii* pneumonitis. *Antibiot Chemother* 30:257–271, 1981.
81. Navin TR, Fontaine RE. Intravenous versus intramuscular administration of pentamidine. *N Engl J Med* 311:1701–1702, 1984.
82. Bennett WM, Muther RS, Parker RA, et al. Drug therapy in renal failure: Dosing guidelines for adults. *Ann Intern Med* 93:62–83, 1980.
83. Conte JE, Chernoff D, Feigal DW, et al. Intravenous or inhaled pentamidine for treating *Pneumocystis carinii* pneumonia in AIDS. *Ann Intern Med* 113:203–209, 1990.
84. Pearson RD, Hewlett EL. Pentamidine for the treatment of *Pneumocystis carinii* pneumonia and other protozoal diseases. *Ann Intern Med* 103:782–786, 1985.
85. Soo Hoo GW, Mohsenifar Z, Meyer RD. Inhaled or intravenous pentamidine therapy for *Pneumocystis carinii* pneumonia in AIDS. *Ann Intern Med* 113:195–202, 1990.
86. Wharton JM, Coleman D, Wofsy C, et al. Trimethoprim-sulfamethoxazole or pentamidine for *Pneumocystis carinii* pneumonia in the acquired im-

munodeficiency syndrome: A prospective randomized trial. *Ann Intern Med* 105:37–44, 1986.

87. Lachaal M, Venuto RC. Nephrotoxicity and hyperkalemia in patients with acquired immunodeficiency syndrome treated with pentamidine. *Am J Med* 87:260–263, 1989.

88. Polsky B, Dryjanski J, Whimbey E, et al. Severe neutropenia during pentamidine treatment of *Pneumocystis carinii* pneumonia in patients with acquired immunodeficiency syndrome—New York City. *MMWR* 33:65–67, 1984.

89. Bouchard Ph, Sai P, Reach G, et al. Diabetes mellitus following pentamidine-induced hypoglycemia in humans. *Diabetes* 31:40–45, 1982.

90. Gordin FM, Simon GL, Wofsy CB, Mills J. Adverse reactions to trimethoprim-sulfamethoxazole in patients with the acquired immunodeficiency syndrome. *Ann Intern Med* 100:495–499, 1984.

91. Carr A, et al. Clinical and laboratory markers of hypersensitivity to trimethoprim-sulfamethoxazole in patients with *Pneumocystis carinii* pneumonia and AIDS. *J Infect Dis* 167:180–185, 1993.

92. Caumes E, et al. Effect of corticosteroids on the incidence of adverse cutaneous reactions to trimethoprim-sulfamethoxazole during treatment of AIDS-associated *Pneumocystis carinii* pneumonia. *Clin Infect Dis* 18:319–323, 1994.

93. Gibbons RB, Lindauer JA. Successful treatment of *Pneumocystis carinii* pneumonia with trimethoprim-sulfamethoxazole in hypersensitive AIDS patients. *JAMA* 253:1259–1260, 1985.

94. Finegold I. Oral desensitization to trimethoprim-sulfamethoxazole in a patient with acquired immunodeficiency syndrome. *Allergy Clin Immunol* 78:905–908, 1986.

95. Absar N, Daneshvar H, Beall G. Desensitization to trimethoprim-sulfamethoxazole in HIV-infected patients. *J Allergy Clin Immunol* 93:1001–1005, 1994.

96. Lau WK, Young LS. Trimethoprim-sulfamethoxazole treatment of *Pneumocystis carinii* pneumonia in adults. *N Engl J Med* 295:716–718, 1976.

97. Sattler FR, Cowan R, Nielsen D, et al. Trimethoprim-sulfamethoxazole compared with pentamidine for the treatment of *Pneumocystis carinii* pneumonia in the acquired immunodeficiency syndrome: A prospective, noncrossover study. *Ann Intern Med* 109:280–287, 1988.

98. Klein NC, et al. Trimethoprim-sulfamethoxazole versus pentamidine for *Pneumocystis carinii* pneumonia in AIDS patients: Results of a large prospective randomized treatment trial. *AIDS* 6:301–305, 1992.

99. Kluge RM, Spaulding DM, Spain AJ. Combination of pentamidine and trimethoprim-sulfamethoxazole in the therapy of *Pneumocystis carinii* pneumonia in rats. *Antimicrob Agents Chemother* 13:975–978, 1978.

100. Mills J, Leoung G, Medina I, et al. Dapsone treatment of *Pneumocystis carinii* pneumonia in the acquired immunodeficiency syndrome. *Antimicrob Agents Chemother* 32:1057–1060, 1988.

101. Leoung GS, Mills J, Hopewell PC, et al. Dapsone-trimethoprim for *Pneumocystis carinii* pneumonia in the acquired immunodeficiency syndrome. *Ann Intern Med* 105:45–48, 1986.

102. Medina I, Mills J, Leoung G, et al. Oral therapy for *Pneumocystis carinii* pneumonia in the acquired immunodeficiency syndrome: A controlled trial of trimethoprim-sulfamethoxazole versus trimethoprim-dapsone. *N Engl J Med* 323:776–782, 1990.

103. Toma E. Clindamycin/primaquine for treatment of *Pneumocystis carinii* pneumonia in AIDS. *Eur J Clin Microbiol Infect Dis* 10:210–213, 1991.

104. Black JR, Feinberg J, Murphy RL, et al. Clindamycin and primaquine as primary treatment for mild and moderately severe *Pneumocystis carinii* pneumonia in patients with AIDS. *Eur J Clin Microbiol Infect Dis* 10:204–207, 1991.

105. Ruf B, Rohde I, Pohle HD. Efficacy of clindamycin/primaquine versus trimethoprim/sulfamethoxazole in primary treatment of *Pneumocystis carinii* pneumonia. *Eur J Clin Microbiol Infect Dis* 10:207–210, 1991.

106. Noskin GA, et al. Salvage therapy with clindamycin-primaquine for *Pneumocystis carinii* pneumonia. *Clin Infect Dis* 14:183–188, 1992.

107. Corkery KJ, Luce JM, Montgomery AB. Aerosolized pentamidine for treatment and prophylaxis of *Pneumocystis carinii* pneumonia: An update. *Respir Care* 33:676–685, 1988.

108. Falloon J, Kovacs J, Hughes W, et al. A preliminary evaluation of 566C80 for the treatment of pneumocystis pneumonia in patients with the acquired immunodeficiency syndrome. *N Engl J Med* 325:1534–1538, 1991.

109. Hughes W, et al. Comparison of atovaquone (566C80) with trimethoprim-sulfamethoxazole to treat *Pneumocystis carinii* pneumonia in patients with AIDS. *N Engl J Med* 328:1521–1527, 1993.

110. Dohn MN, et al. Oral atovaquone compared with intravenous pentamidine for *Pneumocystis carinii* pneumonia in patients with AIDS. Atovaquone Study Group. *Ann Intern Med* 121:174–180, 1994.

111. Allegra CJ, Chabner BA, Tuazon CU, et al. Trimetrexate for the treatment of *Pneumocystis carinii* pneumonia in patients with acquired immunodeficiency syndrome. *N Engl J Med* 317:978–985, 1987.

112. Sattler FR, Allegra CJ, Verdegem, TD, et al. Trimetrexate-leucovorin dosage evaluation study for treatment of *Pneumocystis carinii* pneumonia. *J Infect Dis* 161:91–96, 1990.

113. Sattler FR, et al. Trimetrexate with leucovorin versus trimethoprim-sulfamethoxazole for moderate to severe episodes of *Pneumocystis carinii* pneumonia in patients with AIDS: A prospective, controlled multicenter investigation of the AIDS Clinical Trials Group Protocol 029/031. *J Infect Dis* 170:165–172, 1994.

114. Clement M, Edison R, Turner J, et al. Corticosteroids as adjunctive therapy in severe *Pneumocystis carinii* pneumonia: A prospective placebo-controlled trial. *Am Rev Respir Dis* 139:A250, 1989.

115. Montaner JSG, Lawson LM, Levitt N, et al. Corticosteroids prevent early deterioration in patients with moderately severe *Pneumocystis carinii* pneumonia and the acquired immunodeficiency syndrome (AIDS). *Ann Intern Med* 113:14–20, 1990.

116. Gagnon S, Boota AM, Fischl MA, et al. Corticosteroids as adjunctive therapy for severe *Pneumocystis carinii* pneumonia in the acquired immunodeficiency syndrome. *N Engl J Med* 323:1444–1450, 1990.

117. Bozzette SA, Sattler FR, Chiu J, et al. A controlled trial of early adjunc-

tive treatment with corticosteroids for *Pneumocystis carinii* pneumonia in the acquired immunodeficiency syndrome. *N Engl J Med* 323:1451–1457, 1990.

118. Gill PS, Loureiro C, Bernstein-Singer M, et al. Clinical effect of glucocorticoids on Kaposi sarcoma related to the acquired immunodeficiency syndrome (AIDS). *Ann Intern Med* 110:937–940, 1989.

119. Real FX, Krown SE, Koziner B. Steroid-related development of Kaposi's sarcoma in a homosexual man with Burkitt's lymphoma. *Am J Med* 80:119–122, 1986.

120. Lambertus MW, Goetz MB, Murthy AR, Mathisen GE. Complications of corticosteroid therapy in patients with the acquired immunodeficiency syndrome and *Pneumocystis carinii* pneumonia. *Chest* 98:38–43, 1990.

121. Jones BE, et al. Tuberculosis in patients with HIV-infection who receive corticosteroids for presumed *Pneumocystis carinii* pneumonia. *Am J Respir Crit Care Med* 149:1686–1688, 1994.

122. National Institutes of Health—University of California expert panel for corticosteroids as adjunctive therapy for pneumocystis pneumonia. Special report: consensus statement on the use of corticosteroids as adjunctive therapy for pneumocystis pneumonia in the acquired immunodeficiency syndrome. *N Engl J Med* 323:1500–1504, 1990.

123. Hughes WT, Kuhn S, Chaudhary S, et al. Successful chemoprophylaxis for *Pneumocystis carinii* pneumonitis. *N Engl J Med* 297:1419–1426, 1977.

124. Hughes WT, Rivera GK, Schell MJ, et al. Successful intermittent chemoprophylaxis for *Pneumocystis carinii* pneumonitis. *N Engl J Med* 316:1627–1632, 1987.

125. Masur H, Ognibene FP, Yarchoan R, et al. CD4 counts as predictors of opportunistic pneumonias in human immunodeficiency virus (HIV) infection. *Ann Intern Med* 111:223–231, 1989.

126. Phair J, Munoz A, Detels R, et al. The risk of *Pneumocystis carinii* pneumonia among men infected with human immunodeficiency virus type I. *N Engl J Med* 322:161–165, 1990.

127. Fischl MA, Dickinson GM, La Voie L. Safety and efficacy of sulfamethoxazole and trimethoprim chemoprophylaxis for *Pneumocystis carinii* pneumonia in AIDS. *JAMA* 259:1185–1189, 1988.

128. Wormser GP, Horowitz HW, Duncanson FP, et al. Low-dose intermittent trimethoprim-sulfamethoxazole for prevention of *Pneumocystis carinii* pneumonia in patients with human immunodeficiency virus infection. *Arch Intern Med* 151:688–692, 1991.

129. Ruskin J, LaRiviere M. Low-dose co-trimoxazole for prevention of *Pneumocystis carinii* pneumonia in human immunodeficiency virus disease. *Lancet* 337:468–471, 1991.

130. Hirschel B, Lazzarin A, Chopard P, et al. A controlled study of inhaled pentamidine for primary prevention of *Pneumocystis carinii* pneumonia. *N Engl J Med* 324:1079–1083, 1991.

131. Montaner JSG, Lawson LM, Geravais A, et al. Aerosol pentamidine for secondary prophylaxis of AIDS-related *Pneumocystis carinii* pneumonia: A randomized, placebo-controlled study. *Ann Intern Med* 114:948–953, 1991.

132. Leoung GS, Feigal DW, Montgomery AB, et al. Aerosolized pentamidine

for prophylaxis against *Pneumocystis carinii* pneumonia: The San Francisco Community Prophylaxis Trial. *N Engl J Med* 323:769–775, 1990.

133. Golden JA, et al. A randomized comparison of once monthly or twice monthly high-dose aerosol pentamidine prophylaxis. *Chest* 104:743–750, 1993.

134. Cheung TW, et al. Intramuscular pentamidine for the prevention of *Pneumocystis carinii* pneumonia in patients infected with human immunodeficiency virus. *Clin Infect Dis* 16:22–25, 1993.

135. Metroka CE, Braun N, Josefberg H, et al. Successful chemoprophylaxis for *Pneumocystis carinii* pneumonia with dapsone in patients with AIDS and ARC. Fourth International Conference on AIDS, Stockholm, June 1988.

136. Metroka CE, Jacobus D, Lewis N. Successful chemoprophylaxis for pneumocystis with dapsone or Bactrim. Fifth International Conference on AIDS, Montreal, June 1989.

137. Hughes WT, Kennedy W, Dugdale M, et al. Prevention of *Pneumocystis carinii* pneumonitis in AIDS patients with weekly dapsone. *Lancet* 336:1066, 1990.

138. Lavelle J, Falloon J, Morgan A, et al. Weekly dapsone and dapsone/pyrimethamine for PCP prophylaxis. Seventh International Conference on AIDS, Florence, June 1991.

139. Edelson PJ, Metroka CE, Friedman-Kien AF. Dapsone, trimethoprim-sulfamethoxazole, and the acquired immunodeficiency syndrome. *Ann Intern Med* 103:963, 1985.

140. Jorde UP, Horowitz HW, Wormser GP. Utility of dapsone for prophylaxis of *Pneumocystis carinii* pneumonia in trimethoprim-sulfamethoxazole–intolerant, HIV-infected individuals. *AIDS* 7:355–359, 1993.

141. Pertel P, Hirtschtick R. Adverse reactions to dapsone in persons infected with human immunodeficiency virus. *Clin Infect Dis* 18:630–632, 1994.

142. Gottlieb MS, Knight S, Mitsuyasu R, et al. Prophylaxis of *Pneumocystis carinii* infection in AIDS with pyrimethamine-sulfadoxine. *Lancet* 2:398–399, 1984.

143. Madoff LC, Scavuzzo D, Roberts RB. Fansidar secondary prophylaxis of *Pneumocystis carinii* pneumonia in AIDS patients. *Clin Research* 34:524A, 1986.

144. Fischl MA, Dickinson GM. Fansidar prophylaxis of *Pneumocystis* pneumonia in the acquired immunodeficiency syndrome. *Ann Intern Med* 105:629, 1986.

145. Centers for Disease Control. Fansidar-associated fatal reaction in an HIV-infected man. *MMWR* 37:571–577, 1988.

146. Heald A, Flepp M, Chave JP, et al. Treatment for cerebral toxoplasmosis protects against *Pneumocystis carinii* pneumonia in patients with AIDS. *Ann Intern Med* 115:760–763, 1991.

147. Fischl MA, Richman DD, Grieco MH, et al. The efficacy of azidothymidine (AZT) in the treatment of patients with AIDS and AIDS-related complex: A double-blind, placebo-controlled trial. *N Engl J Med* 317:185–191, 1987.

148. Montgomery AB, Leoung GS, Wardlaw LA, et al. Effect of zidovudine on mortality rates and *Pneumocystis carinii* (PCP) incidence in AIDS and ARC patients on aerosol pentamidine. *Am Rev Respir Dis* 139:A250, 1989.

149. Campbell SSW, Carrow MJ, Gold JWM, et al. Comparison of second

episodes of *Pneumocystis carinii* pneumonia between AIDS patients treated and not treated with AZT. Fourth International Conference on AIDS, Stockholm, June 1988.

150. Causey DM, Leedom JM, Melancon H. Major opportunistic infections in AIDS patients after eight to one hundred weeks of zidovudine (ZDV) therapy. Fourth International Conference on AIDS, Stockholm, June 1988.

151. Girard PM, Landman R, Gaudebout C, et al. Prevention of *Pneumocystis carinii* pneumonia relapse by pentamidine aerosol in zidovudine-treated AIDS patients. *Lancet* I:1348–1353, 1989.

152. Andrews JC, McManus M, Rogers G, et al. Clinical benefits of concurrent administration of zidovudine and therapy for the suppression of *Pneumocystis carinii*. Fourth International Conference on AIDS, Stockholm, June 1988.

153. Hardy WD, et al. A controlled trial of trimethoprim-sulfamethoxazole or aerolized pentamidine for secondary prophylaxis of *Pneumocystis carinii* pneumonia in patients with the acquired immunodeficiency syndrome. *N Engl J Med* 327:1842–1848, 1992.

154. Schneider MME, et al. A controlled trial of aerosolized pentamidine or trimethoprim-sulfamethoxazole as primary prophylaxis against *Pneumocystis carinii* pneumonia in patients with human immunodeficiency virus infection. *N Engl J Med* 327:1836–1841, 1992.

155. Bozzette SA, et al. A randomized trial of three antipneumocystis agents in patients with advanced human immunodeficiency virus infection. *N Engl J Med* 332:693–669, 1995.

156. Blum RN, et al. Comparative trial of dapsone versus trimethoprim/sulfamethoxazole for primary prophylaxis of *Pneumocystis carinii* pneumonia. *J Acquir Immune Defic Syndr* 5:341–347, 1992.

157. Martin MA, et al. A comparison of the effectiveness of three regimens in the prevention of *Pneumocystis carinii* pneumonia in human immunodeficiency virus–infected patients. *Arch Intern Med* 152:523–528, 1992.

158. Podzamczer D, et al. Thrice-weekly co-trimoxazole is better than weekly dapsone-pyrimethamine for the primary prevention of *Pneumocystis carinii* pneumonia in HIV-infected patients. *AIDS* 7:501–506, 1993.

159. Slavin NA, et al. Oral dapsone versus nebulized pentamidine for *Pneumocystis carinii* prophylaxis: An open randomized prospective trial to assess efficacy and haematological toxicity. *AIDS* 6:1169–1174, 1992.

160. Torres RA, et al. Randomized trial of dapsone and aerosolized pentamidine for the prophylaxis of *Pneumocystis carinii* pneumonia and toxoplasmic encephalitis. *Am J Med* 95:573–583, 1993.

161. Girard PM, et al. Dapsone-pyrimethamine compared with aerosolized pentamidine as primary prophylaxis against *Pneumocystis carinii* and toxoplasmosis in HIV-infection. The PRIO Study Group. *N Engl J Med* 328:1514–1520, 1993.

162. Chaisson RE, et al. Pneumocystis prophylaxis and survival in patients with advanced human immunodeficiency virus infection treated with zidovudine. *Arch Intern Med* 152:2009–2013, 1992.

163. Carr A, et al. Low-dose trimethoprim-sulfamethoxazole prophylaxis for toxoplasmic encephalitis in patients with AIDS. *Ann Intern Med* 117:106–111, 1992.

164. May T, et al. Trimethoprim-sulfamethoxazole versus aerosolized pentamidine for primary prophylaxis of *Pneumocystis carinii* pneumonia: A prospective, randomized, controlled clinical trial. LFPMI Study Group. Ligue Française de Prevention des Maladies Infestieuses. *J Acquir Immune Defic Syndr* 7:457–462, 1994.
165. Centers for Disease Control. Recommendations for prophylaxis against *Pneumocystis carinii* pneumonia for adults and adolescents infected with human immunodeficiency virus. *MMWR* 41(RR-4):1–11, 1992.
166. Centers for Disease Control. USPHS/IDSA guidelines for the prevention of opportunistic infections in persons with human immunodeficiency virus: A summary. *MMWR* 44(RR-8):1–34, 1995.

Mycobacterial Infections *20*

Harrison W. Farber, Thomas W. Barber

Mycobacteria are responsible for an increasing proportion of the opportunistic infections associated with HIV disease. *Mycobacterium tuberculosis* and *M. avium-intracellulare* (also known as *M. avium* complex [MAC]) are the most common pathogens, although other species such as *Mycobacterium kansasii* and, perhaps, *Mycobacterium gordonae* may also infect patients with advanced HIV disease [1–3].

Mycobacterium tuberculosis

Epidemiology

Earlier projections that tuberculosis (TB) might be eliminated by the year 2010 have been replaced by increasing concerns that the disease may become the "plague of the 1990s." These fears have been fostered by the potential for rapid spread of TB within susceptible populations, the laxity with which infection control measures are often applied, and the emergence of multidrug-resistant strains [4].

Tuberculosis is unevenly distributed in the United States. Population groups that are known to have a high incidence of TB include blacks, Latinos, Alaskan natives, prisoners, alcoholics, injection drug users (IDUs), the homeless, the elderly, and foreign-born persons from areas with a high prevalence of TB, including the Caribbean basin, Africa, and Asia [5]. The long-standing downward trend in morbidity from TB in the United States reversed and began to rise in the mid-1980s [6]. Current epidemiologic evidence suggests that this resurgence is largely related to the HIV epidemic [7–9].

The greatest increase in reported TB cases has occurred in cities with large numbers of AIDS patients and in population groups with the highest rates of TB [8, 10–15]. For example, in New York City, the incidence of TB has increased by 68 percent over the past decade. A prospective study of 520 IDUs on methadone maintenance found that, while 20 percent of both the HIV-positive and HIV-negative groups had a positive TB skin test (purified protein derivative, or PPD), all 8 subsequent cases of active TB were in HIV-infected individuals [16]. Seven of the eight patients with active TB had a positive PPD, and none had received isoniazid (INH) prophylaxis. In a San Francisco study, a greater percentage of HIV-positive heterosexual IDUs were noted to have TB compared to HIV-positive homosexual, non-IDU control subjects [17]. The increased risk of active TB in Haitians with AIDS appears related to the high prevalence of latent tuberculous infection in this population [8, 18]. In Massachusetts, 33 percent of patients with AIDS and TB are foreign born compared to 3.5 percent of those with AIDS alone [19]. The HIV seropositivity rate in patients from US tuberculosis clinics varies widely, from as high as 46 percent in New York City to as low as 0.3 percent in Honolulu [20] (Table 20-1).

The overall prevalence of TB in HIV-infected patients ranges from 5 to 35 percent, with affected individuals more likely to be male, African-American, Haitian, or Latino. Extrapulmonary TB has increased six-fold compared to pulmonary TB, reflecting its common association with HIV infection [8, 11, 12, 17]; approximately 25 percent of extrapulmonary TB is related to HIV disease, and over 50 percent of the TB that complicates AIDS is extrapulmonary [20]. HIV-infected patients with a positive PPD have an extremely high risk of developing active TB (8% annually vs. 10% lifetime in immunocompetent persons), and clinical disease may develop within months of exposure [16, 21].

There is evidence that HIV-infected individuals are not only predisposed to activation of latent TB but also to acquisition of new infection [22]. Tuberculosis in such patients frequently progresses rapidly to active disease and may be fulminant [20]. There are also data based on molecular biology techniques, which demonstrate that previously infected

Table 20-1 *HIV seropositivity prevalence in patients attending TB clinics in US cities*

City	Total	HIV seropositivity (%)	
		US born	Foreign born
New York	46.0	57.4	31.4
Boston	26.6	30.9	24.6
Miami	23.5	28.5	19.5
Dallas	8.6	11.2	4.6
Chicago	2.4	1.3	1.8
Cleveland	1.7	2.3	0.0
Los Angeles	6.2	13.0	3.3
Honolulu	0.3	0.3	0.0
All cities	3.4	11.2	2.9

patients may become reinfected with a second, sometimes drug-resistant, tuberculous strain [23].

Clinical Manifestations

Before being included in the AIDS case definition, the diagnosis of TB usually coincided with or preceded that of AIDS, suggesting the existence of early defects in cell-mediated immunity [8, 13, 15]. It has also been suggested that the development of TB in HIV-infected individuals may accelerate the course of immunodeficiency [24].

In general, the clinical manifestations of TB are determined by the stage of HIV disease [20, 25] (Table 20-2). These may include fever, night sweats, weight loss, and cough, and there is often evidence of dissemination to extrapulmonary sites, including the lymph nodes, liver, bone marrow, and central nervous system [17, 26–28]. Studies demonstrate that 35 to 65 percent of patients with TB and AIDS have extrapulmonary involvement, and 16 to 23 percent have isolated extrapulmonary disease [8, 17, 18, 26, 27]. The chest x-ray (CXR) most often reveals diffuse or miliary infiltrates, focal infiltrates in upper or lower lung fields, and/or mediastinal or hilar adenopathy, but may be normal in up to 10 percent of patients [26, 27, 29, 30]. Compared to HIV-seronegative patients with TB, the CXR in HIV-infected patients is much less likely to show typical cavitary lesions, apical scarring, or pleural effusions [26, 27, 29, 30]. Rapidly evolving radiographic abnormalities generally indicate a pulmonary process other than TB.

Diagnosis

Tuberculosis is more difficult to identify in HIV-infected patients than in the general population, with diagnosis often delayed because of atypical clinical presentations, negative sputum smears, and cutaneous anergy [4]. As HIV infection progresses and cellular immunity declines, the PPD often becomes nonreactive, and CXR findings are more nonspecific. Positive sputum smears for acid-fast bacilli (AFB) occur in 31 to 82 percent of TB cases associated with HIV disease, with sensitiv-

Table 20-2 *Manifestations of active tuberculosis in patients with HIV disease*

	Early (CD4 cell count > 500/mm³)	*Late (CD4 cell count < 200/mm³)*
PPD	Usually positive	Usually negative
Adenopathy	Unusual	Common
Pulmonary distribution	Upper lobe	Lower and middle lobe
Cavitation	Often present	Typically absent
Extrapulmonary disease	10–15% of cases	≥ 50% of cases

ity decreasing in more severely immunocompromised individuals and tissue biopsy specimens less frequently demonstrating granulomas [31, 32]. However, in the appropriate clinical setting, lymph node, bone marrow, or brain biopsy may be diagnostic [13, 32, 33]. Blood cultures using a lysis-centrifugation system are positive in 26 to 42 percent of HIV-infected patients with TB and should be performed whenever disseminated disease is suspected [32, 34, 35]. Because of the difficulty in establishing an early definitive diagnosis, TB should be considered in any HIV-seropositive patient with pulmonary symptoms, and individuals in whom there is a high index of suspicion of TB should be treated with antimycobacterial therapy pending culture results.

Prognosis

Tuberculosis, both pulmonary and extrapulmonary, is one of the more treatable infectious complications in HIV-infected patients, even in those with severe immunodeficiency [17, 18, 27, 36, 37]. Poor outcome is usually associated with medication noncompliance or the presence of disseminated disease [38]. The response to treatment and median survival of HIV-infected patients with pansensitive strains of TB are not significantly different compared to individuals who are not HIV-infected [39, 40]. However, TB caused by organisms resistant to INH and rifampin is notable for its poor response to treatment with standard drug regimens [41].

Of great concern are outbreaks of multidrug-resistant TB (MDR-TB) in HIV-infected patients initially reported from hospitals and prisons in Miami and New York City [4, 42–45]. Multidrug-resistant TB strains are defined as those that are resistant to at least two first-line antituberculous medications, usually INH and rifampin, although resistance to other agents has also been described [4]. Most patients with MDR-TB had advanced immunodeficiency, and the majority died within 4 months of diagnosis. Several cases were apparently transmitted to health care workers. In many patients, diagnosis was delayed because of unusual clinical presentations, and, in all of the hospitals, AFB isolation precautions were inadequate. In 1991, MDR-TB was found in 3.5 percent of cultures from 35 counties in 13 states. However, there is uneven distribution in the United States; for example, New York City has reported 61 percent of US MDR-TB cases [46].

Management

Treatment should be instituted whenever there is a high index of suspicion of TB or whenever AFB are found in a specimen from an HIV-infected patient (Table 20-3). Because untreated TB is potentially fatal and is transmissible to others, all patients with HIV disease and suspected mycobacterial infection should receive empiric treatment that is

Table 20-3 *Tuberculosis treatment regimens for the HIV-infected patient*

Clinical situation*	Treatment
Initial therapy	
INH resistance unlikely	INH, RIF, PZA
INH resistance likely	INH, RIF, PZA, EMB or STREP
MDR-TB likely	INH, RIF, PZA, 2 others
Therapy after culture results	
Sensitive organism	INH, RIF, PZA (2 mo), then INH, RIF (7 mo) or 6 mo post negative culture (whichever longer)
INH resistance or INH intolerance	RIF, EMB, PZA (18 mo) or 12 mo post negative culture (whichever longer)
RIF intolerance	INH, PZA, EMB (18–24 mo) or 12 mo post negative culture (whichever longer)
MDR-TB	Based on sensitivity (duration unknown)

INH = isoniazid; RIF = rifampin; PZA = pyrazinamide; EMB = ethambutol; STREP = streptomycin; MDR-TB = multidrug-resistant TB.
*See text for specific recommendations and drug dosages.

effective against *M. tuberculosis* [7]. The recent development of DNA probes has expedited the task of distinguishing *M. tuberculosis* from atypical mycobacteria, permitting earlier definitive diagnosis [47]. Pending culture results, initial therapy in this era of multidrug resistance should consist of INH (300 mg/day), rifampin (600 mg/day), pyrazinamide (25 mg/kg/day), and ethambutol (15 mg/kg/day) or streptomycin (15 mg/kg/day) [41]. Note that ethambutol or streptomycin is included in the initial drug regimen unless there is little possibility of resistance (< 4% primary resistance to INH in the community) and the patient has had no previous treatment with antituberculous medications, is not from a country with a high prevalence of drug resistance, and has not been exposed to a drug-resistant case. If MDR-TB is suspected, patients should be treated with a regimen containing INH, rifampin, pyrazinamide, and at least two other drugs to which the mycobacterial strain is likely susceptible based on local drug sensitivity patterns [4, 42]. Drug susceptibility testing should be performed on all isolates and therapy adjusted once culture results are available [48].

The optimal duration of TB therapy in HIV-infected patients is unknown. Current recommendations are for 9 to 12 months (at least 6 months after sputum sterilization) in patients with INH-sensitive strains and 18 months (at least 12 months after sputum sterilization) in patients with INH-resistant strains. Following completion of therapy, some authors recommend continuing INH monotherapy indefinitely [49]. In some studies of HIV-infected patients, a higher rate of adverse reactions to antimycobacterial agents, especially rifampin, has been reported [17, 37]. Liver function tests should be closely monitored during therapy, and dosage adjustment of coadministered drugs that are metabolized in the liver may be necessary.

Prevention

Available evidence indicates that chemoprophylaxis is effective in preventing TB in HIV-infected patients [50–52]. The high rate of active disease and public health concerns make this aspect of management a priority. All HIV-infected patients should have an intermediate-strength (5TU) PPD placed with appropriate controls [53]; induration of 5 mm or more is considered positive. The suggestion has been made that lowering the threshold for a positive PPD to 2 mm induration in HIV-infected IDUs may help identify additional patients who have been exposed to TB [54].

Assuming no contraindications, HIV-infected patients with a positive PPD should receive INH prophylaxis for one year regardless of age once active TB has been excluded [7, 53]. HIV-infected individuals who are anergic on skin testing and at high risk for TB, including IDUs, the homeless, past or current prison inmates, or patients from an endemic area, should also receive chemoprophylaxis [7, 53]. HIV-infected patients with a history of positive PPD who have never been treated with INH or with CXR abnormalities suggestive of prior TB, and close contacts of active cases, should receive prophylaxis as well [7, 53]. Twice-weekly INH (15 mg/kg) can be substituted for daily therapy in patients whose treatment can be supervised. For individuals unable to take INH or when INH resistance is suspected, rifampin can be given instead [55]. An alternative regimen of rifampin and pyrazinamide given for 2 months is currently under investigation [56]. All patients with HIV infection who have a negative PPD should be regularly screened with repeat skin tests for new exposure to TB. Routine administration of a second PPD dose for booster effect is not recommended because of its low utility [57].

HIV-infected patients who are exposed to persons with MDR-TB pose a special problem [58]. Although the appropriate prophylactic regimen is unknown, ethambutol and pyrazinamide, with or without a fluoroquinolone, are currently recommended. This regimen should be given for at least 1 year.

Mycobacterium avium Complex

Epidemiology

Mycobacterium avium and *M. intracellulare* are closely related species of nontuberculous or "atypical" mycobacteria, often classified together as

M. avium-intracellulare or *M. avium* complex. HIV seropositivity with disseminated nontuberculous mycobacterial infection constitutes an AIDS-defining diagnosis. MAC accounted for 96.1 percent of such infections in patients with AIDS reported to the Centers for Disease Control between 1981 and 1987 [59].

Before the emergence of HIV, disseminated MAC infection occurred rarely and almost exclusively in individuals with defective cell-mediated immunity. MAC has also been reported to cause lymphadenitis in children and chronic lung infection in adults with underlying obstructive pulmonary disease [60, 61]. Disseminated MAC infection occurs in HIV-infected patients of all risk groups, ages, and races who are at an advanced stage of immunodeficiency (CD4 lymphocyte count < 100/mm^3) [62–64]. The disease has been diagnosed antemortem in approximately 25 percent of AIDS patients and identified at autopsy in up to 50 percent [65, 66].

Retrospective studies suggest that the time from AIDS diagnosis to development of disseminated MAC infection has increased since the mid-1980s, a trend that is related to the widespread administration of antiretroviral therapy, pneumocystis prophylaxis, and effective treatment of opportunistic infections [67]. Prospective data show that most, if not all, patients with AIDS who do not die from another HIV-related complication will ultimately acquire MAC infection [68].

Patients with AIDS are more likely to develop infection with *M. avium* than *M. intracellulare*, while non-AIDS patients are just as likely to become infected with either species [69–71]. MAC is distributed widely in the environment and has been isolated from a number of wild and domestic animals [68]. Suspected modes of exposure to the organism include inhalation or ingestion of contaminated water, soil, dust, and animal products. Acquisition of MAC from hospital water supplies by HIV-infected inpatients has been documented [72]. It is not known whether person-to-person transmission occurs.

Clinical Manifestations

Disseminated MAC infection produces a nonspecific constellation of symptoms, including fever, night sweats, fatigue, malaise, anorexia, weight loss, abdominal pain, and diarrhea. A malabsorption syndrome has been correlated pathologically with MAC infiltration of the small bowel. Pulmonary symptoms are uncommon. Physical examination reveals cachexia, often with palpable adenopathy and hepatosplenomegaly. Most patients have anemia, thrombocytopenia, leukopenia, and increased liver function tests, especially serum alkaline phosphatase [73]. It is estimated that patients with advanced HIV disease and this clinical profile in whom *Pneumocystis carinii* pneumonia, CMV infection, and infectious diarrhea have been excluded are more than 70 percent likely to have disseminated MAC infection [74].

Diagnosis

Diagnosis of disseminated MAC infection is established by a positive culture of blood or, less often, another body fluid or tissue, such as bone marrow, liver, or lymph node [75]. Blood should be cultured in lysis-centrifugation tubes or using an in vitro radiometric technique. These blood culture systems are highly sensitive, and two blood cultures are almost always sufficient to detect MAC bacteremia [76, 77].

Sputum and stool cultures may reveal MAC but do not dependably indicate or predict disseminated disease [78]. Histopathologic examination of biopsy specimens often shows macrophages, many AFB, and a minimal inflammatory response, with poorly formed epithelioid granulomas and little tissue necrosis or fibrosis [75]. Definitive diagnosis of MAC infection cannot be based solely on histology. Tuberculosis should always be considered in the differential diagnosis of a positive AFB stain pending culture results.

Prognosis

Disseminated MAC infection is associated with profound immunodeficiency and usually preceded by one or more AIDS-defining illnesses [79]. Untreated MAC infection appears to shorten survival by approximately 6 months [59, 80]. In one study, the median survival time for patients with disseminated MAC infection who did not receive antimycobacterial therapy was 4 months, significantly shorter than that in AIDS patients who received treatment for MAC (median survival 8 months) and in matched control subjects with AIDS but without MAC infection (median survival 11 months) [81]. More recent reports have confirmed that MAC infection is associated with increased mortality and that antimicrobial therapy improves survival [82, 83].

Management

Early reports of treatment for disseminated MAC infection in patients with AIDS were disappointing, but a number of more recent studies evaluating various multidrug regimens with newer agents demonstrate that prolonged therapy may result in the clearing of bacteremia and improvement in constitutional symptoms [62, 63, 84, 85]. Treatment-limiting drug toxicity is common. Isolates of MAC are often resistant in vitro to first-line antituberculous agents, but this finding does not consistently correlate with clinical outcome.

Most conventional regimens include two to five agents selected from the drugs known to have activity against some isolates of MAC. The most commonly used agents include clarithromycin, azithromycin, rifampin, rifabutin, clofazimine, ethambutol, ciprofloxacin, and amikacin (Table 20-4). Various combinations of these drugs have been studied in small groups of patients, but there is limited consensus

Table 20-4 *Drugs used in the treatment of MAC infection*

Drug	Dosage	Major toxicities
Clarithromycin	500–1,000 mg PO bid	Gastrointestinal intolerance Hepatotoxicity Rash Headache Dizziness Reversible hearing loss
Azithromycin	500–1,000 mg PO qd	Gastrointestinal intolerance Hepatotoxicity Rash Headache Dizziness Reversible hearing loss
Rifampin[a]	600 mg PO qd	Gastrointestinal intolerance Hepatotoxicity Rash Orange discoloration of secretions
Rifabutin[a,b]	300–600 mg PO qd	Gastrointestinal intolerance Hepatotoxicity Rash Orange discoloration of secretions Uveitis
Clofazimine	50–100 mg PO qd	Gastrointestinal intolerance Abdominal pain Hepatotoxicity Skin discoloration
Ethambutol	15–25 mg/kg PO qd	Optic neuritis Rash Gastrointestinal intolerance Hepatotoxicity
Ciprofloxacin	500–750 mg PO qd	Gastrointestinal intolerance Neurotoxicity Rash
Amikacin	7.5 mg/kg q12–24h IM or IV	Nephrotoxicity Ototoxicity

[a]This agent may affect the serum levels of coadministered drugs that are hepatically metabolized.
[b]This agent in the dose of 300 mg/day has been shown to be effective in the prophylaxis of MAC infection. See text for details.

regarding the optimal regimen. Pending the results of ongoing prospective controlled clinical trials, many clinicians currently use macrolide antibiotic, such as clarithromycin or azithromycin, in combination with one or more other agents chosen to minimize toxicity and drug interactions. The medial regimen may need to be modified over time depending on the severity of the patient's illness and response to therapy. Monotherapy should be discouraged because of the likelihood that selection of resistant mutants or coinfecting MAC strains may ensue [86, 87]. Improvement in constitutional symptoms, abdominal pain, and diarrhea usually requires at least several weeks of therapy. Complex multidrug regimens used for initial therapy can often be simplified to include two or three medications once symptoms of disseminated MAC disease have abated. If tolerated, treatment is generally continued for the remainder of the patient's life.

Prevention

Knowledge of the ecology and risk factors for acquisition of MAC are inadequate to support specific recommendations for avoidance of infection.

Two placebo-controlled trials with identical design have demonstrated that rifabutin is an effective agent for prophylaxis of disseminated MAC disease in HIV-infected patients with CD4 cell counts of 200/mm^3 or less, reducing the rate of MAC bacteremia by 50 percent without significant drug toxicity [88]. Although reduced mortality was not demonstrated, there was a trend toward prolonged survival. Surprisingly, MAC isolates from patients receiving rifabutin therapy in whom MAC bacteremia developed were not resistant to the drug in vitro. Several recent preliminary studies suggest that clarithromycin is also effective for primary prevention of MAC infection [89–91].

Based on the results of these studies, the Food and Drug Administration approved rifabutin for prophylaxis of MAC bacteremia in persons with AIDS, and a Public Health Service Task Force recommended that individuals with HIV infection and CD4 cell counts below 100/mm^3 be given rifabutin [92]. More recent guidelines advocate consideration of rifabutin prophylaxis in persons with CD4 counts less than 75/mm^3 [92a]. However, several investigators have reported a probable association between rifabutin therapy and uveitis [93–95]. It is also possible that the widespread use of rifabutin may increase the prevalence of rifamycin resistance among a variety of bacteria, including *M. tuberculosis*. Finally, there are concerns about interaction between rifabutin and many drugs used in the treatment of advanced HIV disease, including clarithromycin, fluconazole, zidovudine, methadone, and others [96, 97]. Clinicians who prescribe rifabutin should consider these issues while awaiting further data on other options for MAC prophylaxis.

References

1. Scherer R, Sable R, Sonnenberg M, et al. Disseminated infection with *Mycobacterium kansasii* in the acquired immunodeficiency syndrome. *Ann Intern Med* 105:710–712, 1986.
2. Levine B, Chaisson RE. *Mycobacterium kansasii*: A cause of treatable pulmonary disease associated with advanced human immunodeficiency virus infection. *Ann Intern Med* 114:861–868, 1991.
3. Barber TW, Craven DE, Farber HW. *Mycobacterium gordonae*: A possible opportunistic respiratory tract pathogen in patients with advanced human immunodeficiency virus, type 1 infection. *Chest* 100:716–720, 1991.
4. Davey RT, Jr. Mycobacterial disease in HIV-1 infection: Recent therapeutic advances. In HC Lane (moderator), Recent advances in the management of AIDS-related opportunistic infections. *Ann Intern Med* 120:945–955, 1994.
5. Centers for Disease Control. Guidelines for preventing the transmission of tuberculosis in health-care settings, with special focus on HIV-related issues. *MMWR* 39:1–29, 1990.
6. Centers for Disease Control. Update: Tuberculosis elimination—United States. *MMWR* 39:153–156, 1990.
7. Centers for Disease Control. Tuberculosis and human immunodeficiency virus infection: Recommendations of the advisory committee for the elimination of tuberculosis (ACET). *MMWR* 38:236–250, 1989.
8. Rieder HL, Cauthen GM, Bloch AB, et al. Tuberculosis and acquired immunodeficiency syndrome—Florida. *Arch Intern Med* 149:1268–1273, 1989.
9. Chaisson RE, Slutkin G. Tuberculosis and human immunodeficiency virus infection. *J Infect Dis* 159:96–99, 1989.
10. Centers for Disease Control. Tuberculosis—United States, 1985—and the possible impact of the human lymphotropic virus type III/lymphadenopathy-associated virus infection. *MMWR* 35:74–76, 1986.
11. Centers for Disease Control. Tuberculosis and acquired immunodeficiency syndrome—New York City. *MMWR* 36:785–790, 1987.
12. Bloch AB, Reider HL, Kelly GD, et al. The epidemiology of tuberculosis in the United States. *Semin Respir Infect* 4:157–170, 1989.
13. Barnes PF, Bloch AB, Davidson PT, Snider DE, Jr. Tuberculosis in patients with human immunodeficiency virus infection. *N Engl J Med* 324:1644–1650, 1991.
14. Pitchenik AE, Fertel D, Bloch AB. Mycobacterial disease; epidemiology, diagnosis, treatment, and prevention. *Clin Chest Med* 9:425–441, 1988.
15. FitzGerald JM, Grzybowski S, Allen EA. The impact of human immunodeficiency virus infection on tuberculosis and its control. *Chest* 100:191–200, 1991.
16. Selwyn PA, Hartel D, Lewis VA, et al. A prospective study of the risk of tuberculosis among intravenous drug users with human immunodeficiency virus infection. *N Engl J Med* 320:545–550, 1989.

17. Chaisson RE, Schecter GF, Theuer CP, et al. Tuberculosis in patients with the acquired immunodeficiency syndrome: Clinical features, response to therapy, and survival. *Am Rev Respir Dis* 136:570–574, 1987.

18. Pitchenik AE, Burr J, Suarez M, et al. Human T-cell lymphotrophic (virus-III) seropositivity and related disease among 71 nonconsecutive patients in whom tuberculosis was diagnosed. *Am Rev Respir Dis* 135:875–879, 1987.

19. Bernardo J, Murray C, Taylor J, et al. Epidemiology of tuberculosis (TB) and HIV infection in the homeless—Boston, 1989 (abstract). *Am Rev Respir Dis* 141:A260, 1990.

20. Haas DW, Des Prez RM. Tuberculosis and acquired immunodeficiency syndrome: A historical perspective on recent developments. *Am J Med* 96:439–450, 1994.

21. Daley CL, et al. An outbreak of tuberculosis with accelerated progression among persons infected with the human immunodeficiency virus. *N Engl J Med* 326:231–235, 1992.

22. Small PM, et al. The epidemiology of tuberculosis: A population-based model using conventional and molecular methods. *N Engl J Med* 330:1703–1709, 1994.

23. Small PM, et al. Exogenous reinfection with multidrug-resistant *Mycobacterium tuberculosis* in patients with advanced HIV infection. *N Engl J Med* 328:1137–1144, 1993.

24. Wallis RS, et al. Influence of tuberculosis on human immunodeficiency virus: Enhanced cytokine expression and elevated beta-2-microglobulin in HIV-1–associated tuberculosis. *J Infect Dis* 167:43–48, 1993.

25. Jones B, et al. Relationship of the manifestations of tuberculosis to CD4 cell counts in patients with human immunodeficiency virus infection. *Am Rev Respir Dis* 148:1292–1297, 1993.

26. Theuer CP, Hopewell PC, Elias D, et al. Human immunodeficiency virus infection in tuberculosis patients. *J Infect Dis* 162:8–12, 1990.

27. Pitchenik AE, Cole C, Russell BW, et al. Tuberculosis, atypical mycobacteriosis, and the acquired immunodeficiency syndrome among Haitian and non-Haitian patients in south Florida. *Ann Intern Med* 101:610–615, 1984.

28. Berenguer J, et al. Tuberculous meningitis in patients infected with the human immunodeficiency virus. *N Engl J Med* 326:668–672, 1992.

29. Pitchenik AE, Rubinson HA. The radiographic appearance of tuberculosis in patients with the acquired immune deficiency syndrome (AIDS) and pre-AIDS. *Am Rev Respir Dis* 131:393–396, 1985.

30. Colebunders RE, Ryder RW, Nzilambi N, et al. HIV infection in patients with tuberculosis in Kinshasa, Zaire. *Am Rev Respir Dis* 139:1082–1085, 1989.

31. Klein NC, Duncanson FP, Lenox TH, III, et al. Use of mycobacterial smears in the diagnosis of pulmonary tuberculosis in AIDS/ARC patients. *Chest* 95:1190–1192, 1989.

32. Kramer F, Modilevsky T, Waliany AR, et al. Delayed diagnosis of tuberculosis in patients with human immunodeficiency virus infection. *Am J Med* 89:451–456, 1990.

33. Bouchama A, Zuheir Al-Kawi M, Kanaan I, et al. Brain biopsy in tuberculoma: The risks and benefits. *Neurosurgery* 28:405–409, 1991.

34. Shafer RW, Goldberg R, Sierra M, Glatt AE. Frequency of *Mycobacterium tuberculosis* bacteremia in patients with tuberculosis in an area endemic for AIDS. *Am Rev Respir Dis* 140:1611–1613, 1989.

35. Barber TW, Craven DE, McCabe WR. Bacteremia due to *Mycobacterium tuberculosis* in patients with human immunodeficiency virus infection. *Medicine (Baltimore)* 69:375–383, 1990.

36. Louie E, Rice L, Holzmann RS. Tuberculosis in non-Haitian patients with the acquired immuno-deficiency syndrome. *Chest* 90:542–545, 1986.

37. Small PM, Schecter GF, Goodman PC, et al. Treatment of tuberculosis in patients with advanced human immunodeficiency virus infection. *N Engl J Med* 324:289–294, 1991.

38. Chaisson RE, Hopewell PC. Survival after active tuberculosis in patients with HIV infection (abstract). *Am Rev Respir Dir* 142:259A, 1990.

39. Stoneburner R. Survival in a cohort of human immunodeficiency virus–infected tuberculosis patients in New York City. *Ann Intern Med* 152:2033–2037, 1992.

40. Jones BE, Otaya M, Antoniskis D, et al. A prospective evaluation of antituberculous therapy in patients with HIV infection. *Am J Respir Crit Care Med* 150:1499–1502, 1994.

41. Bass JB, Jr, Farer LS, Hopewell PC, et al. Treatment of tuberculosis and tuberculosis infection in adults and children. *Am J Respir Crit Care Med* 149:1359–1374, 1994.

42. Centers for Disease Control. Nosocomial transmission of multidrug-resistant tuberculosis among HIV-infected persons—Florida and New York, 1988–1991. *MMWR* 40:586–591, 1991.

43. Edlin BR, et al. An outbreak of multidrug-resistant tuberculosis among hospitalized patients with the acquired immunodeficiency syndrome. *N Eng J Med* 326:1514–1521, 1992.

44. Fischl MA, et al. An outbreak of tuberculosis caused by multiple-drug-resistant tubercle bacilli among patients with HIV infection. *Ann Intern Med* 117:177–183, 1992.

45. Fischl MA, et al. Clinical presentation and outcome of patients with HIV infection and tuberculosis caused by multiple-drug-resistant bacilli. *Ann Intern Med* 117:184–190, 1992.

46. Bloch AB, Cauthen GM, Onorato IM, et al. Nationwide survey of drug-resistant tuberculosis in the United States. *JAMA* 271:665–671, 1994.

47. Good RC, Mastro TD. The modern mycobacteriology laboratory: How it can help the clinician. *Clin Chest Med* 10:315–322, 1989.

48. American Thoracic Society. Diagnostic standards and classification of tuberculosis. *Am Rev Respir Dis* 142:725–735, 1990.

49. American Thoracic Society. Mycobacterioses and the acquired immuno-deficiency syndrome. *Am Rev Respir Dir* 136:492–496, 1987.

50. Selwyn PA, et al. High risk of active tuberculosis in HIV-infected drug users with cutaneous anergy. *JAMA* 268:504–509, 1992.

51. Pape JW, Jean SS, Ho JL, et al. Effect of isoniazid prophylaxis on incidence

of active tuberculosis and progression of HIV infection. *Lancet* 342:268–272, 1993.

52. Moreno S, et al. Risk of developing tuberculosis among anergic patients infected with HIV. *Ann Intern Med* 119:194–198, 1993.
53. Centers for Disease Control. Screening for tuberculosis and tuberculosis infection in high-risk populations and the use of preventive therapy for tuberculosis infection in the United States: Recommendations of the Advisory Committee for Elimination of Tuberculosis. *MMWR* 39:(RR-8):1–12, 1990.
54. Graham NWH, et al. Prevalence of tuberculin positivity and skin test anergy in HIV-1-seropositive and -seronegative intravenous drug users. *JAMA* 267:369–373, 1992.
55. Gallant JE, Moore RD, Chaisson RE. Prophylaxis for opportunistic infections in patients with HIV infection. *Ann Intern Med* 120:932–944, 1994.
56. Lecoeur HF, Truffot-Pernot C, Grosset JH. Experimental short-course preventive therapy of tuberculosis with rifampin and pyrazinamide. *Am Rev Respir Dir* 140:1189–1193, 1989.
57. Webster CT, et al. Two-stage tuberculin skin testing in individuals with human immunodeficiency virus infection. *Am J Respir Crit Care Med* 151:805–808, 1995.
58. Management of persons exposed to multi-drug resistant tuberculosis. *MMWR.* 41:61–71, 1992.
59. Horsburgh CR, Selik RM. The epidemiology of disseminated nontuberculous mycobacterial infection in the acquired immunodeficiency syndrome (AIDS). *Am Rev Respir Dir* 139:4–7, 1989.
60. Kinsella JP, Culver K, Jeffrey RB, et al. Extensive cervical lymphadenitis due to *Mycobacterium avium-intracellulare*. *Pediatr Infect Dis* 6:289–291, 1987.
61. Rozenzweig DY, Schlueter DP. Spectrum of clinical disease in pulmonary infection with *Mycobacterium avium-intracellulare*. *Rev Infect Dis* 3:1046–1051, 1981.
62. Hoy J, Mitch A, Sandland M, et al. Quadruple-drug therapy for *Mycobacterium avium-intracellulare* bacteremia in AIDS patients. *J Infect Dis* 161:801–805, 1990.
63. Chiu J, Nussbaum J, Bozzette S, et al. Treatment of disseminated *Mycobacterium avium* complex infection in AIDS with amikacin, ethambutol, rifampin, and ciprofloxacin. *Ann Intern Med* 113:358–361, 1990.
64. Nightingale SD, et al. Incidence of *Mycobacterium avium-intracellulare* complex bacteremia in human immunodeficiency virus–positive patients. *J Infect Dis* 165:1082–1085, 1992.
65. Wallace JM, Hannah JB. *Mycobacterium avium* complex infection in patients with the acquired immunodeficiency syndrome: A clinicopathologic study. *Chest* 93:926–931, 1988.
66. Hawkins CC, Gold JUM, Whimby E, et al. *Mycobacterium avium* complex infections in patients with the acquired immunodeficiency syndrome. *Ann Intern Med* 105:184–188, 1986.
67. Havlik JA, Horsburgh CR, Metchock B, et al. Disseminated *Mycobacterium avium* complex infection: Clinical and epidemiologic trends. *J Infect Dis* 165:577–580, 1992.

68. Iseman MC, Corpe RF, O'Brien RJ, et al. Disease due to *Mycobacterium avium-intracellulare*. *Chest* 87:139S–149S, 1985.

69. Guthertz LS, Damsker B, Bottone EJ, et al. *Mycobacterium avium* and *Mycobacterium intracellulare* infections in patients with and without AIDS. *J Infect Dis* 160:1037–1041, 1989.

70. Horsburgh CR, Chon DL, Roberts RB, et al. *Mycobacterium avium-Mycobacterium intracellulare* isolates from patients with or without acquired immunodeficiency syndrome. *Antimicrob Agents Chemother* 30:955–957, 1986.

71. Yakrus MA, Good RC. Geographic distribution, frequency, and specimen source of *Mycobacterium avium* complex serotypes isolated from patients with acquired immunodeficiency syndrome. *J Clin Microbiol* 28:926–929, 1990.

72. von Reyn CF, Maslow JN, Barber TW, et al. Persistent colonisation of potable water as a source of *Mycobacterium avium* infection in AIDS. *Lancet* 343:1137–1141, 1994.

73. Horsburgh CR. *Mycobacterium avium* complex infection in the acquired immunodeficiency syndrome. *N Engl J Med* 324:1332–1338, 1991.

74. Young LS. *Mycobacterium avium* complex infection. *J Infect Dis* 157:863–867, 1988.

75. Klatt EC, Jensen DF, Meyer PR. Pathology of *Mycobacterium avium-intracellulare* infection in acquired immunodeficiency syndrome. *Hum Pathol* 18:709–714, 1987.

76. Yagupsky P, Menegus MA. Cumulative positivity rates of multiple blood cultures for *Mycobacterium avium-intracellulare* and *Cryptococcus neoformans* in patients with the acquired immunodeficiency syndrome. *Arch Pathol Lab Med* 114:923–925, 1990.

77. Wong B, Edwards FF, Kiehn TE, et al. Continuous high-grade *Mycobacterium avium-intracellulare* bacteremia in patients with the acquired immune deficiency syndrome. *Am J Med* 78:35–40, 1985.

78. Havlik JA, et al. A prospective evaluation of *Mycobacterium avium* complex colonization of the respiratory and gastrointestinal tracts of persons with human immunodeficiency virus infection. *J Infect Dis* 168:1045–1048, 1993.

79. Modilevsky T, Sattler FR, Barnes PF. Mycobacterial disease in patients with human immunodeficiency virus infection. *Arch Intern Med* 149:2201–2205, 1989.

80. Jacobson MA, et al. Natural history of disseminated *Mycobacterium avium* complex infection in AIDS. *J Infect Dis* 164:994–998, 1991.

81. Horsburgh CR, Havlik JA, Ellis DA, et al. Survival of patients with acquired immune deficiency syndrome and disseminated *Mycobacterium avium* complex infection with and without antimycobacterial chemotherapy. *Am Rev Respir Dis* 144:557–559, 1991.

82. Horsburgh CR, et al. Predictors of survival in patients with AIDS and disseminated *Mycobacterium avium* complex disease. *J Infect Dis* 170:573–577, 1994.

83. Chin DP, et al. The impact of *Mycobacterium avium* complex and its treat-

ment on survival of AIDS patients: A prospective study. *J Infect Dis* 170:578–584, 1994.

84. Agins BC, et al. Effect of combined therapy with ansamycin, clofazimine, ethambutol, and isoniazid for *Mycobacterium avium* infection in patients with AIDS. *J Infect Dis* 159:784–787, 1989.

85. Kemper CA, et al. Treatment of *Mycobacterium avium* complex bacteremia in AIDS with a four-drug oral regimen. *Ann Intern Med* 116:466–472, 1992.

86. Dautzenburg B, Truffot C, Legris S, et al. Activity of clarithromycin against *Mycobacterium avium* infection in patients with the acquired immune deficiency syndrome: A controlled clinical trial. *Am Rev Respir Dis* 144:564–569, 1991.

87. Young LS, Wiviott L, Wu M, et al. Azithromycin for treatment of *Mycobacterium avium-intracellulare* complex infection in patients with AIDS. *Lancet* 338:1107–1109, 1991.

88. Nightingale S, Cameron DW, Gordin FM, et al. Two controlled trials of rifabutin prophylaxis against *Mycobacterium avium* complex infection in AIDS. *N Engl J Med* 329:828–833, 1993.

89. Pierce M, Heifets L, Crampton S. Clarithromycin for the prevention of *Mycobacterium avium* complex in AIDS. Tenth International Conference on AIDS. Yokohama, Japan, August 1994.

90. Oualls J, Salvato P, Thompson C. *Mycobacterium avium* complex prevention: Clarithromycin versus rifabutin. Tenth International Conference on AIDS. Yokohama, Japan, August 1994.

91. Hellinger JA, Cohen CJ, Mazzullo J. Clarithromycin for the prevention of *Mycobacterium avium* complex in AIDS. Tenth International Conference on AIDS. Yokohama, Japan, August 1994.

92. Masur H, and the Public Health Service Task Force on Prophylaxis and Therapy for *Mycobacterium avium* complex. Recommendations on prophylaxis and therapy for disseminated *Mycobacterium avium* complex disease in patients infected with the human immunodeficiency virus. *N Engl J Med* 329:898–904, 1993.

92a. Centers for Disease Control. USPHS/IDSA guidelines for the prevention of opportuistic infections in persons infected with human immunodeficiency virus: A summary. *MMWR* 44(RR-8):1–34, 1995.

93. Shafran SD, Deschenes J, Miller M, et al. Uveitis and pseudojaundice during a regimen of clarithromycin, rifabutin and ethambutol (letter) *N Engl J Med* 330:438–439, 1994.

94. Frank MO, Graham MB, Wispelwey B. Rifabutin and uveitis (letter). *N Engl J Med* 330:868, 1994.

95. Fuller JD, Stanfield LED, Craven DE. Rifabutin prophylaxis and uveitis (letter). *N Engl J Med* 330:1315–1316, 1994.

96. The DATRI 001 Study Group. Clarithromycin plus rifabutin for MAC prophylaxis: Evidence for a drug interaction (abstract). First National Conference on Human Retroviruses and Related Infections. Washington, DC, October 13, 1993.

97. Narano PK, et al. Fluconazole and enhanced effect of rifabutin prophylaxis (letter). *N Engl J Med* 330:1316, 1994.

Cryptococcosis 21

Alan M. Sugar, Carol A. Saunders

Meningitis is the most serious manifestation of infection with the yeast-like organism *Cryptococcus neoformans*. This ubiquitous fungus can cause disease in normal hosts, as well as in those with immunodeficiency [1]. Several reviews of cryptococcosis in AIDS have been published, and there is continuing controversy over the optimal management of patients with acute cryptococcal meningitis [2–7]. This chapter reviews clinical issues related to cryptococcosis and presents an approach to diagnosis and treatment of the disease in patients with AIDS.

Epidemiology

Cryptococcus neoformans is found in all areas of the world; cryptococcosis is not a geographically restricted disease, such as histoplasmosis and coccidioidomycosis. The fungus grows well in soil, especially when enriched with bird droppings. However, it is uncertain if there is a relationship between exposure to birds and clinical disease in patients with AIDS. In Africa, Swinne and associates [8] reported that cultures of dust obtained from 50 percent of the houses of HIV-infected patients with cryptococcosis grew *C. neoformans*, compared to only 20 percent of dust cultures from randomly selected houses in the same area. Moreover, 40 percent of the patients with cryptococcosis claimed contact with pigeons, and pigeon coops frequently harbored the fungus. They suggested that contaminated house dust or exposure to pigeons was a risk factor for cryptococcosis, but similar associations have not been identified in North America.

Cryptococcus neoformans is the second most commonly isolated fungal pathogen in AIDS patients. Cryptococcosis was a well-recognized, albeit much less frequent, disease before the advent of AIDS. Patients with impaired cell-mediated immunity resulting from lymphoma or corticosteroid use are at risk for development of the disease, but patients with no known immunologic abnormalities may also develop cryptococcal infection. Under usual circumstances, *C. neoformans* is introduced into the body through the lungs; person-to-person transmission does not occur.

Clinical Manifestations

Pneumonia sometimes occurs as an early manifestation of cryptococcosis. In a review of 18 patients with cryptococcal meningitis, we found that 14 (78%) had respiratory symptoms during the 4-month period before the development of meningitis, as compared with 4 of 16 (25%) in the 4 months following [9]. Three patients were found to have cryptococcal pneumonia at the time they presented with meningitis.

Most patients with cryptococcal meningitis do not have clinically evident pneumonia. In immunocompetent persons, cryptococcal pneumonia usually resolves spontaneously [10]. However, in immunosuppressed patients, dissemination to extrapulmonary sites is frequent, and specific antifungal treatment is necessary. *Cryptococcus neoformans* has a propensity to spread to the central nervous system, but infection of skin, bone, lymph nodes, heart, and other sites has been described as well (see Fig. 10-3).

The clinical manifestations of cryptococcal meningitis are variable, ranging from fever and mild constitutional symptoms to seizures and coma. It most often presents insidiously, with symptoms developing over several weeks. The disease has a tendency to wax and wane; symptoms may be initially dismissed as trivial or thought indicative of another process. Patients with cryptococcal meningitis often complain of headache, nausea, and vomiting, reflecting increased intracranial pressure [11]. Photophobia may occur, and signs suggestive of meningeal irritation are sometimes found. Changes in personality and alterations in level of consciousness have also been described.

As more experience has been gained in managing cryptococcal meningitis in the patient with AIDS, significant complications have been recognized. One such finding is the sudden onset of visual loss, which occurs in approximately 2 percent of cryptococcal meningitis cases [12–14]. The pathogenesis of this condition is unknown but may be related to increased intracranial pressure or fungal invasion of the optic nerve or visual centers in the brain. Corticosteroid therapy has been used empirically, but its efficacy is uncertain [14].

Diagnosis

The diagnosis of cryptococcal infection should be considered in the patient with advanced HIV disease who presents with neurologic or respiratory complaints. A history and physical examination is performed initially, with particular attention to the patient's neurologic status and to other possible sites of dissemination (Table 21-1). The patient with suspected cryptococcal meningitis should then undergo lumbar puncture; if papilledema or focal neurologic deficits are present, a computed tomography (CT) or magnetic resonance imaging (MRI) scan of the brain should be done first. Since cryptococcal infection of the central nervous system involves the brain parenchyma as well as meninges, CT or MRI scan may show mass lesions, even in the absence of focal neurologic findings. Cerebrospinal fluid (CSF) should be sent for India ink examination, fungal culture, and cryptococcal antigen assay, in addition to the usual studies. Cryptococcal meningitis in AIDS is usually characterized by a large number of organisms in the CSF and a minimal host inflammatory response. Organisms are readily observed under the microscope, even in uncentrifuged specimens.

The most immediate method for diagnosing cryptococcal meningitis is mixing CSF or its sediment with India ink. A drop of CSF is placed on the microscope slide adjacent to a drop of India ink, and a cover slip is then positioned over them. A positive test shows clearly demarcated circular organisms with a smooth perimeter, a surrounding clear zone (capsule), and a visible internal anatomy (organelles) (Plate 20). False-positive India ink preparations occur when host white blood cells are

Table 21-1 *Evaluation of the patient with cryptococcosis*

History
    Antecedent respiratory symptoms
    Fever, malaise, anorexia
    Headache
    Visual disturbances
    Change in personality or behavior

Physical examination
    Pneumonia
    Focal neurologic abnormalities
    Altered mental status
    Papilledema
    Skin lesions

Laboratory tests
    Cerebrospinal fluid analysis
        Opening pressure
        Cell count, glucose, protein
        India ink preparation
        Culture
        Cryptococcal antigen
    CT or MRI scan of brain
    Serum cryptococcal antigen
    Blood and sputum cultures

confused with the fungus. White blood cells typically have a hazy and poorly demarcated periphery, and no internal structures are seen. Occasionally, adjacent cells touch, giving the appearance of budding yeast.

Capsule-deficient *C. neoformans* has been described in patients with AIDS. The meaning of this observation is not clear and may merely reflect rapid growth of the organism with less time for each yeast to produce capsular material. An alternative hypothesis is that relatively avirulent environmental isolates, not normally encapsulated, may cause disease in sufficiently immunocompromised hosts.

The cryptococcal antigen latex agglutination test remains an important tool for the diagnosis of cryptococcosis. This assay detects the presence of cryptococcal polysaccharide in serum or CSF using antibody-coated particles to trap the antigen. In studies of patients without HIV infection, cryptococcal antigen titers have been useful prognostically, as well as diagnostically [15, 16]. However, in AIDS patients, extraordinarily high titers have been noted, and unpredictable fluctuations in serum titer may occur during the course of treatment, as may false-positive tests. Thus, the measurement of serum cryptococcal antigen titers to monitor therapy is of limited usefulness in this population. In a recent retrospective examination of the utility of serial determinations of cryptococcal antigen, Powderly and associates [17] observed no correlation between therapeutic outcome and changes in serum titers in patients with AIDS. On the other hand, CSF antigen titers that were unchanged or increased correlated with failure of primary therapy. This was especially true in those whose baseline CSF titer was 1:8 or greater. Similarly a rise in CSF antigen titer during maintenance therapy was associated with relapse of the disease.

The mainstay for diagnosis of cryptococcoccosis is the CSF culture. Since the organism enters the body through the lungs and disseminates hematogenously, sputum and blood cultures should also be performed. *Cryptococcus neoformans* readily grows in standard blood culture media, provided that the bottles have been vented to room air, as well as on blood agar. Within 2 to 5 days, yeast-like colonies are generally visible. Definitive microbiologic identification relies on the organism producing a brownish color when cultured on birdseed agar, a result of its intrinsic phenol oxidase activity and the production of melanin.

Management

In the AIDS patient, treatment of cryptococcal meningitis can be divided into two phases: (1) primary or acute therapy, and (2) secondary or maintenance therapy.

Primary Therapy

In the largest study to date, a collaborative effort of the Mycoses Study Group (MSG), AIDS Clinical Trials Group (ACTG), and independent physicians, amphotericin B, in a dose of at least 0.3 mg/kg/day, was compared to fluconazole, initial dose of 200 mg per day, with escalation to 400 mg per day if the patient did not respond [18]. After 10 weeks of therapy, treatment was successful in only 40 percent of amphotericin-B–treated patients and 34 percent of fluconazole-treated patients. Approximately 25 percent of patients in both treatment groups were classified as clinical responders, but their CSF could not be sterilized.

Evidence derived from this study suggests that it is critical to stratify patients into risk groups before embarking on any treatment course. Altered mental status was predictive of poor outcome. A CSF cryptococcal antigen titer greater than 1:1,024 and CSF white blood cell count less than 20/mm^3, reflecting high fungal burden and little host inflammatory response, were also important negative prognostic indicators. Over 90 percent of patients without these findings responded to therapy with either amphotericin B or fluconazole. In contrast, in patients with these findings, mortality was high for treatment both with amphotericin B (33%) and fluconazole (44%).

Thus, in patients with no predictors of poor outcome, either amphotericin B or fluconazole therapy is reasonable. Based on information from several studies in AIDS patients, CSF cultures show no growth after approximately 1 month in patients treated with amphotericin B and after 2 months with fluconazole. In patients with negative prognostic indicators, response to therapy is poor and mortality is high. For this group, consideration should be given to using high doses of amphotericin B with or without flucytosine. Many investigators recommend reduced doses of flucytosine (75–100 mg/kg/day in four divided doses vs. the usual dose of 150 mg/kg/day) in patients with AIDS. However, even at these doses, the hematologic toxicity of flucytosine may still be significant in this patient population.

There may be some benefit in using higher doses of fluconazole for primary therapy. Haubrich and associates [19] reported a series of eight patients who had received fluconazole, 800 mg per day. Five of six patients with meningitis had resolution of clinical symptoms, and all six had negative CSF cultures by day 82 (median, 21 days). This compares favorably with the median time to CSF culture sterility of 62 days in patients treated with 200 mg/day of fluconazole and 42 days in patients treated with amphotericin B. These therapeutic results are especially encouraging given that two of the six patients with cryptococcal meningitis had abnormal mental status when therapy was begun, four had CSF white blood cell counts of less than 20/mm^3, and three had CSF antigen titers greater than 1:1,024, all of which are traditional indicators of poor prognosis.

The combination of fluconazole and flucytosine has also been successfully used for primary therapy of cryptococcal meningitis in HIV-infected patients [20]. However, gastrointestinal and hematologic toxicity was relatively common. Milefchik and associates [21] reported on 36 patients treated for more than 3 months with fluconazole, 800 to 1,600 mg per day with or without flucytosine. In contrast to other series, the response rate of patients treated with fluconazole alone was less than 40 percent but increased remarkably to over 70 percent when flucytosine, 150 mg/kg/day, was added.

In a series of open, noncomparative studies, itraconazole has been reported to be effective in patients with cryptococcal meningitis and other forms of cryptococcosis [21–24]. However, because of important drug interactions and decreased absorption if itraconazole is not administered with food, its role in the management of HIV-related cryptococcal infection is presently unclear [25, 26] (Table 21-2). Of note, one recent randomized study of itraconazole compared to fluconazole performed by the MSG and ACTG was prematurely stopped because of a greater number of relapses in the itraconazole group.

The optimal duration of primary therapy has not been well defined. Ideally, there should be resolution of symptoms and signs of disease and no evidence of growth of the fungus from infected sites. Six to 10 weeks of therapy, and sometimes more, is generally administered before maintenance therapy is begun [16]. Persistence of *C. neoformans* in the prostate has been described and hypothesized as a potential source of reinfection following successful treatment of meningitis [27]. It may be prudent to culture urine and prostatic secretions before and after primary therapy for cryptococcosis.

Table 21-2 *Potential drug interactions with itraconazole*

Drug	Interaction
Didanosine (ddI)	Buffer in tablet formulation of ddI results in decreased itraconazole absorption
Antacids	Decreases itraconazole absorption
H$_2$ blockers	Decreases itraconazole absorption
Cyclosporine	Increases serum cyclosporine concentration
Rifampin	Cannot be taken while patient is receiving itraconazole; serum itraconazole levels are undetectable even up to 1 month following discontinuation of rifampin
Isoniazid	Decreases serum itraconazole concentration
Digoxin	Increases serum digoxin concentration
Phenytoin	Increases serum phenytoin concentration and decreases serum itraconazole concentration
Oral hypoglycemics	Enhanced hypoglycemic effect
Oral anticoagulants	Enhanced anticoagulant effect

Maintenance Therapy

HIV-infected patients with cryptococcal meningitis require lifelong maintenance antifungal therapy. Two open-label studies have been performed to evaluate the role of fluconazole as suppressive therapy for cryptococcal meningitis in AIDS patients [28, 29]. Both have shown that the relapse rate in patients treated with this drug can be decreased to about 10 percent, compared to 50 to 90 percent in those not receiving suppressive therapy. Subsequently, a placebo-controlled trial and a large multicenter study have confirmed fluconazole as the drug of choice for maintenance therapy of cryptococcal meningitis [30, 31]. A dose of 200 mg per day is adequate in most instances.

Monitoring Patients

Once patients have clinically improved on primary therapy, they should be evaluated every 4 to 6 weeks for symptoms and signs of relapse and toxicity related to treatment. Because the first evidence for relapse is often a positive culture, lumbar puncture with CSF culture is recommended on a periodic basis in patients with headache or other neurologic symptoms. Routine lumbar puncture is not indicated during primary therapy, since a negative CSF culture within the first month is unusual regardless of the drug used. Fluctuations in CSF cryptococcal antigen titers usually have no correlation with the disease course, and clinicians should not rely on titers to determine patient management. Rather, such decisions should be based on clinical parameters and CSF culture results.

Specific Treatment Recommendations

Amphotericin B, at a dose of 0.6 to 1.0 mg/kg/day, is the preferred drug in severely ill patients (Table 21-3). The addition of flucytosine, 75 to 150 mg/kg/day in four divided doses, can also be considered if the capacity for monitoring flucytosine serum concentrations is available. As discussed above, the role of high-dose fluconazole in primary therapy is uncertain.

In patients without mental status changes or focal neurologic deficits, the choice of appropriate primary therapy is even less clear. Fluconazole may be preferable to amphotericin B because of its ease of administration. It can be given as a single oral dose of 400 mg/day. On the basis of anecdotal reports, this dose should probably be continued for at least 10 weeks following the first negative CSF culture. Drug interactions with fluconazole are common (Table 21-4), but, in most cases, there is no need for determination of fluconazole serum concentrations.

Fluconazole in a dose of 200 mg per day is the drug of choice for maintenance therapy. Most patients do well on this regimen, although

Table 21-3 *Antifungal therapy for cryptococcosis*

Drug	Usual dose	Comments
Amphotericin B	Primary Rx: 0.6–1.0 mg/kg/day IV	Lower doses, especially when used alone, have not been very effective
	Maintenance Rx: not usually recommended	Combination with flucytosine may improve results, but the large randomized study evaluating this approach is not yet completed
		Patients should be kept well hydrated
		Nonsteroidal antiinflammatory drugs (e.g., ibuprofen) may decrease chills, rigors, and fevers caused by amphotericin B
		Use of lipid-associated amphotericin B formulations is investigational*
Fluconazole	Primary Rx: 400–1,600 mg PO qd	See Table 21-4 for drug interactions
		Combination with flucytosine may improve response, but general recommendations cannot yet be made
	Maintenance Rx: 200 mg PO qd	Measurement of serum fluconazole concentrations may be indicated in selected cases
Itraconazole	Primary Rx: 200 mg PO bid	See Table 21-2 for drug interactions
		It is important to follow serum itraconazole concentrations; failures have been observed when concentrations fall below 5 µg/ml as measured by bioassay
	Maintenance Rx: 200 mg PO qd or bid	
Flucytosine	Primary Rx: 75–150 mg/kg/day PO	Doses lower than the traditionally recommended 150 mg/kg/day may be efficacious and less toxic than "full dose" therapy
	Maintenance Rx: not recommended	Measurement of serum flucytosine concentrations and maintenance at 25–75 µg/ml may decrease toxicity

*RJ Coker et al. Treatment of cryptococcosis with liposomal amphotericin B in 23 patients with AIDS. *AIDS* 7:829–835, 1993.

Table 21-4 *Potential drug interactions with fluconazole*

Drug	Interaction
Zidovudine	Increases serum zidovudine concentration
Cyclosporine	Increases serum cyclosporine concentration
Rifampin	Enhances metabolism of fluconazole, possibly lowering serum concentration; monitoring serum fluconazole levels may be necessary
Isoniazid	Possible decrease in serum fluconazole concentration
Phenytoin	Increases serum phenytoin concentration

a small number will relapse. Patients with relapsing infection can be managed by switching from fluconazole to amphotericin B or by increasing the dose of fluconazole to 600 to 800 mg or more per day in those who cannot tolerate amphotericin B. Itraconazole can be used as an alternate agent.

Prognosis

Most AIDS patients respond well to therapy for an initial episode of cryptococcal meningitis, but relapse is frequent. From studies in the pre-AIDS era, we know that patients with positive India ink smears after completion of therapy, those with high CSF cryptococcal antigen titers, and those with cultures positive for *C. neoformans* at extraneural sites are all at high risk of relapse. Since these characteristics are found in the majority of AIDS patients with cryptococcal infection, all such individuals should be placed on chronic maintenance therapy.

The overall prognosis for AIDS patients with cryptococcosis is guarded. In a retrospective series, Chuck and Sande [6] found mean survival to be approximately 8 months in those receiving long-term antifungal treatment and 5 months in those not receiving maintenance therapy. Similarly, in another retrospective review, mean survival time for the 47 of 68 who died was 5 months [5]. Bozzette and associates [30] found that about two-thirds of their patients died after a mean of approximately 9 months. This was true whether placebo or fluconazole was used during the maintenance phase of treatment.

Prevention

There are no currently recognized means for preventing acquisition of cryptococcal infection. As the organism is ubiquitous, it is not feasible to limit exposure. Moreover, some of the cryptococcal disease occurring in patients with AIDS may represent reactivation of previously acquired infection. Although preliminary evidence suggests that fluconazole may be useful in the prevention of systemic fungal infections [32, 33], it is not recommended routinely for primary prophylaxis at this time [34].

References

1. Diamond RD. *Cryptococcus neoformans*. In GL Mandell, RG Douglas, Jr, JE Bennett (eds), *Principles and Practice of Infectious Diseases* (3rd ed). New York: Churchill Livingstone, 1990.
2. Kovacs JA, Kovacs AA, Polis M, et al. Cryptococcosis in the acquired immunodeficiency syndrome. *Ann Intern Med* 103:533–538, 1985.

3. Zuger A, Louie E, Holzman RS, et al. Cryptococcal disease in patients with the acquired immunodeficiency syndrome. *Ann Intern Med* 104:234–240, 1986.

4. Dismukes WE. Cryptococcal meningitis in patients with AIDS. *J Infect Dis* 157:624–628, 1988.

5. Clark RA, Greer D, Atkinson W, et al. Spectrum of *Cryptococcus neoformans* infection in 68 patients infected with human immunodeficiency virus. *Rev Infect Dis* 12:768–778, 1990.

6. Chuck SL, Sande MA. Infections with *Cryptococcus neoformans* in the acquired immunodeficiency syndrome. *N Engl J Med* 321:794–799, 1989.

7. Sugar AM, Stern JJ, Dupont B. Overview: Treatment of cryptococcal meningitis. *Rev Infect Dis* 12:S338–S348, 1990.

8. Swinne D, Deppner M, Maniratunga S, et al. AIDS-associated cryptococcosis in Bujumbura, Burundi: An epidemiological study. *J Med Vet Mycol* 29:25–30, 1991.

9. Driver J, Saunders CA, Sugar AM. Cryptococcal pneumonia in AIDS: Is cryptococcal meningitis preceded by clinically recognizable pneumonia? *J Acquir Immune Defic Syndr* In press.

10. Kerkering TM, Duma RJ, Shadomy S. The evolution of pulmonary cryptococcosis: Clinical implications from a study of 41 patients with and without compromising host factors. *Ann Intern Med* 94:611–616, 1981.

11. Denning DW, Armstrong RW, Lewis BH, Stevens DA. Elevated cerebrospinal fluid pressures in patients with cryptococcal meningitis and acquired immunodeficiency syndrome. *Am J Med* 91:267–272, 1991.

12. Cohen DB, Glasgow BJ. Bilateral optic nerve cryptococcosis in sudden blindness in patients with acquired immune deficiency syndrome. *Ophthalmology* 100:1689–1694, 1993.

13. Kestelyn P, Taelman H, Bogaerts J, et al. Ophthalmic manifestations of *Cryptococcus neoformans* in patients with the acquired immunodeficiency syndrome. *Am J Ophthalmol* 116:721–727, 1993.

14. Rex JH, Larsen RA, Dismukes WE, et al. Catastrophic visual loss due to *Cryptococcus neoformans* meningitis. *Medicine (Baltimore)* 72:207–224, 1993.

15. Diamond RD, Bennett JE. Prognostic factors in cryptococcal meningitis: A study of 111 cases. *Ann Intern Med* 80:176–181, 1974.

16. Dismukes WE, Cloud G, Gallis HA, et al. Treatment of cryptococcal meningitis with combination amphotericin B and flucytosine for four as compared with six weeks. *N Engl J Med* 317:334–341, 1987.

17. Powderly WG, Cloud GA, Dismukes WE, Saag MS. Measurement of cryptococcal antigen in serum and cerebrospinal fluid: Value in the management of AIDS-associated cryptococcal meningitis. *Clin Infect Dis* 18:789–792, 1994.

18. Saag MS, Powderly WG, Cloud GA, et al. Treatment of acute AIDS-associated cryptococcal meningitis with amphotericin B or fluconazole: Results of a randomized clinical trial. *N Engl J Med* 326:83–89, 1992.

19. Haubrich RH, Haghighat D, Bozzette SA, et al, California Collaborative Treatment Group. High-dose fluconazole for treatment of cryptococcal disease in patients with human immunodeficiency virus infection. *J Infect Dis* 170:238–242, 1994.

20. Larsen RA, et al. Fluconazole combined with flucytosine for treatment of cryptococcal meningitis in patients with AIDS. *Clin Infect Dis* 19:741–745, 1994.

21. Milefchik E, Leal M, Haubrich R, et al. High dose fluconazole with and without flucytosine for AIDS associated cryptococcal meningitis. Ninth International Conference on AIDS. Berlin, June 1993.

22. Denning DW, Tucker RM, Hanson LH, et al. Itraconazole therapy for cryptococcal meningitis and cryptococcosis. *Arch Intern Med* 149:2301–2308, 1989.

23. Denning DM, Tucker RM, Hanson LH, Stevens DA. Itraconazole in opportunistic mycoses: Cryptococcosis and aspergillosis. *J Am Acad Dermatol* 23:602–607, 1990.

24. Cauwenbergh G. Cryptococcal meningitis—the place of itraconazole. *Mycoses* 36:221–228, 1993.

25. Van Peer A, Woestenborghs R, Heykants J, et al. The effects of food and dose on the oral systemic availability of itraconazole in healthy subjects. *Eur J Clin Pharmacol* 36:423–426, 1989.

26. Zimmermann T, Yeates RA, Laufen H, et al. Influence of concomitant food intake on the oral absorption of two triazole antifungal agents, itraconazole and fluconazole. *Eur J Clin Pharmacol* 46:147–150, 1994.

27. Larsens RA, Bozzette S, McCutchan JA, et al. Persistent *Cryptococcus neoformans* infection of the prostate after successful treatment of meningitis. *Ann Intern Med* 111:125–128, 1989.

28. Stern JJ, Hartman BJ, Sharkey P, et al. Oral fluconazole therapy for patients with acquired immunodeficiency syndrome and cryptococcosis: Experience with 22 patients. *Am J Med* 85:477–480, 1988.

29. Sugar AM, Saunders C. Oral fluconazole as suppressive therapy of disseminated cryptococcosis in patients with acquired immunodeficiency syndrome. *Am J Med* 85:481–489, 1988.

30. Bozzette SA, Larsen RA, Chiu J, et al. A placebo-controlled trial of maintenance therapy with fluconazole after treatment of cryptococcal meningitis in the acquired immunodeficiency syndrome. *N Engl J Med* 324:580–584, 1991.

31. Powderly WG, et al. A controlled trial of fluconazole or amphotericin B to prevent relapse of cryptococcal meningitis in patients with the acquired immunodeficiency syndrome. *N Engl J Med* 326:793–798, 1992.

32. Nightingale SD, et al. Primary prophylaxis with fluconazole against systemic fungal infections in HIV-positive patients. *AIDS* 6:191–194, 1992.

33. Powderly WG, et al. A randomized trial comparing fluconazole with clotrimazole troches for the prevention of fungal infections in patients with advanced human immunodeficiency virus infection. *N Engl J Med* 332:700–705, 1995.

34. Centers for Disease Control. USPHS/IDSA guidelines for the prevention of opportuistic infections in persons infected with human immunodeficiency virus: A summary. *MMWR* 44(RR-8):1–34, 1995.

Toxoplasmosis

22

Judith S. Currier, Carol A. Sulis

Toxoplasmosis is a common central nervous system (CNS) infection in patients with advanced HIV disease and an AIDS-defining diagnosis, accounting for approximately 15 percent of all CNS infections [1–9]. Patients are said to have latent infection with *Toxoplasma gondii* when antibody is present but there are no clinical manifestations. Between 20 and 47 percent of HIV-infected patients with serologic evidence of *T. gondii* infection will develop symptomatic disease [10–12].

Epidemiology

Toxoplasma gondii is an obligate intracellular parasite with worldwide distribution. Developmental forms include the oocyst, trophozoite, and tissue cyst. Organisms reproduce sexually in the intestinal mucosa of cats, the only definitive host, to form oocysts, which are excreted in the stool. Humans are infected following ingestion of oocysts from dried cat feces or tissue cysts from contaminated food, especially undercooked meat. Serologic evidence of toxoplasmosis is found in 15 to 70 percent of the United States population and increases with age. High rates are associated with tropical climate, poor sanitary conditions, and prevalence of cats.

Pathogenesis

Following the ingestion of *T. gondii*, trophozoites disseminate throughout the body via the lymphatics and bloodstream. Organisms invade nucleated cells and multiply, resulting in cell death and progressive tissue necrosis [13]. In the immunocompetent patient, host defenses, including T lymphocytes, activated macrophages, gamma-interferon, and type-specific antibody, generally control the primary infection. Most organisms are killed, and the remainder encyst and become latent. Cysts, containing several thousand slowly growing organisms, may develop in any tissue but are especially common in the CNS, myocardium, and skeletal muscle. Through an unknown mechanism, HIV-induced immunosuppression permits reactivation and dissemination of latent infection, producing symptomatic disease [5]. Animal studies suggest that the development of encephalitis during chronic infection may be related to strain-specific virulence factors [14].

Congenital toxoplasmosis occurs following transplacental passage of parasites during acute infection in the pregnant woman. Transplacental transmission of toxoplasmosis may also occur during latent infection in women who are severely immunosuppressed. A case report described four children congenitally infected with both toxoplasmosis and HIV [15]. One of the HIV-infected mothers had symptomatic reactivation of toxoplasmic encephalitis at the time of delivery; the others had a positive *Toxoplasma* serology but no clinical history of toxoplasmosis. The authors postulated that the mothers had either persistent or intermittent parasitemia during gestation.

Clinical Manifestations

In the normal host, most primary *T. gondii* infection is either subclinical or produces a mild, self-limited illness characterized by fever, malaise, and regional adenopathy. Encephalitis is the most common clinical manifestation of toxoplasmosis in HIV disease; pneumonitis and chorioretinitis have been described less frequently.

Toxoplasmic encephalitis often presents with focal or generalized neurologic abnormalities. A prodrome of frontal headache, low-grade fever, lethargy, and confusion or disorientation is common. Focal findings, including seizure activity or a stroke syndrome, may occur as toxoplasmic lesions become necrotic and the surrounding brain edematous; meningismus is infrequent. Other symptoms reported include diplopia, homonymous hemianopsia, blindness, unsteady gait, conus medullaris syndrome, myoclonus, tremor, personality change, hallucinations, and syncope. Without treatment, rapid neurologic deterioration may ensue, followed by coma and death. Even with effective therapy, mean survival following diagnosis is usually less than 1 year [16–19].

Pneumonitis caused by *T. gondii* may be difficult to distinguish from *Pneumocystis carinii* pneumonia (PCP) [20–25]. Toxoplasmic pneumonitis should be considered when a patient presents with fever, cough, and dyspnea, and induced sputum fails to demonstrate pneumocysts. Chest radiograph may show diffuse interstitial infiltrates or a reticulonodular pattern. The diagnosis of pulmonary toxoplasmosis can be made by identification of *T. gondii* in bronchoalveolar lavage fluid stained with Giemsa [23].

Reports of severe disseminated extraneural toxoplasmosis have become more frequent in recent years [23–27]. Clinical manifestations reflect the organ system involved and may include fever, maculopapular rash, generalized adenopathy, and hepatosplenomegaly. Some patients have presented with sepsis syndrome and extremely high serum lactate dehydrogenase levels [25]. Cases of toxoplasmosis involving the testes, gut, heart, and eye have also been reported [26–31].

Eye involvement with *T. gondii* presents as a necrotizing chorioretinitis that may be difficult to distinguish from cytomegalovirus infection [27–31]. The most common symptoms are decreased visual acuity and eye pain. Fluffy white or yellow exudates without hemorrhage, usually with ill-defined borders, are seen on funduscopic examination [31].

Diagnosis

Primary infection with *T. gondii* in the normal host generally results in seroconversion. Antibody is measured by the Sabin-Feldman dye exclusion test or with an indirect fluorescent antibody (IFA) test. The peak level of immunoglobulin G (IgG) is usually 1:1,000 or greater. Immunoglobulin G levels gradually fall, but a low level of antibody (1:16–1:64) persists for years. Although serologic tests are helpful in screening, their use to diagnose active toxoplasmosis in HIV-infected patients is controversial [32–34]. Because toxoplasmosis in this population usually results from reactivation of latent infection, serum immunoglobulin M (IgM) *Toxoplasma* antibodies are not present. Serum IgG antibodies are often detectable, but fewer than one-third of patients achieve the high titers indicative of active infection. Many clinicians obtain a serum IgG *Toxoplasma* antibody assay as part of the initial laboratory evaluation in HIV disease; a positive test will identify patients who are at risk for development of toxoplasmosis and who may benefit from prophylaxis. However, a negative test does not exclude the possibility of toxoplasmic encephalitis [35]. The clinical significance of *Toxoplasma* antibody in cerebrospinal fluid has not been established [10].

Presumptive diagnosis of toxoplasmic encephalitis is based on the combination of clinical manifestations, neuroradiologic findings, and response to empiric therapy [1]. Head computed tomography (CT) scan is usually abnormal, revealing one or more hypodense lesions that enhance in a ring or nodular pattern following the administration of contrast [2, 3] (see Fig. 17-3). Lesions are often located in the basal ganglia but may be scattered throughout the brain parenchyma [2, 3, 10, 36–40]. Magnetic resonance imaging (MRI) is generally more sensitive than CT for detecting cerebral toxoplasmosis. The typical finding on MRI scan is a localized high signal abnormality on T2-weighted imaging [35].

Empiric antimicrobial therapy is usually instituted when a patient presents with neurologic abnormalities and is found to have CT or MRI scan findings consistent with toxoplasmic encephalitis. Follow-up neuroradiologic examination demonstrating improvement of lesions within 10 to 14 days following initiation of specific therapy further supports the diagnosis [1, 3, 5]. Absence of improvement suggests an alternative disease process and is an indication for brain biopsy [39, 41].

Definitive diagnosis of toxoplasmosis requires demonstration of free or intracellular trophozoites in tissue, nucleated cells, or body fluids. Even with the use of special stains, trophozoites are difficult to identify on histologic evaluation because of their small size and location at the periphery of necrotic lesions, where they are surrounded by inflammatory debris and mononuclear cells (Fig. 22-1). Nonspecific pathologic findings in the brain range from focal necrotic abscesses to diffuse meningoencephalitis. Identification of cyst forms or isolation (culture) of organisms from tissue proves prior infection but may not reflect an active disease process. The usefulness of alternative diagnostic modalities, including DNA probes, *Toxoplasma* tissue culture methods, and a *Toxoplasma*-specific antigen test, is being evaluated [26, 40, 42].

Figure 22-1. Brain biopsy showing *Toxoplasma gondii* encephalitis. (From MN Amin. Acquired immunodeficiency syndrome: The spectrum of disease. *Fam Pract Recert* 9:84–118, 1987.)

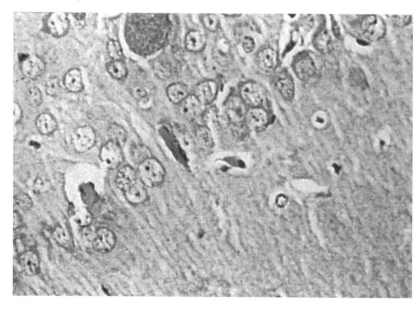

Other neurologic conditions in the HIV-infected patient may present in a manner similar to that of CNS toxoplasmosis. Differential diagnosis of toxoplasmic encephalitis includes cryptococcal meningitis, mycobacterial infection, syphilis, pyogenic brain abscess, progressive multifocal leukoencephalopathy, viral encephalitis, Kaposi's sarcoma, and primary CNS lymphoma.

Treatment

A combination of pyrimethamine and sulfadiazine is the treatment of choice for toxoplasmosis [18, 43, 44] (Table 22-1). This regimen inhibits replication of the trophozoite by blocking folate metabolism, but the drugs do not kill the trophozoite and have no effect on encysted organisms. Toxicity of pyrimethamine may include neutropenia and thrombocytopenia; the oral administration of folinic acid may minimize its myelosuppressive effect. Pyrimethamine is teratogenic and should not be used in pregnant women. Possible side effects of sulfadiazine include fever, rash, and nephrolithiasis. Clindamycin with pyrimethamine is an effective alternative regimen for patients who are intolerant of sulfadiazine [45–48].

Azithromycin, clarithromycin, or atovaquone used in combination with pyrimethamine may also be effective for the treatment of *T. gondii* [49–53]. The optimal doses of these drugs have not yet been defined, and their use should be limited to patients intolerant of standard regimens or on research protocols.

High-dose combination primary therapy is generally continued for 4 to 6 weeks, with drug dosages titrated to minimize toxicity. Corticosteroids can be used adjunctively if there is evidence of cerebral edema [5, 44]. Maintenance therapy using reduced doses of the same agents is continued indefinitely. Recurrent symptoms during maintenance therapy may reflect reactivation of toxoplasmosis or signify a new neurologic process. In this setting, primary therapy should be reinstituted until a diagnostic evaluation has been completed.

Prevention

HIV-infected individuals who are seronegative for toxoplasmosis should avoid exposure to infective forms of *T. gondii*. Meat should be frozen to –20°C or cooked to 60°C to kill tissue cysts [45]. Pet cats should remain indoors to avoid contact with potentially infected wild animals and should not be fed raw meat products, although the overall risk of acquiring toxoplasmosis from exposure to cats appears to be low [54]. Litter boxes should be cleaned regularly using gloved hands; oocysts

Table 22-1 *Treatment of toxoplasmic encephalitis*

Drug	Primary therapy	Maintenance therapy[a]
First choice		
Pyrimethamine[b]	100–200 mg loading dose, then 50–100 mg PO qd	25–50 mg PO qd *or* 0.25 mg/kg PO 2×/wk
and		
Sulfadiazine[c]	1–2 gm PO qid (100 mg/ kg/day)	500 mg–1.0 gm PO qid *or* 75 mg/kg PO 2×/wk
plus		
Folinic acid[d]	5–10 mg PO/IM/IV qd	5–10 mg PO qd
Second choice		
Pyrimethamine	100–200 mg loading dose, then 50–100 mg PO qd	25–50 mg PO qd *or* 0.25 mg/kg PO 2×/wk
and		
Clindamycin[e]	600–1,200 mg q6–8h, IV or PO	300–450 mg PO q6–8h
plus		
Folinic acid	5–10 mg PO qd	5–10 mg PO qd
Alternatives[f]		
Pyrimethamine and folinic acid *plus* one of the following: Azithromycin[g] Clarithromycin[g] Atovaquone[h]	Same doses as above	

[a]Optimal doses have not been established in HIV-infected patients.
[b]Side effects—occasional: blood dyscrasias, folic acid deficiency; rare: rash, vomiting, convulsions, shock.
[c]Side effects—frequent: rash, photosensitivity, drug fever; occasional: renal toxicity, hepatotoxicity, Stevens-Johnson syndrome, blood dyscrasias, hemolytic anemia, vasculitis; rare: myopia, pseudomembranous colitis, crystalluria with stone formation.
[d]The dose should be titrated to minimize bone marrow toxicity; doses as high as 50 mg/day are sometimes required.
[e]Side effects—frequent: diarrhea, allergic reactions; occasional: pseudomembranous colitis; rare: blood dyscrasias, hepatotoxicity.
[f]The use of these agents is currently under investigation, and their optimal doses have not been determined.
[g]Side effects: gastrointestinal intolerance, hepatotoxicity.
[h]Side effects: rash, gastrointestinal intolerance, headache.

require 1 to 21 days to undergo sporogony and become infectious. Other areas where cats may defecate (e.g., sandboxes, moist soil) should be avoided.

Data from both prospective and retrospective studies support the use of prophylaxis for toxoplasmosis in patients with antibody to *T. gondii* in the setting of advanced HIV disease [55–64] (Table 22-2). In two large

Table 22-2 *Prevention of toxoplasmosis*

Drug	Dosage
First choice	
Trimethoprim-sulfamethoxazole	1 DS tab PO qd
Alternatives	
Trimethoprim-sulfamethoxazole	1 DS tab PO 3×/wk or 1 SS tab qd
Pyrimethamine	50 mg PO every wk
plus	
Dapsone	50 mg PO qd

DS = double-strength; SS = single-strength.

prospective trials comparing trimethoprim-sulfamethoxazole (TMP-SMX) and aerosol pentamidine (AP) for PCP prophylaxis, the vast majority of patients in whom toxoplasmosis developed were receiving AP [57, 58]. The combination of pyrimethamine and dapsone also appears to be effective in preventing toxoplasmosis [61, 62]. Prophylaxis with pyrimethamine alone at a dose of 25 mg per week is not beneficial [63]. Other agents with activity against toxoplasmosis that may be useful include pyrimethamine-sulfadoxine (Fansidar), azithromycin, clarithromycin, and atovaquone.

References

1. Centers for Disease Control. Revision of the CDC surveillance case definition for acquired immunodeficiency syndrome. *MMWR* 36 (suppl):1–15, 1987.
2. Levy RM, Bredesen DE, Rosenblum ML. Neurological manifestations of the acquired immunodeficiency syndrome (AIDS): Experience at UCSF and review of the literature. *J Neurosurg* 62:475–495, 1985.
3. Post MJD, Kursunoglu SJ, Hensley GT, et al. Craniel CT in acquired immunodeficiency syndrome: Spectrum of diseases and optimal contrast enhancement technique. *Am J Radiol* 145:929–940, 1985.
4. Levy RM, Bredesen DE. Central nervous system dysfunction in acquired immunodeficiency syndrome. *J Acquir Immune Defic Syndr* 1:41–64, 1988.
5. Israelski DM, Remington JS. Toxoplasmic encephalitis in patients with AIDS. *Infect Dis Clin North Am* 2:429–445, 1988.
6. Elder GA, Sever JL. Neurologic disorders associated with AIDS retroviral infection. *Rev Infect Dis* 10:286–302, 1988.
7. Esiri MM, Scaravilli F, Millard PR, Harcourt-Webster JN. Neuropathology of HIV infection in haemophiliacs: Comparative necropsy study. *Br Med J* 299:1312–1315, 1989.
8. Lingappa JR, Sande MA. Toxoplasmosis. In PT Cohen, MA Sande, PA Volberding (eds), *The AIDS Knowledge Base* (2nd ed). Boston: Little, Brown, 1994. Pp 6.19.1–6.19.22.

9. Laughon BE, Allaudeen HS, Becker JM, et al. Summary of the workshop on future directions in discovery and development of therapeutic agents for opportunistic infections associated with AIDS. *J Infect Dis* 164:244–251, 1991.

10. Luft BJ, Remington JS. Toxoplasmic encephalitis. *J Infect Dis* 157:1–6, 1988.

11. Grant IH, Gold JWM, Rosenblum, et al. *Toxoplasma gondii* serology in HIV-infected patients: The development of central nervous system toxoplasmosis in AIDS. *AIDS* 4:519–521, 1990.

12. Zangerle R, Allerberger F, Pohl P, et al. High risk of developing toxoplasmic encephalitis in AIDS patients seropositive for *Toxoplasma gondii*. *Med Microbiol Immunol* 180:59–66, 1991.

13. Werk R. How does *Toxoplasma gondii* enter host cells? *Rev Infect Dis* 7:449–457, 1985.

14. Suzuki Y, Conley FK, Remington JS. Differences in virulence and development of encephalitis during chronic infection vary with the strain of *Toxoplasma gondii*. *J Infect Dis* 159:790–794, 1989.

15. Mitchell CD, Erlich SS, Mastrucci MT, et al. Congenital toxoplasmosis occurring in infants perinatally infected with human immunodeficiency virus 1. *Pediatr Infect Dis J* 9:512–518, 1990.

16. Engstrom JW, Lowenstein DH, Bredesen DE. Cerebral infarctions and transient neurologic deficits associated with acquired immunodeficiency syndrome. *Am J Med* 86:528–532, 1989.

17. Overhage JM, Greist A, Brown DR. Conus medullaris syndrome resulting from *Toxoplasma gondii* infection in a patient with the acquired immunodeficiency syndrome. *Am J Med* 89:814–815, 1990.

18. Haverkos HW. Assessment of therapy for toxoplasma encephalitis. *Am J Med* 82:907–914, 1987.

19. Turner BJ, Markson LE, McKee L, et al. The AIDS-defining diagnosis and subsequent complications: A survival based severity index. *J Acquir Immune Defic Syndr* 4:1059–1071, 1991.

20. Schnapp LM, Geaghan SM, Campagna A, et al. *Toxoplasma gondii* pneumonitis in patients infected with the human immunodeficiency virus. *Arch Intern Med* 152:1073–1077, 1992.

21. Oksenhendler E, Cadranel J, Sarfati C, et al. *Toxoplasma gondii* pneumonia in patients with the acquired immunodeficiency syndrome. *Am J Med* 88 (suppl 5) :18–21, 1990.

22. Pomeroy C, Filice GA. Pulmonary toxoplasmosis: A review. *Clin Infect Dis* 14:863–870, 1992.

23. Tschirart D, Klatt EC. Disseminated toxoplasmosis in the acquired immunodeficiency syndrome. *Arch Pathol Lab Med* 112:1237–1241, 1988.

24. Garcia LW, Hemphill RB, Marasco WA, Ciano PS. Acquired immunodeficiency syndrome with disseminated toxoplasmosis presenting as an acute pulmonary and gastrointestinal illness. *Arch Pathol Lab Med* 115:459–463, 1991.

25. Pugin J, Vanhems P, Hirschel B, et al. Extreme elevations of serum lactic dehydrogenase differentiating pulmonary toxoplasmosis from pneumocystis pneumonia (letter). *N Engl J Med* 326:1226, 1992.

26. Israelski DM, Skowron G, Leventhal JP, et al. *Toxoplasma* peritonitis in a

patient with acquired immunodeficiency syndrome. *Arch Intern Med* 148:1655–1657, 1988.

27. Gagliuso DJ, Teich SA, Friedman AH, Orellana J. Ocular toxoplasmosis in AIDS patients. *Trans Am Ophthalmol Soc* 88:63–88, 1990.

28. Cappell MS, Mikhail N, Ortega A. Toxoplasma myocarditis in AIDS (letter). *Am Heart J* 123:1728–1729, 1992.

29. Pauwels A, Meyohas MC, Eliaszewicz M, et al. Toxoplasma colitis in the acquired immunodeficiency syndrome. *Am J Gastroenterol* 87:518–519, 1992.

30. Crider SR, Hortsman WG, Massey GS. *Toxoplasma* orchitis: Report of a case and a review of the literature. *Am J Med* 85:421–424, 1988.

31. Cochereau-Massin I, LeHoang P, Lautier-Frau M, et al. Ocular toxoplasmosis in human immunodeficiency virus–infected patients. *Am J Ophthalmol* 114:130–135, 1992.

32. Potasman I, Resnick L, Luft BJ, Remington JA. Intrathecal production of antibodies against *Toxoplasma gondii* in patients with toxoplasmic encephalitis and the acquired immunodeficiency syndrome (AIDS). *Ann Intern Med* 108:49–51, 1988.

33. Stepick-Biek P, Thulliez P, Araujo FG, Remington JS. IgA antibodies for diagnosis of acute congenital and acquired toxoplasmosis. *J Infect Dis* 162:270–273, 1990.

34. Hedman K, Lappalainen M, Seppaia I, Makela O. Recent primary toxoplasma infection indicated by a low avidity of specific IgG. *J Infect Dis* 159:736–740, 1989.

35. Porter SB, Sande MA. Toxoplasmosis of the central nervous system in the acquired immunodeficiency syndrome. *N Engl J Med* 327:1643–1648, 1992.

36. Ciricillo SF, Rosenblum ML. Use of CT and MR imaging to distinguish intracranial lesions and to define the need for biopsy in AIDS patients. *J Neurosurg* 73:720–724, 1990.

37. Levy RM, Rosenbloom S, Perrett LV. Neuroradiological findings in the acquired immunodeficiency syndrome (AIDS): A review of 200 cases. *Am J Radiol* 147:977–983, 1986.

38. Levy RM, Mills CM, Posin JP, et al. The efficacy and clinical impact of brain imaging in neurologically symptomatic AIDS patients: A prospective CT/MRI study. *J Acquir Immune Defic Syndr* 3:461–471, 1990.

39. Cohn JA, McMeeking A, Cohen W, et al. Evaluation of the policy of empiric treatment of suspected *Toxoplasma* encephalitis in patients with the acquired immunodeficiency syndrome. *Am J Med* 86:521–527, 1989.

40. Tirard V, Niel G, Rosenheim M, et al. Diagnosis of toxoplasmosis in patients with AIDS by isolation of the parasite from the blood (letter). *N Engl J Med* 324:634, 1991.

41. Cimino C, Lipton RB, Williams A, et al. The evaluation of patients with human immunodeficiency virus–related disorders and brain mass lesions. *Arch Intern Med* 151:1381–1384, 1991.

42. Weiss LM, Udem SA, Salgo M, et al. Sensitive and specific detection of *Toxoplasma* DNA in an experimental murine model: Use of *Toxoplasma gondii*–specific cDNA and the polymerase chain reaction. *J Infect Dis* 163:180–186, 1991.

43. Leport C, Raffi F, Matheron S, et al. Treatment of central nervous system toxoplasmosis with pyrimethamine/sulfadiazine combination in 35 patients with the acquired immunodeficiency syndrome: Efficacy of long-term continuous therapy. *Am J Med* 84:94–100, 1988.

44. Wong SY, Remington JS. Toxoplasmosis in the Setting of AIDS. In S Broder, TC Merigan, D Bolognesi (eds), *Textbook of AIDS Medicine*. Baltimore: Williams & Wilkins, 1994. Pp 223–257.

45. Dannemann BR, Israelski DM, Remington JS. Treatment of toxoplasmic encephalitis with intravenous clindamycin. *Arch Intern Med* 148:2477–2482, 1988.

46. Dannemann B, McCutchan JA, Israelski D, et al. Treatment of toxoplasmic encephalitis in patients with AIDS. A randomized trial comparing pyrimethamine plus clindamycin to pyrimethamine plus sulfadiazine. *Ann Intern Med* 116:33–43, 1992.

47. Luft BJ, et al. Toxoplasmic encephalitis in patients with the acquired immunodeficiency syndrome. *N Engl J Med* 329:995–1000, 1993.

48. Leport C, Bastuji-Garin S, Perronne C, et al. An open study of the pyrimethamine-clindamycin combination in AIDS patients with brain toxoplasmosis. *J Infect Dis* 160:557–558, 1989.

49. Chang HR, Pechere JCF. In vitro effects of four macrolides (roxithromycin, spiramycin, azithromycin [CP-62, 993], and A-56268) on *Toxoplasma gondii*. *Antimicrob Agents Chemother* 32:524–529, 1988.

50. Huskinson-Mark J, Araujo FG, Remington JS. Evaluation of the effect of drugs on the cyst form of *Toxoplasma gondii*. *J Infect Dis* 164:170–177, 1991.

51. Hughes WT, Kennedy W, Shenep JL, et al. Safety and pharmacokinetics of 566C80, a hydroxynaphthoquinone with anti-*Pneumocystis carinii* activity: A phase 1 study in human immunodeficiency virus (HIV)-infected men. *J Infect Dis* 163:843–848, 1991.

52. Kovacs JA. Efficacy of atovaquone in treatment of toxoplasmosis in patients with AIDS. *Lancet* 340:637–638, 1992.

53. Farthing C, Rendel M, Currie B, Seidlin M. Azithromycin for cerebral toxoplasmosis. *Lancet* 339:437–438, 1992.

54. Wallace MR, et al. Cats and toxoplasmosis risk in HIV-infected adults. *JAMA* 269:76–77, 1993.

55. Gallant JE, Moore RD, Chaisson RE. Prophylaxis for opportunistic infections in patients with HIV infection. *Ann Intern Med* 120:932–944, 1994.

56. Torres RA, Barr M, Thorn M, et al. Randomized trial of dapsone and aerosolized pentamidine for the prophylaxis of *Pneumocystis carinii* pneumonia and toxoplasmic encephalitis. *Am J Med* 95:573–583, 1993.

57. Hardy WD, Feinberg J, Finkelstein DM, et al. A controlled trial of trimethoprim-sulfamethoxazole or aerosolized pentamidine for secondary prophylaxis of *Pneumocystis carinii* pneumonia in patients with the acquired immunodeficiency syndrome. AIDS Clinical Trials Group Protocol 021. *N Engl J Med* 327:1842–1848, 1992.

58. Schneider MM, Hoepelman AI, Eeftinck Schattenkerk JK, et al. A controlled trial of aerosolized pentamidine or trimethoprim-sulfamethoxazole as primary prophylaxis against *Pneumocystis carinii* pneumonia in patients with human immunodeficiency virus infection. *N Engl J Med* 327:1836–1841, 1992.

59. Carr A, Tindall B, Brew BJ, et al. Low-dose trimethoprim-sulfamethoxazole prophylaxis for toxoplasmic encephalitis in patients with AIDS. *Ann Intern Med* 117:106–111, 1992.
60. O'Farrell N, Bradbeer C, Fitt S, et al. Cerebral toxoplasmosis and cotrimoxazole prophylaxis (letter). *Lancet* 337:986, 1991.
61. Girard PM, Landman R, Gaudebout C, et al. Dapsone-pyrimethamine compared with aerosolized pentamidine as primary prophylaxis against *Pneumocystis carinii* pneumonia and toxoplasmosis in HIV infection. *N Engl J Med* 328:1514–1520, 1993.
62. Clotet B, Sirera G, Romeau J, et al. Twice-weekly dapsone-pyrimethamine for preventing PCP and cerebral toxoplasmosis. *AIDS* 5:601–602, 1991.
63. Jacobson MA, Besch CL, Child C, et al. Primary prophylaxis with pyrimethamine for toxoplasmic encephalitis in patients with advanced human immunodeficiency virus disease: Results of a randomized trial. *J Infect Dis* 169:384–394, 1994.
64. Centers for Disease Control. USPHS/IDSA guidelines for the prevention of opportuistic infections in persons infected with human immunodeficiency virus: A summary. *MMWR* 44(RR-8):1–34, 1995.

Syphilis 23

Helen M. Jacoby, Judith L. Steinberg

Epidemiology

Significant changes have occurred in the epidemiology of syphilis over the past two decades. After a period of relative stability in the 1960s and most of the 1970s, rates of primary and secondary syphilis in the United States rose in the 1980s, especially among homosexual men [1]. In the late 1980s, the United States experienced a sharp increase in new cases of syphilis, with the incidence rising 75 percent, to 20 cases per 100,000 persons, representing the highest rate since 1949 [2]. During this period, rates of primary and secondary syphilis for black men increased from 69 to 156 per 100,000 (126%) and for black women from 35 to 116 per 100,000 (231%) [2]. Since 1990, the incidence of primary and secondary syphilis has declined somewhat from these very high rates, especially in homosexual men [3]. The epidemiology of syphilis has paralleled that of the AIDS epidemic over time, with increasing involvement of drug users, heterosexuals, and minorities [4–6].

Many retrospective studies have related HIV seropositivity to historical or serologic evidence of syphilis and other genital ulcer diseases [7–13]. For example, among patients in a Baltimore clinic for sexually transmitted disease (STD), the HIV seroprevalence rate was 24.3 percent in those with positive syphilis serologies compared to 3.5 percent in those with nonreactive tests [14]. Prospective studies have linked both the presence of genital ulcer disease and primary or secondary syphilis with HIV seroconversion [15–17]. One report also described an association between genital ulcer disease in HIV-infected men and the transmission of HIV to their female partners [18].

Syphilis and HIV infection are related epidemiologically in several important ways [19, 20]: (1) Both diseases are acquired through high-risk sexual behaviors; (2) genital ulceration appears to be a significant factor in the transmission and acquisition of HIV; (3) HIV infection may increase susceptibility to other STDs, including syphilis; and (4) HIV infection may alter the clinical presentation, disease severity, and treatment response of syphilis.

Clinical Manifestations

Our current knowledge of syphilis in the context of HIV disease is based on numerous case reports and series but few prospective data. These cases have suggested that HIV-infected patients with syphilis may have atypical clinical presentations, altered serologic response to infection, an increased frequency of neurosyphilis, and an inadequate clinical response to standard therapy. Given that cell-mediated immunity is important in the host response to syphilis, it is understandable that HIV infection might affect its course [21–23]. However, clinical experience suggests that most HIV-infected patients with syphilis have typical disease manifestations [24–26]. (Fig. 23-1; see Plate 13).

Whether concurrent HIV infection predisposes to unusual or very severe cases of syphilis is not entirely clear. Two retrospective studies found no difference in the clinical manifestations or stage at presentation of syphilis in HIV-positive patients compared to seronegative control subjects [25, 26]. However, a recent case-control study found that HIV-infected patients presented more often with secondary syphi-

Figure 23-1. Primary syphilitic chancre. (Courtesy of Upjohn Company, Kalamazoo, MI.)

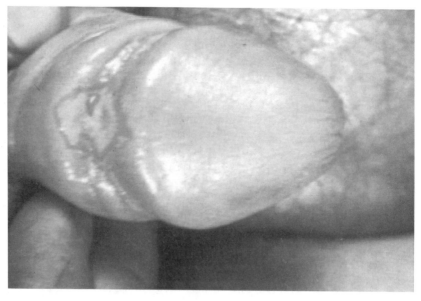

lis and were more likely to have persistent chancres [27]. Case reports of unusual manifestations of syphilis in association with HIV disease have included fever of unknown origin, gastritis, polyarthritis, intraoral gumma, cervical adenitis, pneumonitis with hepatitis, and lues maligna—a rare form of secondary syphilis manifested by skin ulcerations and severe constitutional symptoms [28–37].

Serologic Response

There have been case reports of delayed serologic response and unusually high nontreponemal titers (rapid plasma reagin [RPR], Venereal Disease Research Laboratory [VDRL]) in patients coinfected with HIV and syphilis [25, 26, 38, 39]. However, two studies suggested that, in most instances, the serologic response to syphilis in HIV-infected patients is preserved and comparable to that of seronegative control subjects [39, 40]. Increased nontreponemal titers may be a manifestation of the polyclonal B-cell activation that occurs in HIV disease. An extremely high antibody titer can result in the prozone phenomenon, in which the nontreponemal titer is falsely negative but retesting of the sample after dilution gives a positive result [41]. Some studies of HIV-infected patients have also documented the loss of treponemal test (FTA-abs, MHA-TP) reactivity in HIV-infected patients, which may be related to immune deficiency [42, 43]. An increased frequency of false-positive serologic tests for syphilis in HIV disease has also been described [44].

Neurosyphilis

Central nervous system (CNS) infection is common in the early stages of syphilis and usually asymptomatic. Early investigators documented CNS involvement in up to 13 percent of patients with primary syphilis and 40 percent of those with secondary syphilis [45]. Lukehart and associates [46] isolated *Treponema pallidum* from the cerebrospinal fluid (CSF) in 30 percent of patients with primary and secondary syphilis. The rate of CNS involvement was not related to HIV serostatus.

The significance of early asymptomatic CNS syphilis is unclear; only 5 to 10 percent of untreated HIV-negative patients develop clinically recognizable neurosyphilis [39]. The currently recommended therapy for early and latent syphilis, benzathine penicillin G, does not achieve treponemicidal levels in the CSF [47, 48]. However, despite this observation, progression to neurosyphilis rarely occurs following standard treatment of seronegative patients [39].

The importance of an intact immune system in preventing neurosyphilis is underscored by evidence that neurologic involvement appears to develop more quickly and perhaps more frequently in HIV disease. A recent prospective study found that 9.1 percent of 33 HIV-infected patients with latent syphilis who underwent lumbar puncture had positive CSF VDRL titers [49]. In a similar study, Berger [50] found that 1.8 percent of asymptomatic HIV-infected patients had a positive CSF VDRL on screening lumbar puncture.

Certain manifestations of neurosyphilis appear to be especially common in HIV disease. Katz and colleagues [51] compared HIV-infected patients with neurosyphilis to seronegative control subjects and found more cases of syphilitic meningitis and ophthalmic syphilis in the seropositive group, although statistical significance was not achieved. In addition, the HIV-positive group was more likely to have concurrent features of secondary syphilis.

Clinical features of early neurosyphilis appear to be more commonly associated with HIV infection than those of late neurosyphilis, such as tabes dorsalis, paresis, and dementia. Of 40 cases of neurosyphilis in HIV-infected patients reported in the literature before 1990, 5 had asymptomatic disease, 23 had acute syphilitic meningitis with or without cranial nerve dysfunction, 11 had meningovascular syphilis, and 1 had general paresis [39, 52].

Numerous case reports have documented the unusually rapid development of neurosyphilis with a wide variety of clinical presentations in HIV-positive individuals. Cases of cerebral gumma, cranial nerve abnormalities, meningovascular disease, necrotizing encephalitis, tabes dorsalis, meningomyelitis, lumbosacral polyradiculopathy, otosyphilis, and ocular disease have been described [53–63].

Diagnosis

All HIV-positive persons should be screened regularly for syphilis, and, conversely, HIV testing should be encouraged for patients with newly diagnosed syphilis. Both nontreponemal and treponemal tests are generally reliable for the diagnosis of syphilis in HIV disease [39, 40, 64]. However, if the clinical suspicion for syphilis is high and serologic tests are negative, the nontreponemal titer should be rechecked after dilution of the sample to rule out the prozone effect. In difficult cases, consideration should also be given to alternative diagnostic techniques such as biopsy, dark-field examination, or direct fluorescent antibody staining [64].

Authorities agree that HIV-infected patients with latent syphilis should undergo lumbar puncture to rule out neurologic involvement [64]. In addition, some experts believe that any HIV-positive person with syphilis should have an examination of the CSF performed, regardless of the stage of syphilis [39, 64]. However, interpretation of the results of the CSF analysis in this setting can be problematic.

Neurosyphilis is often characterized by an increased CSF protein level, pleocytosis, and a positive CSF VDRL [65]. The CSF VDRL is extremely specific, but not very sensitive, for neurosyphilis; a positive CSF VDRL alone is sufficient to make the diagnosis [1]. Treponemal tests, such as the FTA-abs, performed on the CSF are sensitive for neurosyphilis but result in too many false-positive tests to be useful in clinical practice [66]. Unfortunately, abnormal CSF findings are common in HIV-infected persons in general, possibly as a result of HIV involvement of the CNS [67, 68]. Given the poor sensitivity of the CSF VDRL, HIV-infected patients with syphilis and an abnormal CSF analysis should probably be treated for presumptive neurosyphilis.

Prognosis

Several reports have documented a poor clinical response to standard antibiotic therapy for syphilis in HIV-infected patients. Telzak and colleagues [69] found that HIV-positive individuals with primary syphilis were significantly less likely than seronegative control subjects to have a fourfold or greater RPR test decrease or seroreversion within 6 months of treatment. Thirty-three and 38 percent of HIV-infected patients with neurosyphilis reviewed by Katz and Berger [70] and Musher [52], respectively, had been previously treated for syphilis; other authors have reported similar results [71, 72]. Lukehart and associates [46] found that three HIV-infected patients treated for secondary syphilis with 2.4 million units (mIU) benzathine penicillin G did not clear the CSF of spirochetes or improve other CSF parameters. More recently, Gordon and colleagues [73] described their experience treating 11 HIV-infected patients with neurosyphilis, 5 of whom had relapsed after previous treatment for early syphilis. All patients were given benzathine penicillin G, 18 to 24 mIU per day for 10 days. Despite this, one person relapsed with meningovascular syphilis 6 months after treatment; the others had resolution or stabilization of their clinical manifestations, but three had persistently abnormal CSF, and three did not have a significant decline of their serum RPR titers after 6 months. Only one small retrospective study showed no difference in the response to treatment for syphilis between HIV-positive and seronegative patients [26].

Management

The most recent Centers for Disease Control (CDC) guidelines for the treatment of syphilis are presented in Table 23-1 [64]. As part of its recommendations, the CDC adds two caveats regarding HIV-infected patients: First, penicillin regimens should be used whenever possible for all stages of syphilis. If necessary, patients can be desensitized and

Table 23-1 *CDC guidelines for the treatment of syphilis*

Primary, secondary, and early latent (< 1 yr duration) syphilis
Recommended regimen: 2.4 mIU benzathine penicillin G IM once
Doxycycline, 100 mg PO bid × 2 wk, if penicillin allergic

Late latent (> 1 yr duration) and cardiovascular syphilis
Recommended regimen: 2.4 mIU benzathine penicillin G IM weekly × 3 wk
(total 7.2 mIU)
Doxycycline, 100 mg PO bid × 4 wk, if penicillin allergic

Neurosyphilis*
Recommended regimen: 12–24 mIU aqueous penicillin G IV daily × 10–14
days
Alternative: 2.4 mIU procaine penicillin IM daily plus 50 mg probenecid PO
qid × 10–14 days
If patient is penicillin allergic, skin test and desensitize as necessary

---

*Note: Following completion of a neurosyphilis regimen, many authorities recommend
the administration of 2.4 mIU benzathine penicillin G weekly × 3 wk.
Source: Adapted from Centers for Disease Control, 1993 Sexually transmitted diseases
treatment guidelines. *MMWR* 42 (RR-14):27–46, 1993.

treated with penicillin. Second, no modification of therapy for syphilis
is recommended in HIV-infected patients. However, in all cases, careful follow-up is necessary to ensure adequacy of treatment.

Some authorities disagree with these recommendations and have
advocated the use of higher doses of benzathine penicillin G. Fiumara
[74] has recommended a regimen of 2.4 mIU benzathine penicillin G
administered weekly for 2 weeks (total dose 4.8 mIU) for all patients
with early syphilis, including those with HIV disease. Others have advocated treating HIV-infected patients with early syphilis with a total
dose of 7.2 mIU benzathine penicillin G: 2.4 mIU administered weekly
for 3 weeks or 1.2 mIU twice a week for 3 consecutive weeks [39, 75,
76]. Tramont [77] has suggested that neurosyphilis regimens should be
used for all HIV-infected individuals with syphilis, regardless of its stage.
Whether higher doses of penicillin are more effective than standard
therapy in HIV disease is not known, but relapses have been reported
even with this more aggressive treatment [73].

Several alternative antibiotic regimens aimed at increasing CSF drug
levels have been proposed. These include: (1) 1.2 mIU procaine penicillin intramuscularly daily for 10 to 14 days, (2) the use of high-dose
oral amoxicillin (up to 6 gm/day), (3) the addition of probenecid to
penicillin regimens, (4) the addition of oral penicillin or amoxicillin to
benzathine penicillin G regimens, and (5) the use of ceftriaxone [78].
Clinical studies have documented the efficacy of ceftriaxone in the
treatment of incubating and early syphilis [79, 80]. However, Dowell
and coworkers [78] found a 23 percent failure rate when they treated

43 HIV-infected patients who had latent syphilis or neurosyphilis with 10 to 14 days of ceftriaxone.

Close observation is therefore necessary following treatment of HIV-infected patients with syphilis. The CDC recommends clinical and serologic follow-up at 1, 2, 3, 6, 9, and 12 months [64]. Others have recommended obtaining nontreponemal tests on a monthly basis for at least the first 6 months [24]. An adequate response to therapy is defined as a fourfold decline in nontreponemal antibody titer by 3 months for primary and secondary syphilis [64]. If this does not occur or if there is a sustained rise in nontreponemal antibody titer, then reevaluation with lumbar puncture is indicated, followed by retreatment [64]. The same is true if, after treatment of latent syphilis, there is a sustained fourfold rise in nontreponemal antibody titer or if an initially high titer (> 1:32) fails to decline over a period of 12 to 24 months.

Of note, a recent study showed that the usual serologic response to treatment of syphilis may be slower than that described above [81]. Romanowski and associates [81] found that successful treatment of primary and secondary syphilis results in a four- and eightfold decline in RPR titer by 6 and 12 months, respectively. A fourfold decline in titer was seen by 12 to 24 months in patients treated for early latent syphilis. Thus, the standard criteria to assess response of early syphilis to therapy may be too stringent.

Recommendations for the follow-up and expected CSF response of patients treated for neurosyphilis vary [64, 82, 83]. According to Simon [82] and Swartz [83], repeat CSF examinations should be performed at 3 to 6 months after treatment and at 6-month intervals thereafter for 2 years or until the CSF cell count and protein level return to normal. An adequate therapeutic response is defined as a normal CSF cell count and a falling protein level (if it was initially increased) at 6 months after treatment. The CSF VDRL titer generally declines but may not become nonreactive. If the CSF cell count is not normal by 3 to 6 months or, if having normalized, the cell count rises, retreatment is necessary. Swartz [83] suggests annual lumbar puncture for several years after the normalization of CSF values. The CDC recommends consideration of retreatment if the CSF cell count does not decline by 6 months or if the count has not normalized by 2 years [64]. However, given the frequency of CSF abnormalities in HIV-infected patients without syphilis and of neurologic disease in AIDS, changes in these nonspecific parameters may not be useful in assessing therapeutic response [67, 68].

Prevention

The prevention and control of syphilis and other STDs require primary, secondary, and tertiary strategies [84]. Disease avoidance (primary prevention) includes health education and interventions to promote safer sexual behaviors. Because the acquisition of syphilis and HIV infection are behaviorally related, such primary prevention strategies may affect the occurrence of both diseases.

The prevention of disease sequelae and transmission of infection (secondary prevention) requires early diagnosis and treatment, including screening of high-risk individuals and partner notification. Targeted syphilis screening and treatment in locations such as crack houses or jails may be necessary to improve the efficacy of these efforts [85–87].

Tertiary prevention (efforts to minimize the effects of disease sequelae) may be especially important in HIV-infected patients with syphilis. This includes intensive antibiotic therapy as described previously, with repeated follow-up evaluations. Some clinicians have suggested that suppressive therapy may be indicated to prevent relapse of syphilis in HIV-infected patients. Musher [52] argues against this, citing that neurologic relapse is rare when three doses of benzathine penicillin are used and chronic oral therapy is unlikely to achieve significant levels in the CSF.

References

1. Hook EW, Marra CM. Acquired syphilis in adults. *N Engl J Med* 326:1060–1069, 1992.
2. Centers for Disease Control. Primary and secondary syphilis—United States, 1981–1990. *MMWR* 40:314–315, 321–323, 1991.
3. Centers for Disease Control. Summary of notifiable diseases, United States, 1992. *MMWR* 41:52–55, 1992.
4. Rolfs RT, Goldberg M, Sharrar RG. Risk factors for syphilis: Cocaine use and prostitution. *Am J Public Health* 80:853–857, 1990.
5. Minkoff HL, McCalla S, Delke I, et al. The relationship of cocaine use to syphilis and human immunodeficiency virus infections among inner city parturient women. *Am J Obstet Gynecol* 163:521–526, 1990.
6. Centers for Disease Control. The HIV/AIDS epidemic: The first 10 years. *MMWR* 40:357–363, 369, 1991.
7. Kreiss JK, Koech D, Plummer FA, et al. AIDS virus infection in Nairobi prostitutes: Spread of the epidemic to east Africa. *N Engl J Med* 314:414–418, 1986.
8. Quinn TC, Glasser D, Cannon RO, et al. Human immunodeficiency virus infection among patients attending clinics for sexually transmitted diseases. *N Engl J Med* 318:197–203, 1988.
9. Stamm WE, Handsfield HH, Rompalo AM, et al. The association between genital ulcer disease and acquisition of HIV infection in homosexual men. *JAMA* 260:1429–1433, 1988.
10. Greenblatt RM, Lukehart SA, Plummer FA, et al. Genital ulceration as a risk factor for human immunodeficiency virus infection. *AIDS* 2:47–50, 1988.
11. Simonsen JN, Cameron DW, Gakinya MN, et al. Human immunodefi-

ciency virus infection among men with sexually transmitted disease: Experience from a center in Africa. *N Engl J Med* 319:274–278, 1988.

12. Evans BA, McLean KA, Dawson SG, et al. Trends in sexual behavior and risk factors for HIV infection among homosexual men, 1984–7. *Br Med J* 298:215–218, 1989.

13. Harkess JR, Kudlac J, Istre GR. Syphilis, human immunodeficiency virus infection, and targeting prevention. *South Med J* 83:1253–1255, 1990.

14. Quinn TC, Cannon RO, Glasser D, et al. The association of syphilis with risk of human immunodeficiency virus infection in patients attending sexually transmitted disease clinics. *Arch Intern Med* 150:1297–1302, 1990.

15. Plummer FA, Simonsen JN, Cameron DW, et al. Cofactors in male-female sexual transmission of human immunodeficiency virus type 1. *J Infect Dis* 163:233–239, 1991.

16. Cameron DW, Simonsen JN, D'Costa LJ, et al. Female to male transmission of human immunodeficiency virus type 1: Risk factors for seroconversion in men. *Lancet* 2:403–407, 1989.

17. Otten MW, Zaidi AA, Peterman TA, et al. High rate of HIV seroconversion among patients attending urban sexually transmitted disease clinics. *AIDS* 8:549–553, 1994.

18. Latif AS, Katzenstein DA, Bassett MT, et al. Genital ulcers and transmission of HIV among couples in Zimbabwe. *AIDS* 3:519–523, 1989.

19. Clottey C, Dallabetta G. Sexually transmitted diseases and human immunodeficiency virus. Epidemiologic synergy? *Infect Dis Clin North Am* 7:753–770, 1993.

20. Wasserheit JN. Epidemiological synergy. Interrelationships between human immunodeficiency virus infection and other sexually transmitted diseases. *Sex Transm Dis* 19:61–77, 1992.

21. Lukehart SA, Baker-Zander SA, Sell S. Characterization of lymphocyte responsiveness in early experimental syphilis. I. *In vitro* response to mitogens and *Treponema pallidum* antigens. *J Immunol* 124:454–460, 1980.

22. Lukehart SA, Baker-Zander SA, Lloyd RM, Sell S. Characterization of lymphocyte responsiveness in early experimental syphilis: Nature of cellular infiltration and *Treponema pallidum* distribution in testicular infection. *J Immunol* 124:461–467, 1980.

23. Pavia CS, Folds JD, Baseman JB. Cell-mediated immunity during syphilis: A review. *Br J Vener Dis* 54:144–150, 1978.

24. Hook EW, III. Syphilis and HIV infection. *J Infect Dis* 160:530–534, 1989.

25. Hutchinson CM, Rompalo AM, Reichart CA, Hook EW, III. Characteristics of patients with syphilis attending Baltimore STD clinics. *Arch Intern Med* 151:511–516, 1991.

26. Gourevitch MN, Selwyn PA, Davenny K, et al. Effects of HIV infection on the serologic manifestations and response to treatment of syphilis in intravenous drug users. *Ann Intern Med* 118:350–355, 1993.

27. Hutchinson CM, Hook EW, Shepherd M, et al. Altered clinical presentation of early syphilis in patients with human immunodeficiency virus infection. *Ann Intern Med* 121:94–99, 1994.

28. Gregory N, Sanchez M, Buchness MR. The spectrum of syphilis in pa-

tients with human immunodeficiency virus infection. *J Am Acad Dermatol* 22:1061–1067, 1990.

29. Radolf JD, Kaplan RP. Unusual manifestations of secondary syphilis and abnormal humoral immune response to *Treponema pallidum* antigens in a homosexual man with asymptomatic human immunodeficiency virus infection. *J Am Acad Dermatol* 18:423–428, 1988.

30. Cusini M, Zerboni R, Mauratori S, et al. Atypical early syphilis in an HIV-infected homosexual male. *Dermatologica* 177:300–304, 1988.

31. Chung WM, Pien FD, Grekin JL. Syphilis: A cause of fever of unknown origin. *Cutis* 31:537–540, 1983.

32. Kasmin F, Reddy S, Mathur-Wagh U. Syphilitic gastritis in an HIV-infected individual. *Am J Gastroenterol* 87:1820–1822, 1992.

33. Burgoyne M, Agudelo C, Pisko E. Chronic syphilitic polyarthritis mimicking systemic lupus erythematosus/rheumatoid arthritis as the initial presentation of human immunodeficiency virus infection. *J Rheumatol* 19:313–315, 1992.

34. Kearns G, Pogrel MA, Honda G. Intraoral tertiary syphilis (gumma) in a human immunodeficiency virus–positive man: A case report. *J Oral Maxillofac Surg* 51:85–88, 1993.

35. Heller H, Fromowitz F, Fuhrer J. Luetic cervical adenitis in patients with human immunodeficiency virus type 1 infection. *Arch Otolaryngol Head Neck Surg* 118:757–758, 1992.

36. Dooley DP, Tomski S. Syphilitic pneumonitis in an HIV-infected patient. *Chest* 105:629–631, 1994.

37. Shulkin D, Tripoli L, Abell E. Lues maligna in a patient with human immunodeficiency virus infection. *Am J Med* 85:425–427, 1988.

38. Hicks CB, Benson PM, Lupton GP, Tramont EC. Seronegative secondary syphilis in a patient infected with the human immunodeficiency virus (HIV) with Kaposi's sarcoma. *Ann Intern Med* 107:492–495, 1988.

39. Musher DM, Hamill RJ, Baughn RE. Effect of human immunodeficiency virus (HIV) infection on the course of syphilis and on the response to treatment. *Ann Intern Med* 113:872–881, 1990.

40. Terry PM, Page ML, Goldmeier LD. Are serological tests of value in diagnosing and monitoring response to treatment of syphilis in patients infected with human immunodeficiency virus? *Genitourin Med* 64:219–222, 1988.

41. Jurado RL, Campbell J, Martin PD. Prozone phenomenon in secondary syphilis: Has its time arrived? *Arch Intern Med* 153:2496–2498, 1993.

42. Haas JS, Bolan G, Larsen SA, et al. Sensitivity of treponemal tests for detecting prior treated syphilis during human immunodeficiency virus infection. *J Infect Dis* 162:862–866, 1990.

43. Johnson PDR, Graves SR, Stewart L, et al. Specific syphilis serological tests may become negative in HIV infection. *AIDS* 5:419–423, 1991.

44. Rompalo AM, et al. Association of biologic false-positive reactions for syphilis with human immunodeficiency virus infection. *J Infect Dis* 165:1124–1126, 1992.

45. Mills CH. Routine examination of the cerebro-spinal fluid in syphilis: Its value in regard to more accurate knowledge, prognosis, and treatment. *Br Med J* 2:527–532, 1927.

46. Lukehart SA, Hook EW, Baker-Zander SA, et al. Invasion of the central nervous system by *Treponema pallidum*: Implications for diagnosis and treatment. *Ann Intern Med* 109:855–862, 1988.
47. Mohr JA, Griffiths W, Jackson R, et al. Neurosyphilis and penicillin levels in cerebrospinal fluid. *JAMA* 236:2208–2209, 1976.
48. Dunlop EMC, Al-Egaily SS, Houang ET. Penicillin levels in blood and CSF achieved by treatment of syphilis. *JAMA* 241:2538–2540, 1979.
49. Holtom PD, Larsen RA, Leal ME, et al. Prevalence of neurosyphilis in human immunodeficiency virus–infected patients with latent syphilis. *Am J Med* 93:9–12, 1992.
50. Berger JR. Neurosyphilis in human immunodeficiency virus type 1–seropositive individuals. *Arch Neurol* 48:700-702, 1991.
51. Katz DA, Berger JR, Duncan RC. Neurosyphilis. A comparative study of the effects of infection with human immunodeficiency virus. *Arch Neurol* 50:243–249, 1993.
52. Musher DM. Syphilis, neurosyphilis, penicillin, and AIDS. *J Infect Dis* 163:1201–1206, 1991.
53. Horowitz HW, Valsamis MP, Wicher V, et al. Brief report: Cerebral syphilitic gumma confirmed by the polymerase chain reaction in a man with human immunodeficiency virus infection. *N Engl J Med* 331:1488–1491, 1994.
54. Morgella S, Laufer H. Quaternary neurosyphilis in a Haitian man with human immunodeficiency virus infection. *Hum Pathol* 20:808–811, 1989.
55. Calderon W, Douville H, Nigro M, et al. Concomitant syphilitic and HIV infection: A case report. *Acta Neurologica* 12:132–137, 1990.
56. Strom T, Schneck SA. Syphilitic meningomyelitis. *Neurology* 41:325–326, 1991.
57. Lanska MJ, Lanska DJ, Schmidley JW. Syphilitic polyradiculopathy in an HIV-positive man. *Neurology* 38:1297–1301, 1988.
58. Smith ME, Canalis RF. Otologic manifestations of AIDS: The otosyphilis connection. *Laryngoscope* 99:365–372, 1989.
59. Passo MS, Rosenbaum JT. Ocular syphilis in patients with human immunodeficiency virus infection. *Am J Ophthalmol* 106:1–6, 1988.
60. Zambrano W, Perez GM, Smith JL. Acute syphilitic blindness in AIDS. *J Clin Neuro Ophthalmol* 7:1–5, 1987.
61. McLeish WM, Pulido JS, Holland S, et al. The ocular manifestations of syphilis in the human immunodeficiency virus type 1-infected host. *Ophthalmology* 97:196–203, 1990.
62. Levy JH, Liss RA, Maguire AM. Neurosyphilis and ocular syphilis in patients with concurrent human immunodeficiency virus infection. *Retina* 9:175–180, 1989.
63. Tamesis RR, Foster CS. Ocular syphilis. *Ophthalmology* 97:1281–1287, 1990.
64. Centers for Disease Control and Prevention. 1993 sexually transmitted diseases treatment guidelines. *MMWR* 42 RR-14:27–46, 1993.
65. Wolters EC, Hische EAH, Tutuarima JA, et al. Central nervous system involvement in early and late syphilis: The problem of asymptomatic neurosyphilis. *J Neurol Sci* 88:29–39, 1988.
66. Tomberlin MG, Holtom PD, Owens JL, Larsen RA. Evaluation of

neurosyphilis in human immunodeficiency virus-infected individuals. *Clin Infect Dis* 18:288–294, 1994.

67. Hollander H. Cerebrospinal fluid normalities and abnormalities in individuals infected with human immunodeficiency virus. *J Infect Dis* 158:855–858, 1988.

68. Appleman ME, Marxhall DW, Brey RL, et al. Cerebrospinal fluid abnormalities in patients without AIDS who are seropositive for the human immunodeficiency virus. *J Infect Dis* 158:193–199, 1988.

69. Telzak EE, Zweig Greenberg MS, Harrison J, et al. Syphilis treatment response in HIV-infected individuals. *AIDS* 5:591–595, 1991.

70. Katz DA, Berger JR. Neurosyphilis in acquired immunodeficiency syndrome. *Arch Neurol* 46:895–898, 1989.

71. Johns DR, Tierney M, Felsenstein D. Alteration in the natural history of neurosyphilis by concurrent infection with the human immunodeficiency virus. *N Engl J Med* 316:1569–1572, 1987.

72. Berry CD, Hooton TM, Collier AC, Lukehart SA. Neurologic relapse after benzathine penicillin therapy for secondary syphilis in a patient with HIV infection. *N Engl J Med* 316:1587–1589, 1987.

73. Gordon SM, Eaton ME, George R, et al. The response of symptomatic neurosyphilis to high-dose intravenous penicillin G in patients with human immunodeficiency virus infection. *N Engl J Med* 331:1469–1473, 1994.

74. Fiumara N. Human immunodeficiency virus infection and syphilis. *J Am Acad Dermatol* 21:141–142, 1989.

75. Felman YM. Recent developments in the diagnosis and treatment of sexually transmitted diseases: Infectious syphilis and acquired immunodeficiency syndrome. *Cutis* 44:288–290, 1989.

76. Manganoni AM, Graifemberghi S, Facchetti F, et al. Effectiveness of penicillin G benzathine therapy for primary and secondary syphilis in HIV infection. *J Am Acad Dermatol* 23:1185–1186, 1990.

77. Tramont EC. Syphilis in the AIDS era. *N Engl J Med* 316:1600–1601, 1987.

78. Dowell ME, et al. Response of latent syphilis or neurosyphilis to ceftriaxone therapy in persons infected with human immunodeficiency virus. *Am J Med* 93:481–488, 1992.

79. Hook EW, III, Roddy RE, Handsfield HH. Ceftriaxone therapy for incubating and early syphilis. *J Infect Dis* 158:881–884, 1988.

80. Schofer H, Vogt HJ, Milbrodt R. Ceftriaxone for the treatment of primary and secondary syphilis. *Chemotherapy* 35:140–145, 1989.

81. Romanowski B, Sutherland R, Fick GH, et al. Serologic response to treatment of infectious syphilis. *Ann Intern Med* 114:1005–1009, 1991.

82. Simon RP. Neurosyphilis. *Arch Neurol* 42:606–613, 1985.

83. Swartz MN. Neurosyphilis. In KK Holmes, P Mardh, PF Sparling, et al (eds), *Sexually Transmitted Diseases* (2nd ed). New York: McGraw-Hill, 1990. Pp 231–246.

84. Report of the NIAID Study Group on integrated behavioral research for prevention and control of sexually transmitted diseases. *Sex Transm Dis* 17:200–210, 1990.

85. Andrus JK, Fleming DW, Harger DR, et al. Partner notification: Can it control epidemic syphilis? *Ann Intern Med* 112:539–543, 1990.

86. Centers for Disease Control. Epidemic early syphilis—Escambia County, Florida, 1987 and July 1989-June 1990. *MMWR* 40:323–325, 1991.
87. Centers for Disease Control. Alternative case-finding methods in a crack-related syphilis epidemic—Philadelphia. *MMWR* 40:77–80, 1991.

Cytomegalovirus Infection   24

David Ives

Cytomegalovirus (CMV) is the most common cause of life-threatening viral infection in patients with HIV disease [1]. Retinitis, leading to blindness; gastrointestinal disease, resulting in wasting, diarrhea, obstruction, or perforation; and central nervous system involvement, with flaccid paralysis or encephalitis, are all manifestations of CMV infection.

Ganciclovir and foscarnet have proved to be effective therapies for CMV infection in patients with AIDS [2–4]. However, many therapeutic problems remain. Relapsing infection, the absence of effective host immunity, other complicating opportunistic diseases, and drug toxicity make management of CMV infection a significant challenge.

Epidemiology

Both CMV and HIV can be transmitted sexually, through blood product transfusion or contaminated drug injection paraphernalia, and vertically from mother to child. The prevalence of antibody to CMV varies widely in different populations [5]. Antibody to CMV is present in up to 90 percent of homosexual men and female prostitutes, and in over half of women who attend sexually transmitted disease clinics in the United States [6, 7]. The likelihood of CMV infection in a person is proportional to their number of prior sexual partners or blood transfusions [8]. HIV-infected patients with hemophilia have high prevalence rates for antibody to CMV [9].

Clinical Manifestations

Cytomegalovirus disease in adults generally results from reactivation of latent infection in the setting of advanced HIV disease (CD4 count less than 100/mm³) [10, 11]. Although hemorrhagic necrotizing retinitis is the most common clinical manifestation, virtually any organ can be affected. The gastrointestinal tract, including the liver, gallbladder, and pancreas, is the second most frequent site of CMV infection [12–17]. Cytomegalovirus neurologic disease, including chronic meningo-encephalitis and polyradiculopathy, accounts for an increasing number of cases [18, 19]. Pneumonitis and adrenalitis have also been described but remain uncommon.

Retinitis

Cytomegalovirus retinitis is the most frequent cause of ocular disease among HIV-infected patients, affecting approximately 20 to 40 percent during the course of their illness [20, 21]. The incidence of CMV retinitis rises with declining CD4 cell count [10, 11] (Fig. 24-1). Without treatment, CMV retinitis progresses to macular involvement and blindness in the majority of patients.

Cytomegalovirus retinitis can be divided into "non–sight-threatening" and "sight-threatening" disease, the former affecting the periph-

Figure 24-1. Kaplan-Meier estimate of proportions of patients developing CMV disease by baseline CD4 cell count: solid line, < 0.05 × 10⁹/liter; dotted line, 0.05– 0.099 × 10⁹/liter; dashed line, ≥ 0.1 × 10⁹/liter. Difference between lower line and two upper lines was significant by log-rank test ($P < .001$); difference between two upper lines was not significant ($P > .05$). (From JE Gallant et al. Incidence and natural history of cytomegalovirus disease in patients with advanced immunodeficiency virus disease treated with zidovudine. *J Infect Dis* 166:1223–1227, 1992.)

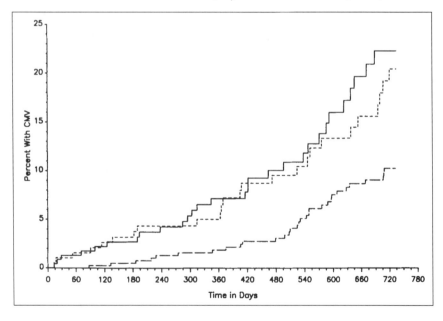

ery of the retina and the latter involving areas near the fovea or optic disk [22]. Cytomegalovirus retinitis generally presents unilaterally but frequently spreads to the other eye; early disease is often asymptomatic. On funduscopic examination, CMV lesions appear as small, multifocal, yellow-white patches with a granular appearance, located contiguous to blood vessels (Plate 8). Hemorrhage is a distinctive feature of CMV retinitis and helps differentiate it from cotton-wool spots (Plate 7). Retinitis that can be visualized using a direct ophthalmoscope through an undilated pupil should be considered sight-threatening and warrants immediate diagnostic confirmation by an ophthalmologist.

Gastrointestinal Disease

Cytomegalovirus can cause ulcerative lesions throughout the gastrointestinal tract and is one of the most common causes of cholangiopathy in patients with AIDS [23, 24]. The incidence of CMV gastrointestinal disease varies widely, depending on the population studied and criteria used for diagnosis [12, 25]. Of the CMV gastrointestinal disease syndromes, esophagitis and colitis are most frequent.

Esophagitis

Esophagitis generally presents with odynophagia (87%), although dysphagia and substernal or midepigastric pain are also commonly described [13]. In one case series, symptoms persisted a median of 4 weeks, with a range of 2 weeks to 24 months, before diagnosis [13]. Candidal and CMV esophagitis cannot be distinguished clinically, and CMV infection should be considered in the differential diagnosis of esophageal symptoms in advanced HIV disease when empiric antifungal therapy is not successful [26]. On endoscopic examination, CMV esophageal ulcers are usually single or few in number, large and shallow [13]. Patients with esophageal biopsies showing evidence of both candidal and CMV infections will frequently respond to antifungal therapy [26].

Colitis

Cytomegalovirus colitis may present either as chronic persistent diarrhea with wasting or as fulminant diarrhea with fever and sometimes perforation [14, 27, 28]. Patients with CMV colitis often have fever (80%), weight loss (89% with a median loss of 8.9 kg), and cramping abdominal pain (64%) [14]. Unfortunately, the clinical characteristics of CMV colitis are not distinguishable from other common causes of diarrhea in patients with AIDS [14, 29]. On endoscopy, the colonic mucosa appears completely normal in 25 percent of patients, with patchy (41%) or diffuse (34%) areas of inflammation and ulceration in the remainder. Cytomegalovirus colitis is frequently associated with retinal disease [14].

Other Gastrointestinal Syndromes

Cytomegalovirus infection has been implicated as a cause of dilated cholangiopathy of AIDS [24, 30]. Acalculous cholecystitis, pancreatitis, and hepatitis resulting from CMV infection have also been reported [15, 16, 31].

Pneumonitis

In an extensive review of the pulmonary complications of HIV disease, CMV was described as a contributing pathogen in 17 percent of cases and the sole pathogen in 4 percent [32]. When CMV is found on transbronchial biopsy in a patient with interstitial pneumonitis, it should be considered pathogenic.

Central Nervous System Disease

Cytomegalovirus is commonly found in the central nervous system (CNS) on autopsy of patients with AIDS [33, 34]. Polyradiculopathy with flaccid paralysis resulting from CMV is an increasingly recognized syndrome that can have devastating impact on a patient's quality of life and independence [18, 35]. Lumbar puncture may reveal findings easily confused with bacterial meningitis, including marked pleocytosis with a polymorphonuclear cell predominance, increased protein level, and low or normal glucose level [30, 36]. Culture for CMV is positive less than 50 percent of the time. In advanced cases, cerebrospinal fluid lymphocytes may show CMV intranuclear inclusions. The use of polymerase chain reaction testing has recently made it possible to identify CMV DNA in the cerebrospinal fluid of patients with suspected CNS infection [37, 38].

Two other distinct entities, mononeuritis multiplex and painful peripheral neuropathy, have also been attributed to CMV infection in patients with HIV disease [19].

Other Syndromes

Cytomegalovirus adrenal disease is a common finding on autopsy of AIDS patients, but clinical adrenal insufficiency is rare [39]. Other more unusual complications of CMV infection include skin involvement, pericarditis, cystitis, and thrombophlebitis [40–43].

Diagnosis

Histology

The varied manifestations of CMV infection and the difficulty in distinguishing them from other complications of HIV disease mandate that tissue be obtained for histologic examination whenever possible. The major exception to this rule is CMV retinitis, the diagnosis of which remains clinical. Histologic diagnosis of CMV infection requires the presence of characteristic "owl's eye" cells, with cytomegaly and large intranuclear or intracytoplasmic inclusions surrounded by a halo. Recent advances with polymerase chain reaction and immunoperoxidase testing have been used to clarify the diagnosis of CMV infection in some instances.

Serology

Because of the high rate of prior CMV infection among patients with HIV disease, the presence of antibody does not increase the probability that a clinical syndrome is caused by CMV. The potential loss of CMV antibody response in advanced HIV disease compromises the clinical utility of this test.

Culture

Positive CMV cultures from urine, blood, or bronchoalveolar lavage fluid are common in the absence of clinical disease. In a prospective evaluation of the usefulness of screening blood and urine cultures for CMV in patients likely to develop symptomatic disease, the predictive value was only 35 percent for a positive blood culture and 28 percent for a positive urine culture [44]. Furthermore, only 45 percent of patients with documented CMV disease had a positive blood culture [44]. Given the expense and time required, there is currently no indication for routine cultures as part of the initial clinical assessment of patients with suspected CMV infection. The role of urine culture in monitoring antiviral therapy is discussed below.

Management

The goal of treatment for CMV disease in patients with AIDS is to suppress active inflammation with a course of high-dose primary or induction therapy and then, in cases of retinitis, to prevent relapse with chronic maintenance therapy (Table 24-1). The use of long-term treatment for CMV disease other than retinitis is controversial (see below).

The cornerstones of management of CMV infection are the two currently approved antiviral agents, ganciclovir and foscarnet. Ganciclovir is a guanosine analogue that is an inactive prodrug, requiring phosphorylation to ganciclovir triphosphate in order to be activated [45]. Foscarnet is a pyrophosphate analogue that is structurally similar to phosphonoacetic acid. Foscarnet prevents pyrophosphate exchange, thereby inhibiting CMV DNA chain elongation catalyzed by DNA

Table 24-1 *Dosing and toxicity of therapies for cytomegalovirus infection*

Drug	Route	Dose	Toxicity
Ganciclovir			
Induction	IV	5 mg/kg q12h	Neutropenia
			Anemia
Maintenance	IV	5 mg/kg qd	Thrombocytopenia
		5–7 days/wk	Nausea/diarrhea
	PO	1 gm tid	Less neutropenia
			than IV
	Intravitreal implant		No systemic toxicity
	(experimental)		
Foscarnet			
Induction	IV	60 mg/kg q8h	Azotemia
		90 mg/kg q12h	Hypocalcemia
			Hypophosphatemia
Maintenance	IV	90–120 mg/kg qd	Hypomagnesemia
			Anemia
			Nausea
			Seizure

polymerase [46]. Since foscarnet binds directly to viral DNA polymerase, it is active against thymidine kinase–deficient CMV mutants [47]. Foscarnet is also a potent inhibitor of HIV reverse transcriptase [48].

Retinitis

Ganciclovir Induction Therapy

For treatment of retinitis, induction therapy with ganciclovir should be instituted at 5 mg/kg intravenously twice a day for 14 to 21 days in patients with normal renal function. Patients with leukopenia may require cytokine support or interruption of other myelosuppressive agents to tolerate induction doses. Ganciclovir induction controls retinitis in 70 to 90 percent of cases [2, 49, 50]. A follow-up ophthalmologic examination is performed after completion of induction therapy to determine if the clinical response has been adequate and whether maintenance therapy can begin. Zidovudine (ZDV) should not be administered during induction therapy because of its combined bone marrow toxicity with ganciclovir. A complete blood cell count is performed twice a week to monitor for neutropenia and thrombocytopenia.

Ganciclovir Maintenance Therapy

The dosage of ganciclovir for maintenance therapy is 5 mg/kg intravenously given once a day. Monthly ophthalmologic examinations during maintenance therapy permit early detection of relapsing CMV disease.

Cytomegalovirus retinitis that relapses should be managed with a course of reinduction ganciclovir or by switching to foscarnet. During maintenance therapy, ZDV can be restarted, and a complete blood count should be performed every 1 to 4 weeks. A positive urine culture for CMV during ganciclovir maintenance therapy suggests that viral resistance has developed.

Foscarnet Induction Therapy

The dosage of foscarnet currently recommended for induction therapy is 180 mg/kg/day intravenously given in divided doses every 8 hours for 14 days. Induction therapy controls retinitis in up to 90 percent of patients [3, 4]. An every-12-hour induction regimen has been used successfully in France with similar results and has gained wide acceptance in the United States [51]. The dose of foscarnet must be adjusted for creatinine clearance in accordance with the nomogram in the package insert. Failure to reduce the drug dosage for declining renal function is a common cause of toxicity during foscarnet administration.

Before initiation of foscarnet therapy, the creatinine clearance should be determined, and any preexisting hypocalcemia or hypomagnesemia should be corrected (Table 24-2). Intravenous infusion of 500 to 750 ml normal saline per dose should be given before or during the drug infusion to reduce renal toxicity. Foscarnet administration requires an infusion pump for delivery of the drug at a fixed rate. The time required for daily induction therapy with hydration may be as long as 6 hours. The concurrent use of intravenous pentamidine and foscarnet is not recommended because of an increase in the risk of seizure.

Foscarnet Maintenance Therapy

The dose of foscarnet for maintenance therapy is 90 to 120 mg/kg/day. In several studies, maintenance therapy with foscarnet delayed progression of retinitis by about 60 days [3, 4]. Volume expansion with normal saline should be given before each foscarnet dose during maintenance therapy.

Follow-up ophthalmologic examinations for patients receiving foscarnet maintenance therapy should be performed using the same schedule as for patients being treated with ganciclovir. Relapse of retinitis can be treated with a repeat course of induction therapy and a return to maintenance dosage once the disease is controlled. Patients who have had multiple relapses of retinitis while on maintenance therapy at 90 mg/kg/day may benefit from maintenance at a dose of 120 mg/kg/day. However, this higher dose may be associated with an increased frequency of side effects.

The most serious toxicities of foscarnet are renal failure and seizures. Serum creatinine, calcium, magnesium, and albumin should be moni-

Table 24-2 *Monitoring foscarnet therapy**

Test	Frequency	Action
Prior to induction		
Serum creatinine Ca++, Mg++, CBC, 24-hr urine and calculation of Crcl	Once	Adjust Ca++, Mg++ into "high normal" range
Patient weight		Calculate foscarnet dose using nomogram
Induction therapy		
Serum creatinine	TIW	Recalculate foscarnet dose if creatinine ↑ 0.2 mg/dl or 10%
Serum Ca++, Mg++	TIW	Replace as necessary to keep in normal range (corrected for alb)
Weight	Weekly	Adjust dose if weight changes by ≥ 10%
Maintenance therapy		
24-hr urine and calculation of Crcl	At start and monthly	Use for dose calculation and compare to estimated Crcl
Serum creatinine, Ca++, Mg++, weight	Weekly	Recalculate foscarnet dose if creatinine ↑ 0.2 mg/dl or 10%

Crcl = creatinine clearance; TIW = three times per week; alb = albumin.
*If in doubt about patient's renal function or fluid status, hold foscarnet. If diarrhea or other cause of dehydration develops, recheck renal function immediately and recalculate dose.

tored one to three times per week during the induction phase and two to four times per month during maintenance (Table 24-2). A 24-hour urine collection for creatinine clearance is recommended once per month to ensure that the serum creatinine remains an accurate indicator of renal function.

Gastrointestinal Disease

The dose of ganciclovir for induction therapy in patients with CMV gastrointestinal disease is identical to that used for retinitis (5 mg/kg every 12 hours for 14 to 21 days). The resolution of gastrointestinal symptoms, odynophagia or diarrhea, should be the primary determinant of the success of induction therapy [52]; it is not necessary to repeat an endoscopy. A placebo-controlled trial of ganciclovir for CMV colitis showed an improvement in diarrhea after 14 days of therapy [50]. Failure of symptoms to respond to induction therapy should prompt diagnostic evaluation for other pathogens.

The need for maintenance therapy for CMV disease of the gastrointestinal tract has not been established by clinical trials. However, if the clinical presentation is fulminant or if relapse occurs soon after cessation of treatment, maintenance therapy should be considered. All patients with established CMV gastrointestinal disease should be referred for ophthalmologic examination to rule out concurrent retinitis before the need for maintenance therapy is determined.

Foscarnet has been shown to be effective as initial treatment of CMV gastrointestinal disease and as "salvage" therapy when there is lack of response to ganciclovir [53, 54]. Improvement of symptoms often occurs within 2 weeks of beginning induction therapy [51].

Cytomegalovirus-associated cholangiopathy is generally unresponsive to antiviral therapy if biliary duct dilation is present. Papillotomy or cholecystectomy may offer effective palliation.

Other Organ System Involvement

There is little information on the efficacy of treatment for CMV pneumonitis associated with HIV disease. Induction doses of therapy with either ganciclovir or foscarnet should be initiated if the diagnosis is confirmed. As with CMV gastrointestinal disease, a search for evidence of retinitis should be completed before a decision about maintenance therapy is made.

In patients who have undergone organ or bone marrow transplantation, CMV pneumonitis is a common complication, with a high mortality in the absence of specific treatment. Several uncontrolled studies have demonstrated improved survival in bone marrow transplant patients with CMV pneumonitis following treatment with ganciclovir and CMV immunoglobulin [55, 56]. However, the applicability of this therapeutic approach to HIV-infected patients with CMV pneumonitis is uncertain.

Treatment of CMV polyradiculopathy has been disappointing. Four studies, each involving small numbers of patients, have evaluated ganciclovir for the management of peripheral CMV neurologic syndromes [36, 57–59]. Of note, all of the patients whose conditions improved or stabilized were treated early in the course of their disease. One report claimed no benefit with ganciclovir [60]. In another study, seven patients with CMV mononeuritis were managed with ganciclovir, and three responded [17]. Anecdotal evidence also suggests that treatment of CMV meningoencephalitis with ganciclovir is sometimes beneficial [61].

Ganciclovir Toxicity

The most common side effect of ganciclovir is neutropenia. During induction therapy, 10 to 40 percent of patients treated with ganciclovir develop neutropenia, as defined by an absolute neutrophil count (ANC) of less than 1,000/µl [1]. Neutropenia is exacerbated by the use of other myelosuppressive drugs, such as ZDV, pyrimethamine, and trimethoprim-sulfamethoxazole. When neutropenia develops in a patient who is being treated with ganciclovir, the clinician has four options: (1) discontinue other myelosuppressive agents, (2) switch to foscarnet, (3) institute supportive therapy with a cytokine, or (4) reduce the dose of ganciclovir.

Option one, discontinuing other myelosuppressive agents, may temporarily reduce the overall bone marrow suppressant effect, but neutropenia often recurs. Option two, switching to foscarnet maintenance therapy, offers the advantage of a proven CMV therapy without impact on the neutrophil count. If there is no evidence of progression of CMV disease while the patient is receiving ganciclovir, then reinduction with foscarnet is not required, and the patient can be started on maintenance therapy. Option three, supportive therapy with a cytokine, will allow ganciclovir therapy to be continued in most patients. In general, granulocyte colony-stimulating factor (G-CSF) is associated with a lower incidence of side effects than granulocyte-macrophage colony-stimulating factor (GM-CSF), but both are effective in increasing the neutrophil count [62, 63]. Dose of the cytokine should be titrated individually for each patient, beginning with 1 µg/kg subcutaneously daily to maintain an ANC over 500/µl (Table 24-3). The fourth option, lowering the dose of ganciclovir, results in reduced serum levels and should be considered only as a last resort, as CMV retinitis may be more likely to progress.

Foscarnet Toxicity

The most common side effects of foscarnet are renal failure and electrolyte abnormalities [3, 4]. Severe hypocalcemia or hypomagnesemia may contribute to the increased incidence of seizure activity in these patients. Anemia is a frequent finding during prolonged foscarnet therapy. Nausea and penile ulcerations have also been reported.

Transient, reversible increases in serum creatinine are commonly seen after the third week of foscarnet therapy. Renal dysfunction may be minimized with aggressive volume support and careful drug dose adjustment. If renal impairment cannot be managed with foscarnet dose reduction, consideration should be given to switching therapy to ganciclovir. In a study comparing ganciclovir and foscarnet for initial therapy of CMV retinitis, mild renal insufficiency (creatinine clearance

Table 24-3 *Cytokine usage guidelines*

	Start of GCV	*Induction therapy*	*Maintenance*
GCV dose	5 mg/kg q12h	5 mg/kg q12h	5 mg/kg qd
ANC to start cytokine	1,500	1,500	750
Target ANC		1,000	1,000
Cytokine dose	1 µg/kg/day	Adjust weekly	Adjust weekly
ZDV	Hold	Hold	Restart

GCV = ganciclovir; ANC = absolute neutrophil count; ZDV = zidovudine.

< 1.2 ml/min/kg) at study entry contributed to an increased mortality among patients randomly assigned to receive foscarnet [64].

Hypocalcemia or hypomagnesemia can be managed with oral or, when necessary, intravenous replacement therapy. Patients should be instructed to immediately report symptoms of hypocalcemia, such as numbness and tingling around the mouth or muscle twitching.

Penile ulcerations appear to be a direct toxic effect of foscarnet on the skin of the penis and may be more common in men who are uncircumcised. Interruption of foscarnet therapy until the ulceration heals and reinstitution with careful attention to cleaning any residual urine from under the foreskin may reduce ulcer formation.

Alternative Delivery Systems for Ganciclovir

The requirement for daily intravenous administration, with its associated increased risk of catheter-related sepsis, and the systemic toxicity of ganciclovir have led to the search for alternative ways to deliver the medication. Two methods, intravitreal administration and oral dosing, are currently under investigation.

Intravitreal ganciclovir, delivered by intermittent injection, has been used with some success for several years, but the need for frequent administration makes the procedure unattractive to many patients [65]. More recently, a sustained-release ganciclovir implant has been reported to result in prolonged therapeutic levels of ganciclovir in the eye, no systemic toxicity, and a favorable clinical response; randomized trials are ongoing [66].

Oral ganciclovir has also been evaluated. Results from a randomized trial comparing oral with intravenous ganciclovir for maintenance therapy of peripheral retinitis showed similar clinical efficacy when patients received 3 weeks of induction therapy [67]. However, subjects randomized to oral ganciclovir had a greater number of new CMV lesions in the previously unaffected eye. In both the oral and intravenous groups, there was a marked decrease in the number of subjects with positive urine cultures for CMV, indicating that both preparations decrease replication of the virus. Subjects receiving oral ganciclovir had a lower incidence of neutropenia and intravascular catheter infections. Preliminary information suggests that oral ganciclovir may be effective in preventing CMV infection in patients with advanced HIV disease [67a], and clinical trials are continuing. The drug has recently been approved by the Food and Drug Administration for maintenance therapy of CMV retinitis.

Choosing Between Ganciclovir and Foscarnet for Initial Management of Cytomegalovirus Disease

The choice between ganciclovir and foscarnet for initial treatment of CMV disease poses a dilemma (Table 24-4). Both agents have been

Table 24-4 *Choosing between ganciclovir (GCV) and foscarnet (FOS)*

This table recreates the clinical decision-making process involved in choosing anti-CMV therapy for a patient with newly diagnosed CMV retinitis. It assumes that ganciclovir and foscarnet are equally effective at treating the disease.

Read each question carefully and choose the answer that best fits the patient's condition.

To start: Answer question 1; use a pointer to find the place on the line equal to the points suggested next to the answer you chose.

Move down the diagram in a series of steps, following a vertical line between each question, and add or subtract points with each answer.

If the total reaches either **–10 or +10, STOP**.

The point total at the end suggests which agent to use. You can go back and try answering the questions differently to see how the recommendation changes.

History, clinical situation, or laboratory value	Answers and points	GCV ↓ FOS (scale –10, –5, 0, +5, +10)
1. Seizure disorder?	No = 0; distant = –5; active* = –10	
2. Creatinine?	< 1.0 = 0; 1.5 = –4; > 2.0 = –8*	
3. Absolute neutrophil count (in thousands)?	> 3 = 0; < 1.5 = +5; < 1.0 = +8	
4. Cytokine available and affordable?	Yes = 0; no = +5	
5. Requires other nephrotoxins?	Yes = –7; no = 0	
6. Requires pyrimethamine, other bone marrow suppressor?	Yes = +3; no = 0	
7. Difficult to manage fluid status?	Yes = –5; no = 0	
8. Anti-HIV therapy?	None = +5; ZDV > 1yr = +3; ddI or ddC = 0	
9. Patient preference?	GCV = –3; none = 0; FOS = +3	

ZDV = zidovudine; ddI = didanosine; ddC = zalcitabine, formerly dideoxycytidine.
*Foscarnet is contraindicated in patients with seizure disorder or serum creatinine > 2.4 mg/dl.

shown to be effective but toxic, and both require intravenous administration. Recent reports have suggested that foscarnet may have a positive effect on overall survival. Studies of the Ocular Complications of AIDS Research Group (SOCA) demonstrated a longer median survival (12.6 vs. 8.5 months) for patients with CMV retinitis randomly assigned to treatment with foscarnet compared to ganciclovir [64]

(Fig. 24-2). This survival advantage was not explained by the higher percentage of patients on the foscarnet arm who were able to tolerate ZDV. In another study, an AIDS Clinical Trials Group study compared three different doses (60 mg/kg/day, 90 mg/kg/day, and 120 mg/kg/day) for maintenance therapy of CMV retinitis. Subjects randomized to the 120-mg/kg maintenance dose of foscarnet had a significantly longer median survival compared with those given the 90-mg/kg dose (336 vs. 157 days) [68].

Ganciclovir is the drug of choice in patients with a history of seizures, impaired renal function, or cardiomyopathy, and those who require other nephrotoxic agents. Foscarnet should be selected in patients with a low white blood cell count, particularly those who cannot re-

Figure 24-2. Kaplan-Meier curves showing the cumulative probability of mortality among patients assigned to foscarnet or ganciclovir for CMV retinitis. Mortality was significantly higher in the ganciclovir group ($P = .006$ by the log-rank test). The number of patients at risk at each time point are shown at the bottom of the figure. (From Studies of the Ocular Complications of AIDS Research Group, in collaboration with the AIDS Clinical Trials Group. Mortality in patients with the acquired immunodeficiency syndrome treated with either foscarnet or ganciclovir for cytomegalovirus retinitis. *N Engl J Med* 326:213–220, 1992. Reprinted by permission of the New England Journal of Medicine.)

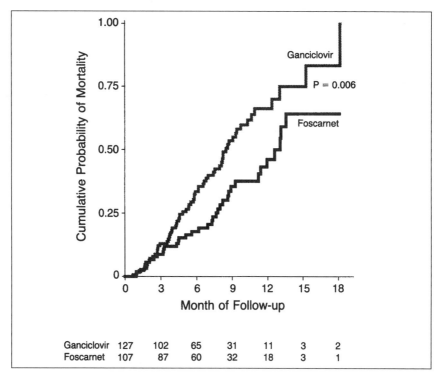

ceive adjunctive colony-stimulating factor therapy; thrombocytopenia; or documented resistance to ganciclovir.

Combination Therapy with Ganciclovir and Foscarnet

Ganciclovir and foscarnet are synergistic against CMV in vitro, and there are reports of both alternating and combination regimens for the treatment of CMV retinitis [69–72]. In general, alternating regimens have been used to reduce drug toxicity, and combinations to manage refractory disease. Dieterich and associates [73] recently reported successful treatment of retinitis unresponsive to ganciclovir or foscarnet alone when the agents were administered concurrently. Of 10 patients who had failed both monotherapies, 9 improved on combination induction therapy at the full dose for each agent.

Future Directions

Ganciclovir and foscarnet are both effective agents for the treatment of CMV infection associated with HIV disease. However, their toxicities are substantial and frequently lead to dose reduction or interruption of therapy. Oral ganciclovir and sustained-release intravitreal ganciclovir implants are among the more exciting areas of active research. In addition, HPMPC, an intravenous anti-CMV nucleotide analogue that is dosed only once every 2 weeks for maintenance therapy, is currently in phase I/II clinical trials with encouraging preliminary results.

Prevention

Preliminary data suggest that oral ganciclovir may have a role in the primary prophylaxis of CMV disease, but additional studies are ongoing [67a]. High-dose oral acyclovir failed as a preventive agent in a double-blind, placebo-controlled trial [74]. Surveillance ophthalmologic examination should be encouraged on a regular basis for HIV-infected patients at risk for CMV disease in order to detect early retinitis.

References

1. Crumpacker CL, Heath-Chiozzi M. Overview of cytomegalovirus infections in HIV-infected patients: Current therapies and future strategies. *J Acquir Immune Defic Syndr* 4(suppl):S1–S5, 1991.
2. Collaborative DHPG Treatment Study Group. Treatment of serious cytomegalovirus infections with 9-(1,3-dihydroxy-2-propoxymethyl)guanine

in patients with AIDS and other immunodeficiencies. *N Engl J Med* 314:801–805, 1986.

3. Walmsley SL, Chew E, Read SE, et al. Treatment of cytomegalovirus retinitis with trisodium phosphonoformate hexahydrate (foscarnet). *J Infect Dis* 157:569–572, 1988.

4. Jacobson MA, O'Donnel JJ, Mills J. Foscarnet treatment of cytomegalovirus retinitis in patients with the acquired immunodeficiency syndrome. *Antimicrob Agents Chemother* 33:736–741, 1989.

5. Ho M. Epidemiology of cytomegalovirus infections. *Rev Infect Dis* 12 (Suppl 7):S701–710, 1990.

6. Drew WL, Mintz L, Miner RC, et al. Prevalence of cytomegalovirus infection in homosexual men. *J Infect Dis* 150:330–333, 1984.

7. Willmott FE. Cytomegalovirus in female patients attending a VD clinic. *Br J Vener Dis* 51:278–280, 1975.

8. Chandler SH, Alexander ER, Holmes KK. Epidemiology of cytomegalovirus infection in a heterogeneous population of pregnant women. *J Infect Dis* 152:249–256, 1985.

9. Webster A, Lee CA, Cook DG, et al. Cytomegalovirus infections and progression towards AIDS in haemophiliacs with human immunodeficiency virus. *Lancet* 2:63–66, 1989.

10. Gallant JE, Moore RD, Richman DD, et al. Incidence and natural history of cytomegalovirus disease in patients with advanced immunodeficiency virus disease treated with zidovudine. *J Infect Dis* 166:1223–1227, 1992.

11. Pertel P, Hirshtick R, Phair J, et al. Risk of developing cytomegalovirus retinitis in persons infected with the human immunodeficiency virus. *Acquir Immune Defic Syndr* 5:1069–1074, 1992.

12. Puy-Montbrun T, Ganasia R, Lemarchand N, et al. Anal ulcerations due to cytomegalovirus in patients with AIDS. Report of six cases. *Dis Colon Rectum* 33:1041–1043, 1990.

13. Wilcox CM, Dielh DL, Cello, JP, et al. Cytomegalovirus esophagitis in patients with AIDS: A clinical, endoscopic, and pathologic correlation. *Ann Intern Med* 113:589–593, 1990.

14. Dieterich DT, Rahmin M. Cytomegalovirus colitis in AIDS: Presentation in 44 patients and review of the literature. *J Acquir Immune Defic Syndr* 4 (suppl 1):S29–S35, 1990.

15. Aaron JS, Wynter CD, Kitron OC, Simko V. Cytomegalovirus associated with acalculous cholecystitis in a patient with acquired immune deficiency syndrome. *Am J Gastroenterol* 83:879–881, 1988.

16. Wilcox CM, Forsmark CE, Grenell JH, et al. Cytomegalovirus-associated acute pancreatic disease in patients with acquired immunodeficiency syndrome. *Gastroenterology* 99:263–267, 1990.

17. Benhamou Y, Caumes E, Gerosa Y, et al. AIDS-related cholangiopathy—critical analysis of prospective series of 26 patients. *Dig Dis Sci* 38:1113–1118, 1993.

18. Eidelberg D, Sotrel A, Vogel H, et al. Progressive polyradiculopathy in acquired immune deficiency syndrome. *Neurology* 36:912–916, 1986.

19. Fuller GN. Cytomegalovirus and the peripheral nervous system in AIDS. *J Acquir Immune Defic Syndr* 5 (suppl):S33–S36, 1992.

20. Jacobson MA, Mills J. Serious cytomegalovirus disease in the acquired immunodeficiency syndrome (AIDS): Clinical findings, 24. Diagnosis and treatment. *Ann Intern Med* 108:585–594, 1988.
21. Drew WL. Cytomegalovirus infection in patients with AIDS. *J Infect Dis* 158:449–546, 1988.
22. Spector SA, Weingeist T, Pollard RB, et al. A randomized, controlled study of intravenous ganciclovir therapy for cytomegalovirus peripheral retinitis in patients with AIDS. *J Infect Dis* 168:557–563, 1993.
23. Goodgame RW. Gastrointestinal cytomegalovirus disease. *Ann Intern Med* 19:924–935, 1993.
24. Cello JP. Acquired immunodeficiency syndrome cholangiopathy: Spectrum of disease. *Am J Med* 86:539–546, 1989.
25. Smith PD, Lane HC, Gill VJ, et al. Intestinal infections in patients with the acquired immunodeficiency syndrome. *Ann Intern Med* 108:328–334, 1988.
26. Laine L, Bonacini M, Sattler F, et al. Cytomegalovirus and *Candida* esophagitis in patients with AIDS. *J Acquir Immune Defic Syndr* 5:605–609, 1992.
27. Rich JD, Crawford JM, Kazanjian SN, et al. Discrete gastrointestinal mass lesions caused by cytomegalovirus in patients with AIDS: Report of three cases and review. *Clin Infect Dis* 15:609–614, 1992.
28. Kram HB, Shoemaker WC. Intestinal perforation due to cytomegalovirus infection in patients with AIDS. *Dis Colon Rectum* 33:1037–1040, 1990.
29. Kotler DP. Cytomegalovirus colitis and wasting. *J Acquir Immune Defic Syndr* 4 (Suppl 1):S29–S35, 1991.
30. Cholestasis and disseminated cytomegalovirus disease in patients with acquired immunodeficiency syndrome. *Am J Med* 84:218–224, 1988.
31. Vieco PT, Rochon L, Lisbona A. Multifocal cytomegalovirus-associated hepatic lesions simulating metastases in AIDS. *Radiology* 176:123–124, 1990.
32. Murray JF, Felton CP, Garay SM et al. Pulmonary complications of the acquired immunodeficiency syndrome: Report of the National Heart, Lung, and Blood Institute workshop. *N Engl J Med* 310:162–168, 1985.
33. Snider W, Simpson D, Nielsen S, et al. Neurologic complications of the acquired immunodeficiency syndrome: Analysis of 50 patients. *Ann Neurol* 14:403–418, 1983.
34. Klatt E, Shibata D. Cytomegalovirus infection in the acquired immunodeficiency syndrome: Clinical and autopsy findings. *Arch Pathol Lab Med* 112:540–543, 1988.
35. Gozlan J, Salord J, Roullet E, et al. Rapid detection of cytomegalovirus DNA in cerebrospinal fluid in AIDS patients with neurologic disorders. *J Infect Dis* 166:1416–1421, 1992.
36. Miller RG, Storey JR, Greco CM. Ganciclovir in the treatment of progressive AIDS-related polyradiculopathy. *Neurology* 40:569–574, 1990.
37. Wolf DG, Spector SA. Diagnosis of human cytomegalovirus central nervous system disease in AIDS patients by DNA amplification from cerebrospinal fluid. *J Infect Dis* 166:1412–1415, 1992.
38. Cinque P, Vago L, Brytting M, et al. Cytomegalovirus infection of the central nervous system in patients with AIDS: Diagnosis by DNA amplification from cerebrospinal fluid. *J Infect Dis* 166:1408–1411, 1992.

39. Pulakhandam U, Dincsoy HP. Cytomegalovirus adrenalitis and adrenal insufficiency in AIDS. *Am J Clin Pathol* 93:651–656, 1990.
40. Bournerias I, Boosnic S, Patey O, et al. Unusual cutaneous cytomegalovirus involvement in patients with acquired immunodeficiency syndrome. *Arch Dermatol* 125:1243–1246, 1989.
41. Nathan PE, Arusra EL, Zappi M. Pericarditis with tamponade due to cytomegalovirus in the acquired immunodeficiency syndrome. *Chest* 99:765–766, 1991.
42. Peterson P, Stahl-Bayliss CM. Cytomegalovirus thrombophlebitis after successful DHPG therapy. *Ann Intern Med* 106:632–633, 1987.
43. Benson MC, Kaplan MS, O'Toole K, Romagnoli M. A report of cytomegalovirus cystitis and review of the genitourinary manifestations of the acquired immunodeficiency syndrome. *J Urol* 140:153–154, 1988.
44. Zurlo JJ, O'Neill D, Polis M. Lack of clinical utility of cytomegalovirus blood and urine cultures in patients with HIV infection. *Ann Intern Med* 118:12–17, 1993.
45. Tocci MJ, Livelli TJ, Perry HC, et al. Effects of nucleoside analogue 2'-nor-2'-deoxyquanosine on human cytomegalovirus replication. *Antimicrob Agents Chemother* 25:247–252, 1984.
46. Crumpacker CS. Mechanism of action of foscarnet against viral polymerase. *Am J Med* 92 (suppl 2A):3S-7S, 1992.
47. Stanat SC, Reardon JE, Erice A, et al. Ganciclovir resistant CMV clinical isolates mode of resistance to ganciclovir. *Antimicrob Agents Chemother* 35:2191–2197, 1991.
48. Sandstrom EG, Kaplan JC, Byington RE, Hirsch MS. Inhibition of human T-cell lymphotropic virus type III in vitro by phosphonoformate. *Lancet* 1(8444):1480-1482, 1985.
49. Jabs DA, Newman C, DeBustros S. Treatment of cytomegalovirus retinitis with ganciclovir. *Ophthalmology.* 94:815–823, 1987.
50. Laskin OL, Stahl-Baylis CM, Kalman CM, et al. Use of ganciclovir to treat serious cytomegalovirus infections in patients with AIDS. *J Infect Dis* 155:323–327, 1987.
51. Katlama C, Dohin E, Caumes E, et al. Foscarnet induction therapy for cytomegalovirus retinitis in AIDS: Comparison of twice daily and three-times-daily regimens. *J Acquir Immune Defic Syndr* 5 (suppl):S18–S24, 1992.
52. Dieterich DT, Kotler DP, Busch DF et al. Ganciclovir treatment of cytomegalovirus colitis in AIDS: A randomized, double-blind, placebo controlled multicenter study. *J Infect Dis* 67:278–282, 1993.
53. Dieterich DT, Poles MA, Dicker M, et al. Foscarnet treatment of cytomegalovirus gastrointestinal infections in acquired immunodeficiency syndrome patients who have failed ganciclovir induction. *Am J Gastroenterol* 88:542–548, 1993.
54. Nelson MR, Connolly GM, Hawkins DA, et al. Foscarnet in the treatment of cytomegalovirus infection of the esophagus and colon in patients with acquired immune deficiency syndrome. *Am J Gastroenterol* 86:876–881, 1991.
55. Emanuel D, Cunningham L, Jules-Elysee K, et al. Cytomegalovirus pneumonia after bone marrow transplantation successfully treated with the

combination of ganciclovir and high-dose intravenous immune globulin. *Ann Intern Med* 109:777–782, 1988.

56. Reed E, Bowden R, Dnadliker P, et al. Treatment of cytomegalovirus pneumonia with ganciclovir and intravenous cytomegalovirus immuno-globulin in patients with bone marrow transplants. *Ann Intern Med* 109:783–788, 1988.

57. Graveleau P, Perol R, Chapman A. Regression of cauda equina syndrome in AIDS patients being treated with ganciclovir. *Lancet* 1:511–512, 1989.

58. Fuller GN, Gill SK, Gulioff RJ, et al. Ganciclovir for lumbosacral polyradiculopathy in AIDS. *Lancet* 1:48–49, 1990.

59. Kim VS, Hollander H. Polyradiculopathy due to cytomegalovirus: Report of two cases in which improvement occurred after prolonged therapy and review of the literature. *Clin Infect Dis* 17:32–37, 1993.

60. Jacobson MA, Mills J, Rush J, et al. Failure of antiviral therapy for acquired immunodeficiency syndrome related cytomegalovirus myelitis. *Arch Neurol* 45:1090–1092, 1988.

61. Enting R, deGans J, Reiss P, et al. Ganciclovir/foscarnet for cytomegalovirus meningoencephalitis in AIDS. *Lancet* 340:559–560, 1992.

62. Hardy DW. Combined ganciclovir and recombinant human granulocyte-macrophage colony-stimulating factor in the treatment of cytomegalovirus retinitis in AIDS patients. *J Acquir Immune Defic Syndr* 4 (suppl):S22–S28, 1991.

63. Miles SA, Mitsuyasu RT, Moreno J, et al. Combined therapy with recombinant granulocyte-stimulating factor and erythropoietin decreases hematologic toxicity from zidovudine. *Blood* 77:2109–2117, 1991.

64. Studies of the Ocular Complications of AIDS Research Group, in collaboration with the AIDS Clinical Trials Group. Mortality in patients with the acquired immunodeficiency syndrome treated with either foscarnet or ganciclovir for cytomegalovirus retinitis. *N Engl J Med* 326:213–220, 1992.

65. Henry K, Cantrill H, Fletcher C, et al. Use of intravitreal ganciclovir (dihydroxypropoxymethyl guanine) for cytomegalovirus retinitis in patients with AIDS. *Am J Ophthalmol* 103:17–23, 1987.

66. Sanborn GE, Anand R, Torti RE, et al. Sustained-release ganciclovir therapy for treatment of cytomegalovirus retinitis. *Arch Ophthalmol* 110:188–195, 1992.

67. Crumpacker C and the Collaborative Oral Ganciclovir Study Group. Oral vs intravenous ganciclovir as maintenance treatment of newly diagnosed CMV retinitis (abstract). Presented at the First National Conference on Human Retroviruses and Related Infections, Washington, DC, 1993.

67a. Second Annual National Conference on Human Retroviruses and Related Infections. Washington, DC, January 1995.

68. Jacobson M, Causey D, Polsky B, et al. A dose-ranging study of daily maintenance intravenous foscarnet therapy for cytomegalovirus retinitis in AIDS. *J Infect Dis* 168:444–448, 1993.

69. Manischewitz JF, Quinnan GV, Lane C, et al. Synergistic effects of ganciclovir and foscarnet on cytomegalovirus replication in vitro. *Antimicrob Agents Chemother* 34:373–375, 1990.

70. Peters M, Bagmann F, Grunewald T, et al. Safety and efficacy of combined and alternating ganciclovir and foscarnet in acute and maintenance

therapy for CMV infection in HIV positive patients. Eighth International Conference on AIDS. Amsterdam, July 1992.

71. Stoehr A, Plettenberg A, Wassmuth R, et al. Combination induction therapy for CMV-disease in AIDS-patients with half dose foscarnet and ganciclovir. Ninth International Conference on AIDS. Berlin, June 1993.

72. Jacobson MA, et al. Randomized phase I trial of two different combination foscarnet and ganciclovir chronic maintenance therapy regimens for AIDS patients with cytomegalovirus retinitis: ARTG protocol 151. *J Infect Dis* 170:189–195, 1994.

73. Dieterich DT, Poles MA, Lew EA, et al. Concurrent use of ganciclovir and foscarnet to treat cytomegalovirus infection in AIDS patients. *J Infect Dis* 167:1184–1188, 1993.

74. Youle MS, et al. Effects of high-dose oral acyclovir on herpesvirus disease and survival in patients with advanced HIV disease. A double-blind, placebo-controlled study. *AIDS* 5:641–650, 1994.

Herpes Simplex and Varicella-Zoster Virus Infections

25

Carol A. Sulis

Primary or recurrent infection with herpes simplex virus (HSV) and varicella-zoster virus (VZV) is common in HIV disease. Illness is often more severe, more invasive, and of longer duration than in the immunocompetent host. Both viruses cause painful mucocutaneous lesions and may disseminate, with significant visceral involvement [1–3].

Herpes Simplex Virus

Epidemiology

Herpes simplex virus is ubiquitous. Primary infection occurs 2 to 12 days after the introduction of infectious secretions into the oral cavity (HSV-1), genital area (HSV-2), skin, or eye. Thirty to fifty percent of adults have antibody to HSV, with a higher prevalence in certain populations, including male homosexuals, urbanites, and those from developing countries. Anal or perianal HSV-2 infection, with autoinoculation to thigh and hand, is especially common among male homosexuals. Up to 90 percent of women who are seropositive for HSV-2 deny a history of genital herpes. Twenty-five percent of women presenting with what they describe as their first episode of genital HSV infection have serologic evidence of prior exposure [4–6]. Recurrent HSV infection, usually due to reactivation of latent virus, occurs with variable frequency and severity. Rarely, recurrence is the result of exogenous reinfection. Several studies noted an association between genital HSV infection and acquisition of HIV [6–10]. Others clarified the mechanisms by which acute and reactivated HSV infection induces HIV expression, modifying and potentially accelerating the course of disease [11–13].

Pathogenesis

Herpes simplex virus replicates in, then lyses, epithelial cells. The characteristic thin-walled vesicle on an erythematous base is the result of a local inflammatory response. Histologic examination reveals multinucleated giant cells, marked edema, and Cowdry type A intranuclear inclusions. As nerve endings become infected, the virus is transported intraaxonally to ganglia, where it remains latent. In the normal host, infection is contained locally by cell-mediated immunity, with only a minor contribution from neutralizing antibody [14, 15]. With reactivation, the virus moves back along sensory nerves to the skin [16]. In neonates and immunocompromised hosts, viremia and visceral dissemination may ensue.

Clinical Manifestations

Primary Infection
In the normal host, primary HSV-1 infection generally occurs during childhood and is asymptomatic. Some children have gingivostomatitis, characterized by fever, leukocytosis, intensely painful oral lesions, and foul breath. Vesicles begin on the buccal or gingival mucosa or tongue, coalesce, and rupture, leaving ulcers with an erythematous margin and a white-yellow necrotic membrane. The course varies in severity and duration but is generally self-limited, with complete healing within 2 weeks. Differential diagnosis include aphthous stomatitis, Stevens-Johnson syndrome, and herpangina. Adolescents with symptomatic primary HSV-1 infection often have constitutional symptoms, exudative pharyngitis, cervical adenopathy, headache, and leukocytosis. HSV-1 infection of the eye may cause acute, self-limited keratoconjunctivitis or progress to corneal ulceration with scarring. Herpetic "whitlow" is an infection of the skin, usually the finger.

Primary infection with HSV-2 usually occurs during adolescence or adulthood. It is manifested by constitutional symptoms and exquisitely tender vesicular lesions in the genital area. Vesicles ulcerate rapidly and become covered with a grayish-white exudate, requiring several weeks to heal completely. HSV-2 is a common cause of nongonococcal proctitis in sexually active homosexual men. Symptoms of primary perianal/rectal HSV-2 infection include painful ulcers and tenesmus associated with constitutional symptoms. Difficulty in urinating, constipation, sacral paresthesias, radiculopathy, impotence, and neurogenic bladder occur less frequently. In the normal host, disease is usually self-limited [16, 17]. Chronic aggressive perianal HSV infection was among the first opportunistic diseases described with AIDS [18].

Perianal ulcers may occur without true proctitis; lesions coalesce, extend along the gluteal crease resembling a decubitus ulcer or anal fissure, and may become superinfected [19].

Reactivation Infection

Herpes labialis ("cold sore" or "fever blister") is the most common presentation of recurrent HSV-1 infection. Patients describe several hours of burning, tingling, itching, or localized hyperesthesia or pain before eruption of lesions at the mucocutaneous junction of the lip. In the normal host, recurrent HSV-1 rarely involves oral mucosa. Painful vesicles appear, ulcerate, crust within 48 hours, and heal in 8 to 10 days. Recurrent HSV-1 infection in the context of HIV disease manifests more like primary infection [20, 21]. Oral ulcers may progress to frank gingivostomatitis, with extensive tissue destruction and prolonged viral shedding. Orolabial recurrences increase in frequency and severity as immunosuppression worsens. Mucocutaneous HSV infection that persists longer than 4 weeks in an HIV-infected patient fulfills the Centers for Disease Control (CDC) case definition for AIDS [22]. In the normal host, recurrent HSV-2 genital disease is associated with milder systemic symptoms and less extensive local involvement compared to first attacks [16, 17, 23]. HIV-infected patients may have prolonged formation of new, exquisitely painful lesions, continued tissue destruction, and persistent viral shedding (see Plate 9).

Encephalitis is a rare complication of primary or recurrent infection with HSV-1 or HSV-2 [24]. Headache, meningismus, and personality changes may develop gradually, or the onset may be abrupt, with fever, headache, nausea, and rapidly progressive neurologic abnormalities, including altered mental status, cranial nerve deficits, aphasia, and seizures. Rarely, aseptic meningitis complicates primary HSV-2 genital infection.

In the HIV-infected patient, diagnosis of herpetic esophagitis, tracheobronchitis, or pneumonia meets the CDC AIDS case definition [22]. Herpes simplex virus esophagitis is manifested by retrosternal pain and odynophagia; bacterial or fungal superinfection of ulcers may occur [25]. HIV-infected patients do not have an increased frequency of the more unusual syndromes caused by HSV, such as erythema multiforme, hepatitis, monoarticular arthritis, adrenal necrosis, and glomerulonephritis.

Diagnosis

Although the presence of HSV infection is often determined clinically, isolation of virus is required for definitive diagnosis. Optimally, fluid should be cultured from an intact vesicle or the epithelial cells scraped from the base of a freshly unroofed ulcer. Because as many as 15 percent of normal adults shed HSV in oral or genital secretions, a positive culture from these sites may not reflect active disease. Specimens can be stored for a few hours at 4°C but should be inoculated as soon as possible into tissue culture. Cytopathic changes induced by HSV are generally seen within 24 to 48 hours. Tzanck smear of specimens is prepared with Wright's, Gram's, or Papanicolaou's stains. Multinucleated giant cells and intranuclear inclusions, suggestive of HSV infection, can also be seen with VZV. Most commercially available immunoassays are not sufficiently sensitive or specific to be diagnostically useful, and the utility of polymerase chain reaction testing is currently under investigation [26–28].

Esophagitis occurs commonly in the AIDS patient. Neither symptoms nor the finding of cobblestone mucosa on barium swallow study permits differentiation between candidal, viral (HSV, cytomegalovirus), and malignant (Kaposi's sarcoma) esophagitis. Definitive diagnosis requires endoscopic visualization with biopsy and culture [25, 29]. Dendritic corneal ulcers that stain with fluorescein in a patient with keratitis strongly suggest HSV infection but can also be caused by VZV. Herpes simplex virus infection of the skin can be distinguished from VZV by the absence of dermatomal distribution and by culture. Definitive diagnosis of HSV encephalitis requires brain biopsy, as the virus cannot be cultured from cerebrospinal fluid [24, 28, 30–32]. Histopathologic findings seen in the normal host, such as hemorrhagic cortical necrosis and lymphocytic infiltration, may be sparse or absent in the AIDS patient.

Treatment

The antiviral drug acyclovir, a nucleoside analogue, is currently the treatment of choice for HSV infection [2, 6, 23, 33–40]. Acyclovir penetrates virus-infected cells, undergoes monophosphorylation by virus-specific thymidine kinase, and is phosphorylated to an active triphosphate by cellular enzymes. The activated drug selectively inhibits viral DNA polymerase, causing early termination of DNA chain synthesis. Acyclovir distributes into all tissues including the central nervous system. It is cleared by the kidney and has a half-life of 2 to 3 hours; the dose must be adjusted for patients with renal insufficiency. Acyclovir is available in topical, oral, and intravenous preparations. Route, dosage, and duration of therapy depend on the type and severity of HSV infection (Table 25-1).

Topical acyclovir is not effective for recurrent herpes labialis but is occasionally useful in primary genital HSV infection [36, 41]. Oral acyclovir in a dose of 200 to 400 mg five times a day is indicated for mucocutaneous disease associated with HIV infection. Anecdotal reports that larger doses are more effective in this population are currently under investigation [39, 40]. Therapy is continued until all lesions have crusted, usually 7 to 10 days; there are no data available to support longer regimens. Intravenous acyclovir should be used in

Table 25-1 *Treatment of HSV and VZV infections associated with HIV disease*

HSV infection	
Primary or recurrent mucocutaneous disease	Acyclovir, 200–400 mg PO q4h while awake × 7 days[a,b]
Extensive mucocutaneous disease or disseminated infection	Acyclovir, 5 mg/kg IV q8h × 7–14 days
Encephalitis	Acyclovir, 10 mg/kg IV q8h × 14–21 days
Prevention of relapse	Oral acyclovir at reduced dose
Infection with acyclovir-resistant HSV strain	Topical trifluridine 5% or foscarnet,[c] 40 mg/kg IV q8h
VZV infection	
Localized infection (shingles)	Acyclovir, 800 mg PO q4h while awake × 7 days[a]
Disseminated infection (cutaneous or visceral)	Acyclovir, 10 mg/kg IV q8h × 7–14 days
Prevention of relapse	No therapy indicated
Infection with acyclovir-resistant VZV stain	Foscarnet,[c] 40 mg/kg IV q8h

[a]Side effects of acyclovir—frequent: phlebitis (IV preparation); occasional: headache, rash, gastrointestinal intolerance, vertigo, renal dysfunction, bone marrow depression, hepatic dysfunction; rare: encephalopathy.
[b]Dose of acyclovir should be decreased in the presence of renal dysfunction.
[c]See Chap. 24 for additional information.

patients with severe mucocutaneous HSV disease; involvement of viscera, such as brain, eye, or esophagus; or neurologic complications, such as transverse myelitis or atonic bladder. Patients with suspected HSV encephalitis should be treated empirically with intravenous acyclovir; brain biopsy is generally not necessary [28, 31, 32, 42]. Ocular HSV infection is treated with trifluridine. Acyclovir cannot eliminate latent virus from ganglia, and severe, prolonged, and frequent recurrences may occur after discontinuation of therapy [37, 38, 43].

Acyclovir-resistant strains of HSV with thymidine kinase or DNA polymerase mutations are being reported with increasing frequency; viral culture and sensitivity testing should be performed in patients whose symptoms do not improve with standard therapy [44–54]. In most reports, acyclovir-resistant HSV isolates have been sensitive to either foscarnet or vidarabine and may also respond to treatment with HPMPC, an acyclic nucleoside phosphonate analogue [55–57], or topical trifluridine. Foscarnet is a pyrophosphate analogue that directly inhibits DNA polymerase. Side effects are common and include fever, malaise, dizziness, mental status changes, renal insufficiency, alterations in serum calcium, magnesium, and phosphorus levels, anemia, and leukopenia [40, 58]. Rare cases of painful penile ulceration have been reported [58]. Vidarabine, which is activated to a triphosphate by cellular enzymes, also inhibits viral DNA polymerase, but is generally less active than acyclovir against HSV and has numerous side effects. The combined administration of zidovudine and acyclovir for the treatment of HIV infection is currently being evaluated in clinical trials, but there are insufficient data to determine if such therapy is more effective than acyclovir alone for the treatment of HSV [59]. Studies examining systemic beta-interferon, topical 15% idoxuridine in 80% dimethyl sulfoxide (DMSO), topical 3% edoxudine cream, topical alpha-interferon (10^6 IU/gm with 1% nonoxynol-9 in 3.5% methylcellulose), and foscarnet cream for the treatment of HSV infection have been promising [60–63]. Trials evaluating trifluridine as treatment for acyclovir-resistant HSV infection are in progress [64, 65].

Prevention

There is no evidence that primary prophylaxis against HSV is effective in HIV-infected patients. The efficacy of secondary prophylaxis is being evaluated, but it appears that AIDS patients who have frequently recurrent or chronic HSV infection benefit from suppressive acyclovir therapy [23, 39, 40, 66–68]. Recurrence during treatment may represent the development of viral resistance. Patients who are receiving long-term acyclovir therapy should be warned that discontinuation of the drug may be associated with a severe exacerbation of their condition. Condom use is effective in preventing the spread of HSV infection. Health care workers should avoid contact with potentially infectious lesions by wearing gloves or employing barrier precautions, and patients with extensive herpetic lesions should be isolated. No effective vaccine is available for the prevention of HSV infection.

Varicella-Zoster Virus

Herpes zoster (shingles) is a dermatomal cutaneous eruption caused by reactivation of the VZV. This virus remains latent in sensory ganglia after infection with varicella (chickenpox). While chickenpox is generally a mild disease in children, visceral dissemination occurs in one-third of normal adults and develops at an even higher frequency in immunocompromised hosts [70]. Since 90 percent of adults have prior infection with VZV, most HIV-infected patients are not at risk for primary VZV infection [71–73].

Epidemiology

The overall annual incidence of zoster is 3.4 in 1,000, with the highest rates in the elderly and immunosuppressed. Zoster occurs with an increased frequency in patients throughout the spectrum of HIV infection, and recurrences are common [74–81]. Immunosuppression predisposes to systemic and central nervous system dissemination. Zoster does not appear to be an independent predictor of HIV disease progression [75].

Pathogenesis

Studies have clarified the mechanism of viral dissemination during primary varicella infection in normal children, as well as VZV reactivation in adult cancer patients and HIV-infected children [82–86]. Few data are available regarding primary, recurrent, and disseminated VZV infection in adults with HIV disease.

Clinical Manifestations

Shingles occurs when latent VZV is reactivated, travels along the peripheral sensory nerve, and seeds the skin. Most patients have a prodrome of dermatomal pain (sometimes mistaken as visceral in origin), itching, or paresthesias several days before eruption of the characteristic vesicular rash. The rash begins as erythematous macules, and clustered vesicles appear over the next 24 hours (see Plate 10). Lesions dry during the first week and crust during the second week; residual scarring is variable. While zoster may affect any of the cranial nerves, involvement of the first branch of the trigeminal nerve is most common. Acute retinal necrosis may occur as a complication of ophthalmic zoster [87–91]. Facial palsy, with the loss of taste on the anterior two thirds of the tongue, is seen both with otic zoster (Ramsay Hunt syndrome) and C2–3 (cervical collar) zoster. Segmental weakness, sometimes associated with zoster of the extremities or trunk, corresponds to the involved cutaneous dermatome(s).

Zoster may occur recurrently and with more frequent cutaneous and visceral dissemination in HIV-infected patients [70, 77–79, 92–95]. Acyclovir-resistant virus has been isolated from skin lesions in patients with VZV infection who are maintained on chronic oral acyclovir prophylaxis [96–100]. Mild diffuse meningoencephalitis sometimes accompanies acute zoster. A more severe form with delirium and cerebrospinal fluid pleocytosis has been described 3 to 8 days after the onset of chickenpox and 1 to 2 weeks after the onset of zoster [101–103]. Focal VZV encephalitis is a rare complication seen primarily in the immunosuppressed host. It is characterized by cerebral white matter lesions that resemble progressive multifocal leukoencephalopathy. Onset may be months after the cutaneous rash, and definitive diagnosis requires brain biopsy. Myelitis is a late complication of VZV infection that is sometimes seen in the immunosuppressed patient, usually presenting with bladder dysfunction, transient mild asymmetry of reflexes, and lower-extremity weakness or sensory deficits [104]. Cerebral vasculitis has also been described in association with VZV infection [105].

Diagnosis

Clinical diagnosis of zoster is based on the presence of a dermatomal vesicular rash and a positive Tzanck smear. Definitive diagnosis requires direct culture or immunohistochemical stain of biopsied tissue. Serologic tests are not diagnostically helpful. The use of polymerase chain reaction testing is under investigation [87, 100].

Treatment

The main goals of therapy for VZV infection are to abort cutaneous infection and prevent dissemination. Acyclovir is the treatment of choice [33, 106, 107] (see Table 25-1). Small trials evaluated the efficacy of acyclovir in the treatment of primary varicella in normal adults and immunocompromised children, varicella pneumonia in normal adults, and acute zoster [108–113]. Although clinical experience suggests that acyclovir is effective for the treatment of shingles in HIV-infected patients, this has not been demonstrated in a controlled clinical trial.

Standard doses of oral acyclovir do not achieve sufficient serum levels to inhibit VZV in tissue culture. A higher dose (800 mg five times a day) is generally necessary for satisfactory clinical response but may be associated with gastrointestinal toxicity. Acyclovir resistance is a concern, especially in patients treated for an extended period of time [114, 115]. Several uncontrolled studies of patients with cutaneous acyclovir-resistant zoster described healing in response to foscarnet administration [56]. Zoster lesions may become secondarily infected and require antibiotic or antifungal therapy; necrotic lesions sometimes need debridement.

Intravenous acyclovir is recommended for VZV infection that is severe, disseminated, or associated with local complications [116, 117]. Patients treated with intravenous acyclovir have reduced new lesion formation, shorter duration of viral shedding, and a lower incidence of dissemination [118]. The optimal duration of therapy is unknown. The question of whether corticosteroids decrease the incidence of postherpetic neuralgia in the normal host is controversial [119, 120]. HIV-infected patients, because of their relatively young age, appear to have a low frequency of postherpetic neuralgia. In this population, empiric steroid use is generally discouraged because of its potential immunosuppressive effect.

Prevention

There have been no studies on the use of antiviral therapy to prevent primary or recurrent varicella-zoster infection. Varicella-zoster virus is easily spread, and isolation with the use of barrier precautions is strongly recommended to prevent nosocomial transmission, especially on wards with immunocompromised patients [121–123]. Vaccination with live attenuated VZV has been shown to be safe and effective in preventing severe or fatal infection in children with leukemia [124, 125]. However, the vaccine is less immunogenic in adults, and its safety and efficacy in HIV-infected patients are unknown. The CDC recommends that varicella-zoster immune globulin (VZIG) be given to susceptible immunocompromised hosts within 96 hours of exposure to VZV, although its benefit in preventing or modifying infection in this population is uncertain.

References

1. Armstrong D, Gold JWM, Dryjanski J, et al. Treatment of infections in patients with the acquired immunodeficiency syndrome. *Ann Intern Med* 103:738–743, 1985.
2. Drew WL, Buhles W, Erlich KS, et al. Herpes virus infections (cytomegalovirus, herpes simplex virus, varicella zoster virus): How to use gancyclovir (DHPG) and acyclovir. *Infect Dis Clin North Am* 2:495–509, 1988.
3. Quinnan GV, Masur H, Rook AH, et al. Herpes virus infections in the acquired immunodeficiency syndrome. *JAMA* 252:72–77, 1984.
4. Breinig MK, Kingsley LA, Armstrong JA, et al. Epidemiology of genital herpes in Pittsburgh: Serologic, sexual, and racial correlates of apparent and inapparent herpes simplex infections. *J Infect Dis* 162:299–305, 1990.
5. Lafferty WE, Coombs RW, Benedetti J, et al. Recurrences after oral and genital herpes simplex virus infection. *N Engl J Med* 316:1444–1449, 1987.
6. Mertz GJ. Genital herpes simplex virus infections. *Med Clin North Am* 74:1433–1454, 1990.
7. Holmberg SD, Stewart JA, Gerber AR, et al. Prior herpes simplex virus type 2 infection as a risk factor for HIV infection. *JAMA* 259:1048–1050, 1988.
8. Stamm WE, Handsfield HH, Rompalo AM, et al. The association between genital ulcer disease and acquisition of HIV infection in homosexual men. *JAMA* 260:1429–1433, 1988.
9. Kuiken CL, van Griensven GJP, de Vroome EMM, Coutinho RA. Risk factors and changes in sexual behavior in male homosexuals who seroconverted for human immunodeficiency virus antibodies. *Am J Epidemiol* 132:523–530, 1990.
10. Keet IPM, Lee FK, van Griensven GJP, et al. Herpes simplex virus type 2 and other genital ulcerative infections as a risk factor for HIV-1 acquisition. *Genitourin Med* 66:330–333, 1990.
11. Stevens JG. Human herpesviruses: A consideration of the latent state. *Microbiol Rev* 53:318–332, 1989.
12. Laurence J. Molecular interactions among herpesviruses and human immunodeficiency viruses. *J Infect Dis* 162:338–346, 1990.
13. Heng MC, Heng SY, Allen SG. Co-infection and synergy of human immunodeficiency virus-1 and herpes simplex virus-1. *Lancet* 343:255–258, 1994.
14. Kohl S. Role of antibody-dependent cellular cytotoxicity in defense against herpes simplex virus infections. *Rev Infect Dis* 13:108–114, 1991.
15. Mester JC, Glorioso JC, Rouse BT. Protection against zosteriform spread of herpes simplex virus by monoclonal antibodies. *J Infect Dis* 163:263–269, 1991.

16. Corey L, Spear PG. Infections with herpes simplex viruses. *N Engl J Med* 314:686–691, 749–757, 1986.
17. Corey L, Adams HG, Brown ZA, et al. Genital herpes simplex virus infections: Clinical manifestations, course, and complications. *Ann Intern Med* 98:958–972, 1983.
18. Siegal FP, Lopez C, Manner GS, et al. Severe acquired immunodeficiency in male homosexuals manifested by chronic perianal ulcerative herpes simplex lesions. *N Engl J Med* 305:1439–1444, 1981.
19. Goodell SE, Quinn TC, Mkrtichian E, et al. Herpes simplex virus proctitis in homosexual men: Clinical, sigmoidoscopic, and histopathological features. *N Engl J Med* 308:868–871, 1983.
20. Safrin S, Ashley R, Houlihan C, et al. Clinical and serologic features of herpes simplex virus infection in patients with AIDS. *AIDS* 5:1107–1110, 1991.
21. Grossman ME, Stevens AW, Cohen PR. Brief report: Herpetic geometric glossitis. *N Engl J Med* 329:1859–1860, 1993.
22. Centers for Disease Control. Revision of the CDC surveillance case definition for acquired immunodeficiency syndrome. *MMWR* 36 (suppl):1–15, 1987.
23. Mertz GJ. Diagnosis and treatment of genital herpes infections. *Infect Dis Clin North Am* 1:341–366, 1987.
24. Nahmias AJ, Whitley RJ, Visintine AN, et al. Herpes simplex virus type 2 encephalitis: Laboratory evaluations and their diagnostic significance. *J Infect Dis* 146:829–836, 1982.
25. Gould E, Kory WP, Raskin JB, et al. Esophageal biopsy findings in the acquired immunodeficiency syndrome (AIDS): Clinicopathologic correlation in 20 patients. *South Med J* 81:1392–1395, 1988.
26. Ashley R, Cent A, Maggs V, et al. Inability of enzyme immunoassays to discriminate between infections with herpes simplex virus types 1 and 2. *Ann Intern Med* 115:520–526, 1991.
27. Cone RW, Hobson AC, Palmer J, et al. Extended duration of herpes simplex virus in DNA in genital lesions detected by the polymerase chain reaction. *J Infect Dis* 164:757–760, 1991.
28. Guffond T, Dewilde A, Lobert P, et al. Significance and clinical relevance of the detection of herpes simplex virus DNA by the polymerase chain reaction in cerebrospinal fluid from patients with presumed encephalitis. *Clin Infect Dis* 18:744–749, 1994.
29. Bonacini M, Young T, Laine L. The causes of esophageal symptoms in human immunodeficiency virus infection. *Arch Intern Med* 151:1567–1572, 1991.
30. Kahlon J, Chatterjee S, Lakeman FD, et al. Detection of antibodies to herpes simplex virus in the cerebrospinal fluid of patients with herpes simplex encephalitis. *J Infect Dis* 155:38–44, 1987.
31. Soong S, Watson NE, Caddell GR, et al. Use of brain biopsy for diagnostic evaluation of patients with suspected herpes simplex encephalitis: A statistical model and its clinical implications. *J Infect Dis* 163:17–22, 1991.
32. Quintiliani R, Levitz RE. Herpes simplex encephalitis: The case against brain biopsy (letter). *J Infect Dis* 164:426, 1991.

33. Dorsky DI, Crumpacker CS. Drugs five years later: Acyclovir. *Ann Intern Med* 107:859–874, 1987.
34. Stone KM, Whittington WL. Treatment of genital herpes. *Rev Infect Dis* 12 (suppl):S610–S619, 1990.
35. Spruance SL, Stewart JCB, Rowe NH, et al. Treatment of recurrent herpes simplex labialis with oral acyclovir. *J Infect Dis* 161:185–190, 1990.
36. Whitley RJ, Levin M, Barton N, et al. Infections caused by herpes simplex virus in the immunocompromised host: Natural history and topical acyclovir therapy. *J Infect Dis* 150:323–329, 1984.
37. Nusinoff-Lehrman S, Douglas JM, Corey L, et al. Recurrent genital herpes and suppressive oral acyclovir therapy: Relation between clinical outcome and in-vitro sensitivity. *Ann Intern Med* 104:786–790, 1986.
38. Thin RN. Management of genital herpes simplex infections. *Am J Med* 85(2A):3–6, 1988.
39. Shepp DH, Newton BA, Dandliker PS, et al. Oral acyclovir therapy for mucocutaneous herpes simplex virus infections in immunocompromised marrow transplant recipients. *Ann Intern Med* 102:783–785, 1985.
40. Straus SE, Seidlin M, Takiff H, et al. Oral acyclovir to suppress recurring herpes simplex virus infections in immunodeficient patients. *Ann Intern Med* 100:522–524, 1984.
41. Spruance SL, Freeman DJ, Stewart JCB, et al. The natural history of ultraviolet radiation–induced herpes simplex labialis and response to therapy with peroral and topical formulations of acyclovir. *J Infect Dis* 163:728–734, 1991.
42. Whitley RJ, Alford CA, Hirsch MS, et al. Vidarabine versus acyclovir therapy in herpes simplex encephalitis. *N Engl J Med* 314:144–149, 1986.
43. Fife KH, Crumpacker CS, Mertz GJ, et al. Recurrence and resistance patterns of herpes simplex virus following cessation of ≥6 years of chronic suppression with acyclovir. *J Infect Dis* 169:1338–1341, 1994.
44. Sacks SL, Wanklin RJ, Reece DE, et al. Progressive esophagitis from acyclovir-resistant herpes simplex: Clinical roles for DNA polymerase mutants and viral heterogeneity? *Ann Intern Med* 111:893–899, 1989.
45. Birch CJ, Tachedjian G, Doherty RR, et al. Altered sensitivity to antiviral drugs of herpes simplex virus isolates from a patient with acquired immunodeficiency syndrome. *J Infect Dis* 162:731–734, 1990.
46. Ljungman P, Ellis MN, Hackman RC, et al. Acyclovir-resistant herpes simplex virus causing pneumonia after marrow transplantation. *J Infect Dis* 162:244–248, 1990.
47. Gateley A, Gander RM, Johnson PC, et al. Herpes simplex virus type 2 meningoencephalitis resistant to acyclovir in a patient with AIDS. *J Infect Dis* 161:711–715, 1990.
48. Englund JA, Zimmerman ME, Swierkosz EM, et al. Herpes simplex virus resistant to acyclovir: A study in a tertiary care center. *Ann Intern Med* 112:416–422, 1990.
49. Chatis PA, Miller CH, Schrager LE, Crumpacker CS. Successful treatment with foscarnet of an acyclovir-resistant mucocutaneous infection with herpes simplex virus in a patient with acquired immunodeficiency syndrome. *N Engl J Med* 320:297–300, 1989.

50. Erlich KS, Mills J, Chatis P, et al. Acyclovir-resistant herpes simplex virus infections in patients with the acquired immunodeficiency syndrome. *N Engl J Med* 320:293–296, 1989.

51. Safrin S, Assaykeen T, Follansbee S, Mills J. Foscarnet therapy for acyclovir-resistant mucocutaneous herpes simplex virus infection in 26 AIDS patients: Preliminary data. *J Infect Dis* 161:1078–1084, 1990.

52. Safrin S, Crumpacker C, Chatis P, et al. A controlled trial comparing foscarnet with vidarabine for acyclovir-resistant mucocutaneous herpes simplex in the acquired immunodeficiency syndrome. *N Engl J Med* 325:551–555, 1991.

53. Kost RG, Hill EL, Tigges M, Straus SE. Brief report: Recurrent acyclovir-resistant genital herpes in an immunocompetent patient. *N Engl J Med* 329:1777–1782, 1993.

54. Safrin S, Elbeik T, Mills J. A rapid screen test for in vitro susceptibility of clinical herpes simplex virus isolates. *J Infect Dis* 169:879–882, 1994.

55. Safrin S, Kemmerly S, Plotkin B, et al. Foscarnet-resistant herpes simplex virus infection in patients with AIDS. *J Infect Dis* 169:193–196, 1994.

56. Balfour HH, et al. Management of acyclovir-resistant herpes simplex and varicella-zoster virus infections. *J Acquir Immune Defic Syndr* 7:254–260, 1994.

57. Lalezari JP, Drew WL, Glutzer E, et al. Treatment with intravenous (S)-1-[3-hydroxy-2-(phosphonylmethoxy)propyl]-cytosine of acyclovir-resistant mucocutaneous infection with herpes simplex virus in a patient with AIDS. *J Infect Dis* 170:570–572, 1994.

58. Gross AS, Dretler RH. Foscarnet-induced penile ulcer in an uncircumcised patient with AIDS (letter). *Clin Infect Dis* 17:1076–1077, 1993.

59. Cooper DA, Pedersen C, Aiuti F, et al. The efficacy and safety of zidovudine with or without acyclovir in the treatment of patients with AIDS-related complex. *AIDS* 5:933–943, 1991.

60. Spruance SL, Stewart JCB, Freeman DJ, et al. Early application of topical 15% idoxuridine in dimethyl sulfoxide shortens the course of herpes simplex labialis: A multicenter placebo-controlled trial. *J Infect Dis* 161:191–197, 1990.

61. Sacks SL, Tyrrell LD, Lawee D, et al. Randomized, double-blind, placebo-controlled, clinic initiated Canadian multicenter trial of topical edoxudine 3% cream in the treatment of recurrent genital herpes. *J Infect Dis* 164:665–672, 1991.

62. Sacks SL, Varner TL, Davies KS, et al. Randomized, double-blind, placebo-controlled, patient initiated study of topical high- and low-dose interferon-alpha with nonoxynol-9 in the treatment of recurrent genital herpes. *J Infect Dis* 161:692–698, 1990.

63. Sacks SL, Portnoy J, Lawee D, et al. Clinical course of recurrent genital herpes and treatment with foscarnet cream: Results of a Canadian multicenter trial. *J Infect Dis* 155:178–186, 1987.

64. Snoeck R, Andrei G, De Clercq E, et al. A new topical treatment for resistant herpes simplex infections (letter). *N Engl J Med* 329:968–969, 1993.

65. Kessler IA, et al. Treatment of acyclovir-resistant mucocutaneous herpes simplex virus infection in patients with AIDS: Open label pilot study of

topical trifluridine (abstract). Eighth International Conference on AIDS, Amsterdam, July 1992.

66. Kaplowitz LG, Baker D, Gelb L, et al. Prolonged continuous acyclovir treatment of normal adults with frequently recurring genital herpes simplex virus infection. *JAMA* 265:747–751, 1991.

67. Klein RS. Prophylaxis of opportunistic infections in individuals infected with HIV. *AIDS* 3 (suppl 1):S161–S173, 1989.

68. Gold D, Corey L. Acyclovir prophylaxis for herpes simplex virus infection. *Antimicrob Agents Chemother* 31:361–367, 1987.

69. Mertz GJ, Ashley R, Burke RL, et al. Double-blind, placebo-controlled trial of a herpes simplex virus type 2 glycoprotein vaccine in persons at high risk for genital herpes infection. *J Infect Dis* 161:653–660, 1990.

70. Cohen PR, Beltrani VP, Grossman ME. Disseminated herpes zoster in patients with human immunodeficiency virus infection. *Am J Med* 84:1076–1080, 1988.

71. Dolin R, Reichman RC, Mazur MH, et al. Herpes zoster and varicella infections in immunosuppressed patients. *Ann Intern Med* 89:375–388, 1978.

72. Straus SE (moderator). Varicella-zoster virus infection: Biology, natural history, treatment, and prevention. *Ann Intern Med* 108:221–237, 1988.

73. Weller TH. Varicella and herpes zoster: Changing concepts of the natural history, control, and importance of a not-so-benign virus. *N Engl J Med* 309:1362–1368, 1434–1440, 1983.

74. Buchbinder SP, Katz MH, Hessol NA, et al. Herpes zoster and human immunodeficiency virus infection. *J Infect Dis* 166:1153–1156, 1992.

75. Rogues AM, Dupon M, Ladner J, et al. Herpes zoster and human immunodeficiency virus infection: A cohort study of 101 coinfected patients (letter). *J Infect Dis* 168:245, 1993.

76. Glesby MJ, Moore RD, Chaisson RE, the Zidovudine Epidemiology Study Group. Herpes zoster in patients with advanced human immunodeficiency virus infection treated with zidovudine. *J Infect Dis* 168:1264–1268, 1993.

77. Colebunders R, Mann JM, Francis H, et al. Herpes zoster in African patients: A clinical predictor of human immunodeficiency virus infection. *J Infect Dis* 157:314–318, 1988.

78. Cone LA, Schiffman MA. Herpes zoster and the acquired immunodeficiency syndrome (letter). *Ann Intern Med* 100:462, 1984.

79. Van de Perre P, Bakkers E, Batungwanayo J, et al. Herpes zoster in African patients: An early manifestation of HIV infection. *Scand J Infect Dis* 20:277–282, 1988.

80. Friedman-Kien AE, Lafleur FL, Gendler E, et al. Herpes zoster: A possible early clinical sign for the development of acquired immunodeficiency syndrome in high risk individuals. *J Am Acad Dermatol* 14:1023–1028, 1986.

81. Melbye M, Grossman RJ, Goedert JJ, et al. Risk of AIDS after herpes zoster. *Lancet* 1:728–730, 1987.

82. Asano Y, Itakura N, Kajita Y, et al. Severity of viremia and clinical findings in children with varicella. *J Infect Dis* 161:1095–1098, 1990.

83. Rusthoven JJ, Ahlgren P, Elhakim T, et al. Varicella-zoster infection in adult cancer patients. *Arch Intern Med* 148:1561–1566, 1988.

84. Jura E, Chadwick EG, Josephs SH, et al. Varicella-zoster virus infections

in children infected with human immunodeficiency virus. *Pediatr Infect Dis J* 8:586–590, 1989.

85. Patterson LE, Butler KM, Edwards MS. Clinical herpes zoster shortly following primary varicella in two HIV-infected children. *Clin Pediatr* 28:354, 1989.

86. Koropchak CM, Graham G, Palmer J, et al. Investigation of varicella-zoster virus infection by polymerase chain reaction in the immunocompetent host with acute varicella. *J Infect Dis* 163:1016–1022, 1991.

87. Chess J, Marcus DM. Zoster-related bilateral acute retinal necrosis syndrome as presenting sign in AIDS. *Ann Ophthalmol* 20:431–435, 438, 1988.

88. Sandor E, Croxson TS, Millman A, et al. Herpes zoster ophthalmicus in patients at risk for AIDS (letter). *N Engl J Med* 310:1118–1119, 1984.

89. Sandor E, Croxson TS, Millman A, et al. Herpes zoster ophthalmicus in patients at risk for the acquired immunodeficiency syndrome (AIDS). *Am J Ophthalmol* 101:153–155, 1986.

90. Cole EL, Meisler DM, Calabrese LM, et al. Herpes zoster ophthalmicus and acquired immune deficiency syndrome. *Arch Ophthalmol* 102:1027–1029, 1984.

91. Rousseau F, Perronne C, Raguin G, et al. Necrotizing retinitis and cerebral vasculitis due to varicella-zoster virus in patients infected with the human immunodeficiency virus (letter). *Clin Infect Dis* 17:943–944, 1993.

92. Gilson IH, Barnett JH, Conant MA, et al. Disseminated ecthymatous herpes varicella-zoster virus infection in patients with acquired immunodeficiency syndrome. *J Am Acad Dermatol* 20:637–642, 1989.

93. Gilden DH, Murray RS, Wellish M, et al. Chronic progressive varicella-zoster virus encephalitis in an AIDS patient. *Neurology* 38:1150–1153, 1988.

94. Perronne C, Lazanas M, Leport C, et al. Varicella in patients infected with the human immunodeficiency virus. *Arch Dermatol* 126:1033–1036, 1990.

95. Anderson DR, Schwartz J, Hunter NJ, et al. Varicella hepatitis: A fatal case in a previously healthy, immunocompetent adult. *Arch Intern Med* 154:2101–2106, 1994.

96. Jacobson MA, Berger TG, Fikrig S, et al. Acyclovir-resistant varicella zoster virus infection after chronic oral acyclovir therapy in patients with acquired immunodeficiency syndrome (AIDS). *Ann Intern Med* 112:187–191, 1990.

97. Hoppenjans WB, Bibler MR, Orme RL, Solinger AM. Prolonged cutaneous herpes zoster in acquired immunodeficiency syndrome. *Arch Dermatol* 126:1048–1050, 1990.

98. Disler RS, Dover JS. Chronic localized herpes zoster in the acquired immunodeficiency syndrome. *Arch Dermatol* 126:1105–1106, 1990.

99. Safrin S, Berger TG, Gilson I, et al. Foscarnet therapy in five patients with AIDS and acyclovir-resistant varicella-zoster virus infection. *Ann Intern Med* 115:19–21, 1991.

100. Boivin G, Edelman CK, Pedneault L, et al. Phenotypic and genotypic characterization of acyclovir-resistant varicella-zoster viruses isolated from persons with AIDS. *J Infect Dis* 170:68–75, 1994.

101. Jemsek J, Greenberg SB, Taber L, et al. Herpes zoster–associated encephalitis: Clinicopathologic report of 12 cases and a review of the literature. *Medicine (Baltimore)* 62:81–97, 1983.

102. Rostad SW, Olson K, McDougall J, et al. Transsynaptic spread of varicella zoster virus through the visual system: A mechanism of viral dissemination in the central nervous system. *Hum Pathol* 20:174–179, 1989.
103. Ryder JW, Croen K, Kleinschmidt-De-Masters BK, et al. Progressive encephalitis three months after resolution of cutaneous zoster in a patient with AIDS. *Ann Neurol* 19:182–188, 1986.
104. Gomez-Tortosa E, Gadea I, Gegundez MI, et al. Development of myelopathy before herpes zoster rash in a patient with AIDS. *Clin Infect Dis* 18:810–812, 1994.
105. Verghese A, Sugar AM. Herpes zoster ophthalmicus and granulomatous angiitis: An ill-appreciated cause of stroke. *J Am Geriatr Soc* 34:309–312, 1986.
106. Shepp DH, Dandliker PS, Meyers JD. Treatment of varicella zoster virus infection in severely immunocompromised patients. *N Engl J Med* 314:208–212, 1986.
107. Straus SE. The management of varicella and zoster infections. *Infect Dis Clin North Am* 1:367–383, 1987.
108. Feder HM. Treatment of adult chickenpox with oral acyclovir. *Arch Intern Med* 150:2061–2065, 1990.
109. Nyerges G, Meszner Z, Gyarmati E, Kerpel-Fronius S. Acyclovir prevents dissemination of varicella in immunocompromised children. *J Infect Dis* 157:309–313, 1988.
110. Haake DA, Zakowski PC, Haake DL, Bryson YL. Early treatment with acyclovir for varicella pneumonia in otherwise healthy adults: Retrospective controlled study and review. *Rev Infect Dis* 12:788–798, 1990.
111. Huff JC, Bean B, Balfour HH, et al. Therapy of herpes zoster with oral acyclovir. *Am J Med* 85 (suppl 2A):84–89, 1988.
112. Wood MJ, Ogan PH, McKendrick MW, et al. Efficacy of oral acyclovir treatment of acute herpes zoster. *Am J Med* 85 (suppl 2A):79–84, 1988.
113. McKendrick MW, McGill JI, White JE, et al. Oral acyclovir and herpes zoster. *Br Med J* 293:1529–1532, 1986.
114. Pahwa S, Biron K, Lim W, et al. Continuous varicella-zoster infection associated with acyclovir resistance in a child with AIDS. *JAMA* 260:2879–2882, 1988.
115. Snoeck R, Gerard M, Sadzot-Delvaux C, et al. Meningoradiculoneuritis due to acyclovir-resistant varicella-zoster virus in a patient with AIDS (letter). *J Infect Dis* 168:1330–1331, 1993.
116. Seiff SR, Margolis T, Graham SH, O'Donnell JJ. Use of intravenous acyclovir for treatment of herpes zoster ophthalmicus in patients at risk for AIDS. *Ann Ophthalmol* 20:480–482, 1988.
117. Schulman JA, Peyman GA. Management of viral retinitis. *Ophthalmic Surg* 19:876–884, 1988.
118. Balfour HH, Bean B, Laskin OL, et al. Acyclovir halts progression of herpes zoster in immunocompromised patients. *N Engl J Med* 308:1448–1453, 1983.
119. Gilden DH. Herpes zoster with postherpetic neuralgia—persisting pain and frustration. *N Engl J Med* 330:932–934, 1994.
120. Wood MJ, Johnson RW, McKendrick MW, et al. A randomized trial of acyclovir for 7 days or 21 days with and without prednisolone for treatment of acute herpes zoster. *N Engl J Med* 330:896–900, 1994.

121. Josephson A, Gombert ME. Airborne transmission of nosocomial varicella from localized zoster. *J Infect Dis* 158:238–241, 1988.
122. Sawyer MH, Chamberlin CJ, Wu YN, et al. Detection of varicella-zoster virus DNA in air samples from hospital rooms. *J Infect Dis* 169:91–94, 1994.
123. Connelly BL, Stanberry LR, Bernstein DI. Detection of varicella-zoster virus DNA in nasopharyngeal secretions of immune household contacts of varicella. *J Infect Dis* 168:1253–1255, 1993.
124. Gershon AA, Steinberg SP, National Institute of Allergy and Infectious Diseases Varicella Vaccine Study Group. Live attenuated varicella vaccine: Protection in healthy adults compared with leukemic children. *J Infect Dis* 161:661–666, 1990.
125. Lawrence R, Gershon AA, Holzman R, Steinberg SP, NIAID Varicella Vaccine Collaborative Study Group. The risk of zoster after varicella vaccination in children with leukemia. *N Engl J Med* 318:543–548, 1988.

Candidiasis 26

Carol A. Sulis

Candidiasis, a mucocutaneous infection caused by the fungus *Candida albicans* and other species, commonly occurs in patients with HIV disease.

Epidemiology

Candida species are ubiquitous. In the normal host, the fungi colonize the skin, mucosa, and gastrointestinal tract, and they are probably transmitted from person to person without an environmental reservoir. Colonization at all sites is increased by the use of antibiotic and corticosteroid therapies.

Pathogenesis

Candida attach to tissues using fungal synthetic products such as "adhesin." Infection occurs when the skin or mucosa is disrupted; the adherent *Candida* organisms then invade the superficial epithelium or disseminate hematogenously. In the normal host, polymorphonuclear leukocytes and cellular immune mechanisms limit the extent and severity of infection. Disseminated infection is associated with neutropenia, and an increased incidence of mucocutaneous disease occurs in the context of defective cell-mediated immunity. While HIV-induced suppression of the immune system facilitates candidal infection, there are also data suggesting that candidiasis may induce T- and B-lymphocyte defects that enhance bacterial superinfection [1, 2]. New or unusually virulent candidal strains have not been associated with HIV disease [3, 4].

Clinical Manifestations

Mucocutaneous Infection

Thrush, the most common fungal disease in HIV-infected patients, was described early in the epidemic and is independently predictive of progression to AIDS [5–8]. The likelihood of thrush, which generally develops in patients with CD4 counts less than 500/mm^3, increases as the CD4 count declines [9]. The most frequent manifestation of candidiasis is white patches or "pseudomembranes" on the tongue or oral mucosa (see Plate 1). Removal of this material leaves an erythematous base that may ooze or bleed. Clinical variants include an atrophic form (smooth red patches anywhere in the mouth), *Candida* leukoplakia (firm, adherent white patches that are difficult to remove), and angular cheilitis (erythematous fissures at the corner of the mouth) [10]. Thrush may be asymptomatic or present with pain or a bad taste in the mouth [11]. Oral hairy leukoplakia is distinguished from thrush by its papilliform appearance and location on the lateral aspect of the tongue (see Plate 3).

Candidal esophagitis is a frequent AIDS-defining diagnosis, occurring most often when the CD4 count is below 100/mm^3 [12–18]. Patients may complain of dysphagia, retrosternal pain, and odynophagia. Odynophagia associated with herpes simplex virus or cytomegalovirus esophagitis is generally more severe than with candidiasis [18–20].

Recurrent or chronic vulvovaginal candidiasis is a common early manifestation of HIV infection in women, although it may occur in immunocompetent hosts as well [15, 21, 22]. Occasional cases of cutaneous and gastrointestinal infection with *C. albicans* have also been described with HIV disease, but dissemination is uncommon in the absence of other predisposing factors [23]. Candidal balanitis, cystitis, intertrigo, and paronychia do not appear to occur with increased frequency in the context of HIV infection [22, 24].

Hematogenously Disseminated Candidiasis

Candidal endophthalmitis, meningitis, brain abscess, endocarditis, pneumonia, and infections of the liver and kidney are unusual in HIV-infected patients; other risk factors, such as neutropenia, diabetes mellitus, intravascular lines, and high-dose corticosteroid therapy, are generally present [24–29]. Diagnosis of candidiasis of the trachea, bronchi, or lungs meets the Centers for Disease Control case definition for AIDS, although these conditions are relatively rare [13].

Diagnosis

Mucocutaneous lesions should be scraped, and the specimen suspended in 10% potassium hydroxide (KOH). This preparation, which dissolves squamous cells and leukocytes, is examined microscopically for the presence of hyphae, pseudohyphae, and budding yeast. Neither symptoms nor radiographic appearance of "cobblestone mucosa" on barium swallow study are sufficient to differentiate candidal esophagitis (> 50% of cases) from viral infection or malignancy. Definitive diagnosis of candidal esophagitis requires the demonstration of tissue-invasive mycelia on endoscopic biopsy, although a presumptive diagnosis can be made if odynophagia and thrush are present [13, 18, 19, 30–33]. Disseminated candidal infection may be extremely difficult to document and requires biopsy evidence of tissue invasion or isolation of fungus from a normally sterile body site. Positive blood cultures may reflect a removable intravascular focus of candidal infection, such as a central venous line, or indicate disseminated candidiasis [34, 35]. Skin tests and serologic studies for candidal antibody or antigen show inconsistent results and are not recommended for diagnosis.

Treatment

Superficial mucous membrane infection may respond to topical therapy with nystatin, a polyene antifungal drug that is available in oral suspension, or clotrimazole, an imidazole available in troche form (Table 26-1). Vaginal and cutaneous infections generally resolve with antifungal creams. If mucocutaneous candidal infection fails to improve on topical therapy or if esophagitis is suspected because of the presence of odynophagia, treatment with ketoconazole or fluconazole, which are oral azoles, is indicated. While mycotic "cure" is infrequent with any of these agents, clinical symptoms usually remit with treatment. Resistance to each of the drugs has been described with prolonged use [9].

Ketoconazole is metabolized by the liver [36], and absorption requires an acid pH, with levels greatly diminished in achlorhydric patients and those receiving H_2 blockers or antacids. Ketoconazole has been associated with hepatic necrosis, interference with oral anticoagulants, and inhibition of steroidogenesis [37–40]. Patients receiving ketoconazole or other azole antifungal agents should not be treated concurrently with the antihistamines terfenadine or astemizole because of an increased risk of serious cardiac dysrhythmias [41]. Ketoconazole is embryotoxic in animals and is contraindicated in pregnancy.

Table 26-1 *Treatment of candidiasis associated with HIV disease*

Type of infection	Treatment
Thrush	Nystatin suspension swish and swallow, 5 ml five times/day *or* Clotrimazole troche, 10 mg five times/day
Cutaneous infection	Clotrimazole cream
Vaginitis	Clotrimazole cream or troches
Oral, cutaneous, or vulvovaginal infection, refractory to topical therapy or frequently recurrent	Ketoconazole, 200 mg PO qd *or* Fluconazole, 50–100 mg PO qd
Esophagitis	Ketoconazole, 200–400 mg PO qd *or* Fluconazole, 100–200 mg PO qd
Fungemia or disseminated infection	Amphotericin B, 0.6 mg/kg/day IV

Treatment of mucocutaneous candidal infection with ketoconazole is usually continued for 1 to 2 weeks, although longer regimens are sometimes required. Experience suggests that maintenance therapy is often necessary to prevent recurrence; antimicrobial resistance and the emergence of other fungal pathogens may occur over time [31, 42–44]. In HIV-infected patients with odynophagia, endoscopy is generally reserved for those situations in which the patient fails to respond to empiric antifungal therapy.

Fluconazole is indicated in HIV-infected patients with mucocutaneous candidiasis who do not respond to topical therapy or ketoconazole [18, 45–48]. Clinical trials comparing fluconazole to ketoconazole suggest equal or superior efficacy and fewer side effects for fluconazole with similar relapse rates [49–56]. Most (80%) of the drug is excreted unchanged by the kidney. Common side effects of fluconazole include nausea, vomiting, and mildly increased serum transaminases. A number of important drug interactions have been reported, including increased serum levels of phenobarbital and cyclosporine, and potentiation of warfarin and oral sulfonylureas; a decreased serum level of fluconazole has been noted when the agent is given with rifampin [49]. Because its effect on the fetus is uncertain, the use of fluconazole should be avoided during pregnancy. Itraconazole, which is similar to fluconazole in its high bioavailability, predominant renal excretion, and low toxicity, also appears to be effective therapy for candidal infection.

Disseminated candidiasis requires treatment with intravenous amphotericin B, a polyene antifungal agent. The optimal duration of therapy is unknown, and its use is associated with significant toxicity, including fever, chills, thrombophlebitis, and renal dysfunction. There is no evidence that the addition of flucytosine to amphotericin is beneficial in the treatment of disseminated candidiasis in HIV-infected patients [57].

Prognosis and Prevention

Because *Candida* is a commensal organism, mucocutaneous infection can be expected to recur in the immunocompromised host unless antimicrobial prophylaxis is maintained. Recurrent disease may be the result of failure to eradicate the pathogen or acquisition of new infection; it is more frequent in HIV-infected patients with advanced immunodeficiency [58–61]. While fluconazole appears useful in the prevention of systemic fungal infections, it is not recommended for primary prophylaxis in most patients [61a, 61b]. Data are inadequate to determine the impact of prophylactic therapy on the development of fungal resistance [48, 62–70]. Nosocomial transmission of fungal pathogens is uncommon. Isolating patients with candidal infection is unnecessary; however, health care workers are urged to employ barrier techniques and thorough hand washing to avoid cross-contamination.

References

1. Baldwin GC, et al. Human immunodeficiency virus causes mononuclear phagocyte dysfunction. *Proc Natl Acad Sci USA* 87:3933–3937, 1990.
2. Crislip MA, Edwards JE. Candidiasis. *Infect Dis Clin North Am* 3:103–133, 1989.
3. Whelan WL, Kirsch DR, Kwon-Chung KJ, et al. *Candida albicans* in patients with the acquired immunodeficiency syndrome: Absence of a novel or hypervirulent strain. *J Infect Dis* 162:513–518, 1990.
4. Powderly WG, Robinson K, Keath EJ. Molecular typing of *Candida albicans* isolated from oral lesions of HIV-infected individuals. *AIDS* 6:81–84, 1992.
5. Barone R, Ficarra G, Gaglioti D, et al. Prevalence of oral lesions among HIV-infected intravenous drug abusers and other risk groups. *Oral Surg Oral Med Oral Pathol* 69:169–173, 1990.
6. Gottlieb MS, Schroff R, Schanker HM, et al. *Pneumocystis carinii* pneumonia and mucosal candidiasis in previously healthy homosexual men. *N Engl J Med* 305:1425, 1981.
7. Klein RS, Harris CA, Small CB, et al. Oral candidiasis in high-risk patients as the initial manifestation of the acquired immunodeficiency syndrome. *N Engl J Med* 311:354–358, 1984.
8. Murray HW, Godbold JH, Jurica KB, Roberts RB. Progression to AIDS in patients with lymphadenopathy or AIDS-related complex: Reappraisal of risk and predictive factors. *Am J Med* 86:533–538, 1989.
9. Sangeorzan JA, et al. Epidemiology of oral candidiasis in HIV-infected patients: Colonization, infection, treatment and emergence of fluconazole resistance. *Am J Med* 97:339–346, 1994.

10. Ficarra G, Barone R, Gaglioti D, et al. Oral hairy leukoplakia among HIV-positive intravenous drug abusers: A clinicopathologic and ultrastructural study. *Oral Surg Oral Med Oral Pathol* 65:421–426, 1988.
11. Greenspan JS, Greenspan D, Winkler JR. Diagnosis and management of the oral manifestations of HIV infection and AIDS. *Infect Dis Clin North Am* 2:373–385, 1988.
12. Walsh TJ, Hamilton SR, Belitsos N. Esophageal candidiasis: Managing an increasingly prevalent infection. *Postgrad Med* 84:193–205, 1988.
13. Centers for Disease Control. Revision of the surveillance case definition for acquired immunodeficiency syndrome. *MMWR* 36 (suppl):1–15, 1987.
14. Carpenter CCJ, Mayer KH, Fisher A, et al. Natural history of acquired immunodeficiency syndrome in women in Rhode Island. *Am J Med* 86:771–775, 1989.
15. Imam N, et al. Hierarchical pattern of mucosal candida infections in HIV-seropositive women. *Am J Med* 89:142–146, 1990.
16. Pena JM, Martinez-Lopez MA, Arnalich F, et al. Esophageal candidiasis associated with acute infection due to human immunodeficiency virus: Case report and review. *Rev Infect Dis* 13:872–875, 1991.
17. Scott GB, Hutto C, Makuch RW, et al. Survival in children with perinatally acquired human immunodeficiency type 1 infection. *N Engl J Med* 321:1791–1796, 1989.
18. Laine L, Bonacini M. Esophageal disease in human immunodeficiency virus infection. *Arch Intern Med* 154:1577–1582, 1994.
19. Bonacini M, Young T, Laine L. The causes of esophageal symptoms in human immunodeficiency virus infection. *Arch Intern Med* 151:1567–1572, 1991.
20. Agha FP, Lee HH, Nostrant TT. Herpetic esophagitis: A diagnostic challenge in immunocompromised patients. *Am J Gastroenterol* 81:246–253, 1986.
21. Sobel JD. Vaginal infections in adult women. *Med Clin North Am* 74:1573–1602, 1990.
22. Rhoads JL, Wright DC, Redfield RR, Burke DS. Chronic vaginal candidiasis in women with human immunodeficiency virus infection. *JAMA* 257:3105–3107, 1987.
23. Oriba HA, Lo JS, Bergfeld WF. Disseminated cutaneous fungal infection and AIDS. *Cleve Clin J Med* 57:189–191, 1990.
24. Diamond RD. The growing problem of mycoses in patients infected with the human immunodeficiency virus. *Rev Infect Dis* 13:480–486, 1991.
25. Ehni W, Ellison RT. Spontaneous *Candida albicans* meningitis in a patient with the acquired immune deficiency syndrome (letter). *Am J Med* 83:806–807, 1987.
26. Haron E, Feld R, Tuffnell P, et al. Hepatic candidiasis: An increasing problem in immunocompromised patients. *Am J Med* 83:17–26, 1987.
27. Matthews R, Burnie J, Smith D, et al. Candida and AIDS: Evidence for protective antibody. *Lancet* 2:263–266, 1988.
28. Kirpatrick CH. Host factors in defense against fungal infections. *Am J Med* 77:1–12, 1984.
29. Cohen MS, Isturiz RE, Malech HL, et al. Fungal infection in chronic

granulomatous disease: The importance of the phagocyte in defense against fungi. *Am J Med* 71:59–66, 1981.

30. Tavitian A, Raufman J, Rosenthal LE. Oral candidiasis as a marker for esophageal candidiasis in the acquired immunodeficiency syndrome. *Ann Intern Med* 104:54–55, 1986.

31. Tavitian A, Raufman J, Rosenthal LE, et al. Ketoconazole-resistant candida esophagitis in patients with acquired immunodeficiency syndrome. *Gastroenterology* 90:443–445, 1986.

32. Devita VT, Broder S, Fauci AS, et al. Developmental therapeutics and the acquired immunodeficiency syndrome. *Ann Intern Med* 106:568–581, 1987.

33. Bonacini MB, Laine L, Gal AA, et al. Prospective evaluation of blind brushing of the esophagus for *Candida* esophagitis in patients with human immunodeficiency virus infection. *Am J Gastroenterol* 85:385–389, 1990.

34. Ellis CA, Spivack ML. The significance of candidemia. *Ann Intern Med* 67:511–522, 1967.

35. Rinaldi MG. Problems in the diagnosis of invasive fungal diseases. *Rev Infect Dis* 13:493–495, 1991.

36. Sugar AM, Alsip SG, Galgiani JN, et al. Pharmacology and toxicity of high-dose ketoconazole. *Antimicrob Agents Chemother* 31:1874–1878, 1987.

37. Lewis JH, Zimmerman HJ, Benson GD, Ishak KG. Hepatic injury associated with ketoconazole therapy: Analysis of 33 cases. *Gastroenterology* 86:503–513, 1984.

38. Duarte PA, Chow CC, Simons F, Ruskin J. Fatal hepatitis associated with ketoconazole therapy. *Arch Intern Med* 144:1069–1070, 1984.

39. Sonino N. Drug therapy: The use of ketoconazole as an inhibitor of steroid production. *N Engl J Med* 317:812–818, 1987.

40. Smith AG. Potentiation of oral anticoagulants by ketoconazole. *Br Med J* 288:188–189, 1984.

41. Safety of terfenadine and astemizole. *Med Lett Drugs Ther* 34:9–10, 1992.

42. Sobel JD. Recurrent vulvovaginal candidiasis: A prospective study of the efficacy of maintenance ketoconazole therapy. *N Engl J Med* 315:1455–1458, 1986.

43. Korting HC, Ollert M, Georgii A, Froschel M. *In vitro* susceptibilities and biotypes of *Candida albicans* isolates from the oral cavities of patients infected with human immunodeficiency virus. *J Clin Microbiol* 26:2626–2631, 1988.

44. Powderly WG. Mucosal candidiasis caused by non-albicans species of *Candida* in HIV-positive patients. *AIDS* 6:604–605, 1992.

45. Kauffman CA, Bradley SF, Ross SC, Weber DR. Hepatosplenic candidiasis: Successful treatment with fluconazole. *Am J Med* 91:137–141, 1991.

46. Anaissie E, Bodey GP, Kantarjian H, et al. Fluconazole therapy for chronic disseminated candidiasis in patients with leukemia and prior amphotericin B therapy. *Am J Med* 91:142–150, 1991.

47. DeWit S, Goossens H, Clumeck N. Single-dose versus 7 days of fluconazole treatment for oral candidiasis in human immunodeficiency virus-infected patients: A prospective, randomized pilot study (letter). *J Infect Dis* 168:1332–1333, 1993.

48. Sangeorzan JA, Bradley SF, He X, et al. Epidemiology of oral candidiasis

in HIV-infected patients: Colonization, infection, treatment, and emergence of fluconazole resistance. *Am J Med* 97:339–346, 1994.

49. Larsen RA. Azoles and AIDS. *J Infect Dis* 162:727–730, 1990.

50. DeWit S, Weerts D, Goossens H, Clumeck N. Comparison of fluconazole and ketoconazole for oropharyngeal candidiasis in AIDS. *Lancet* 1:746–748, 1989.

51. Meunier F, Aoun M, Gerard M. Therapy for oropharyngeal candidiasis in the immunocompromised host: A randomized double-blind study of fluconazole versus ketoconazole. *Rev Infect Dis* 12 (suppl 3):S364–S368, 1990.

52. Laine L, Conteas C, DeBruin M, Multicenter Study Group. A prospective, randomized trial of fluconazole versus ketoconazole for candida esophagitis. *Gastroenterology* 98:A458, 1990.

53. Dismukes WE. Azole antifungal drugs: Old and new. *Ann Intern Med* 109:177–179, 1988.

54. Hay RJ. Overview of studies of fluconazole in oropharyngeal candidiasis. *Rev Infect Dis* 12 (suppl 3):S334–S337, 1990.

55. Robinson PA, Knirsch AK, Joseph JA. Fluconazole for life-threatening fungal infections in patients who cannot be treated with conventional antifungal agents. *Rev Infect Dis* 12 (suppl 3):S349–S363, 1990.

56. Laine L, et al. Fluconazole compared with ketoconazole for the treatment of candida esophagitis in AIDS. *Ann Intern Med* 117:655–660, 1992.

57. Como JA, Dismukes WE. Oral azole drugs as systemic antifungal therapy. *N Engl J Med* 330:263–272, 1994.

58. Bruatto M, Vidotto V, Marinuzzi G, et al. *Candida albicans* biotypes in human immunodeficiency virus type 1-infected patients with oral candidiasis before and after antifungal therapy. *J Clin Microbiol* 29:726–730, 1991.

59. Powderly WG, Robinson K, Keath EJ. Molecular epidemiology of recurrent oral candidiasis in human immunodeficiency virus-positive patients: Evidence for two patterns of recurrence. *J Infect Dis* 168:463–466, 1993.

60. Van Belkum A, Melchers W, de Pauw BE, et al. Genotypic characterization of sequential *Candida albicans* isolates from fluconazole-treated neutropenic patients. *J Infect Dis* 169:1062–1070, 1994.

61. Berthold P, Stewart J, Cumming C, et al. Candida organisms in dental plaque from AIDS patients (letter). *J Infect Dis* 170:1053–1054, 1994.

61a. Powderly WG, et al. A randomized trial comparing fluconazole with clotrimazole troches for the prevention of fungal infections in patients with advanced immunodeficiency virus infection. *N Engl J Med* 332:700–705, 1995.

61b. Centers for Disease Control. USPHS/IDSA guidelines for the prevention of opportunistic infections in persons infected with human immunodeficiency virus: A summary. *MMWR* 44(RR-8):1–34, 1995.

62. Samonis G, Rolston K, Karl C, et al. Prophylaxis of oropharyngeal candidiasis with fluconazole. *Rev Infect Dis* 12 (suppl 3):S369–S373, 1990.

63. Klein RS. Prophylaxis of opportunistic infections in individuals infected with HIV. *AIDS* 3 (suppl 1):S161–S173, 1989.

64. Boken DJ, Swindells S, Rinaldi MG. Fluconazole-resistant *Candida albicans*. *Clin Infect Dis* 17:1018–1021, 1993.

65. Redding S, Smith J, Farinacci G, et al. Resistance of *Candida albicans* to

fluconazole during treatment of oropharyngeal candidiasis in a patient with AIDS: Documentation by in vitro susceptibility testing and DNA subtype analysis. *Clin Infect Dis* 18:240–242, 1994.

66. Newman SL, Flanigan TP, Fisher A, et al. Clinically significant mucosal candidiasis resistant to fluconazole treatment in patients with AIDS. *Clin Infect Dis* 19:684–686, 1994.

67. Bailey GG, Perry FM, Denning DW, Mandal BK. Fluconazole-resistant candidosis in an HIV cohort. *AIDS* 8:787–792, 1994.

68. White A, Goetz MB. Azole-resistant *Candida albicans*: Report of two cases of resistance to fluconazole and review. *Clin Infect Dis* 19:687–692, 1994.

69. Pfaller MA, Rhine-Chalberg J, Redding SW, et al. Variations in fluconazole susceptibility and electrophoretic karyotype among oral isolates of *Candida albicans* from patients with AIDS and oral candidiasis. *J Clin Microbiol* 32:59–64, 1994.

70. Chavanet P, Lopez J, Grappin M, et al. Cross-sectional study of the susceptibility of *Candida* isolates to antifungal drugs and in vitro–in vivo correlation in HIV-infected patients. *AIDS* 8:945–950, 1994.

Gastrointestinal Parasites *27*

Thomas L. Treadwell

Nearly all HIV-infected patients experience diarrhea sometime during the course of their disease. Opportunistic infections are the most common cause, and specific pathogens can be identified in more than one-half of AIDS patients with persistent diarrhea [1, 2]. Protozoal and cytomegalovirus (CMV) infections account for most of these cases [3].

Several species of protozoa have been associated with acute and chronic diarrhea in HIV disease (Table 27-1). The coccidians, *Cryptosporidium* species and *Isospora belli*, are sporozoans that are taxonomically related to *Toxoplasma gondii* [4]. The oocysts of both organisms are acid-fast. Cryptosporidia are distinguished from *I. belli* by their small size (5–7 microns) compared to the larger, ovoid *I. belli*, which has two sporoblasts (see Plates 17, 18). The presence of chronic diarrhea related to these pathogens meets the Centers for Disease Control case definition criteria for AIDS [5]. Another acid-fast organism, *Cyclospora* species, which is probably a coccidian, has also recently been identified in AIDS patients with persistent diarrhea [6, 7].

Giardia lamblia and *Entamoeba histolytica* are common causes of intestinal infection in homosexual men with or without HIV disease, although many patients who excrete these organisms are asymptomatic [2]. Several species of the intracellular *Microsporidia* species, including *Enterocytozoon bieneusi* and *Septata intestinalis*, have also been implicated as causes of HIV-related diarrhea and biliary tract disease [8, 9]. In addition, several species of "nonpathogenic" intestinal protozoa, including *Blastocystis hominis* and *Dientamoeba fragilis*, have been associated with diarrhea in patients with AIDS, but convincing evidence of causality is lacking [10].

Finally, the nematode *Strongyloides stercoralis*, a ubiquitous parasite in tropical and subtropical areas, can cause diarrhea and overwhelming infestation (hyperinfection syndrome) in patients with a variety of immunosuppressive disorders, including HIV disease [11].

Table 27-1 *Pathogenic intestinal protozoa in HIV disease*

Cryptosporidium species
Isospora belli
Cyclospora species
Giardia lamblia
Entamoeba histolytica
Microsporidia species
    Enterocytozoon bieneusi
    Septata intestinalis
*Blastocystis hominis**
*Dientamoeba fragilis**

*There is some uncertainty as to whether these organisms cause disease.

Epidemiology

Transmission of intestinal protozoal infection usually results from ingestion of fecally contaminated food or water and is more common in developing areas of the world. For example, the incidence of *I. belli* infection in Haitian patients with AIDS is 15 percent, compared to less than 1 percent in the United States [12].

More than one-half of AIDS patients in Africa develop cryptosporidiosis sometime during the course of their disease [13]. Large outbreaks of cryptosporidial infection have also occurred in North America from contaminated surface drinking water [14]. Person-to-person spread of cryptosporidiosis is well documented [15]. This is presumably the result of infected individuals excreting large numbers of oocysts, which are transmitted via the fecal-oral route. Many mammalian species, especially calves, excrete cryptosporidia and may transmit infection to humans, either directly or through contaminated public water supplies [16].

Sexual transmission of *E. histolytica* and giardiasis occurs frequently among homosexual men, although the prevalence of these disorders appears to have declined in recent years. Other protozoal infections have also been reported to be sexually transmitted [2, 17].

Clinical Manifestations

Cryptosporidium, Isospora, Giardia, and *Microsporidia* species generally infect the proximal portion of the small bowel, although cryptosporidia may also result in colonic disease [18]. Patients typically complain of large-volume, nonbloody, watery diarrhea; individuals with cryptosporidiosis often have voluminous bowel movements associated with severe, crampy abdominal pain [3]. Fever and anorexia are unusual. In general, clinical features of the diarrheal illness do not help to distinguish between these parasites.

Most HIV-infected patients with *E. histolytica* have no gastrointestinal symptoms, perhaps due to the presence of nonpathogenic strains. However, symptomatic colitis has also been described [19]. Patients typically report abdominal cramps and diarrhea containing both blood and mucus. The clinical manifestations of amebiasis and giardiasis in patients with HIV infection do not differ from those seen in seronegative homosexual men [3].

Cryptosporidium, Isospora, and *Microsporidia* species have been implicated in HIV-related biliary tract disease, including sclerosing cholangitis and acalculous cholecystitis [20, 21]. Patients with cholangitis generally present with right upper quadrant pain in the setting of advanced HIV disease. The serum alkaline phosphatase level is increased disproportionately to other liver enzymes, but jaundice is rare. Endoscopic retrograde cholangiopancreatography (ERCP) may be necessary to establish the diagnosis.

Diagnosis

Many infectious agents can cause enterocolitis in patients with HIV disease, and multiple pathogens are often involved [2]. A general diagnostic approach to diarrhea is provided in Chapter 12. The diagnosis of protozoal diarrhea is based on identification of the organism in stool or intestinal biopsy specimen (Table 27-2). Protozoal infections are sometimes not associated with the presence of stool leukocytes, but individuals with *I. belli* infection may have fecal Charcot-Leyden crystals [3].

In patients with diarrhea that does not remit within 48 to 72 hours, stool should be submitted for ova and parasite examination in addition to other recommended studies. The optimum number of stool samples for diagnosis of parasitic infection is unknown, but several may be necessary to detect organisms present in low numbers. Obtaining fresh specimens appears to maximize the diagnostic yield. A variety of stain and concentration methods have been described [22]. The detection of coccidia requires the use of acid-fast stain, and clinicians should alert the laboratory if cryptosporidiosis or isosporiasis is suspected. Special stains are also available to identify microsporidia in stool specimens, and the findings of such studies performed in experienced laboratories correlate well with duodenal biopsy results [23].

If examination of several stool specimens does not yield a diagnosis or if diarrhea persists despite specific treatment of an established cause, use of additional diagnostic modalities, such as duodenal aspiration and endoscopic biopsy, may uncover new pathogens, including CMV

Table 27-2 *Gastrointestinal parasites: diagnostics*

Pathogen	Examination	Stain preparation
Cryptosporidium species	Stool	Modified acid-fast
	Duodenal aspirate or small bowel biopsy	Acid-fast or hematoxylin-eosin
Isospora belli	Same as cryptosporidia	Saline or modified acid-fast
Giardia lamblia	Stool	Iodine or trichome
Entamoeba histolytica	Stool	Saline (direct) or trichome
Microsporidia species	Stool	Chromotrope-based
	Small bowel biopsy	Electron microscopy

and microsporidia [3]. Small bowel biopsy may also demonstrate HIV-related histologic changes and be useful in identifying individuals less likely to benefit from enteral feeding [8]. However, many of the infections identified in small bowel biopsy specimens are not amenable to treatment, and patients with newly identified pathogens are often in the late stages of HIV disease. A recent study found no association between endoscopically demonstrated microsporidiosis and diarrhea in patients with HIV infection, casting doubt on the utility of the procedure [24]. Some authors also question its cost-effectiveness in this setting [25].

Sigmoidoscopic or colonoscopic biopsy should be considered if the physician believes that identifying a specific organism could alter management. Biopsy specimens should be cultured and examined for viral inclusions, acid-fast bacilli, and protozoa. Ulcerative lesions may be directly aspirated and examined for the *E. histolytica* trophozoites. In individuals with chronic watery diarrhea and negative results on stool examination, small bowel biopsy offers the greatest yield for detection of cryptosporidia, isospora, giardia, and microsporidia. Although light microscopy may identify many of these protozoa, electron microscopy is considered necessary for recognition and speciation of microsporidia [18].

Prognosis

In patients with AIDS, both the frequency and severity of diarrheal illness correlate with the degree of immunologic dysfunction [8]. This is particularly true for patients with cryptosporidial infection. Fewer than 2 percent of North American patients have symptomatic cryptosporidiosis as a first manifestation of HIV disease [13]. Chronic infection with this pathogen is typically associated with very low CD4 lymphocyte counts and defective secretory immunity, and mortality is high [26]. HIV-infected patients do not usually succumb to cryptosporidiosis itself but often develop other opportunistic diseases as a result of malnutrition and immunodeficiency.

Management

Since patients with cryptosporidiosis and AIDS often have intractable diarrhea, the cornerstone of management is fluid replacement. Oral administration of fluid and electrolyte solutions, often several liters per day, is essential (see Chap. 12), and patients with severe diarrhea may need intravenous fluid replacement. Dietary modification may also improve symptoms. General recommendations include increasing carbohydrate intake and avoiding caffeine, alcohol, dairy products, and fatty foods. The role of parenteral nutrition is controversial [3]. Antiperistaltic agents, such as loperamide and tincture of opium, may temporarily reduce cramps and diarrheal volume in patients with severe cryptosporidial infection.

Paromomycin, an oral aminoglycoside, has been associated with clinical improvement and decreased oocyst excretion in HIV-infected patients with cryptosporidiosis [27, 28]. Initial reports of successful treatment with spiramycin, a macrolide antibiotic, were followed by a study demonstrating no benefit [29]. Many other drugs have also been tried with limited success. Preliminary reports suggest that azithromycin and bovine colostrum may also be effective, but these observations have yet to be confirmed [3]. The use of subcutaneous octreotide, a somatostatin analogue, has resulted in modest improvement in some HIV-infected patients with refractory diarrhea [30]. However, octreotide is expensive, and individuals with a specific cause of chronic diarrhea such as cryptosporidiosis tend to respond less well than those with no identified pathogen.

Isosporiasis is treated with trimethoprim-sulfamethoxazole. There is no proven therapy for microsporidiosis, although clinical improvement on albendazole and metronidazole has been reported in uncontrolled studies [31]. Patients with *S. intestinalis* infection seem to respond best to albendazole. Treatment options for other gastrointestinal parasites are listed in Table 27-3. Patients treated for cryptosporidiosis and isosporiasis may require lifelong suppressive therapy to prevent relapse [27, 32, 33].

Prevention

HIV-infected persons should avoid contact with human and animal feces and should not drink water directly from lakes or rivers [33a]. Outbreaks of cryptosporidiosis have been linked to municipal water supplies. During such times, boiling water for one minute will eliminate the risk of infection.

Table 27-3 *Gastrointestinal parasites: treatment*

Pathogen	Standard therapy	Alternative
Cryptosporidium species*	Paromomycin, 500–750 mg PO qid × 21 days [27, 28]	Azithromycin
*Isospora belli**	Trimethoprim-sulfamethoxazole DS, PO qid × 20 days [32]	Pyrimethamine
Cyclospora species	None proven	Trimethoprim-sulfamethoxazole
Giardia lamblia	Metronidazole, 250 mg PO tid × 5 days	Quinacrine
Entamoeba histolytica (symptomatic)	Metronidazole, 750 mg PO tid × 10 days followed by iodoquinol 650 mg PO tid × 20 days	
Entamoeba histolytica (asymptomatic)	Iodoquinol, 650 mg PO tid × 20 days	Paromomycin
Microsporidia species	None proven	Albendazole Metronidazole
Blastocystis hominis	None proven	Metronidazole
Dientamoeba fragilis	Iodoquinol	Paromomycin
Strongyloides stercoralis	Thiabendazole, 25 mg/kg PO bid × 5–10 days	

*Patients with these infections may require lifelong therapy to prevent relapse.

Patients with protozoal diarrhea shed large numbers of infective oocysts. Health care workers and household contacts should be instructed in the use of enteric precautions, including hand washing, gloves, and disinfectants (e.g., bleach) for contaminated surfaces. Medical equipment should be routinely autoclaved after use. Most, if not all, of the protozoa discussed can be spread sexually; although unproved, limiting unprotected oral-anal sexual practices may reduce the risk of transmission.

Strongyloidiasis

S. stercoralis is unique among nematodes in two respects: Strongyloides can cause autoinfection and persist in the host for many years, and it has the ability to cause overwhelming infection in immunocompromised hosts [11]. However, despite the prevalence of strongyloidiasis in warmer climates of the world, severe infection in patients with HIV disease is relatively uncommon.

The adult strongyloides nematode resides in the submucosa of the proximal small bowel, where it sheds its eggs. Unlike other human nematodes, the eggs hatch in the intestine, producing rhabditiform larvae. These then pass into the stool and, if exposed to soil, establish a free-living adult life cycle. Some of the larvae transform in the gut into larger invasive filariform organisms. These may penetrate normal perianal skin or mucosa, resulting in persistent infection. In immunocompromised hosts, this transformation may accelerate, resulting in widespread dissemination of filariform larvae and secondary bacterial infections [34].

Strongyloidiasis hyperinfection may be difficult to recognize clinically. Some patients develop mucosal ulcerations throughout the intestinal tract and diarrhea; others present with severe gram-negative infection, such as bacteremia, pneumonia, or meningitis, associated with high mortality [34].

Strongyloidiasis should be suspected in an HIV-infected patient from an endemic area, including the southeastern region of the United States, who presents with serious gram-negative bacillary infection. Eosinophilia is sometimes a clue to the diagnosis. Stool examination for larvae is often negative, because the worm only produces a few eggs per day, but the yield may be increased by examining duodenal aspirates or small bowel biopsy specimens. Demonstration of larvae in extraintestinal specimens, including sputum and bronchial washings, is also diagnostic [35, 36]. Therapy with thiabendazole is effective, but relapses are common.

References

1. Greenson JK, Belitsos PC, Yardley JH, et al. Occult enteric infections and duodenal mucosal alterations in chronic diarrhea. *Ann Intern Med* 114:366–372, 1991.
2. Smith PD, Lane HC, Gill VJ, et al. Intestinal infections in patients with the acquired immunodeficiency syndrome (AIDS). *Ann Intern Med* 108:328–333, 1988.
3. Smith PD, Quinn TC, Strober W, et al. Gastrointestinal infections in AIDS. *Ann Intern Med* 116:63–77, 1992.
4. Navin TR, Juranek DD. Cryptosporidiosis. Clinical, epidemiologic, and parasitologic review. *Rev Infect Dis* 6:313–327, 1984.
5. Centers for Disease Control. Revision of the CDC surveillance case definition for acquired immunodeficiency syndrome. *MMWR* 36 (15):1–15, 1987.
6. Ortega YR, Sterling CR, Gilman RH, et al. Cyclospora species—a new protozoan pathogen of humans. *N Engl J Med* 328:1308–1312, 1993.
7. Pope JW, et al. Cyclospora infection in adults infected with HIV. *Ann Intern Med* 121:654–657, 1994.
8. Kotler DP, Francisco A, Clayton F, et al. Small intestinal injury and parasitic diseases in AIDS. *Ann Intern Med* 113:444–449, 1990.
9. Cali A, Kotler DP, Orenstein JM. *Septata intestinalis*, an intestinal

microsporidian associated with chronic diarrhea and dissemination in AIDS patients. *J Eukaryot Microbiol* 40:101–112, 1993.

10. Rolston KVI, Winans R, Rodriquez S. *Blastocystis hominis*: Pathogen or not? *Rev Infect Dis* 11:661–662, 1989.

11. Maayan S, Wormser GP, Widerhorn J, et al. *Strongyloides stercoralis* hyperinfection in a patient with the acquired immune deficiency syndrome. *Am J Med* 83:945–949, 1987.

12. DeHovitz JA, Pape JW, Boncy M, et al. Clinical manifestations and therapy of *Isospora belli* infection in patients with the acquired immunodeficiency syndrome. *N Engl J Med* 315:87–90, 1986.

13. Soave R, Johnson WD. *Cryptosporidium* and *Isospora belli* infections. *J Infect Dis* 157:225–230, 1988.

14. Hayes EB, Matte TD, O'Brien TR, et al. Large community outbreak of cryptosporidiosis due to contamination of a filtered water supply. *N Engl J Med* 320:1372–1376, 1989.

15. Current WL. *Cryptosporidium parvum*: Household transmission. *Ann Intern Med* 120:518–519, 1994.

16. Jokiph L, Jokiph AMM. Timing of symptoms and oocyst excretion in human cryptosporidiosis. *N Engl J Med* 315:1643–1646, 1986.

17. Phillips SC, Mildvan D, William DC, et al. Sexual transmission of enteric protozoa and helminths in a venereal-disease-clinic population. *N Engl J Med* 305:603–606, 1981.

18. Current WL, Owen RL. Cryptosporidiosis and Microsporidiosis. In MJG Farthing, GT Keusch (eds), *Enteric Infection*. New York: Raven, 1989. Pp 223–249.

19. Quinn TC, Stamm WE, Goodell SE, et al. The polymicrobial origin of intestinal infections in homosexual men. *N Engl J Med* 309:576–582, 1983.

20. Pol S, Romana CA, Richard S, et al. *Microsporidia* infection in patients with human immunodeficiency virus and unexplained cholangitis. *N Engl J Med* 328:95–99, 1993.

21. Benatar DA, et al. *Isospora belli* infection associated with acalculous cholecystitis in a patient with AIDS. *Ann Intern Med* 121:663–664, 1994.

22. Ma P. Cryptosporidiosis and Immune Enteropathy: A Review. In JS Remington, MN Swartz (eds), *Current Clinical Topics in Infectious Diseases* (Vol 8). New York: McGraw-Hill, 1987. Pp 99–153.

23. Weber R, Bryan RT, Owen RL, et al. Improved light-microscopical detection of microsporidia spores in stool and duodenal aspirates. *N Engl J Med* 326:161–166, 1992.

24. Rabeneck L, Gyorkey F, Genta RM, et al. The role of *Microsporidia* and the pathogenesis of HIV-related chronic diarrhea. *Ann Intern Med* 119:895–899, 1993.

25. Rene E, Roze C. Diagnosis and Treatment of Gastrointestinal Infections in AIDS. In DP Kotler (ed), *Gastrointestinal and Nutritional Manifestations of AIDS*. New York: Raven, 1991. Pp 65–91.

26. Flanigan T, Whalen C, Turner J, et al. *Cryptosporidium* infection and CD4 counts. *Ann Intern Med* 116:840–842, 1992.

27. Clinton A, et al. Paromomycin for cryptosporidiosis in AIDS: A prospective, double-blind trial. *J Infect Dis* 170:419–424, 1994.

28. Fichtenbaum CJ, Ritchie DJ, Powderly WG. Use of paromomycin for treat-

ment of cryptosporidiosis in patients with AIDS. *Clin Infect Dis* 16:298–300, 1993.

29. Portnoy D, Whiteside ME, Buckley E, et al. Treatment of intestinal cryptosporidiosis with spiramycin. *Ann Intern Med* 101:202–204, 1984.

30. Cello JP, Grendell JH, Basuk P, et al. Effect of octreotide on refractory AIDS-associated diarrhea. *Ann Intern Med* 115:705–710, 1991.

31. Blanshard C, Ellis DS, Tovey DG, et al. Treatment of intestinal microsporidiosis with albendazole in patients with AIDS. *AIDS* 6:311–313, 1992.

32. Pape JW, Verdier RI, Johnson WD. Treatment and prophylaxis of *Isospora belli* infection in patients with the acquired immunodeficiency syndrome. *N Engl J Med* 320:1044–1047, 1989.

33. Weiss LM, Perlman DC, Sherman J, et al. *Isospora belli* infection: Treatment with pyrimethamine. *Ann Intern Med* 109:474–475, 1988.

33a. Centers for Disease Control. USPHS/IDSA guidelines for the prevention of opportunistic infections in persons infected with human immunodeficiency virus: A summary. *MMWR* 44(RR-8):1–34, 1995.

34. Madico G. Treatment of cyclospora infections with cotrimoxazole. *Lancet* 342:122–123, 1993.

35. Longworth D, Weller P. Hyperinfection Syndrome with Strongyloidiasis. In JS Remington, MN Swartz (eds), *Current Clinical Topics in Infectious Diseases* (Vol 7). New York: McGraw-Hill, 1986. Pp 1–25.

36. Schaimber GL, Scheinberg MA. Recovery of *Strongyloides stercoralis* by bronchoalveolar lavage in a patient with the acquired immunodeficiency syndrome. *Am J Med* 87:486, 1989.

Conventional Bacterial Infections 28

Kathleen Bennett, Robert A. Witzburg

Conventional bacterial infections are frequently associated with HIV disease. Recurrent, complicated, or severe bacterial infections may be the first clinical evidence of immunodeficiency in HIV-seropositive persons [1]. Bacterial infections may require repeated hospitalization, therapy with potentially toxic antimicrobial agents, and occasionally, surgical intervention. Early recognition and treatment of conventional bacterial infections may reduce morbidity and mortality (Table 28-1).

Epidemiology

Rolston and associates [2] reported a rate of 31 bacterial infections per 100 HIV-related hospitalizations. In this series of predominantly homosexual men, 90 percent of the infections were nosocomial in origin. In a study by Witt and colleagues [3] from Boston City Hospital, bacterial infections developed significantly more often in injection drug users (IDUs) than in homosexual men (58 vs. 14%). In an autopsy series, Nichols and coworkers [4] reported that bacterial infections were present in 83 percent of cases with HIV disease, were more common than opportunistic infections, and were the sole or contributing cause of death in 37 percent. Selwyn and colleagues [5] demonstrated similar findings in a prospective cohort study of HIV-infected IDUs enrolled in a methadone treatment program in New York City. In this group bacterial infections occurred earlier in the course of the disease (median CD4 lymphocyte count of $318/mm^3$), appeared to predict disease progression, and accounted for substantial morbidity and mortality.

Revised from MA Fagan, RA Witzburg. Conventional Bacterial Infections. In H Libman, RA Witzburg (eds), *HIV Infection: A Clinical Manual* (2nd ed). Boston: Little, Brown, 1993.

Table 28-1 *Management guidelines for bacterial infection in HIV disease*

1. Recommend HIV antibody testing in patients with bacterial infection who are at risk for HIV disease.
2. Obtain blood cultures in all systemically ill-appearing patients. Attempt to identify the source of bacteremia and choose empiric antibiotic therapy based on the pathogens most likely to cause this type of infection.
3. Choose specific antibiotic therapy on the basis of Gram's stain and culture results of body fluids or biopsy material.
4. Identify and correct reversible causes of neutropenia.
5. Use appropriate immunizations as early as possible in the course of HIV disease.

Staphylococcus aureus is the most frequent bacterial pathogen associated with HIV disease, with *Streptococcus pneumoniae* and *Haemophilus influenzae* common as well. *Pseudomonas aeruginosa* and other nosocomial pathogens may also cause infection in patients with advanced immunodeficiency [6].

Pathogenesis

The pathophysiology of bacterial infections associated with HIV disease involves abnormalities in cell-mediated, humoral, and nonspecific immunity [7–10]. Quantitative and functional deficits in CD4 lymphocytes, with diminished cytokine production and impaired macrophage activity, predispose to infection with *Salmonella* species, *Listeria* species, and mycobacteria. Inadequate production of opsonizing antibodies reduces defense against encapsulated organisms, such as *S. pneumoniae* and *H. influenzae* [9, 10]. Neutrophil dysfunction impairs chemotaxis, phagocytosis, and bacterial killing [11]. Loss of integrity of the mucocutaneous barrier in IDUs and in patients undergoing invasive diagnostic and therapeutic procedures increases the risk of aspiration pneumonia and sinusitis (disruption of the upper respiratory tract) and local and disseminated infection with *S. aureus* (disruption of the skin). Frequent hospitalization and exposure to broad-spectrum antibiotics may increase the risk of infection with nosocomial pathogens.

Clinical Syndromes

Bacterial infections common in HIV disease are listed in Table 28-2.

Bacteremia

In a study of community-acquired infection in AIDS patients, Krumholz and associates [12] reported bacteremia as a complication in 5 percent.

Table 28-2 *Common bacterial infections in HIV disease*

Infection	Pathogens	Treatment*	Prevention
Bacteremia	S. aureus Gram-negative rods	Oxacillin Third-generation cephalosporin, aztreonam, or aminoglycoside	Avoid unnecessary intravascular lines
Pneumonia	S. pneumoniae H. influenzae	Penicillin Ampicillin, third-generation cephalosporin, or aztreonam	Appropriate immunizations
Periodontitis	Oral anaerobes	Debridement, curettage, anti-bacterial mouthwash, antibiotics prn	Good preventive dental care
Sinusitis	S. pneumoniae H. influenzae	Ampicillin or TMP-SMX, decongestant, surgical drainage prn	
Gastroenteritis	Salmonella species; Shigella species Campylobacter species Clostridium difficile	TMP-SMX or quinolone Erythromycin Metronidazole or oral vancomycin	Avoid undercooked meats, raw eggs Avoid unnecessary antibiotics
Skin/soft tissue infections Cellulitis/folliculitis	S. aureus	Dicloxacillin or first-generation cephalosporin	Good skin hygiene
Bacillary angiomatosis	Rochalimaea species	Erythromycin	
Pyomyositis	S. aureus	Oxacillin, surgical drainage	

prn = as needed, TMP-SMX = trimethoprim-sulfamethoxazole.
*Choice of specific antibiotic therapy should be based on sensitivity testing and knowledge of the patient's allergy history.

Among 44 episodes of bacteremia, 10 were secondary to pulmonary infections, 8 were associated with infected intravascular catheters, and 7 resulted from cellulitis. In a series from Boston City Hospital, 34 episodes of bacteremia were described in 16 patients [3]. Of 25 community-acquired bacteremic episodes, the majority were caused by S. aureus, S. pneumoniae, or other streptococci. All S. aureus bacteremias occurred in IDUs, with endocarditis being the most common type of infection. Streptococcal bacteremias were associated with either pneumonia or endocarditis. Recent data indicate that HIV-infected IDUs are also at risk for bacteremia with H. influenzae type b [13].

HIV-infected patients with indwelling venous catheters have an increased rate of bacteremia compared to seronegative individuals [14]. In the clinically stable patient, management of a catheter-associated infection can be attempted initially with antibiotic therapy alone, leaving the device in place. However, if the patient is acutely ill or has persistent fever or bacteremia, removal of the intravascular catheter is necessary.

Neutropenia is common in HIV disease, and neutrophil counts below 500/mm^3 have been associated with an increased risk of bacterial infection [15]. Neutropenic patients are prone to infection with staphylococci, enteric gram-negative pathogens such as P. aeruginosa, and fungi [16, 17]. The optimal management of the febrile neutropenic HIV-infected patient is uncertain, but most clinicians start empiric broad-spectrum antibiotic therapy pending culture results. While the role of colony stimulating factors in the prevention and treatment of conventional bacterial infections associated with neutropenia has not been established, their use may be warranted in neutropenic HIV-infected patients who are ill.

As many as 50 percent of bacteremic patients with HIV disease show no evidence of systemic toxicity [12]. In one study, the median duration of fever before diagnosis in patients with S. aureus bacteremia was 6 days [17]. The case fatality rate for community-acquired bacteremia in HIV-infected patients may be as high as 9 percent, with half of the deaths attributable to inappropriate empiric therapy directed against opportunistic pathogens [12].

Pneumonia

Bacterial pulmonary infections are common and frequently severe in HIV disease [18–21]. Recurrent pneumonia (two or more episodes in 1 year) in an HIV-infected patient has been included in the 1993 expanded surveillance case definition of AIDS [22].

Among hospitalized patients with HIV disease, the frequency of bacterial pneumonia may be as high as 50 percent; in one outpatient methadone program, the incidence of bacterial pneumonia was increased fourfold in HIV-seropositive clients [23]. A multicenter prospective study of HIV-infected patients during an 18-month period revealed that the most frequent pulmonary disorder was bacterial pneumonia, with a predilection for IDUs [24]. A retrospective study of 249 patients with HIV infection admitted to an urban hospital demonstrated that bacterial pneumonia was the most common pulmonary complication requiring hospitalization, occurring in 32 percent of patients [25]. Schuchat and associates [26] found that advanced immunodeficiency was associated with a higher incidence of complications from pneumonia, including bacteremia and empyema, as well as increased mortality.

The most common causes of bacterial pneumonia in HIV-infected patients are *S. pneumoniae* and *H. influenzae* [4, 12, 27]. Other frequent bacterial pathogens include *S. aureus*, *Moraxella catarrhalis*, *Klebsiella pneumoniae*, and *P. aeruginosa*. The clinical presentation, similar to that in persons without HIV infection, includes the abrupt onset of fever, productive cough, and pleuritic chest pain. However, atypical radiologic findings are common [19–21]. In patients with advanced HIV disease, the clinical picture may be further complicated by the coexistence of bacterial and opportunistic infections, particularly *Pneumocystis carinii* pneumonia (PCP) [3].

Evaluation of the patient with suspected bacterial pneumonia includes microscopic examination and culture of sputum, chest radiograph, arterial blood gas analysis, and blood cultures. Diagnosis is made by sputum examination and culture in approximately 75 percent of patients; blood cultures identify the pathogen 20 to 40 percent of the time [19, 20, 28]. The syndrome of fever, purulent sputum, and the presence of localized infiltrate on chest radiograph strongly suggests bacterial pneumonia and additional diagnostic tests are generally of little value [29]. However, a lack of response to standard antibiotic therapy indicates the need for further evaluation. Semiquantitative cultures of bronchoalveolar lavage fluid may be a helpful diagnostic tool in lieu of lung biopsy [30].

Upper Aerodigestive Tract Infections

Gingivitis and periodontitis, the result of infection with anaerobic mouth flora, are common and sometimes severe in HIV-infected patients [30]. Management includes local debridement, curettage, antibacterial mouthwash, and antibiotic therapy as needed. Otitis media and sinusitis occur in up to 40 percent of patients with HIV disease and are the presenting illness in 10 percent [31–33]. As in lower respiratory tract infections, the predominant pathogens are *S. pneumoniae* and *H. influenzae*, but *S. aureus*, anaerobes, enteric gram-negative organisms, mycobacteria, and fungi may also play a role [32, 33]. Symptoms of sinusitis often include fever, facial discomfort, headache, and nasal discharge, but may be nonspecific or absent. If necessary, clinical diagnosis can be confirmed with plain radiography; computed tomographic and magnetic resonance imaging scans are useful for identifying posterior sinus involvement. Treatment consists of antibiotic therapy and decongestants. Relapsing or chronic disease is common, often necessitating surgical intervention.

Gastrointestinal Tract and Pelvic Infections

The gastrointestinal (GI) tract is an occasional site of bacterial infection in HIV disease. Dryden and Shanson [34] reviewed causes of diarrhea in 179 HIV-seropositive patients and found nontyphoidal *Salmonella* species in 5, *Campylobacter* species in 4, and *Shigella* species in 1. In a prospective study of 132 AIDS patients with intestinal infection, René and associates [35] reported stool cultures that were positive for *Salmonella* species in 6 patients, *Shigella* species in 1, and *Yersinia* species in 1. Advanced HIV disease does not appear to be a predictor of bacterial diarrhea, but homosexual behavior may increase the risk [35, 36]. In the United States, residence in the Northeast, minority status, and injection drug use predispose to salmonellosis [37].

Invasive bacterial pathogens of the GI tract, including *Salmonella*, *Shigella*, and *Campylobacter* species, may cause severe or prolonged illness in patients with HIV disease. The incidence of salmonellosis is increased 20- to 100-fold in HIV-infected patients [37, 38]. The condition most often presents with fever and constitutional symptoms. Gastrointestinal complaints may be entirely absent, and blood and stool cultures typically grow a nontyphoidal strain of the organism, such as *Salmonella typhimurium* or *Salmonella enteritidis* [37, 39]. The source of bacteremia, which is present in up to 50 percent of patients, is frequently not identified [37, 39–41].

Management of *Salmonella* infection, especially recurrent bacteremia, may be problematic. Initial treatment, based on drug sensitivity testing, consists of a 3-week course of trimethoprim-sulfamethoxazole (TMP-SMX), a third-generation cephalosporin, or a quinolone. However, as many as 50 percent of patients relapse after completion of this regimen, and chronic antibiotic therapy is generally recommended.

Shigella infection usually manifests as fever, abdominal pain and tenderness, and bloody diarrhea, with symptoms slowly escalating for weeks before presentation [42–45]. Identification of the organism may require multiple stool cultures. Shigellemia, rare in the immunocompetent host, is not unusual in HIV-infected patients [44, 45]. A 10- to 14-day course of TMP-SMX or a quinolone, based on sensitivity testing results, is usually adequate to eradicate the organism. Although relapsing infection has been described, it generally responds to retreatment; maintenance therapy is not often necessary [43, 45].

Campylobacter gastroenteritis occurs more frequently in the presence of HIV infection, with the annual incidence reported as high as 519 per 100,000 AIDS patients [46]. Clinical features include fever, diarrhea, and weight loss [47, 48]. Although many cases are self-limited, erythromycin is indicated for treatment of protracted or severe disease. Treatment failure and early relapse secondary to erythromycin resistance have been reported [47, 48]. Lack of clinical response within the first week of treatment or early relapse should prompt a change in therapy to tetracycline or a quinolone.

Clostridium difficile enterocolitis, which may follow the use of any antibiotic agent, appears to occur more often in association with HIV disease [49]. Clindamycin, ampicillin, and cephalosporins are the most common precipitants. Management consists of discontinuation of the antibiotic and administration of metronidazole or oral vancomycin. Relapses may occur after completion of the standard course of therapy.

The increasing number of women with HIV infection has led to an appreciation of gynecologic abnormalities specific to this population. Studies have suggested that pelvic inflammatory disease and tuboovarian abscess occur with greater frequency in women with HIV infection and are more likely to be refractory to therapy [50]. Therapeutic modalities are the same as those for seronegative women; however, more aggressive treatment may be required to effect a clinical response.

Skin and Soft Tissue Infections

Bacterial infections of the skin are a source of considerable morbidity in HIV-infected patients. *S. aureus*, the most common pathogen, has been implicated in cellulitis, ecthyma, bullous impetigo, hidradenitis suppurativa, folliculitis, subcutaneous abscess, and the syndrome of generalized pruritus [51, 52].

Folliculitis presents as multiple, small, erythematous papules and pustules involving the face, trunk, or groin. Staphylococci can be identified by Gram's stain of pus. The condition generally responds to treatment with an oral antistaphylococcal penicillin or cephalosporin; the addition of rifampin may be helpful in refractory cases. Staphylococcal skin infection may occur as a primary event or as a superinfection complicating other dermatologic disorders. In advanced HIV disease, even relatively minor breaks in skin integrity may result in local infection and bacteremia.

Staphylococcal pyomyositis occurs in approximately 1 in 10,000 patients with HIV infection, generally at an advanced stage [53]. This condition presents with fever and localized soft tissue swelling, with the large muscles of the leg most commonly involved. Management consists of surgical drainage and parenteral antibiotic therapy. Relapsing disease has been described.

Bacillary angiomatosis, a newly recognized infectious disorder, involves the skin and viscera [54–57]. The condition most often presents with painless, plaque-like skin lesions that may resemble Kaposi's sarcoma. Visceral involvement manifests as fever, abdominal pain, and progressive hepatic failure. Warthin-Starry staining of biopsy specimens shows bacilli similar to those seen in cat-scratch fever, and DNA studies indicate that the pathogen is a *Rochalimaea* species [56, 57]. Diagnosis of bacillary angiomatosis is based on the clinical presentation and histology. Repeated biopsies are sometimes necessary, and if histopathology fails to establish a diagnosis, polymerase chain reaction and culture may be useful [57]. Skin lesions generally resolve on treatment with erythromycin. Visceral disease may also respond to antibiotic therapy, although relapses have been reported.

Prevention

Primary prevention of infection with some of the most commonly encountered bacterial pathogens may be possible with immunization. The Advisory Committee on Immunization Practices [58] recommends the following immunization protocol directed at the prevention of bacterial infections for all patients with HIV disease: 23-valent pneumococcal vaccine and tetanus toxoid, absorbed (Td). Immunization with *H. influenzae* type b (Hib) conjugate vaccine should also be considered [58].

The pneumococcal serotypes responsible for pneumonia and bacteremia in patients with HIV infection are similar to those in seronegative persons. In a study by Janoff and colleagues [27], 86 percent of the serotypes isolated from patients with HIV infection were included in the 23-valent pneumococcal vaccine. It appears that immunization early in the course of HIV disease, when the patient is asymptomatic and has a relatively high CD4 cell count, is more likely to result in a protective immunologic response. However, some patients will show an antigenic response to immunizations even after the development of AIDS [59–64]. One study suggested that antibody responses after pneumococcal immunization in advanced HIV disease may be improved by the concurrent use of zidovudine [65]. As with immunization directed against pneumococcal infection, the antibody response to Hib vaccine is highly correlated with CD4 count [66]. However, while the risk for *H. influenzae* type b infection is increased in the setting of HIV disease, it is still relatively infrequent [67].

Trimethoprim-sulfamethoxazole administered daily for PCP prophylaxis may also be effective in preventing serious bacterial respiratory infections, but its indiscriminate use could promote the development of resistant organisms [67a].

Patients should be advised to thoroughly cook eggs, chicken, and meat products to prevent infection with *Salmonella*, *Campylobacter*, and *Listeria* organisms. Unpasteurized dairy products should be avoided. Patients should also be instructed in the proper cleansing of hands, utensils, and cutting boards for food preparation [68]. The effectiveness of conventional "modified reverse precautions" for hospitalized neutropenic HIV-infected patients is unknown. It is uncertain whether eradication of cutaneous staphylococcal colonization is beneficial in preventing invasive disease [69].

References

1. Drucker E, Webber MP, McMaster P, Vermund SH. Increasing rate of pneumonia hospitalizations in the Bronx: A sentinel indicator for human immunodeficiency virus. *Int J Epidemiol* 18:926–933, 1989.
2. Rolston KVI, Radentz S, Rodriguez S. Bacterial and fungal infections in patients with the acquired immunodeficiency syndrome. *Cancer Detect Prev* 14:377–381, 1990.
3. Witt DJ, Craven DE, McCabe WR. Bacterial infections in adult patients with the acquired immune deficiency syndrome (AIDS) and AIDS-related complex. *Am J Med* 82:900–906, 1987.
4. Nichols L, et al. Bacterial infections in the acquired immune deficiency syndrome: Clinicopathologic correlations in a series of autopsy cases. *Am J Clin Pathol* 92:787–790, 1989.
5. Selwyn P, Alcabes P, Hartel D, et al. Clinical manifestations and predictors of disease progression in drug users with HIV infection. *N Engl J Med* 327:1697–1703, 1992.
6. Baron AD, Hollander H. *Pseudomonas aeruginosa* bronchopulmonary infection in late human immunodeficiency virus disease. *Am Rev Respir Dis* 148:992–996, 1993.
7. Lane HC, Masur H, Edgar LC, et al. Abnormalities of B-cell activation and immunoregulation in patients with the acquired immunodeficiency syndrome. *N Engl J Med* 309:453–458, 1983.
8. Amman AJ, Schiffman G, Abrams D, et al. B-cell immunodeficiency in acquired immune deficiency syndrome. *JAMA* 251:1447–1449, 1984.
9. Muller F, Rollag H, Froland SS. Reduced oxidative burst responses in monocytes and monocyte-derived macrophages from HIV-infected subjects. *Clin Exp Immunol* 82:10–15, 1990.
10. Barat LM, Craven DE, Steinberg JL, et al. A prospective study of documented fever in patients infected with HIV-1: Diagnosis and outcome in a municipal hospital. Seventh International Conference on AIDS, Florence, June 1991.
11. Murphy PM, Lane HC, Fauci AS, Gallin JI. Impairment of neutrophil bactericidal capacity in patients with AIDS. *J Infect Dis* 158:627–630, 1988.
12. Krumholz HM, Sande MA, Lo B. Community-acquired bacteremia in patients with acquired immunodeficiency syndrome: Clinical presentation, bacteriology, and outcome. *Am J Med* 86:776–779, 1989.
13. Casadevall A, et al. *Hemophilus influenzae* type b bacteremia in adults with AIDS and at risk for AIDS. *Am J Med* 92:587–590, 1992.
14. Raviglione MC, Battan R, Pablos-Mendez A, et al. Infections associated with Hickman catheters in patients with acquired immunodeficiency syndrome. *Am J Med* 86:780–786, 1989.
15. Shaunak S, Bartlett JA. Zidovudine-induced neutropenia: Are we too cautious? *Lancet* 2:91–92, 1989.

16. Kielhofner M, et al. Life-threatening *Pseudomonas aeruginosa* infections in patients with human immunodeficiency virus infection. *Clin Infect Dis* 14:403–411, 1992.
17. Jacobson MA, Gellerman H, Chambers H. *Staphylococcus aureus* bacteremia and recurrent staphylococcal infection in patients with acquired immunodeficiency syndrome and AIDS-related complex. *Am J Med* 85:172–176, 1988.
18. Murata GH, Ault MJ, Meyer RD. Community-acquired bacterial pneumonias in homosexual men: Presumptive evidence for a defect in host resistance. *AIDS Res Hum Retroviruses* 1:379–393, 1984–85.
19. Stover DE, White DA, Romano PA, et al. Spectrum of pulmonary diseases associated with the acquired immune deficiency syndrome. *Am J Med* 78:429–437, 1985.
20. Polsky B, Gold JWM, Whimbey E, et al. Bacterial pneumonia in patients with the acquired immunodeficiency syndrome. *Ann Intern Med* 104:38–41, 1986.
21. Magnenat JL, et al. Mode of presentation and diagnosis of bacterial pneumonia in human immunodeficiency virus–infected patients. *Am Rev Respir Dis* 144:917–922, 1991.
22. Centers for Disease Control. 1993 Revised classification system for HIV infection and expanded case definition for AIDS among adolescents and adults. *MMWR* 41 (RR-17):1–19, 1992.
23. Zuger A. Bacterial infections in AIDS. *AIDS Clin Care* 4:9, 10, 1992.
24. Wallace J, Rao A, Glassroth J, et al. Respiratory illness in persons with HIV infection. *Am Rev Respir Dis* 148:1523–1529, 1993.
25. Ruzi J, Rosen M. The changing spectrum of pulmonary complications of HIV infection (abstract). *Am Rev Respir Dis* 145 (suppl A):820, 1992.
26. Schuchat A, et al. Use of surveillance for invasive pneumococcal disease to estimate the size of the immunosuppressed HIV-infected population. *JAMA* 265:3275–3279, 1991.
27. Janoff E, Brieman R, Daley C, et al. Pneumococcal disease during HIV infection, epidemiologic, clinical, and immunologic perspectives. *Ann Intern Med* 117:314–324, 1992.
28. Levine SJ, White DA, Fels AOS. The incidence and significance of *Staphylococcus aureus* in respiratory cultures from patients infected with the human immunodeficiency virus. *Am Rev Respir Dis* 141:89–93, 1990.
29. Amorosa JK, Nahass RG, Nosher JL, Gocke DJ. Radiologic distinction of pyogenic pulmonary infection from *Pneumocystis carinii* pneumonia in AIDS patients. *Radiology* 175:721–724, 1990.
30. Murray PA, et al. The microbiology of HIV-associated periodontal lesions. *J Clin Periodontol* 16:636–642, 1989.
31. Rothstein SG, Persky MS, Edelman BA, et al. Epiglottitis in AIDS patients. *Laryngoscope* 99:389–392, 1989.
32. Zurlo JJ, et al. Sinusitis in HIV-1 infection. *Am J Med* 93:157–162, 1992.
33. Godofsky EW, et al. Sinusitis in HIV-infected patients: A clinical and radiologic review. *Am J Med* 93:163–170, 1992.
34. Dryden MS, Shanson DC. The microbial causes of diarrhoea in patients infected with the human immunodeficiency virus. *J Infect* 17:107–114, 1988.

35. René E, Marche C, Regnier B, et al. Intestinal infections in patients with acquired immunodeficiency syndrome: A prospective study in 132 patients. *Dig Dis Sci* 34:773–780, 1989.
36. Antony MA, Brandt LJ, Klein RS, Bernstein LH. Infectious diarrhea in patients with AIDS. *Dig Dis Sci* 33:1141–1146, 1988.
37. Levine WC, Buehler JW, Bean NH, Tauxe RV. Epidemiology of nontyphoidal *Salmonella* bacteremia during the human immunodeficiency virus epidemic. *J Infect Dis* 164:81–87, 1991.
38. Celum CL, Chaisson RE, Rutherford GW, et al. Incidence of salmonellosis in patients with AIDS. *J Infect Dis* 156:998–1002, 1987.
39. Glaser JB, Morton-Kute L, Berger SR, et al. Recurrent *Salmonella typhimurium* bacterium associated with the acquired immunodeficiency syndrome. *Ann Intern Med* 102:189–193, 1985.
40. Fischl MA, Dickinson GM, Sinave C, et al. *Salmonella* bacteremia as manifestation of acquired immunodeficiency syndrome. *Arch Intern Med* 146:113–115, 1986.
41. Nadelman RB, Mathur-Wagh U, Yancovitz SR, Mildvan D. *Salmonella* bacteremia associated with the acquired immunodeficiency syndrome (AIDS). *Arch Intern Med* 145:1968–1971, 1985.
42. Simor AE, Poon R, Borczyk A. Chronic *Shigella flexneri* infection preceding development of acquired immunodeficiency syndrome. *J Clin Microbiol* 27:353–355, 1989.
43. Blaser MJ, Hale TL, Formal SB. Recurrent shigellosis complicating human immunodeficiency virus infection: Failure of pre-existing antibodies to confer protection. *Am J Med* 86:105–107, 1989.
44. Mandell W, Neu HC. Shigella bacteremia in adults. *JAMA* 255:3116–3117, 1986.
45. Baskin DH, Lax JD, Barenberg D. Shigella bacteremia in patients with the acquired immune deficiency syndrome. *Am J Gastroenterol* 82:338–341, 1987.
46. Sorvillo FJ, Lieb LE, Waterman SH. Incidence of campylobacteriosis among patients with AIDS in Los Angeles County. *J Acquir Immune Defic Syndr* 4:598–602, 1991.
47. Perlman DM, Ampel NM, Schifman RB, et al. Persistent *Campylobacter jejuni* infections in patients with human immunodeficiency virus (HIV). *Ann Intern Med* 108:540–546, 1988.
48. Bernar E, Roger PM, Carles D, et al. Diarrhea and *Campylobacter* infections in patients infected with the human immunodeficiency virus. *J Infect Dis* 159:143–144, 1989.
49. Hutin Y, et al. Risk factors for *Clostridium difficile*–associated diarrhea in HIV-infected patients. *AIDS* 7:1441–1447, 1993.
50. Hoegsberg B, et al. Sexually transmitted disease and HIV infection among women with pelvic inflammatory disease. *Am J Obstet Gynecol* 163:1135–1139, 1990.
51. Scully M, Berger TG. Pruritis, *Staphylococcus aureus*, and human immunodeficiency virus infection. *Arch Dermatol* 126:684–685, 1990.
52. Duvic M. Staphylococcal infections and the pruritus of AIDS-related complex. *Arch Dermatol* 123:1217–1220, 1987.
53. Schwartzman WA, Lambertus MW, Kennedy CA, Goetz MB. Staphylo-

coccal pyomyositis in patients infected by the human immunodeficiency virus. *Am J Med* 90:595–600, 1991.

54. Schlossberg D, Morad Y, Krouse TB, et al. Culture-proved disseminated cat-scratch disease in acquired immunodeficiency syndrome. *Arch Intern Med* 149:1437–1439, 1989.

55. LeBoit PE, Egbert BM, Stoler MH, et al. Epithelioid haemangioma-like vascular proliferation in AIDS: Manifestation of cat scratch disease bacillus infection? *Lancet* 1:960–963, 1988.

56. Koehler J, Quinn F, Berger T, et al. Isolation of *Rochalimaea* species from cutaneous and osseous lesions of bacillary angiomatosis. *N Engl J Med* 327:1625–1631, 1992.

57. Tappero J, Mohle-Boetani J, Koehler J, et al. The epidemiology of bacillary angiomatosis and bacillary peliosis. *JAMA* 269:770–775, 1993.

58. Recommendation of Advisory Committee on Immunization Practices: Use of vaccines and immune globulins in persons with altered immunocompetence. *MMWR* 42 (RR-4):1–18, 1993.

59. ACIP. Pneumococcal polysaccharide vaccine. *MMWR* 38:64–76, 1989.

60. Huang KL, Ruben FL, Rinaldo CR, et al. Antibody responses after influenza and pneumococcal immunization in HIV-infected homosexual men. *JAMA* 257:2047–2050, 1987.

61. Poland GA, et al. Routine immunization of the HIV-positive asymptomatic patient. *J Gen Intern Med* 5:147–150, 1990.

62. Janoff EN, Douglas JM Jr, Gabriel M, et al. Class-specific antibody response to pneumococcal capsular polysaccharides in men infected with human immunodeficiency virus type 1. *J Infect Dis* 158:983–990, 1988.

63. Rhoads JL, Birx DL, Wright DC, et al. Response to vaccination in HIV seropositive subjects. Third International Conference on AIDS, Washington, DC, 1987.

64. Gallant J, Moore R, Chaisson R. Prophylaxis for opportunistic infections in patients with HIV infection. *Ann Intern Med* 120:932–944, 1994.

65. Glaser J, Volpe S, Aguire A, et al. Zidovudine improves response to pneumococcal vaccine among persons with AIDS and AIDS-related complex. *J Infect Dis* 164:761–764, 1991.

66. Steinhoff M, Auerbach B, Nelson K, et al. Antibody responses to *Haemophilus influenzae* type b vaccine in men with HIV infection. *N Engl J Med* 325:1837–1842, 1991.

67. Steinhart R, Reingold A, Taylor I, et al. Invasive *Haemophilus influenzae* infection in men with HIV infection. *JAMA* 268:3350–3352, 1992.

67a. Centers for Disease Control. USPHS/IDSA guidelines for the prevention of opportunistic infections in persons infected with human immunodeficiency virus: A summary. *MMWR* 44(RR-8):1–34, 1995.

68. Jewett J, Hecht F. Preventive health care for adults with HIV infection. *JAMA* 269:1144–1153, 1993.

69. Ganesh R, Castle D, McGibbon D, et al. Staphylococcal carriage and HIV infection. *Lancet* 2:558, 1989.

Kaposi's Sarcoma 29

Timothy P. Cooley

Kaposi's sarcoma (KS) was first described in 1872 by the Hungarian dermatologist Moritz Kaposi, and before the AIDS epidemic it was a rare tumor [1]. Classic, endemic, acquired, and epidemic forms of KS have been identified. The "classic" form presents with multiple violaceous skin nodules on the lower extremities. It predominates in elderly men of Mediterranean or Eastern European background, has an indolent course, and is frequently associated with hematologic malignancies [2, 3]. The "endemic" form of KS, found in children and young men in equatorial Africa, is more virulent than the classic form [4]. "Acquired" KS occurs in patients treated with immunosuppressive drugs, especially individuals who have received organ transplants [5–7]. "Epidemic" KS associated with HIV infection was first observed among young homosexual men in major urban areas in the United States during the early 1980s [8–15]. Although the histopathology of all forms of KS is virtually identical, the clinical manifestations differ remarkably, with the epidemic form exhibiting a more variable and aggressive course [16, 17].

Pathogenesis

Many studies have attempted to elucidate the pathogenesis of epidemic KS. There is increasing evidence to support the presence of an unidentified, sexually transmitted cofactor that may induce KS in conjunction with HIV infection [18–21]. Surveillance data from the Centers for Disease Control (CDC) indicate that rates for KS are highest among those who acquire HIV sexually. Kaposi's sarcoma was four times more common in HIV-infected women with bisexual partners than in those who had partners with other risk behaviors [18]. Friedman-Kien and Alvin [19] reported seven cases of KS in HIV-seronegative homosexual men; the serostatus of six was confirmed by polymerase chain reaction and p24 antigen studies, suggesting that KS in homosexual men may be caused by a sexually transmitted pathogen other than HIV. Further supporting a role for an infectious agent in the pathophysiology of KS has been the recent identification of herpesvirus-like DNA from KS tissue in people with and without AIDS [22, 22a].

Studies at the National Cancer Institute (NCI) established another possible mechanism for development of KS. Cultured KS cell lines were shown to produce soluble factors promoting the growth of angiogenic lesions in nude mice that were histologically similar to those of KS but genotypically murine [14, 23]. Additional studies demonstrated that KS-derived spindle cells in culture produce a variety of cytokines including basic fibroblast growth factor (bFGF), interleukin-1 (IL-1), -6, and -8, platelet-derived growth factor (PDGF), vascular endothelial growth factor (VEGF), tumor necrosis factor (TNF), and granulocyte-macrophage colony stimulating factor (GM-CSF) [24–26]. It is theorized that these cytokines induce both autocrine and paracrine effects, resulting in further proliferation of spindle cells and the stimulation of tumor angiogenesis [24–26]. Recent reports suggested that bFGF may play a major role in mediating KS cell proliferation induced by IL-1 and oncostatin M [27–29].

Other investigators believe that HIV may play a more direct role in the development of KS. Several studies suggested that the HIV transactivating (*tat*) gene may be important in the induction of KS [30–33]. Transgenic mice bearing the *tat* gene develop KS-like lesions. This effect is linked with male gender, implying hormonal control, and with the expression of *tat* in the skin of the animals. However, *tat* is not expressed by KS itself or by cell lines derived from KS lesions [30, 33]. Tat protein released into tissue culture by HIV-infected cells acts as a vascular cell growth factor, thereby promoting the activation of KS [30, 34]. Recent reports indicated that Tat is generated during acute HIV infection and after transactivation of the gene by mechanisms other than cell death [32, 35].

Epidemiology

Kaposi's sarcoma is 20,000 times more common in patients with AIDS than in the US general population, and the incidence varies greatly among different HIV transmission groups [18, 35]. Approximately 94 percent of epidemic KS has been diagnosed in homosexual or bisexual men; KS develops in 21 percent of homosexual or bisexual men with AIDS [18]. The disease is seen infrequently in AIDS patients with other risk behaviors, occurring in 6 percent of cases from endemic areas, 4 percent of cases related to blood transfusion, and 3 percent of heterosexual injection drug users [18]. Hemophiliacs have very small risk (< 1%) of developing KS [18].

Overall, KS is diagnosed in approximately 15 percent of patients with AIDS at some point during the course of their disease [18, 37]. Analysis of CDC data shows that the percentage of AIDS patients with KS as an indicator disease has declined by 20 percent per year in homosexual men and by 10 percent per year in other HIV risk groups between 1983 and 1988 [18]. A similar study by the San Francisco Department of Health found that the proportion of AIDS patients in whom KS developed declined from 60 to 20 percent between 1981 and 1987 [37]. This finding does not seem to be an artifact of selective underreporting and may reflect changing patterns of behavior among homosexual men, resulting in reduced exposure to sexually transmitted agents [18, 37, 38].

Clinical Manifestations

Epidemic KS has a variable clinical course, ranging from minimal disease presenting as an incidental finding to explosive tumor growth resulting in death [16, 17, 39]. The distribution of cutaneous lesions is more widespread than in other forms of the disease [8, 16, 17]. Most patients have multiple painless, nonpruritic subcutaneous tumor nodules that vary in size from several millimeters to several centimeters in diameter [8–15] (see Plates 15 and 16). Lesions are usually hyperpigmented, brownish-red to purplish-black, and nonblanching. Less commonly, patients have plaque-like lesions, particularly on the soles of the feet and thighs [40]. Exophytic tumor masses with breakdown of overlying skin are infrequent but may occur in areas exposed to trauma [38]. Lymphedema, particularly in the face, genitalia, and lower extremities, is seemingly out of proportion to the extent of cutaneous disease [39].

Extracutaneous spread of KS is common. Lymph node involvement is found in up to 30 percent of AIDS-related KS but is not a poor prognostic sign as it is in African KS [40–42]. Intraoral KS occurs in approximately one-third of patients and is the initial site of disease in about 15 percent [43–47]. Kaposi's sarcoma of the oral cavity affects the mucosa of the hard and soft palates and less commonly, the gingiva, tonsillar pillars, and pharynx (see Plate 5). Complications include superficial ulceration of palatal lesions and dental displacement or bleeding from gingival lesions. The majority of patients with oral KS have lesions elsewhere in the gastrointestinal tract [48].

Gastrointestinal involvement, most common in the stomach and duodenum, is found in 40 percent of KS patients at the time of initial diagnosis and in almost 80 percent at autopsy [49–51]. Gastrointestinal KS is more likely if extensive cutaneous disease is present but has been reported in patients without skin involvement [48, 49, 52]. Diagnosis is generally made by endoscopic visualization of typical red, raised, nonulcerated lesions that vary in size from 0.5 to 2.0 cm in diameter [40]. Because lesions tend to be submucosal, only a minority of biopsy specimens are positive [49]. Gastrointestinal KS sometimes appears as smooth round masses protruding into the intestinal lumen [50, 51, 53]. While demonstrable on contrast barium studies, they are rarely seen on computed tomographic scans.

The clinical presentation of pulmonary KS is often nonspecific. Dyspnea and a nonproductive cough are nearly universal; fever is common but in most cases related to a concomitant infection [54–57]. Pulmonary KS may cause severe symptoms, including bronchospasm and progressive respiratory insufficiency [56, 58–60]. The chest x-ray may be normal or show diffuse bilateral infiltrates in an alveolar, interstitial, mixed alveolar-interstitial, or nodular pattern, as well as pleural effusions [57, 58, 61–67] (see Fig. 11-3). The presence of violaceous endobronchial lesions on bronchoscopy is diagnostic of pulmonary KS; transbronchial biopsy may result in significant bleeding, and crush artifact can make identification of typical histologic results difficult [57–59, 68, 69]. Bronchoscopy fails to provide evidence of KS in up to 30 percent of patients in whom pulmonary involvement is subsequently confirmed by open lung biopsy or autopsy [57, 59, 68, 69]. The majority of patients with pulmonary KS have extensive cutaneous disease at the time of diagnosis [55, 60, 63, 70, 71].

Diagnosis

A 4- to 6-mm punch biopsy of a skin lesion is usually adequate to establish the diagnosis of KS. Fine-needle aspiration biopsy can also be used to evaluate cutaneous or mucosal lesions and lymph nodes [72, 73]. Pathologically, KS is characterized by the proliferation of spindle-shaped cells that form slit-like spaces, which may contain extravasated erythrocytes. Mixed with the spindle cells are fibroblasts, endothelial cells, inflammatory cells, and evidence of neoangiogenesis [8, 74–76].

While diagnosis of cutaneous KS is relatively easy, the detection and documentation of extracutaneous sites of disease can be more difficult. Gastrointestinal and endobronchial lesions can be viewed endoscopically, but biopsies have a low yield [40, 53, 61, 62, 66–71]. KS is frequently thallium avid, and sequential gallium and delayed 3-hour thallium scintigraphy represent a potentially useful noninvasive technique for detecting extracutaneous KS, particularly lymphatic and pulmonary involvement [77–79]. Enhanced thallium uptake with no gallium uptake occurs in areas of biopsy-proved KS; an infectious process is gallium avid and thallium negative, and lymphoma is both thallium avid and gallium avid [78, 80–83].

Prognosis

Until recently, there was no uniform staging system for KS [84]. Studies have shown that early tumor stage and the absence of systemic symptoms correlate closely with increased survival [39, 85–87]. A history of opportunistic infection implies a poor prognosis, with a median survival time of only 7 months [16, 43, 87]. The CD4 cell count is another important prognostic indicator with an 85 percent 1-year survival rate for patients with a CD4 count greater than $300/mm^3$ compared to a 35 percent 1-year survival rate for those with a CD4 count less than $100/mm^3$ [43, 87, 88]. In AIDS patients with KS, mortality may occur as a direct result of tumor progression but is more often related to other complications of HIV disease [40, 89]. A new staging system proposed by the AIDS Clinical Trials Group (ACTG) is intended to be comprehensive and facilitate the evaluation of treatment [89] (Table 29-1). In addition to extent of tumor and presence of constitutional symptoms, this system incorporates immunologic staging by CD4 cell count.

Management

The choice of therapy in epidemic KS is problematic given the variable natural history of the disease. With the exception of pulmonary or gastrointestinal involvement, KS is rarely life threatening, and the goals

Table 29-1 *Staging system for Kaposi's sarcoma*

	Good risk (0) (all of the following)	*Poor risk (1) (any of the following)*
Tumor (T)	Confined to skin and/or lymph nodes and/or minimal oral disease	Tumor-associated edema or ulceration Extensive oral, GI, or other extranodal visceral KS
Immune system (I)	CD4 cells $\geq 200/mm^3$	CD4 cells $< 200/mm^3$
Systemic illness (S)	No history of opportunistic infection or thrush No "B" symptoms Karnofsky performance status $\geq 70\%$	History of opportunistic infection or thrush "B" symptoms present Karnofsky performance status $< 70\%$ Other HIV-related illness (lymphoma, neurologic disease)

Source: Adapted from SE Krown, C Metroka, JC Werntz, AIDS Clinical Trials Group Oncology Committee. Kaposi's sarcoma in the acquired immune deficiency syndrome: A proposal for uniform evaluation, response and staging criteria. *J Clin Oncol* 7:1201–1207, 1989.

of treatment are usually palliative. There are no data to show that the current systemic agents used in the therapy of AIDS-related KS increase survival [16]. However, treatment may result in significant improvement by decreasing the size of cutaneous lesions, alleviating the discomfort associated with edema and ulcerations, and controlling symptoms related to mucosal or visceral involvement.

Local Modalities

Small localized lesions can be surgically excised or removed by electrodesiccation and curettage. Topical application of liquid nitrogen [40] or of all-*trans*-retinoic acid (tRA) [90] has been used successfully to treat localized skin lesions. Individual cutaneous and intraoral lesions can be treated with dilute vinblastine injection, achieving response rates higher than 90 percent [91, 92]. The complications of intralesional chemotherapy include local pain and skin irritation.

Radiation Therapy

Kaposi's sarcoma is a radiosensitive tumor, with response rates of 50 to 85 percent [93]. Radiation therapy is most effective as a palliative measure to relieve localized mass effect and pain, particularly in the lower extremities. The results of palliative radiation therapy for cosmesis are generally not as good as with other treatment modalities, and complete responses are unusual [93]. Optimal dosing schedules have not been established, but doses of 25 to 30 Gray (Gy) generally produce tumor regression [93, 94]. A single fraction of 8 Gy appears to give equivalent results to more prolonged schedules [95]. Acute radiation toxicity, including mucositis, desquamation, and hyperpigmentation, is often disproportionate to the amount of radiation delivered. Local toxicity, especially in the treatment of oropharyngeal lesions, can be so severe that many authorities consider radiation therapy to be a measure of last resort [94, 96, 97].

Interferon

The treatment of KS with interferon has been under study since the early 1980s. The activity of interferon against KS may be mediated by a variety of immunoregulatory, antiproliferative, antiviral, and antiangiogenic mechanisms [98–102]. Initial studies of alpha-interferon revealed a clear dose response of tumor regression, with high doses (> 20 million units) resulting in objective response rates of 10 to 40 percent [102]. Response to therapy correlated with preservation of immune function; nonresponders had a history of previous opportunistic infection and significant constitutional symptoms. Patients with cutaneous KS but no history of opportunistic infection or systemic symptoms have shown tumor response rates of 30 to 50 percent [102–104]. Individuals with CD4 counts of 200/mm³ or higher appear to be more likely to benefit from therapy with alpha-interferon [103], but data regarding the duration of antitumor response are limited [103, 105]. Common side effects include a flu-like syndrome with fevers, chills, and malaise; dose reduction is required in up to one-third of patients because of chronic fatigue, malaise, and neutropenia [102].

Alpha-interferon has been shown to have antiviral effects in vitro and in vivo [106, 107]. While zidovudine (ZDV) alone has been shown to have no effect on KS, recent clinical studies confirmed the in vitro synergistic antiviral and antitumor effects of combined therapy with alpha-interferon and ZDV [108–113]. As with earlier studies, the major dose-limiting toxicity was neutropenia. In an effort to improve the hematologic tolerance of the alpha-interferon/ZDV combination, Krown and associates [114] treated five patients with KS in a phase I trial using recombinant GM-CSF; no reductions in interferon or ZDV doses were required. A phase II study using ZDV, alpha-interferon, and GM-CSF showed significant antitumor response in 50 percent of patients with minimal toxicity [115]. A phase II ACTG study of alpha-interferon in combination with didanosine (ddI), which is not myelosuppressive, is currently underway.

Other interferons and cytokines, including fibroblast-beta-interferon, gamma-interferon, and interleukin-2, have also been evaluated in the treatment of KS [103]. Beta-interferon, which has a substantially higher maximum tolerated dose and less hematologic toxicity than alpha-interferon, had no significant antitumor effect in patients with advanced KS [116]. Clinical trials with gamma-interferon [117, 118] and with interleukin-2 [119] did not demonstrate any benefit, and rapid progression of KS was found when beta-interferon and interleukin-2 were used in combination [120]. Clinical trials evaluating interleukin-4, which suppresses interleukin-6 in vitro [121], in the treatment of KS are ongoing.

Chemotherapy

Systemic chemotherapy may be appropriate for patients with rapidly progressive KS or those with widespread symptomatic disease. Active chemotherapeutic agents include doxorubicin [122–124], vinblastine [125], vincristine [126], bleomycin [127], etoposide (VP-16) [128], and paclitaxel (taxol) [129]. Published studies of single-agent therapy for KS in patients with a wide range of disease involvement have reported response rates of 14 to 76 percent [122–129]. The vinca alkaloids are the most commonly used antineoplastic drugs, with response rates of 26 to 48 percent [125, 126]. When given as low-dose weekly therapy, vincristine and vinblastine are well tolerated, and serious toxicity is infrequent [125, 126]. The major toxicity of vinblastine is myelosuppression, which may require treatment delay, dose reduction, or the use of cytokine growth factors [125]. The most common side effect associated with vincristine is peripheral neuropathy [126]. Particular care must be exercised when giving vincristine to patients with preexisting peripheral neuropathy and to individuals taking ddI, zalcitabine (formerly dideoxycytidine or ddC), or stavudine (d4T). The toxicities of vincristine and vinblastine may be ameliorated by giving the drugs weekly on an alternating basis [130]. Etoposide has a reported response rate of 76 percent [118] but tends to be more myelosuppressive than the vinca alkaloids. An ACTG study investigating the use of prolonged low-dose oral etoposide is currently underway.

Although doxorubicin is highly active as a single agent in the treatment of KS, its use is limited by myelosuppression [122–124]. In an attempt to increase the efficacy and decrease the toxicity of doxorubicin, investigators studied the use of a new liposomal encapsulated formulation of the drug given biweekly [131]. The overall response rate was 92 percent, with a complete response in 7 percent of patients. The most common toxicity was neutropenia, with many individuals requiring use of cytokine growth factors [132]. A clinical trial of liposomal encapsulated daunorubicin administered biweekly had similar results with a comparable toxicity profile [132].

Bleomycin has been given as single-drug therapy [127] but is more commonly used as part of combination chemotherapy regimens. Treatment with vincristine and bleomycin has a reported response rate of 50 percent [133] and may be useful in neutropenic patients who are less likely to tolerate myelosuppressive combination chemotherapy. A recent study of bleomycin given as 72-hour continuous intravenous infusion reported a 65 percent partial response rate with minimal toxicity [134].

Standard doses of cytotoxic chemotherapy in the treatment of advanced KS are associated with severe myelosuppression and frequent development of opportunistic infections [128]. Contrary to earlier experience with high-dose chemotherapy, the use of marrow-sparing agents, such as vincristine and bleomycin, in combination with low doses of myelosuppressive drugs often results in clinical and functional improvement in patients with aggressive cutaneous or visceral disease. The most effective regimen appears to be ABV (doxorubicin at doses of 10–20 mg/m^2, bleomycin, and vincristine), with reported response rates of 45 to 88 percent and a median survival time of 9 months [123, 135]. In a series of patients with symptomatic pulmonary KS, an overall response rate to ABV of 80 percent was reported [54]. Significant neutropenia occurs in 40 to 50 percent of patients, with a 30 percent incidence of opportunistic infections when *Pneumocystis carinii* pneumonia prophylaxis is used [135]. An ACTG study administering ABV, ZDV, and GM-CSF to advanced-stage KS patients demonstrated comparable antitumor responses without significant neutropenia or infectious complications [136]. Another trial using ABV with either ddI or ddC in patients with advanced KS is also under review. The chemotherapy regimen of ABV with liposomal encapsulated doxorubicin substituted for the standard formulation is being evaluated as well.

Noncytotoxic Approaches

Several drugs that may inhibit angiogenesis are now being studied for the treatment of KS. TNP-470 (AGM-1470, *O*-[chloroacetylcarbamoyl] fumagillol), an analogue of the antibiotic fumagillin and platelet factor-4 (PF-4), as well as the anticoagulants xylanopolyhydrogensulfate (pentosan polysulfate) and tecogalan (SPPG), have been reported to inhibit endothelial cell proliferation [137–141] and proliferation of KS-associated spindle cells in vitro [142, 143]. Trials of pentosan have not shown clinical benefit [144, 145]. The intralesional injection of PF-4 has demonstrated some antitumor effect [146], and studies of systemically administered PF-4 are planned. Phase I and II clinical trials of TNP-470 and SPPG are currently in progress.

References

1. Albini A, Mitchell CD, Thompson EW, et al. Invasive activity and chemotactic response to growth factors by Kaposi's sarcoma cells. *J Cell Biochem* 36:369–376, 1988.
2. Auerbach HE, Brooks JJ. Kaposi's sarcoma: Observation and a hypothesis. *Lab Invest* 52:44–46, 1985.
3. Beakstead JH, Wood GS, Fletcher V. Evidence of the origin of Kaposi's sarcoma from lymphatic endothelium. *Am J Pathol* 119:294–299, 1985.
4. Brooks JJ. Kaposi's sarcoma: A reversible hyperplasia. *Lancet* 2:1309–1311, 1986.
5. Burgess WH, Maciag T. The heparin binding (fibroblast) growth factor family of proteins. *Annu Rev Biochem* 58:575–606, 1989.
6. Bussolino F, Wang JM, Delfilippi P, et al. Granulocyte and granulocyte-macrophage colony stimulating factors induce human endothelial cells to migrate and proliferate. *Nature* 337:471–473, 1989.
7. Clark SC, Kamen R. The human hematopoietic colony stimulating factors. *Science* 236:1229–1236, 1987.
8. Friedman-Kien AE. Disseminated Kaposi's sarcoma syndrome in young homosexual men. *J Am Acad Dermatol* 5:468–471, 1981.
9. Centers for Disease Control. Kaposi's sarcoma and pneumocystis pneumonia among homosexual men: New York City and California. *MMWR* 30:305–308, 1981.
10. Hymes KB, Cheung TL, Green JB, et al. Kaposi's sarcoma in homosexual men: A report of eight cases. *Lancet* 2:598, 1981.
11. Friedman-Kien AE, Laubenstein LJ, Rubinstein P, et al. Disseminated Kaposi's sarcoma in homosexual men. *Ann Intern Med* 96:693–700, 1982.
12. Marmor M, Laubenstein L, William DC, et al. Risk factors for Kaposi's sarcoma in homosexual men. *Lancet* 1:1084–1086, 1982.

13. Jaffe HW, Keewhan C, Thomas PA, et al. National case control study of Kaposi's sarcoma and *Pneumocystis carinii* pneumonia in homosexual men: Part 1, epidemiologic results. *Ann Intern Med* 99:145–151, 1983.

14. Drew WL, Miner RC, Ziegler JL, et al. Cytomegalovirus and Kaposi's sarcoma in young homosexual men. *Lancet* 2:125–127, 1982.

15. Urmacher C, Myskowski P, Ochoa M Jr, et al. Outbreak of Kaposi's sarcoma in young homosexual men. *Am J Med* 72:69–75, 1982.

16. Krigel RL, Friedman-Kien AE. Kaposi's Sarcoma. In VT DeVita, S Hellman, SA Rosenberg (eds), *AIDS: Etiology, Diagnosis, Treatment, and Prevention.* Philadelphia: Lippincott, 1988. Pp 245–261.

17. Krown SE. AIDS-associated Kaposi's sarcoma: Pathogenesis, clinical course and treatment. *AIDS* 2:71–80, 1988.

18. Beral V, Peterman TA, Berkelman RL, Jaffe HW. Kaposi's sarcoma among patients with AIDS: A sexually transmitted infection? *Lancet* 335:123–128, 1990.

19. Friedman-Kien AE, Alvin E. Kaposi's sarcoma in HIV-1 seronegative homosexual men (abstract). Sixth International Conference on AIDS, San Francisco, June 1990.

20. Archibald CP, Schechter MT, Craig KJP, et al. Evidence for a sexually transmitted cofactor for Kaposi's sarcoma in a cohort of homosexual men (abstract). Sixth International Conference on AIDS, San Francisco, June 1990.

21. Jacobson LP, Munoz A, Dudlet J, et al. Examination of timing of potential Kaposi's sarcoma cofactor relative to HIV-1 infection (abstract). Sixth International Conference on AIDS, San Francisco, June 1990.

22. Chang Y, et al. Identification of herpes-virus-like DNA sequences in AIDS-associated Kaposi's sarcoma. *Science* 266:1865–1869, 1994.

22a. Moore, PS, Chang Y. Detection of herpesvirus-like DNA sequences in Kaposi's sarcoma in patients with and those without HIV infection. *N Engl J Med* 332:1181–1185, 1995.

23. Drew WL, Mills J, Levy J, et al. Cytomegalovirus infection and abnormal T lymphocyte subset ratios in homosexual men. *Ann Intern Med* 103:61, 1985.

24. Ensoli B, Nakamura S, Salahuddin SZ, et al. AIDS-Kaposi's sarcoma–derived cells express cytokines with autocrine and paracrine growth effects. *Science* 243:223, 1989.

25. Windel K, Marme D, Weich HA. AIDS-associated Kaposi's sarcoma cells in culture express vascular endothelial growth factor. *Biochem Biophys Res Commun* 189:824–831, 1992.

26. Miles SA, Nezair AR, Salazar-Gonzalez JF, et al. AIDS Kaposi sarcoma-derived cells produce and respond to interleukin 6. *Proc Natl Acad Sci USA* 87:4068–4072, 1990.

27. Marx J. Kaposi's sarcoma puzzle begins to yield. *Science* 248:442–443, 1990.

28. Nair BC, DeVico AL, Nakamura S, et al. Identification of a major growth factor for AIDS-Kaposi's sarcoma cells as oncostatin M. *Science* 255:1430–1432, 1992.

29. Miles SA, Martinez-Maza O, Rezai A, et al. Oncostatin M as a potent mitogen for AIDS-Kaposi's sarcoma-derived cells. *Science* 255:1432–1434, 1992.

30. Ensoli B, Barillari G, Salahuddin SZ, et al. *Tat* protein of HIV-1 stimulates growth of cells derived from Kaposi's sarcoma lesions of AIDS patients. *Nature* 345:84–86, 1990.
31. Vogel J, Hinrichs SH, Reynolds RK, et al. The HIV *tat* gene induces dermal lesions resembling Kaposi's sarcoma in transgenic mice. *Nature* 335:606–611, 1988.
32. Ensoli B, Barillari G, Salahuddin SZ, et al. Tat protein of HIV-1 stimulates growth of cells derived from Kaposi's sarcoma lesions of AIDS patients. *Nature* 345:84–86, 1990.
33. Barillari G, Buonaguro L, Fiorelli V, et al. Effects of cytokines from activated immune cells on vascular cell growth and HIV-1 gene expression. *J Immunol* 149:3727–3734, 1992.
34. Corallini A, Altavilla G, Pozzi L, et al. Systemic expression of HIV-1 tat gene in transgenic mice induces endothelial proliferation and tumors of different histotypes. *Cancer Res* 53:107, 1993.
35. Ensoli B, Buonaguro L, Barillari G, et al. Release, uptake and effects of extracellular human immunodeficiency virus type 1 Tat protein on cell growth and viral transactivation. *J Virol* 67:277–287, 1993.
36. Des Jarlais DC, Marmor M, Thomas O, et al. Kaposi's sarcoma among four different AIDS risk groups. *N Engl J Med* 310:1119, 1984.
37. Rutherford GW, Schwarz SK, Lemp GF, et al. The epidemiology of AIDS-related Kaposi's sarcoma in San Francisco. *J Infect Dis* 159:569–572, 1989.
38. Polk BF, Munoz A, Fox R, et al. Decline of Kaposi's sarcoma (KS) among participants in MACS (abstract). Fourth International Conference on AIDS, Stockholm, June 1988.
39. Mitsuyasu RT, Taylor JMG, Glaspy J, Fahey JL. Heterogeneity of epidemic Kaposi's sarcoma: Implications for therapy. *Cancer* 57:1657–1661, 1986.
40. Northfelt DW. Kaposi's Sarcoma: Epidemiology and Clinical Characteristics. In PT Cohen, MA Sande, PA Volberding (eds), *The AIDS Knowledge Base* (2nd ed). Boston: Little, Brown, 1994. Pp 7.1.3–7.1.4.
41. Volberding P. Therapy of Kaposi's sarcoma in AIDS. *Semin Oncol* 11:60–67, 1984.
42. Moskowitz LB, Hensley TG, Gould EW, Weiss SD. Frequency and anatomic distribution of lymphadenopathic Kaposi's sarcoma in the acquired immunodeficiency syndrome: An autopsy series. *Hum Pathol* 16:447–456, 1985.
43. Lozada F, Silverman S, Migliorate C, et al. Oral manifestations of tumor and opportunistic infections in the epidemic of acquired immune deficiency syndrome. *Cancer* 45:4646–4648, 1985.
44. Green T, Beckstead J, Lozada-Nur F, et al. Histopathologic spectrum of oral Kaposi's sarcoma. *Oral Surg Oral Med Oral Pathol* 58:306–314, 1984.
45. Sooy CD. Otolaryngologic manifestations of acquired immunodeficiency syndrome. *West J Med* 141:674, 1984.
46. Gnepp DR, Chandler W, Hyams V. Primary Kaposi's sarcoma of the head and neck. *Ann Intern Med* 100:107–114, 1984.
47. Keeney K, Abaza NA, Tidwel O, Quinn P. Oral Kaposi's sarcoma in acquired immune deficiency syndrome. *J Oral Maxillofac Surg* 45:815–821, 1987.
48. Saltz RK, Kurtz RC, Lightdale CJ, et al. Kaposi's sarcoma. Gastrointesti-

nal involvement correlation with skin findings and immunologic function. *Dig Dis Sci* 29:817–823, 1984.

49. Friedman SL, Wright TL, Altman DF. Gastrointestinal Kaposi's sarcoma in patients with the acquired immune deficiency syndrome: Endoscopic and autopsy findings. *Gastroenterology* 890:102–108, 1985.

50. Rose HS, Balthazar EJ, Megibow AJ, et al. Alimentary tract involvement in Kaposi's sarcoma: Radiographic and endoscopic findings in 25 homosexual men. *Am J Radiol* 139:661–666, 1982.

51. Frager DH, Frager JD, Brandt LJ, et al. Gastrointestinal complications of AIDS: Radiologic features. *Radiology* 158:597–603, 1986.

52. Barrison IG, Foster S, Harris JW, et al. Upper gastrointestinal Kaposi's sarcoma in patients positive for HIV antibody without cutaneous disease. *Br Med J* 296:92–93, 1988.

53. Moon KL, Federle MP, Abrams DI, et al. Kaposi's sarcoma and lymphadenopathy syndrome: Limitations of abdominal CT in acquired immunodeficiency syndrome. *Radiology* 150:479–483, 1984.

54. Gill PS, Alcil B, Colletti P, et al. Pulmonary Kaposi's sarcoma: Clinical findings and results of therapy. *Am J Med* 87:57–61, 1989.

55. Garay SM, Belenko M, Fazzini E, Schinella R. Pulmonary manifestations of Kaposi's sarcoma. *Chest* 91:39–43, 1987.

56. Ognibene FP, Steis RG, Macher AM, et al. Kaposi's sarcoma causing pulmonary infiltrates and respiratory failure in the acquired immunodeficiency syndrome. *Ann Intern Med* 102:471–475, 1985.

57. Meduri GU, Stover DE, Lee M, et al. Pulmonary Kaposi's sarcoma in the acquired immune deficiency syndrome. *Am J Med* 81:11–18, 1986.

58. Kaplan LC, Hopewell PC, Jaffe H, et al. Kaposi's sarcoma involving the lung in patients with the acquired immune deficiency syndrome. *J Acquir Immune Defic Syndr* 1:23–30, 1988.

59. Pitchenik AF, Fischl MA, Saldana MJ. Kaposi's sarcoma of the tracheobronchial tree: Clinical, bronchoscopic and pathologic features. *Chest* 87:122–124, 1985.

60. Kornfeld H, Azelrod JL. Pulmonary presentation of Kaposi's sarcoma in a homosexual patient. *Am Rev Respir Dis* 127:248–249, 1983.

61. Case Records of the Massachusetts General Hospital (Case 1-1990). *N Engl J Med* 322:43–51, 1990.

62. Nyberg DA, Federle MP. AIDS-related Kaposi's sarcoma and lymphoma. *Semin Roentgenol* 22:54–65, 1987.

63. Davis SD, Henschke CI, Chamides BK, Westcott JL. Intrathoracic Kaposi's sarcoma in AIDS patients: Radiographic-pathologic correlation. *Radiology* 163:495–500, 1987.

64. Naidich DP, Tarras M, Garay SM, et al. Kaposi's sarcoma: CT-radiographic correlation. *Chest* 96:723–728, 1989.

65. Sivit CJ, Schwartz AM, Rockoff SD. Kaposi's sarcoma of the lung in AIDS: Radiologic-pathologic analysis. *Am J Radiol* 148:25–28, 1987.

66. Ognibene FP, Shelhamer JH. Kaposi's sarcoma. *Clin Chest Med* 9:459–465, 1988.

67. Kramer EL, Sanger JJ, Garay SM, et al. Gallium scans of the chest in patients with AIDS. *J Nucl Med* 28:1107–1114, 1987.

68. Hanson PJV, Hancourt-Webster JN, Grazzard BG, Collins JV. Fibroscopic

bronchoscopy in the diagnosis of pulmonary Kaposi's sarcoma. *Thorax* 42:269–271, 1987.

69. Lau KY, Rubin A, Littner M, Krauthammer M. Kaposi's sarcoma of the tracheobronchial tree: Clinical, bronchoscopic and pathologic features. *Chest* 89:158–159, 1986.

70. Niedt GW, Schinella RA. Acquired immunodeficiency syndrome: Clinicopathologic study of 56 autopsies. *Arch Pathol Lab Med* 109:727–734, 1985.

71. Bach MC, Bagwell SP, Fanning JP. Primary pulmonary Kaposi's sarcoma in the acquired immunodeficiency syndrome: A cause of persistent pyrexia. *Am J Med* 85:274–275, 1988.

72. Bottles K, McPhaul LW, Volberding P. Fine-needle aspiration biopsy of patients with acquired immunodeficiency syndrome (AIDS): Experience in an outpatient clinic. *Ann Intern Med* 108:42–45, 1988.

73. Hales M, Bottles K, Miller T, et al. Diagnosis of Kaposi's sarcoma by fine-needle aspiration biopsy. *Am J Clin Pathol* 88:20–25, 1987.

74. Reynolds WA, Winkleman RK, Soule EH. Kaposi's sarcoma: A clinicopathologic study with particular reference to its relationship to the reticuloendothelial system. *Medicine (Baltimore)* 44:419–433, 1965.

75. Gottlieb GJ, Ackerman AB. Kaposi's sarcoma: An extensively disseminated form in young homosexual men. *Hum Pathol* 13:882–892, 1982.

76. McNutt NS, Fletcher V, Conant MA. Early lesions of Kaposi's sarcoma in homosexual men: An ultrastructural comparison with other vascular proliferations in skin. *Am J Pathol* 111:62–77, 1983.

77. Lee VW, Rosen MP, Baum A, et al. AIDS-related Kaposi's sarcoma: Findings on thallium-2021 scintigraphy. *Am J Radiol* 151:1233–1235, 1988.

78. Lee VW, Fuller JD, O'Brien MJ, et al. Pulmonary Kaposi sarcoma in patients with AIDS: Scintigraphic diagnosis with sequential thallium and gallium scanning. *Radiology* 180:409–412, 1991.

79. Lee VW, Chen H, Panageas E, et al. Subcutaneous Kaposi's sarcoma: Thallium scan demonstration. *Clin Nucl Med* 15:569–571, 1990.

80. Salvotore M, Canatu L, Porta E. T1-201 as a positive indicator for lung neoplasm: Preliminary experience. *Radiology* 121:487–488, 1976.

81. Tonami N, Shuke N, Yokoyama K, et al. Thallium 201: SPECT in evaluation of suspected lung cancer. *J Nucl Med* 30:997–1004, 1981.

82. Waxman AD, Ramanna L, Said J. Thallium scintigraphy in lymphoma: Relationship to gallium-67 (abstract). *J Nucl Med* 30:915, 1989.

83. Hamada S, Nishimura T, Hayashida K, Uchara T. Intracardiac malignant lymphoma detected by gallium-67 and thallium-201 chloride. *J Nucl Med* 29:1868–1870, 1988.

84. Volberding PA. Moving towards a uniform staging for human immunodeficiency virus–associated Kaposi's sarcoma. *J Clin Oncol* 7:1184–1185, 1989.

85. Krigel RL, Laubenstein LJ, Muggia FM. Kaposi's sarcoma: A new staging classification. *Cancer Treat Rep* 67:531–534, 1983.

86. Mitsuyasu RT, Groopman JE. Biology and therapy of Kaposi's sarcoma. *Semin Oncol* 11:53–59, 1984.

87. Mituyasu RT. Clinical variants and staging of Kaposi's sarcoma. *Semin Oncol* 14 (suppl 3):13–18, 1987.

88. Taylor J, Afrasiabi R, Fahey JL, et al. Prognostically significant classifica-

tion of immune changes in AIDS with Kaposi's sarcoma. *Blood* 67:666–671, 1986.

89. Krown SE, Metroka C, Werntz JC, AIDS Clinical Trials Group Oncology Committee. Kaposi's sarcoma in the acquired immune deficiency syndrome: A proposal for uniform evaluation, response and staging criteria. *J Clin Oncol* 7:1201–1207, 1989.

90. Bonhomme L, Fredj G, Averous S, et al. Topical treatment of epidemic Kaposi's sarcoma with all-*trans*-retinoic acid. *Ann Oncol* 2:234, 1991.

91. Conant MA, Galzagorry G, Illeman M. Intralesional vinblastine (Velban) treatment of lesions of Kaposi's sarcoma (abstract). Fifth International Conference on AIDS, Montreal, June 1989.

92. Epstein J, Lozade-Nur F, McLeod WA, et al. Oral Kaposi's sarcoma in AIDS: Management with intralesional chemotherapy (abstract). Fifth International Conference on AIDS, Montreal, June 1989.

93. Chak LK, Gill PS, Levine AM, et al. Radiation therapy for acquired immunodeficiency syndrome–related Kaposi's sarcoma. *J Clin Oncol* 6:863–867, 1988.

94. Harris JW, Reed TA. Kaposi's Sarcoma in AIDS: The Role of Radiation Therapy. In JM Veath (ed), *Frontiers of Radiation Therapy and Oncology*. Basel: Karger, 1985. Pp 126–132.

95. Quivey JM, Wara WM, Berson AM. Radiotherapy for the treatment of AIDS-related Kaposi's sarcoma: An updated analysis (abstract). Sixth International Conference on AIDS, San Francisco, June 1990.

96. Epstein JB, Lozada-Nur F, McLeod A, Spinelli J. Oral Kaposi's sarcoma in acquired immunodeficiency syndrome. *Cancer* 64:2424–2430, 1989.

97. Cooper JS, Fried PR, Laubenstein LJ. Initial observations of the effect of radiotherapy on epidemic Kaposi's sarcoma. *JAMA* 252:934–935, 1984.

98. Cheeseman SH, Rubin RH, Stewart JA, et al. Controlled clinical trial of prophylactic human-leukocyte interferon in renal transplantation: Effects on cytomegalovirus and herpes simplex viral infections. *N Engl J Med* 300:1345, 1979.

99. Borden EC, Ball LA. Interferons: Biological, cell growth inhibitory and immunological effects. *Prog Hematol* 12:299–339, 1981.

100. Borden EC, Hogan T, Voelkel JG. Comparative antiproliferative activity in vitro of natural interferons alpha and beta for diploid and transformed human cells. *Cancer Res* 42:4948–4953, 1982.

101. Sidky YA, Borden EC. Inhibition of angiogenesis by interferons. Effects on tumor and lymphocyte-induced vascular response. *Cancer Res* 47:5155–5161, 1987.

102. Krown SE. The role of interferon in the therapy of epidemic Kaposi's sarcoma. *Semin Oncol* 14 (suppl 3):27–33, 1987.

103. Krown SE. Interferon and other biologic agents for the treatment of Kaposi's sarcoma. *Hematol Oncol Clin North Am* 5:311–322, 1991.

104. Groopman JE, Scadden DT. Interferon therapy for Kaposi's sarcoma associated with the acquired immunodeficiency syndrome (AIDS). *Ann Intern Med* 110:335–337, 1989.

105. Real FX, Oettgen HF, Krown SE. Kaposi's sarcoma and the acquired immunodeficiency syndrome. Treatment with high and low doses of recombinant leukocyte A interferon. *J Clin Oncol* 4:544–551, 1986.

106. Ho DD, Hartshorn KL, Rota TR, et al. Recombinant human interferon alpha-A suppresses HTLV-III replication in-vitro. *Lancet* 1:602–604, 1985.
107. Lane HC, Kovacs JA, Feinberg J, et al. Antiretroviral effects of interferon-alpha in AIDS-associated Kaposi's sarcoma. *Lancet* 2:1218–1222, 1988.
108. Hartshorn KL, Vogt MW, Chou TC, et al. Synergistic inhibition of human immunodeficiency virus in vitro by azidothymidine and recombinant alpha A interferon. *Antimicrob Agents Chemother* 31:168–172, 1987.
109. de Wit R, Reiss P, Bakker RJM, et al. Lack of activity of zidovudine in AIDS-associated Kaposi's sarcoma. *AIDS* 3:847–850, 1989.
110. Lane CH, Fallon T, Walker RE, et al. Zidovudine in patients with human immunodeficiency virus (HIV) infection and Kaposi's sarcoma. *Ann Intern Med* 111:41–50, 1989.
111. Krown SE, Gold TWM, Niedzwieck D, et al. Interferon-alpha with zidovudine: Safety, tolerance and clinical and virologic effects in patients with Kaposi's sarcoma associated with the acquired immunodeficiency syndrome (AIDS). *Ann Intern Med* 112:812–821, 1990.
112. Fischl MA. Antiretroviral therapy in combination with interferon for AIDS-related Kaposi's sarcoma. *Am J Med* 90 (suppl 4A):2S–8S, 1991.
113. Kovacs JA, Deyton L, Davey R, et al. Combined zidovudine and interferon-alpha therapy in patients with Kaposi's sarcoma and the acquired immunodeficiency syndrome (AIDS). *Ann Intern Med* 111:280–287, 1989.
114. Krown SE, Paredes J, Bundow D, et al. Interferon-alpha, zidovudine, and granulocyte-macrophage colony-stimulating factor: A phase I AIDS Clinical Trials Group study in patients with Kaposi's sarcoma associated with AIDS. *J Clin Oncol* 10:1344–1351, 1992.
115. Scadden DT, Bering HA, Levine JD, et al. Granulocyte-macrophage colony-stimulating factor mitigates the neutropenia of combined interferon alpha and zidovudine treatment of acquired immunodeficiency syndrome–associated Kaposi's sarcoma. *J Clin Oncol* 9:802–808, 1991.
116. Miles SA, Wang H, Cortes J, et al. Beta-interferon therapy in patients with poor-prognosis Kaposi's sarcoma related to the acquired immunodeficiency syndrome (AIDS). *Ann Intern Med* 112:582–589, 1990.
117. Kriegel RL, Odajnyk CM, Laubenstein LH, et al. Therapeutic trial of interferon-gamma in patients with epidemic Kaposi's sarcoma. *J Biol Response Modif* 4:358–364, 1985.
118. Lane HC, Sherwin SA, Masur H, et al. A phase I trial of recombination immune gamma interferon in patients with the acquired immunodeficiency syndrome. *Clin Res* 33:407, 1985.
119. Volberding P, Moody DJ, Beardslee D, et al. Therapy of acquired immune deficiency syndrome with recombinant interleukin-2. *AIDS Res Hum Retroviruses* 3:115–124, 1987.
120. Krigel RL, Padavic SK, Rudolph AR, et al. Exacerbation of epidemic Kaposi's sarcoma with a combination of interleukin-2 and beta-interferon: Results of a phase 2 study. *J Biol Response Modif* 8:359–365, 1989.
121. te Velde AA, Hiijbens RJF, Heige K, et al. Interleukin-4 (IL-4) inhibits secretion of IL-1 beta, tumor necrosis factor alpha, and IL-6 by human monocytes. *Blood* 76:1392–1397, 1990.
122. Gill PS, Akil B, Colletti P, et al. Pulmonary Kaposi's sarcoma: Clinical findings and results of therapy. *Am J Med* 87:57–61, 1989.

123. Gill PS, Rarick M, McCutchan JA, et al. Systemic treatment of AIDS-related Kaposi's sarcoma: Results of a randomized trial. *Am J Med* 90:427–433, 1991.

124. Fischl MA, Krown SE, Boyle KP, et al. Weekly doxorubicin in the treatment of patients with AIDS-related Kaposi's sarcoma. *J Acquir Immune Defic Syndr* 6:259–264, 1993.

125. Volberding PA, Abrams DI, Conant M, et al. Vinblastine therapy for Kaposi's sarcoma in the acquired immunodeficiency syndrome. *Ann Intern Med* 103:335–338, 1985.

126. Mintzer DM, Real FX, Jovino L, et al. Treatment of Kaposi's sarcoma and thrombocytopenia with vincristine in patients with acquired immunodeficiency syndrome. *Ann Intern Med* 102:200–202, 1985.

127. Lassoued K, Clauvel J-P, Katlama C, et al. Treatment of the acquired immune deficiency syndrome–related Kaposi's sarcoma with bleomycin as a single agent. *Cancer* 66:1869–1872, 1990.

128. Laubenstein LJ, Krigel RL, Odajnyk CM, et al. Treatment of Kaposi's sarcoma with etoposide or combination of doxorubicin, bleomycin, and vinblastine. *J Clin Oncol* 2:1115–1120, 1984.

129. Saville MW, Lietzau J, Wilson W, et al. A trial of paclitaxel (taxol) in patient with HIV-associated Kaposi's sarcoma (KS) (abstract). *Proc Am Soc Clin Oncol* 13:54, 1994.

130. Kaplan LD, Abrams D, Volberding PA. Treatment of Kaposi's sarcoma in acquired immunodeficiency syndrome with an alternating vincristine-vinblastine regimen. *Cancer Treat Rep* 70:1121, 1986.

131. Bogner JR, Kronawitter U, Rolinski K, et al. Liposomal doxorubicin in the treatment of advanced AIDS-related Kaposi sarcoma. *J Acquir Immune Defic Syndr* 7:463–468, 1994.

132. Presant CA, Scolaro M, Kennedy P, et al. Liposomal daunorubicin treatment of HIV-associated Kaposi's sarcoma. *Lancet* 341:1242–1243, 1993.

133. Gill PS, Rarick M, Bernstein-Singer M. Treatment of advanced KS using a combination of bleomycin and vincristine. *Am J Clin Oncol* 13:315–319, 1990.

134. Remick SC, Reddy M, Herman D, et al. Continuous infusion bleomycin in AIDS-related Kaposi's sarcoma. *J Clin Oncol* 12:1130–1136, 1994.

135. Gill PS, Rarick MU, Espira B, et al. Advanced acquired immunodeficiency syndrome–related Kaposi's sarcoma: Results of pilot studies using combination chemotherapy. *Cancer* 65:1074–1079, 1990.

136. Gill PS, Bernstein-Singer M, Espina BM, et al. Adriamycin, bleomycin and vincristine chemotherapy with recombinant granulocyte-macrophage colony-stimulating factor in the treatment of AIDS-related Kaposi's sarcoma. *AIDS* 6:1477–1481, 1992.

137. Ingber D, Fujita T, Kishimoto S, et al. Synthetic analogues of fumagillin that inhibit angiogenesis and suppress tumor growth. *Nature* 348:555–557, 1990.

138. Herbert JM, Cottineau M, Driot F, et al. Activity of pentosan polysulphate and derived compounds on vascular endothelial cell proliferation and migration induced by acidic and basic FGF *in vitro*. *Biochem Pharmacol* 37:4281, 1988.

139. Klein-Soyer C, Beretz A, Cazenave J-P, et al. Sulfated polysaccharides

modulate effects of acidic and basic fibroblast growth factors on repair of injured confluent human vascular endothelium. *Arteriosclerosis* 9:147–153, 1989.

140. Maione TE, Gray GS, Petro J, et al. Inhibition of angiogenesis by recombinant human platelet factor-4 and related peptides. *Science* 247:77–79, 1990.
141. Kusaka M, Sudo K, Fujita T, et al. Potent anti-angiogenic action of AGM-1470. Comparison to the fumagillin parent. *Biochem Biophys Res Commun* 174:1070–1076, 1991.
142. Saville MW, Foli A, Broder S, et al. *In vitro* activity of TNP-470, a novel angiogenesis inhibitor in Kaposi's sarcoma (KS)–related spindle cells. *J Cell Biochem Suppl* 17E:22, 1993.
143. Nakamura S, Sakurada SS, Salahuddin Z, et al. Inhibition of development of Kaposi's sarcoma–related lesions by a bacterial cell wall complex. *Science* 255:1437–1440, 1992.
144. Pluda JM, Shay LE, Foli A, et al. Administration of pentosan polysulfate to patients with human immunodeficiency virus-associated Kaposi's sarcoma. *J Natl Cancer Inst* 85:1585–1592, 1993.
145. Schwartsman G, Sander E, Prolla G, et al. Phase II trial of pentosan polysulfate (PPS) in patients with AIDS-related Kaposi's sarcoma. *Proc Am Soc Clin Oncol* 12:54, 1993.
146. Kahn J, Ruiz R, Kerschmann R, et al. A phase 1/2 study of recombinant platelet factor 4 (rPF4) in patients with AIDS related Kaposi's sarcoma (KS) (abstract). *Proc Am Soc Clin Oncol* 12:50, 1993.

AIDS-Related Lymphoma   *30*

Timothy P. Cooley

In 1985, the Centers for Disease Control included systemic high-grade, B-cell, non-Hodgkin's lymphoma (NHL) in HIV-infected patients as a criterion for the diagnosis of AIDS [1]. Currently, NHL develops in about 5 percent of AIDS patients during the course of their disease, generally as a late manifestation [2–4]. It is anticipated that the incidence of lymphoma in this population will continue to rise as HIV-infected patients live longer [3, 4]. Clinical data suggest that patients with symptomatic HIV infection who survive for 3 years on antiretroviral therapy have a high probability of developing NHL [3].

Pathogenesis

Non-Hodgkin's lymphoma has frequently been observed in association with abnormal cell-mediated immunity, such as that occurring with immunosuppressive therapy related to organ transplantation [5, 6]. Circumstantial evidence supports a role for Epstein-Barr virus (EBV) in the etiology of NHL in this setting [7]. Unlike transplant-associated lymphoma but similar to non-African Burkitt's lymphoma, EBV genomes are found in a minority of patients with HIV-related NHL [8]. The precise role of EBV in the development of NHL associated with HIV disease is uncertain.

Although the pathogenesis of HIV-related NHL remains unclear, some of its molecular characteristics have been identified. Chromosomal translocations have been observed in some individuals [9, 10]. These translocations may allow for deregulation of the c-*myc* oncogene, which has been implicated in the malignant transformation of B lymphocytes [11, 12]. The c-*myc* rearrangements in AIDS lymphoma tissue described by investigators are similar to those seen in Burkitt's lymphoma [8]; some researchers demonstrated this finding only in a minority of patients with HIV-related NHL [13, 14].

HIV does not appear to be directly involved in the development of NHL, as the virus is undetectable by Southern blot analysis within B-cell AIDS lymphoma tissue [13, 15, 16]. However, HIV may induce the polyclonal activation of B cells [17] and be involved in the production and release of cytokines and growth factors, such as interleukin-1, -6, and -10, which may stimulate both HIV replication and B-cell proliferation [18–22]. It is currently hypothesized that HIV-related NHL develops from chronic viral antigenic stimulation leading to increased proliferation of B lymphocytes and oncogene rearrangement resulting in malignant transformation [13–16].

Epidemiology

Since the beginning of the HIV epidemic, epidemiologic studies have demonstrated an increased frequency of NHL in a population at high risk for HIV infection: never-married men, aged 25 to 54 years, who live in communities with high AIDS-related mortality [23]. No such increase has been identified among men who have married or in women regardless of marital status. Although never-married men include some heterosexuals, it is assumed that most homosexual men at risk for HIV infection would be in this category.

While the majority of cases of NHL in North America have been identified in homosexual or bisexual men, the disease may occur in patients with any risk behavior [24]. Series from the University of Southern California (USC) and the University of California at San Francisco (UCSF) reported that more than 90 percent of their patients with NHL were male homosexuals [2, 25, 26]. In contrast, a study from New York University found that 19 percent of lymphoma cases occurred in patients with a history of injection drug use [27]. In Italy, 64 percent of patients with HIV-related NHL have a history of injection drug use [28]. Lymphoma has been reported in about 5 percent of HIV-infected hemophiliacs, with a 24- to 29-fold increased incidence compared to the expected rate [29, 30].

Clinical Manifestations

The majority of patients with HIV-related NHL have high-grade, B-cell lymphomas of either B-immunoblastic or small noncleaved type, which may be Burkitt or non-Burkitt variants [25, 31–35]. This pathologic spectrum is most unusual when compared to series of lymphomas before the AIDS epidemic, in which only 4 to 9 percent were of the B-immunoblastic type and 5 to 7 percent were of the small noncleaved type [35, 36].

Nearly all patients with HIV-related NHL present with wide-

spread disease, and 75 percent report constitutional symptoms [14].
The most characteristic clinical feature is the high frequency of
extranodal disease, which is found in up to 85 percent of patients,
compared to a 40 percent incidence in NHL not associated with HIV
disease [2, 5, 6, 26–28, 36–41]. Common sites of involvement include bone marrow (25%), central nervous system (CNS; 32%), gastrointestinal tract (26%), liver (12%), and kidney (9%) [26, 27, 37–41].
Unusual sites of extranodal disease, such as the myocardium and
popliteal fossa, have also been reported [23, 31]. Although primary CNS
lymphoma accounts for up to 25 percent of HIV-related NHL cases,
metastatic brain involvement is unusual in patients with systemic
lymphoma [42–45].

Diagnosis

Diagnosis is made by excisional lymph node biopsy or biopsy of
an involved extranodal site. Routine staging should also include computed tomography (CT) or magnetic resonance imaging (MRI) of
the head, chest, abdomen, and pelvis; gallium scan; lumbar puncture
with cytologic analysis of cerebrospinal fluid; and bone marrow examination. Gastrointestinal symptoms should be investigated
endoscopically.

Prognosis

In a review of patients followed at USC, shortened survival time was
associated with a Karnofsky performance status of less than 70 percent,
a diagnosis of AIDS before the appearance of NHL, and lymphomatous
involvement of bone marrow [40]. The poor prognosis group had a
median survival time of 4 months, compared to 11 months in the group
without these features. A similar analysis performed at UCSF showed
that the total CD4 cell count was the most important predictor of survival: Patients with counts of less than $100/mm^3$ had a median survival time of 4.5 months, compared to 24 months in patients with counts
higher than $100/mm^3$ [2]. Negative predictors of survival also included
a Karnofsky performance status of less than 70 percent and the presence of extranodal disease [2].

Management

Although aggressive combination chemotherapy for high-grade NHL
not associated with HIV disease may be very effective, treatment for
HIV-related NHL has been less successful. Early trials using standard

doses of chemotherapy with regimens, such as COMP (cyclophospha-mide, vincristine, methotrexate, and prednisone) [46], ProMACE-MOPP (prednisone, methotrexate with folinic acid rescue, doxorubicin, cyclo-phosphamide, etoposide, mechlorethamine [nitrogen mustard], vincristine, procarbazine, and prednisone) [47], high-dose cytosine arabinoside (ara-C) and methotrexate [48], and COMET-A (cyclophos-phamide, vincristine, methotrexate, etoposide, high-dose cytosine ara-binoside) [2], had extremely high rates of severe myelosuppression, major opportunistic and bacterial infections, and death. In addition, among patients who responded to therapy, there was a high incidence of CNS relapse [48].

A subsequent study sponsored by the AIDS Clinical Trials Group (ACTG) treated patients with low-dose m-BACOD (methotrexate, folinic acid, bleomycin, doxorubicin, vincristine, and dexamethasone), using CNS prophylaxis with intrathecal ara-C and zidovudine (ZDV) main-tenance after completion of chemotherapy. This regimen produced a complete response rate of 50 percent, with a durable effect in 75 per-cent of complete responders and no CNS relapses reported [49]. The median survival time was 6.5 months, with a median response dura-tion of 15 months among responders. Despite the modified doses of chemotherapy used, significant myelosuppression occurred in 60 per-cent of patients [49]. In a small phase I pilot study, the ACTG subse-quently evaluated the use of standard-dose m-BACOD with recombi-nant granulocyte-macrophage colony stimulating factor (GM-CSF). The regimen had tumor response rates and toxicity comparable to low-dose m-BACOD without evidence of increased HIV replication [50]. An ACTG trial comparing low-dose m-BACOD to standard-dose chemo-therapy with GM-CSF was recently completed in 194 patients [51]. Complete antitumor response was noted in 46% of patients receiving low-dose m-BACOD, with a median survival of 34 weeks, compared to a response rate of 50% and a median survival of 31 weeks in those receiving standard-dose m-BACOD. These differences were not statis-tically significant, and complete response duration was similar in the two treatment groups. The primary cause of death was lymphoma in 56% of patients on low-dose m-BACOD compared with 38% who re-ceived standard-dose m-BACOD. Although the rates of toxicity in the two treatment groups were similar, the severity of hematologic toxicity was greater in the group receiving standard-dose chemotherapy. Based on the results of this trial, current recommendations are to treat newly diagnosed HIV-related NHL with a low-dose chemotherapy regimen.

A randomized trial of CHOP (cyclophosphamide, doxorubicin, vincristine, and prednisone) with or without GM-CSF in 30 patients demonstrated that the severity and duration of neutropenia associated with chemotherapy were significantly reduced in patients who had received GM-CSF [52]. The overall complete response rate was 67 per-cent in both groups. However, in patients receiving GM-CSF, median p24 antigen levels more than doubled from baseline, suggesting stimulation of HIV replication.

The prognosis for patients with relapsing or refractory HIV-related lymphoma is extremely poor, with a median survival time of 2 to 4 months. Alternate chemotherapy regimens such as infusional CDE (cyclophosphamide, doxorubicin, and etoposide) [53] or oral LECP (lomustine, etoposide, cyclophosphamide, procarbazine) [54] are frequently given as salvage therapy, despite the lack of data supporting their use. A number of investigational drugs are also being evaluated in this setting. Methylglyoxal bisguanylhydrazone (MGBG) is an antimetabolite with good CNS penetration, relative lack of myelosuppression, and a long half-life. Investigators [55] reported a durable complete response rate of 14 percent, with mild toxicity consisting primarily of flushing, paresthesias, and nausea. A dose escalation study of anti–B4 (CD19) monoclonal antibody conjugated with ricin (anti–B4 blocked ricin; B4BR) recently reported a complete response rate of 10 percent, with toxicity consisting primarily of mild liver function test abnormalities [56]. Trials combining B4BR with standard chemotherapy regimens are underway.

Primary Central Nervous System Lymphoma

Primary CNS lymphoma accounts for up to 25 percent of HIV-related NHLs [32, 43–45, 57]. The prognosis is extremely poor, with a median survival time of less than 1 month from when the patient first seeks medical attention [43, 44]. The most common symptoms are headache, seizures, cranial nerve palsies, and hemiparesis [43, 44]. However, subtle personality changes and altered mental status may be the only abnormalities on presentation [43].

The clinical and radiologic manifestations of primary CNS lymphoma may be indistinguishable from those of CNS toxoplasmosis [43–45]. On CT and MRI scans, lymphomas appear as isodense or hyperdense space-occupying lesions showing contrast enhancement [44, 58] (see Fig. 17-4). In contrast to CNS toxoplasmosis, lymphomas generally appear as solitary lesions larger than 3 cm involving the cerebrum, cerebellum, basal ganglion, or pons, with varying degrees of edema and mass effect [44, 58]. Sites of lymphomatous involvement within the brain are varied, and any region may be affected [43, 44, 58, 59]. Cerebrospinal fluid abnormalities are found in only 15 to 25 percent of patients [43, 44]. A preliminary study suggested that polymerase chain reaction (PCR) testing of cerebrospinal fluid for EBV DNA may be diagnostically helpful [60], but definitive diagnosis requires brain biopsy [58]. The vast majority of primary CNS lymphomas have immunoblastic or large cell histology [40, 43, 61, 62], with most expressing EBV genomes [14, 61]. Unlike systemic HIV-related NHL, it is uncommon to find small noncleaved cells in primary CNS lymphoma [40, 43, 61, 62]. Standard therapy, which consists of whole-brain irradiation with 30 to 35 Gray (Gy) and a 10-Gy boost to the primary lesion, results in a complete response rate of 50 percent [53]. Despite treatment, the median survival time is short (5.5 months), with the majority of patients dying of opportunistic infections [57, 63].

Hodgkin's Disease

Hodgkin's disease (HD), particularly the mixed cellularity subtype, continues to be reported in HIV-infected patients, with an increased incidence found in homosexual men [64–68]. Hodgkin's disease in this setting is more aggressive than usual, often presenting as stage III or IV disease [64, 69]. There is a high incidence of bone marrow involvement, which is found at the time of diagnosis in 48 percent of HIV-infected patients with HD, compared to 3.5 percent of historical controls [69]. As in HIV-related NHL, other sites of extranodal disease are also common [69]. HIV-related HD is associated with a poor prognosis despite therapy with standard chemotherapeutic regimes such as MOPP (mechlorethamine [nitrogen mustard], vincristine, procarbazine, and prednisone) or ABVD (doxorubicin, bleomycin, vincristine, and dexamethasone) [69]. The survival rate of historical controls, 80 percent at 9 years, contrasts sharply with the 1-year survival rate of 30 percent in HIV-related HD [69, 70]. Poor prognosis appears more closely related to the development of opportunistic infections and profound myelosuppression than to uncontrolled HD [69].

References

1. Centers for Disease Control. Revision of the case definition of acquired immunodeficiency syndrome for national reporting: United States. *Ann Intern Med* 103:402–403, 1985.
2. Kaplan LD, Abrams DI, Feigal E, et al. AIDS associated non-Hodgkin's lymphoma in San Francisco. *JAMA* 261:719–724, 1989.
3. Pluda JM, et al. Development of non-Hodgkin's lymphoma in a cohort of patients with severe human immunodeficiency (HIV) infection on long-term antiretroviral therapy. *Ann Intern Med* 113:276–282, 1990.
4. Moore RD, Kessler H, Richman DD, et al. Non-Hodgkin's lymphoma in patients with advanced HIV infection treated with zidovudine (abstract). Seventh International Conference on AIDS, Florence, June 1991.
5. Hoover R, Fraumeni JF. Risk of cancer in renal transplant patients. *Lancet* 2:55–57, 1973.
6. Frizzera G, Rosai J, Delner LP, et al. Lymphoreticular disorders in primary immunodeficiencies: New finding based on an up-to-date histologic classification of 35 cases. *Cancer* 46:692–699, 1980.

7. Hanto DW, Frizzera G, Purtilo DT, et al. Clinical spectrum of lymphoproliferative disorders in renal transplant recipients and evidence for the role of Epstein Barr virus. *Cancer Res* 41:4253–4261, 1981.

8. Subar M, Neri A, Inghirami G, et al. Frequent c-myc oncogene activation and infrequent presence of Epstein-Barr virus genome in AIDS-associated lymphoma. *Blood* 72:667–671, 1988.

9. Gaidano G, Ballerini P, Gong JZ, et al. p53 Mutations in human lymphoid malignancies: Association with Burkitt lymphoma and chronic lymphocytic leukemia. *Proc Natl Acad Sci USA* 88:5413, 1991.

10. Whang-Peng J, Lee EC, Sieverts H, Magrath IT. Burkitts' lymphoma in AIDS: Cytogenetic study. *Blood* 63:818–822, 1984.

11. Lombardi L, Newcomb EW, Dalla-Favera R. Pathogenesis of Burkitt lymphoma: Expression of an activated c-myc oncogene causes the tumorigenic conversion of EBV infected human B lymphoblasts. *Cell* 49:161–170, 1987.

12. Adams JM, Harris AW, Pinkert CA, et al. The c-myc oncogene driven by immunoglobulin enhancers induces lymphoid malignancy in transgenic mice. *Nature* 318:533–538, 1985.

13. Pelicci PG, Knowles DM, II, Arlin ZA, et al. Multiple monoclonal B cell expansions and c-myc oncogene rearrangements in acquired immune deficiency syndrome–related lymphoproliferative disorders: Implications for lymphomagenesis. *J Exp Med* 164:2049–2060, 1986.

14. Meeker TC, Shiramizu B, Kaplan L, et al. Evidence for molecular subtypes of HIV-associated lymphoma: Division into peripheral monoclonal, polyclonal and central nervous system lymphoma. *AIDS* 5:669–674, 1991.

15. Groopman JE, Sullivan JL, Wong-Staal F, et al. Pathogenesis of B cell lymphoma in a patient with AIDS. *Blood* 67:612–615, 1986.

16. Rechavi G, Ben-Bassat M, Berkowicz M, et al. Molecular analysis of Burkitt's leukemia in two hemophiliac brothers with AIDS. *Blood* 70:1713–1717, 1987.

17. Schnittman SM, Lane HC, Higgins SE, et al. Direct polyclonal activation of human B lymphocytes by the AIDS virus. *Science* 233:1084–1086, 1986.

18. Paul WE. Interleukin 4/B cell stimulatory factor 1: One lymphokine, many functions. *FASEB J* 1:456–461, 1987.

19. Jelinek DF, Lipsky PE. Enhancement of human B cell proliferation and differentiation by tumor necrosis factor-alpha and interleukin 1. *J Immunol* 139:2970–2976, 1987.

20. Jelinek DF, Splawski JB, Lipsky PE. The roles of interleukin-2 and interferon-gamma in human B cell activation, growth and differentiation. *Eur J Immunol* 16:925–932, 1986.

21. Saeland S, Duvert V, Pandraw D, et al. Interleukin-7 induces the proliferation of normal human B cell precursors. *Blood* 78:2229–2238, 1991.

22. Zlotnik A, Morre KW. Interleukin 10. *Cytokine* 3:366–371, 1991.

23. Kristal AR, Nasca PC, Burkett WS, Mikl J. Changes in the epidemiology of non-Hodgkin's lymphoma associated with epidemic human immunodeficiency virus (HIV) infection. *Am J Epidemiol* 128:711–718, 1988.

24. Levine AM. Reactive and Neoplastic Lymphoproliferative Disorders with HIV Infection. In VT DeVita, S Hellman, SA Rosenberg (eds), *AIDS: Etiology, Diagnosis, Treatment and Prevention*. Philadelphia: Lippincott, 1988.

Pp 263–275.

25. Levine AM, Meyer PR, Begandy MK, et al. Development of B-cell lymphoma in homosexual men: Clinical and immunologic findings. *Ann Intern Med* 100:7, 1984.

26. Levine AM, Gill PS, Meyer PR, et al. Retrovirus and malignant lymphoma in homosexual men. *JAMA* 254:1921, 1985.

27. Knowles DM, Chamulak GA, Subar M, et al. Lymphoid neoplasia associated with the acquired immunodeficiency syndrome (AIDS). *Ann Intern Med* 108:744–753, 1988.

28. Monfardini S, Vaccher E, Foa R, et al. AIDS associated non Hodgkin's lymphoma in Italy: Intravenous drug users versus homosexual men. *Ann Oncol* 1:203–211, 1990.

29. Rabin CS, et al. Incidence of lymphomas and other cancers in HIV-infected and HIV-uninfected patients with hemophilia. *JAMA* 267:1090–1094, 1992.

30. Ragni MV, Belle SH, Jaffe RA, et al. Acquired immunodeficiency syndrome–associated non-Hodgkin's lymphoma and other malignancies in patients with hemophilia. *Blood* 81:1889–1897, 1993.

31. Levine AM, Gill PS. AIDS-related malignant lymphoma: Clinical presentation and treatment approaches. *Oncology* 1:41–46, 1987.

32. Ziegler JL, Beckstead JA, Volberding PA, et al. Non-Hodgkin's lymphoma in 90 homosexual men. *N Engl J Med* 311:565–570, 1984.

33. Lukes RJ, Collins RD. Immunologic characterization of human malignant lymphoma. *Cancer* 34:1488, 1974.

34. Non-Hodgkin's Lymphoma Pathologic Classification Project: National Cancer Institute sponsored study of classifications of non-Hodgkin's lymphomas: Summary and description of a working formulation for clinical usage. *Cancer* 49:2112, 1982.

35. Lukes RJ, Parker JW, Taylor CR, et al. Immunologic approach to non-Hodgkin's lymphomas and related leukemias: Analysis of results of multiparameter studies of 425 cases. *Semin Hematol* 15:322–351, 1978.

36. Bermudez MA, Grant KM, Rodvien R, Mendes F. Non-Hodgkin's lymphoma in a population with or at risk for acquired immunodeficiency syndrome: Indications for intensive chemotherapy. *Am J Med* 86:71–76, 1989.

37. Gill PS, Levine AM, Krailo M, et al. AIDS-related malignant lymphoma: Results of prospective treatment trials. *J Clin Oncol* 5:1322, 1987.

38. Kalter SP, Riggs SA, Cabanillas F, et al. Aggressive non-Hodgkin's lymphomas in immunocompromised homosexual males. *Blood* 66:655–659, 1985.

39. Kaplan MH, Susin M, Pahwa SG, et al. Neoplastic complications of HTLV-III infection: Lymphomas and solid tumors. *Am J Med* 82:389–396, 1987.

40. Levine AM, Sullivan-Halley J, Pike MC, et al. HIV-related lymphoma: Prognostic factors predictive of survival. *Cancer* 68:2466–2472, 1991.

41. Lowenthal DA, Straus DJ, Campbell SW, et al. AIDS-related lymphoid neoplasia: The Memorial Hospital Experience. *Cancer* 61:2325–2337, 1988.

42. Jones SE, Faks Z, Bullm M, et al. Non-Hodgkin's lymphoma IV. Clinico-pathologic correlation of 405 cases. *Cancer* 31:806–823, 1973.

43. Gill PS, Levine MA, Meyer PR, et al. Primary CNS lymphoma in homo-

sexual men: Clinical, immunologic, and pathologic features. *Am J Med* 78:742–748, 1985.

44. So YT, Beckstead JH, Davis RL. Primary central nervous system lymphoma in acquired immunodeficiency syndrome: A clinical and pathologic study. *Ann Neurol* 20:556–572, 1986.
45. Rosenblum ML, Levy RM, Bredesen DE, et al. Primary central nervous system lymphomas in patients with AIDS. *Ann Neurol* 23 (suppl):S13–S16, 1988.
46. Odajynk C, Subar M, Dugan M, et al. Clinical features and correlates with immunopathology and molecular biology of a large group of patients with AIDS associated small noncleaved lymphoma (SNCL) (abstract). *Blood* 68:131A, 1986.
47. Dugan M, Subar M, Odajynk C, et al. Intensive multiagent chemotherapy for AIDS related diffuse large cell lymphoma (abstract). *Blood* 68:124A, 1986.
48. Gill PS, Levine AM, Krailo M, et al. AIDS-related malignant lymphoma: Results of prospective trials. *J Clin Oncol* 5:1322–1388, 1987.
49. Levine AM, Wernz JC, Kaplan LD, et al. Low dose chemotherapy with central nervous system prophylaxis and azidothymidine maintenance in AIDS-related lymphoma: A prospective multi-institutional trial. *JAMA* 266:84–88, 1991.
50. Walsh D, Wernt T, Laubenstein L, et al. Phase I study of m-BACOD with GM-CSF in AIDS-associated non-Hodgkin's lymphoma. *J Acquir Immune Defic Syndr* 6:265–271, 1993.
51. Executive summary: Abstract ACTG 142. A Phase III randomized trial of low-dose versus standard-dose m-BACOD chemotherapy with rGM-CSR for treatment of AIDS-associated non-Hodgkin's lymphoma. Washington, DC: National Institute of Allergy and Infectious Diseases, 1995.
52. Kaplan LD, Kahn JO, Crowe S, et al. Clinical and virologic effects of recombinant human granulocyte-macrophage colony stimulating factor in patients receiving chemotherapy for human immunodeficiency virus-associated non-Hodgkin's lymphoma: Results of a randomized trial. *J Clin Oncol* 9:929–940, 1991.
53. Sparano JA, et al. Infusional cyclophosphamide, doxorubicin and etoposide in human immunodeficiency virus- and human T-cell leukemia virus type I-related non-Hodgkin's lymphoma: a highly active regimen. *Blood* 81:2810–2815, 1993.
54. Remick SC, et al. Novel oral combination chemotherapy in the treatment of intermediate-grade and high-grade AIDS-related non-Hodgkin's lymphoma. *J Clin Oncol* 11:1691–1702, 1993.
55. Levine AM, Weiss G, Tulpule A, et al. MGBG: A highly active drug in relapse or refractory AIDS-lymphoma (abstract). *Proc Am Soc Clin Oncol* 13:52, 1994.
56. Tulpule A, Anderson LJJ, Levine AM, et al. Anti-B4 (CD 19) monoclonal antibody, conjugated with ricin (B4-blocked ricin: B4BR) in refractory AIDS-lymphoma. *Proc Am Soc Clin Oncol* 13:52, 1994.
57. Formenti SC, Gill PS, Lean E, et al. Primary central nervous system lymphoma in AIDS. *Cancer* 63:1101–1107, 1989.
58. Gill PS, Graham RA, Boswell W, et al. A comparison of imaging, clinical

and pathologic aspects of space occupying lesions within the brain in patients with acquired immunodeficiency syndrome. *Am J Physiol Imaging* 1:134–139, 1986.

59. Ciricillo SF, Rosenblum ML. Use of CT and MR imaging to distinguish intracranial lesions and to define the need for biopsy in AIDS patients. *J Neurosurg* 73:720–724, 1990.

60. Cinque P, et al. Epstein-Barr virus DNA in cerebrospinal fluid from patients with AIDS-related primary lymphoma of the central nervous system. *Lancet* 342:398–401, 1993.

61. McMahon EM, Glass JD, Hayward SD, et al. Epstein-Barr virus in AIDS-related primary central nervous system lymphoma. *Lancet* 338:969–973, 1991.

62. Goldstein JD, Dickson DW, Moser FG, et al. Primary central nervous system lymphoma in acquired immunodeficiency syndrome: A clinical and pathologic study with results of treatment with radiation. *Cancer* 67:2503–2508, 1991.

63. Baumgartner JE, Rachlin JR, Beckstead JH, et al. Primary central nervous system lymphomas: Natural history and response to radiation therapy in 55 patients with acquired immunodeficiency syndrome. *J Neurosurg* 73:206–211, 1990.

64. Baer D, Anderson ET, Wilkinson LS. Acquired immunodeficiency syndrome in homosexual men with Hodgkin's disease. *Am J Med* 80:738–740, 1986.

65. Unger PD, Stranchen JA. Hodgkin's disease in AIDS-related complex patients. *Cancer* 58:821–825, 1986.

66. Roithmann S, Toledano M, Tourani JM, Andrieu JM. HIV-associated lymphomas (HAL): Report of 160 cases from France (abstract). Sixth International Conference on AIDS, San Francisco, June 1990.

67. Tirelli U, Carbone A, Monfardini S, et al. Malignant tumors in patients with immunodeficiency virus infection: A report of 580 cases. *J Clin Oncol* 7:1582–1583, 1989.

68. Hessol NA, Katz MH, Liu JY, et al. Increased incidence of Hodgkin disease in homosexual men with HIV infection. *Ann Intern Med* 117:309–311, 1992.

69. Ames ED, Conjalka MS, Goldberg AF, et al. Hodgkin's disease and AIDS: Twenty-three new cases and a review of the literature. *Hematol Oncol Clin North Am* 5:343–356, 1991.

70. Colby TV, Hoppe RT, Warnke RA. Hodgkin's disease: A clinicopathologic study of 659 cases. *Cancer* 49:1848–1858, 1981.

Special Topics   IV

Antiretroviral Therapy   *31*

Kevan L. Hartshorn, Timothy P. Cooley

Specific therapy to control viral replication has become a cornerstone in the management of HIV-infected patients. Antiretroviral therapy is undergoing continual evolution, and current recommendations will clearly change over time. Currently, four drugs are approved by the Food and Drug Administration (FDA) for the treatment of HIV infection: zidovudine (ZDV, formerly azidothymidine [AZT]), didanosine (ddI), zalcitabine (formerly dideoxycytidine [ddC]), and stavudine (d4T). Zidovudine has been shown to slow HIV disease progression and enhance survival and is recommended as initial therapy in most patients. Didanosine has been approved in patients who have been on prolonged ZDV therapy, who are intolerant to ZDV, or who have clinical or immunologic evidence of disease progression on ZDV. Zalcitabine is recommended for use alone or in combination with ZDV in patients with advanced HIV disease. Stavudine has been approved for the treatment of patients with advanced HIV disease who have failed or are intolerant to other approved therapies. Lamivudine (3TC), a cytosine analogue, is in clinical trials at this time, as is a promising new class of drugs called protease inhibitors. This chapter reviews these agents and discusses the direction of current research. In addition, a comprehensive strategy for antiretroviral therapy is presented.

Zidovudine

Mechanism of Action and Pharmacology

Zidovudine is a thymidine analogue utilized by retroviral reverse transcriptases, leading to premature termination of the HIV DNA chain [1]. Mammalian DNA polymerases apparently have greater ability to detect and remove the aberrant nucleotide, accounting for the relatively specific effect of ZDV on viral replication. Zidovudine must be converted into a triphosphate derivative in the host cell before it can become incorporated into DNA. The active antiviral compound is not ZDV itself but rather its triphosphate derivative. Pharmacologically, ZDV has the advantages of high oral bioavailability and central nervous system penetration due to lipid solubility. The serum half-life is approximately 1 hour. Trough levels achieved with every 4-hour administration exceed the concentration shown to inhibit HIV replication in vitro. The drug is metabolized principally by glucuronidation in the liver, with a lesser contribution (25%) from direct renal excretion of the active compound. The hepatic metabolite is also handled by the kidney, and marked accumulation occurs with renal failure [2]. Both ZDV and its hepatic metabolite are incompletely removed by dialysis, and probenecid decreases ZDV excretion substantially, probably by its effect on liver glucuronidation and renal excretion.

Clinical Effects

Clinical benefits of ZDV have been documented with respect to survival, immunologic status and incidence of opportunistic infections, neurologic status, HIV-related immune thrombocytopenic purpura (ITP), and decreased vertical transmission.

Zidovudine has been shown to lengthen survival in persons with AIDS or advanced AIDS-related complex (ARC), although this benefit may diminish over time [3]. Zidovudine (250 mg orally every 4 hours) was given in a randomized, placebo-controlled trial involving 160 AIDS patients recently recovered from *Pneumocystis carinii* pneumonia (PCP) and 122 ARC patients considered at high risk for development of AIDS [4]. Despite the relatively short (6 months) duration of the initial trial, a marked improvement in survival was noted in both AIDS and ARC patients who received ZDV; overall, 1 death occurred in the ZDV group, compared to 19 in the placebo group. A significant decrease in the incidence and severity of opportunistic infections was noted in the ZDV group as well. Improved performance status and weight gain were observed, as were increased CD4 lymphocyte counts and regained skin test reactivity. The ZDV-treated ARC group was noted to have a more sustained rise in CD4 counts and greater clinical benefit than the AIDS group.

A substantially larger number of subjects (4,805) with AIDS diagnosed on the basis of prior PCP received ZDV as part of a compassionate-use protocol before drug licensure [5]. A 73 percent survival rate was noted at 44 weeks, which was significantly higher than that of historical controls. In this study, delay in the onset of ZDV therapy after AIDS diagnosis and lower pretreatment performance status were associated with poorer clinical outcome.

Since these early studies, the clinical indications for ZDV have been expanded and refined. In AIDS Clinical Trials Group (ACTG) protocol 002, 524 patients with prior PCP were randomized to treatment with 250 mg of ZDV orally every 4 hours or 200 mg every 4 hours for 4 weeks followed by 100 mg every 4 hours for the remainder of the study [6]. After a median of 2 years of follow-up evaluation, improved survival and reduced rates of neutropenia and anemia were noted in the low-dose group. The effects on CD4 counts and p24 viral antigen levels were similar in both groups. Other studies confirmed the finding that lower-dose ZDV is as effective as and less toxic than the high-dose regimen in advanced HIV disease [7]. Based on these studies, ZDV at a dose of 200 mg three times a day has been recommended for previously untreated persons with symptomatic HIV infection or AIDS.

There is currently no evidence of benefit from ZDV treatment in asymptomatic people with CD4 counts higher than $500/mm^3$. Three placebo-controlled studies evaluated the efficacy of ZDV monotherapy in this population. The European-Australian Collaborative Group enrolled subjects with CD4 counts higher than $400/mm^3$ and randomized them to receive ZDV (1000 mg per day) or placebo [8]. The authors concluded that people treated with ZDV developed fewer early HIV-related complications than did the placebo group, but that progression to ARC or AIDS and survival were not significantly different. The Anglo-French Concorde study [9] included asymptomatic people with CD4 cell counts higher than $500/mm^3$ and found no difference in survival between immediate and deferred treatment with ZDV at a dose of 1000 mg per day. Among persons with CD4 counts higher than $500/mm^3$ enrolled in the ACTG 019 study [10, 11], those randomized to both the low-dose (500 mg per day) and high-dose (1500 mg per day) ZDV arms showed a delay in CD4 cell count decline compared to placebo control subjects. However, no significant differences in progression to ARC or AIDS or survival were identified.

Whether asymptomatic people with CD4 counts between 200 and $500/mm^3$ should be started on ZDV is more controversial. Three large trials evaluated the effect of ZDV compared to placebo in asymptomatic persons with CD4 counts in this range. The ACTG 019 study demonstrated a delay in progression to symptomatic HIV disease but no survival difference between treatment groups [12, 13]. The Concorde trial showed no difference in disease progression or survival [9]. A large observational study by the Multicenter AIDS Cohort Study (MACS) reported a survival advantage for subjects with CD4 counts between 200 and $350/mm^3$ who were treated with ZDV [14, 15]. A detailed quality of life evaluation among study participants in ACTG 019 revealed that adverse events related to ZDV treatment virtually negated any beneficial effect of the medication as compared to placebo [16]. Based on the results of these studies, a National Institutes of Allergy and Infectious Diseases (NIAID) expert panel recommended that treatment for asymptomatic persons with CD4 cell counts of 200 to $500/mm^3$ be individualized, as there is no compelling medical indication to begin ZDV in this setting [17]. Patient preference and other factors, such as the development of symptoms or a significant decline in CD4 count, should guide the decision of whether to start ZDV or monitor the patient off antiretroviral therapy.

For symptomatic patients with CD4 counts between 200 and 500/mm^3, ZDV treatment is recommended based on two placebo-controlled studies, ACTG 016 [18] and the Veterans Affairs Cooperative Study [19], demonstrating a delay in progression to ARC or AIDS. No survival difference was found between treatment groups in either study. At the currently recommended dosage of ZDV, toxicities of therapy are relatively mild in this population (see below). Hence, the benefits in terms of delayed progression of disease and improvement of symptoms generally outweigh the adverse effects of ZDV.

Clinical benefits of ZDV have not been confined to enhancement of immunologic function and general health status. In the original placebo-controlled trial, a subset of patients was studied with respect to cognitive function, and significant improvement was noted in the ZDV group, especially among those with AIDS [4]. Two prospective studies of ZDV in patients with HIV dementia also demonstrated benefit [20, 21]. Three reports showed a positive effect on platelet counts in individuals with HIV-related thrombocytopenia [22–24]. Despite an earlier report that ZDV therapy may not significantly benefit some minorities, recent studies indicate that the medication appears to be effective in women, blacks, Latinos, and injection drug users [25–27].

Zidovudine crosses the placenta and reaches adequate levels in the fetus [28]. Recent results from ACTG 076, a large, randomized placebo-controlled study in HIV-infected pregnant women, showed that antepartum and intrapartum administration of ZDV followed by 6 weeks of ZDV to newborn infants reduced the incidence risk of vertical transmission by two-thirds compared to control subjects (8.3 vs. 25.5%) [29]. The only significant toxicity was decreased hemoglobin in the neonates. As a result of this study, the FDA approved the use of ZDV in pregnancy, with the following dosing recommendations: antepartum—ZDV, 200 mg three times daily to start after gestational age of 14 weeks; intrapartum—ZDV, 2 mg/kg intravenous loading dose followed by continuous intravenous infusion at 1 mg/kg/hr until delivery; and newborn—ZDV syrup, 2 mg/kg every 6 hours for 6 weeks beginning 8 to 12 hours after birth.

The prophylactic use of ZDV after accidental needlestick or mucous membrane exposure to HIV-infected blood is controversial. Despite the absence of data supporting its use in this setting, prophylaxis with ZDV, 200 mg every 4 hours for 28 to 42 days, is offered at many institutions [30].

Toxicity

In general, ZDV is well tolerated. The most frequent complaint among subjects receiving ZDV in clinical trials has been nausea, occurring in 3 to 10 percent. Headaches, insomnia, rash, and malaise have been described as well, although similar rates of these symptoms were observed in placebo groups. One case of Stevens-Johnson syndrome thought to be related to ZDV has been reported [5]. Seizure activity and a single case of lethal neurotoxicity have been attributed to ZDV [5, 31, 32]. Two cases of ZDV overdose have been described, both of which had minimal sequelae [33, 34].

The most common and troublesome toxicities of ZDV are hematologic, notably anemia and neutropenia. In the original randomized trial, anemia occurred significantly more frequently in ZDV recipients, with 21 percent becoming transfusion dependent compared to 4 percent in the placebo group. Neutropenia was described in 16 percent of ZDV recipients compared to 2 percent of those receiving placebo [4]. Another report confirmed that severe, prolonged marrow hypoplasia may result from ZDV therapy [35]. This effect should be distinguished from the nearly universal development of macrocytosis and megaloblastic erythroid changes in the bone marrow, which generally do not portend hematologic deterioration.

The use of lower doses of ZDV has reduced the frequency of hematologic toxicity (Table 31-1). In addition, it has also become clear that HIV-infected patients with minimal symptoms and CD4 cell counts higher than $200/mm^3$ have a substantially reduced incidence of anemia and neutropenia. Despite earlier concerns regarding coadministration of acetaminophen with ZDV, the analgesic does not appear to affect significantly either ZDV clearance or production of its glucuronide conjugate [36].

Recombinant erythropoietin and granulocyte-macrophage colony stimulating factor (GM-CSF) have been demonstrated to ameliorate, respectively, the anemia and the neutropenia associated with ZDV administration [37–40]. Daily subcutaneous erythropoietin has been shown to reduce the transfusion requirement of severely anemic ZDV-treated patients with serum erythropoietin levels of less than 500 mU/ml. Granulocyte colony stimulating factor (G-CSF), unlike GM-CSF, does not appear to enhance HIV replication and, therefore, is generally the

Table 31-1 *Incidence of anemia[a] and neutropenia[b] in ZDV recipients*

HIV disease stage	Incidence by ZDV dosage (% of patients)			
	High dose		Low dose	
	Anemia	Neutropenia	Anemia	Neutropenia
AIDS	39	51	29	37
Symptomatic, not AIDS	5	4		
Asymptomatic	6	6	1	2

[a]Anemia = hemoglobin < 8 gm/dl.
[b]Neutropenia = neutrophil count < $750/mm^3$.
Source: Data from [6, 8, 9, 35].

preferred agent for management of neutropenia [41]. Chemotherapy and other drug treatment, such as trimethoprim-sulfamethoxazole or ganciclovir, may necessitate interruption of ZDV therapy. Table 31-2 presents options for managing hematologic intolerance associated with ZDV administration.

Other adverse events attributable to ZDV include generalized myopathy, cardiomyopathy, and cholestatic hepatitis [42–44]. The incidence of myopathy related to ZDV appears to be highest among patients who received the drug for 12 months, occurring in 1 to 2 percent of those with early HIV infection [39]. Zidovudine myopathy, which manifests as proximal muscle weakness with an increased level of serum creatine phosphokinase (CPK), is sometimes severe. Nonsteroidal anti-inflammatory agents often improve symptoms, but discontinuation of ZDV or institution of corticosteroid therapy, or both, may be necessary. Histologic examination reveals abnormalities in muscle mitochondria, perhaps resulting from ZDV-induced inhibition of gamma-DNA polymerase, which can be differentiated from the immune-mediated myopathy related to HIV infection itself [45].

Viral resistance to ZDV has been described in patients who have received the drug for 6 months or more [46]. In one study, 93 percent of viral isolates from patients on ZDV for 3 years or more were resistant [47]. While the clinical significance of this finding is still being investigated, it appears to correlate independently with HIV disease progression [48–49a]. Syncytium-inducing phenotypes of HIV may also affect the course of disease [50]. Resistance to ZDV does not, in general, extend to the dideoxynucleosides, ddI or ddC, suggesting that switching to a regimen containing one of these agents might be beneficial after several months to a year of treatment with ZDV. Patients with symptomatic HIV infection receiving ZDV who survive for an extended period of time appear to be at increased risk for development of non-Hodgkin's lymphoma [51]. Whether this trend is related to immunosuppression itself or antiretroviral therapy is uncertain.

Table 31-2 *Management options for patients with ZDV intolerance*

Type of intolerance[a]	Treatment options[b]
Anemia requiring transfusion	Administer erythropoietin or change to ddI, ddC, or d4T
Neutropenia	Administer G-CSF, or change to ddI, ddC, or d4T
Nonhematologic	Change to ddI, ddC, or d4T

[a]Whether due to ZDV per se or to the concurrent use of necessary myelosuppressive agents, such as ganciclovir or trimethoprim-sulfamethoxazole.
[b]Dose reduction of ZDV to 100 mg PO tid may ameliorate mild hematologic toxicity, but the clinical efficacy of this regimen is unproved.

Treatment Recommendations

The recommended dose of ZDV is 200 mg orally three times a day. The effects and toxicity of ZDV in the context of renal failure are not well documented, but a dose of 100 mg orally three times a day has been proposed for patients undergoing dialysis [52]. The frequency of follow-up evaluation depends on the stage of HIV disease and preexisting hematologic abnormalities. The annual cost of ZDV therapy is approximately $3,200. An indigent patient assistance program is available through the Burroughs Wellcome Company (telephone: 1-800-722-9294).

Didanosine

Mechanism of Action and Pharmacology

The mechanism of action of ddI is similar to that of ZDV [1]. Didanosine is converted into dideoxyadenosine (ddA), which is then phosphorylated to form the active compound ddATP. Since this nucleotide lacks a hydroxyl group in the 3' position, it, like ZDV and ddC, results in HIV reverse transcriptase inhibition and viral DNA chain termination. Renal handling of ddI accounts for about 50 percent of total body clearance. It is not yet clear what effect renal or hepatic dysfunction has on the toxicology of ddI, and current recommendations include a proviso that dose reductions should be considered in these settings.

Clinical Effects

Three phase I studies of ddI have now been completed [53–55]. The agent was shown to have anti-HIV activity in vivo, to increase CD4 cell counts, and to have early clinical benefit when administered orally once or twice a day. Didanosine appears to be free of hematologic toxicity and was associated with a significant increase in hemoglobin level in one trial [54].

Kahn and coworkers [56] reported the results of ACTG 116B/117, in which the role of ddI in patients with advanced HIV disease who had previously been treated with ZDV was evaluated. This multicenter, double-blind study involved 913 subjects who had received ZDV for at least 16 weeks. Participants had AIDS, ARC with CD4 counts of 300/mm³ or less, or asymptomatic HIV infection with CD4 counts of 200/mm³ or less. Subjects were randomly assigned to receive ZDV, 600 mg per day; ddI, 750 mg per day; or ddI, 500 mg per day. After a mean follow-up period of 55 weeks, significantly more new AIDS-defining events occurred in the ZDV group than in the 500-mg ddI group; death rates in the two groups were comparable. The efficacy of ddI was unrelated to the duration of previous ZDV therapy. Increases in CD4 cell count and decreases in p24 antigen level were more pronounced in both ddI groups than in patients who continued to receive ZDV. Similar results were reported by Spruance and colleagues [57]. Hence, changing from ZDV to ddI is a reasonable choice in patients previously treated with ZDV in whom there is significant disease progression or ZDV intolerance.

Data on the use of ddI as initial antiretroviral therapy are limited. Two large placebo-controlled studies compared ZDV and ddI as initial treatment in persons with CD4 counts less than $500/mm^3$. ACTG 116, which studied patients with CD4 counts less than $300/mm^3$, found the two drugs to be essentially equivalent [58]. In subset analyses, ZDV was more effective than ddI in persons with no history of ZDV therapy, while ddI was more effective among those who had previously received ZDV for as long as 4 months [58]. An Italian study [59] of people with ARC showed similar results.

Toxicity

The major dose-limiting toxicities of ddI are pancreatitis and peripheral neuropathy. Pancreatitis occurred in 9 percent of subjects in the phase I trials who were receiving the currently recommended dose of ddI. Didanosine-related pancreatitis can be fatal when not recognized promptly. If abdominal pain, nausea, vomiting, or a significantly increased serum amylase level occurs in association with ddI treatment, the drug should be discontinued pending full clinical assessment. The incidence of ddI-associated pancreatitis is higher (30%) in patients with a history of pancreatitis and in those with advanced HIV disease. Individuals with alcoholism, hypertriglyceridemia, or concurrent use of intravenous pentamidine may also be more prone to this complication. Peripheral neuropathy, characterized by numbness, tingling, and pain in the feet and hands, occurred in approximately 3 percent of subjects in phase I trials who were receiving the currently recommended dose of ddI. In the ACTG 116B/117 trial, neuropathy was no more frequent in the ddI group (approximately 14% incidence) than in the group receiving ZDV [56]. Neuropathic symptoms related to ddI are reversible if identified early, and evidence of significant neuropathy should prompt discontinuation of ddI therapy.

Other toxicities of ddI include increased serum uric acid level at higher doses, diarrhea (more frequent with the powder than the tablet preparation), and restlessness. One case of fatal hepatic failure related to ddI has been described [60]. Didanosine preparations contain acid-buffering components, and ketoconazole, dapsone, and ciprofloxacin, which require gastric acid for absorption, should not be taken within 2 hours of administration.

Drug resistance has been noted in HIV isolates from patients treated with ddI [61]. Didanosine resistance results from mutations in viral reverse transcriptase that differ from those conferring ZDV resistance.

Isolates of HIV with resistance to ddI have been described among patients who had discontinued ZDV for 6 to 12 months, as well as in those who had never received ZDV [61, 62]. An initial report suggested that the presence of a ddI resistance mutation in the context of ZDV resistance increased HIV sensitivity to ZDV [61]. A subsequent study demonstrated that the development of ddI resistance does not invariably attenuate ZDV resistance [62].

Treatment Recommendations

Didanosine is available in buffered 25- and 100-mg tablets, which must be chewed completely or predissolved in water, and powder form. It should be administered on an empty stomach and is dosed in adults according to body weight. In patients 60 kg or more, the dose is 200 mg orally twice a day in tablet form, or 250 mg orally twice a day of powder dissolved in 4 ounces of water. In patients less than 60 kg, the dose is 125 mg orally twice a day in tablet form, or 167 mg orally twice a day of powder dissolved in 4 ounces of water. The approximate annual cost of ddI is $2,200. Bristol-Myers Squibb offers an assistance program for uninsured patients (telephone: 1-800-426-7644).

Zalcitabine

Zalcitabine is another dideoxynucleotide that is the subject of active clinical investigation. Initial trials of this agent employed higher doses than are currently being studied or recommended, and a prohibitive incidence of painful, severe peripheral neuropathy was noted, despite significant antiretroviral effect and minimal hematologic toxicity [63]. Recent trials using lower doses showed that antiretroviral effect is preserved, with reduced neurotoxicity [64]. However, ddC does not penetrate into the spinal fluid as well as ZDV, which may limit its usefulness in the treatment of HIV-related encephalopathy.

Preliminary data from ACTG 114 indicate that ddC is inferior to ZDV as monotherapy in the initial treatment of HIV infection [65]. In a study of patients with advanced HIV disease who were receiving ZDV, switching to ddC was no more effective than continuing ZDV therapy [66]. Results from ACTG 155, a double-blind trial that randomized subjects with CD4 cell counts less than $300/mm^3$ and long-term ZDV use to receive ZDV, ddC, or ZDV with ddC indicated that ddC alone or in combination with ZDV did not confer an advantage over continuing ZDV [67]. However, subgroup analysis identified a 45 percent decrease in disease progression among people with entry CD4 counts of $150/mm^3$ or higher receiving combination therapy compared to those receiving ZDV alone [67]. An open-label trial comparing ddI with ddC after intolerance to ZDV found that ddI and ddC had equivalent efficacy [68]. These results suggest that the choice between ddC and ddI as monotherapy in this setting should be dictated by their side effect profiles [69]. Results of several small trials of ZDV combined with ddI or ddC revealed no pharmacokinetic interactions between these agents and indicated that, based on immunologic parameters, combination therapy may be superior to ZDV alone [70–72]. However, no clinical advantage of this regimen has been documented [9].

The recommended dose of ddC is 0.750 mg three times a day, whether as monotherapy or given in conjunction with ZDV. Its annual cost is approximately $2,600. Toxicities of ddC include peripheral neuropathy, gastrointestinal intolerance, and mucosal ulcerations. Hoffmann-LaRoche offers a patient assistance program (telephone: 1-800-526-6367).

Stavudine

Stavudine (2',3'-didehydro-3'-deoxythymidine or d4T) is a thymidine analogue that inhibits HIV replication in a manner similar to ZDV. A phase I study of d4T [73] determined a maximum tolerated dose of 2.0 mg/kg/day, with toxicities including painful peripheral neuropathy and asymptomatic increased hepatic transaminase levels. A subsequent parallel track program of HIV-infected patients with CD4 cell counts less than 300/mm³ who were intolerant to or had failed treatment with ZDV or ddI randomized subjects to receive a dose of either 10 mg or 20 mg twice daily. An intention-to-treat analysis demonstrated the same 40-week survival rate (79%) in the two groups [73]. An ongoing phase III randomized, double-blind trial compares d4T to ZDV in HIV-infected adults with CD4 cell counts of 50 to 500/mm³ and at least 6 months of prior ZDV treatment. An interim analysis of the study data demonstrated that after 12 weeks, there was a mean rise in CD4 counts of 20/mm³ among subjects in the d4T arm compared to a mean drop of 20/mm³ in the ZDV arm [74]. The incidence of peripheral neuropathy was higher in patients receiving d4T than in those taking ZDV (15 vs. 6%) [74]. To date, results from clinical trials of d4T have not demonstrated a delay in the clinical progression of HIV disease or improved survival. Long-term use of d4T has not been associated with the development of significant viral resistance [75].

The recommended dose of d4T is 40 mg twice daily for patients weighing 60 kg or more, and 30 mg twice daily for those less than 60 kg. Zidovudine may block activation of d4T and should not be given concurrently. The annual cost of d4T is approximately $2,750. Bristol-Myers Squibb offers a patient assistance program (telephone: 1-800-426-7644).

Lamivudine

Lamivudine (2'-deoxy-3'-thiacytidine or 3TC) is a cytosine analogue and reverse transcriptase inhibitor that is currently in clinical trial evaluation. Phase I studies of 3TC [76, 77] described toxicities, including neutropenia, macrocytosis without anemia, vasculitis, and peripheral neuropathy, but did not define a maximum tolerated dose. Transient increases in CD4 count and decreases in p24 antigen titer were reported [76, 77]. The effect of 3TC monotherapy on the clinical course of HIV infection is unknown. Preliminary reports indicate that combination therapy with ZDV and 3TC is associated with substantial, persistent increases in CD4 cell counts and decreases in HIV RNA as measured by polymerase chain reaction, although the clinical efficacy of this regimen has not yet been established [78, 79]. Lamivudine is available from Glaxo through a parallel track program (telephone: 1-800-248-9757).

Future Directions in Antiretroviral Therapy

Current research is focused on development of different classes of reverse transcriptase inhibitors, as well as identification of compounds that might act as inhibitors of other parts of the viral life cycle. Much interest has been generated recently in a new class of drugs called protease inhibitors and their possible role when used with reverse transcriptase inhibitors in the treatment of HIV infection. Phase II studies of saquinavir [80], indinavir, and other protease inhibitors in combination with nucleoside analogues are ongoing.

While soluble CD4 inhibits HIV replication in vitro by preventing virus attachment to the cell, its effects have been marginal in vivo [81]. Methods of conjugating CD4 to other molecules are being explored [82]. Inhibitors of the HIV *tat* gene, antisense DNA, and ribozymes have in vitro activity and may translate into clinically useful compounds. Alpha-interferon administered subcutaneously has been shown to have antiretroviral effect in patients with early HIV infection or Kaposi's sarcoma, although its usual toxicities, including flu-like syndrome and mild bone marrow suppression, have also been observed [83]. Intermittent dosing of interleukin-2 has recently been demonstrated to improve immunologic function in HIV-infected patients with CD4 counts above $200/mm^3$, but drug toxicity was common [84]. Inosine pranobex was found to significantly delay progression to AIDS in a randomized, placebo-controlled trial [85]. This agent is believed to function as an immunomodulator, although its precise mechanism of action is not well defined [86].

Combination antiretroviral therapy may offer the best hope for control of HIV disease [87]. Alpha- and beta-interferons synergistically inhibit HIV when used in combination with ZDV or other reverse transcriptase inhibitors [88]. Pilot studies evaluating combination therapy with ZDV and alpha-interferon [89–92] demonstrated increased CD4 cell counts without clear effect on clinical progression.

Several small clinical trials of ZDV and high-dose acyclovir [93–96] failed to demonstrate a benefit over ZDV alone. However, a large European-Australian study [97] reported improved survival in subjects randomized to receive ZDV and high-dose acyclovir compared to ZDV monotherapy. The survival advantage occurred despite a lack of significant differences in CD4 cell count changes or progression of HIV disease. A retrospective analysis of data from the Multicenter AIDS Cohort Study has confirmed this finding in patients receiving a median daily dose of 600–800 mg of acyclovir [98]. High-dose acyclovir alone has also been shown to prolong life in patients with advanced HIV disease [99].

The number of completed clinical trials using combinations of nucleoside analogues is small. Concurrent use of ZDV and ddI is associated with decreased plasma viremia [100] and increased CD4 cell counts [71] compared to monotherapy, but the clinical implications of these findings are not clear. Results from ACTG 175, a recently completed study comparing ZDV and ddI monotherapies to ZDV with ddI and ZDV with ddC in persons with CD4 cell counts of 200 to 500/mm^3 may provide important insights into the future role of combination therapy with nucleoside analogues.

Nonnucleoside reverse transcriptase inhibitors have anti-HIV activity in vivo, although viral resistance develops rapidly [101–103]. Several drugs in this class, including L-697, 661 [104], BI-RG 0587 (nevirapine) [105], U-87201E (atevirdine) [106], and U-90152S (delavirdine) [107] demonstrated antiviral effect in phase I and II trials. The rapid emergence of resistance has stopped further development of L-697,661 [104]. However, nevirapine, atevirdine, and delavirdine continue to be studied in combination with ZDV or ddI in ongoing phase II and III studies. The results of several clinical trials of combination therapy using nucleoside and nonnucleoside reverse transcriptase inhibitors are awaited with interest and may lead to new therapeutic recommendations over the next few years.

Recommendations for Antiretroviral Therapy

For newly diagnosed patients with HIV infection, assessment of clinical status and CD4 lymphocyte count should guide management [17] (Table 31-3). If the patient is asymptomatic and has a CD4 count higher than 500/mm^3, no antiretroviral therapy is recommended, but follow-up evaluation should be performed at least every 6 months. If the patient

Table 31-3 *Recommendations for antiretroviral therapy*

CD4 cell count/ clinical setting	Treatment	Laboratory monitoring
> 500/mm^3	None	CD4 count q6mo
200–500/mm^3, symptomatic	ZDV, 200 mg PO tid	CBC q1–3mo, chemistries q3mo, CD4 count q3mo
200–500/mm^3, asymptomatic	ZDV as above *or* No therapy	As above CD4 count q3mo
< 200/mm^3	ZDV as above*	CBC q1–3mo, chemistries q3mo, CD4 count q3mo
Disease progression on ZDV	Change to monotherapy with ddI, ddC, d4T, or 3TC *or* combination therapy with ZDV and ddI *or* ZDV and ddC *or* ZDV and 3TC	CBC q1–3mo, chemistries q3mo, CD4 count q3mo
ZDV intolerance	See Table 31-2	See Table 31-2

*Consider addition of acyclovir in advanced HIV disease (see text).

has a CD4 count of 200 to 500/mm^3 and HIV-related symptoms, ZDV therapy should be offered. If the patient has a CD4 count between 200 and 500/mm^3 and is asymptomatic, either initiating ZDV or holding therapy until there is clinical or immunologic progression is reasonable. Knowledge of the patient's preference and philosophy about taking medication is important in making this decision. Zidovudine is recommended for HIV-infected patients with CD4 counts less than 200/mm^3, although its role in end-stage HIV disease is not as well established.

Once ZDV therapy is started, complete blood cell counts should be obtained at follow-up visits to monitor for hematologic toxicity; hepatic and renal function and the serum CPK level should also be checked periodically. If drug intolerance develops, ZDV can be restarted at a reduced dose (100 mg orally three times a day), or ddI or ddC can be substituted provided the patient does not have a history of pancreatitis or severe neuropathy (see Table 31-2). In patients receiving ddI, serum amylase levels should be monitored in addition to hepatic and renal function tests. If ZDV is continued and there is evidence of disease progression manifested by significant symptoms or decline in CD4 cell count to 200/mm^3 or less, ddI or ddC should be substituted. The choice between these two agents is based primarily on their toxicity profiles. Monotherapy with d4T or 3TC represents an additional therapeutic option for patients who cannot tolerate ZDV, ddI, or ddC, or who develop disease progression with these drugs. The combination of ZDV with ddI, ddC, or 3TC may provide another alternative for the treatment of patients whose disease has progressed while on ZDV alone. However, because of the possible increased risk of drug toxicity in advanced HIV disease [65] and insufficient evidence of clinical benefit, the routine use of combination antiretroviral therapy outside of clinical trials cannot be strongly advocated at this time. While acyclovir may confer a survival advantage in some patients, especially those with advanced HIV disease, its specific role in management is as yet undefined [99].

References

1. Yarchoan R, Mitsuya H, Myers CE, et al. Clinical pharmacology of 3'-azido-2'3'-dideoxythymidine and related dideoxynucleosides. *N Engl J Med* 321:726–738, 1989.
2. Laskin OL, DeMiranda P, Blum MR. Azidothymidine steady-state pharmacokinetics in patients with AIDS and AIDS-related complex. *J Infect Dis* 159:8745–8747, 1989.
3. Lundgren JD, et al. Comparison of long-term prognosis of patients with AIDS treated and not treated with zidovudine. *JAMA* 271:1088–1092, 1994.
4. Fischl MA, Richman DD, Grieco MH, et al. The efficacy of AZT in the treatment of patients with AIDS and AIDS-related complex. *N Engl J Med* 317:185–191, 1987.
5. Kirk TC, Doi P, Andrews E, et al. Survival experience among patients with AIDS receiving zidovudine. *JAMA* 260:3009–3053, 1988.
6. Fischl MA, Parker CB, Pettinelli C, et al. A randomized controlled trial of a reduced daily dose of zidovudine in patients with the acquired immunodeficiency syndrome. *N Engl J Med* 323:1009–1014, 1990.
7. Nordic Medical Research Council's HIV Therapy Group. Double-blind dose-response study of zidovudine in AIDS and advanced HIV infection. *Br Med J* 304:13–17, 1992.
8. Cooper DA, Gatell JM, Kroon S, et al. Zidovudine in persons with asymptomatic HIV infection and CD4 cell counts greater than 400 per cubic millimeter. *N Engl J Med* 329:297–303, 1993.
9. Concorde Coordinating Committee. Concorde: MRC/ANRS randomised double-blind controlled trial of immediate and deferred zidovudine in symptom-free HIV infection. *Lancet* 343:871–881, 1994.
10. National Institutes of AIDS and Infectious Diseases. Executive summary: Preliminary results of ACTG 019: CD4 cell counts >500/mm^3. August 4, 1994.
11. Volberding PA, et al. A comparison of immediate with deferred zidovudine therapy for asymptomatic HIV-infected adults with CD4 cell counts of 500 or more per cubic millimeter. *N Engl J Med* 333:401–407, 1995.
12. Volberding PA, Lagakos SW, Koch MA, et al. Zidovudine in asymptomatic human immunodeficiency virus infection. *N Engl J Med* 322:941–949, 1990.

13. Volberding PA, et al. The duration of zidovudine benefit in persons with asymptomatic HIV infection. *JAMA* 272:437–442, 1994.
14. Graham NM, Piantadosi S, Park LP, et al. CD4+ lymphocyte response to zidovudine as a predictor of AIDS-free time and survival time. *J Acquir Immune Defic Syndr* 6:1258–1266, 1993.
15. Graham NM, Zeger SL, Park LP, et al. The effects on survival of early treatment of human immunodeficiency virus infection. *N Engl J Med* 326:1037–1042, 1992.
16. Lenderking WR, Gelber RD, Cotton DJ, et al. Evaluation of the quality of life associated with zidovudine treatment in asymptomatic human immunodeficiency virus infection. *N Engl J Med* 330:738–743, 1994.
17. Sande MA, Carpenter CCJ, Cobbs CG, et al. Antiretroviral therapy for adult HIV-infected patients. Recommendations from a state-of-the-art conference. *JAMA* 270:2583–2589, 1993.
18. Fischl MA, Richman D, Hansen N, et al. The safety and efficacy of zidovudine (AZT) in the treatment of subjects with mildly symptomatic human immunodeficiency virus type 1 (HIV) infection. *Ann Intern Med* 112:727–737, 1990.
19. Hamilton JD, Hartigan PM, Simberkoff MS, et al. A controlled trial of early versus late treatment with zidovudine in symptomatic human immunodeficiency virus infection: Results of the Veterans Affairs Cooperative Study. *N Engl J Med* 326:437–443, 1992.
20. Yarchoan R, Berg G, Brouwers P, et al. Response of HIV associated neurological disease to AZT. *Lancet* 1:132–135, 1987.
21. Sidtis JJ, Gatsonis C, Price RW, et al. Zidovudine treatment of the AIDS dementia complex: Results of a placebo-controlled trial. AIDS Clinical Trials Group. *Ann Neurol* 33:343–349, 1993.
22. Hymes KB, Greene JB, Karpatkin S. The effect of azidothymidine on HIV-related thrombocytopenia. *N Engl J Med* 318:516–517, 1988.
23. Gottlieb MS, Wolfe PR, Chafey S. Case report: Response of AIDS-related thrombocytopenia to intravenous and oral azidothymidine (3'-azido-3'-deoxythymidine). *AIDS Res Hum Retroviruses* 3:109, 1987.
24. The Swiss Group for Clinical Studies on AIDS. Zidovudine for the treatment of thrombocytopenia associated with HIV. *Ann Intern Med* 109:718–721, 1988.
25. Lagakos S, Fischl MA, Stein DS, et al. Effects of zidovudine therapy in minority and other subpopulations with early HIV infection. *JAMA* 266:2709–2712, 1991.
26. Easterbrook PJ, Kervly JC, Creagh-Kirk T, et al. Racial and ethnic differences in outcome in zidovudine-treated patients with advanced HIV disease. *JAMA* 266:2713–2718, 1991.
27. Selwyn PA, Alcabes P, Hartel D, et al. Clinical manifestations and predictors of disease progression in drug users with human immunodeficiency virus infection. *N Engl J Med* 327:1697–1703, 1992.
28. Pons JC, Taburet AM, Singlas E, et al. Placental passage of azidothymidine (AZT) during the second trimester of pregnancy: Study by direct fetal blood sampling under ultrasound. *Eur J Obstet Gynecol Reprod Biol* 40:229–231, 1991.

29. Connor EM, et al. Reduction of maternal-infant transmission of HIV-1 with zidovudine treatment. *N Engl J Med* 331:1173–1180, 1994.

30. Centers for Disease Control. Public Health Service statement on management of occupational exposure to human immunodeficiency virus, including considerations regarding zidovudine postexposure use. *MMWR* 39:1–14, 1990.

31. Richman DD, Fischl MA, Frieco MH, et al. The toxicity of AZT in the treatment of patients with AIDS and AIDS-related complex. *N Engl J Med* 317:192–197, 1987.

32. Hagler DN, Frame PT. AZT neurotoxicity. *Lancet* 2:1392–1393, 1986.

33. Spear JB, Kessler HA, Nusinoff-Lehrman S, de Miranda P. Zidovudine overdosage. *Ann Intern Med* 109:76–77, 1988.

34. Pickus OB. Overdose of zidovudine. *N Engl J Med* 318:1206, 1988.

35. Gill PS, Rarick M, Brynes RK, et al. AZT associated bone marrow failure in AIDS. *Ann Intern Med* 107:502–505, 1987.

36. Sattler FR, Ko R, Antoniskis D, et al. Acetaminophen does not impair clearance of zidovudine. *Ann Intern Med* 114:937–940, 1991.

37. Fischl M, Galpin JE, Levine JD, et al. Recombinant human erythropoietin for patients with AIDS treated with zidovudine. *N Engl J Med* 322:1488–1493, 1990.

38. Pluda JM, Yarchoan R, Smith PD, et al. Subcutaneous recombinant granulocyte-macrophage colony-stimulating factor used as a single agent and in an alternating regimen with azidothymidine in leukopenic patients with severe human immunodeficiency virus infection. *Blood* 76:463–472, 1990.

39. Groopman JE, Mitsuyasu RT, DeLeo MJ, et al. Effect of recombinant human granulocyte-macrophage colony-stimulating factor on myelopoiesis in the acquired immunodeficiency syndrome. *N Engl J Med* 317:593–598, 1987.

40. Grossberg HS, Bonnem EM, Buhles WC. GM-CSF with ganciclovir for the treatment of CMV retinitis in AIDS. *N Engl J Med* 320:1560, 1989.

41. Miles SA, Mitsuyasu RT, Moreno J, et al. Combined therapy with granulocyte colony-stimulating factor and erythropoietin decreases hematologic toxicity from zidovudine. *Blood* 77:2109–2117, 1990.

42. Bessen LJ, Greene JB, Louie E, et al. Severe polymyositis-like syndrome associated with zidovudine therapy of AIDS and ARC. *N Engl J Med* 318:708, 1988.

43. Herskowitz A, et al. Cardiomyopathy associated with antiretroviral therapy in patients with HIV infection: A report of six cases. *Ann Intern Med* 116:311–313, 1992.

44. Dubin G, Braffman MN. Zidovudine-induced hepatotoxicity. *Ann Intern Med* 110:85–86, 1989.

45. Dalakas MC, Illa I, Pezeshkpour GH, et al. Mitochondrial myopathy caused by long-term zidovudine therapy. *N Engl J Med* 322:1098–1105, 1990.

46. Richman DD. Zidovudine resistance of human immunodeficiency virus. *Rev Infect Dis* 12 (suppl):S506–S512, 1990.

47. Land S, et al. Incidence of zidovudine-resistant human immunodeficiency virus isolated from patients before, during, and after therapy. *J Infect Dis* 166:1139–1142, 1992.

48. Montaner JSG, et al. Clinical correlates of in vitro HIV-1 resistance to

zidovudine: Results of the Multicentre Canadian AZT Trial. *AIDS* 7:189–196, 1993.

49. D'Aquilla RT, et al. Zidovudine resistance and HIV-1 disease progression during antiretroviral therapy. *Ann Intern Med* 122:401–408, 1995.

49a. Japour AJ, et al. Prevalence and clinical significance of zidovudine resistance mutations in human immunodeficiency virus isolated from patients after long-term zidovudine treatment. *J Infect Dis* 171:1172–1179, 1995.

50. St. Clair MH, et al. Zidovudine resistance, syncytium-inducing phenotype, and HIV disease progression in a case-control study. *J Acquir Immune Defic Syndr* 6:891–897, 1993.

51. Pluda JM, et al. Development of non-Hodgkin lymphoma in a cohort of patients with severe human immunodeficiency virus (HIV) therapy on long-term antiretroviral therapy. *Ann Intern Med* 113:276–282, 1990.

52. Deray G, Diquet B, Martinez F, et al. Pharmacokinetics of zidovudine in a patient on maintenance hemodialysis. *N Engl J Med* 319:1606–1607, 1988.

53. Lambert JS, Seidlin M, Reichman RC, et al. 2'3'-Dideoxyinosine (ddI) in patients with the acquired immunodeficiency syndrome or AIDS-related complex. *N Engl J Med* 322:1333–1340, 1990.

54. Cooley TP, Kunches LM, Saunders CA, et al. Once-daily administration of 2'3'-dideoxyinosine (ddI) in patients with the acquired immunodeficiency syndrome or AIDS-related complex. *N Engl J Med* 322:1340–1345, 1990.

55. Yarchoan R, Mitsuya H, Thomas RV, et al. In vivo activity against HIV and favorable toxicity profile of 2'3'-dideoxyinosine. *Science* 245:412–415, 1989.

56. Kahn JO, Lagakos SW, Richman DD, et al. A controlled trial comparing continued zidovudine with didanosine in human immunodeficiency virus infection. *N Engl J Med* 327:581–587, 1992.

57. Spruance SL, Pavia AT, Peterson D, et al. Didanosine compared with continuation of zidovudine in HIV-infected patients with signs of clinical deterioration while receiving zidovudine. *Ann Intern Med* 120:360–368, 1994.

58. Dolin R, Amato D, Fischl M, et al. Efficacy of didanosine (ddI) versus zidovudine (ZDV) in patients with no or ≤ 16 weeks of prior ZDV therapy (abstract). Ninth International Conference on AIDS, Berlin, June, 1993.

59. Vella S, Floridia M, Tomino C, et al. Comparative evaluation of AZT and ddI in previously untreated patients with early or advanced ARC: Preliminary results of the Italian randomized multicenter study ISS-902 (abstract). Eighth International Conference on AIDS, Amsterdam, July, 1992.

60. Lai KK, Gang DL, Zawacki JK, Cooley TP. Fulminant hepatic failure associated with 2'3'-dideoxyinosine (ddI). *Ann Intern Med* 115:283–284, 1991.

61. St. Clair MH, Martin JL, Tudor-Williams G, et al. Resistance to ddI and sensitivity to AZT induced by a mutation in HIV-1 reverse transcriptase. *Science* 253:1557–1559, 1991.

62. Eron JJ, Chow Y-K, Caliendo AM, et al. pol Mutations conferring zidovudine and didanosine resistance with different effects in vitro yield multiply resistant human immunodeficiency virus type 1 isolates in vivo. *Antimicrob Agents Chemother* 37:1480–1487, 1993.

63. Merigen TC, Skowron G, Bozzette SA, et al. Circulating p24 antigen lev-

els and responses to dideoxycytidine in human immunodeficiency virus (HIV) infections. *Ann Intern Med* 110:189–194, 1989.

64. Broder S. Proceedings of a symposium. Dideoxycytidine (ddC): A potent antiretroviral agent for human immunodeficiency virus infection. *Am J Med* 88 (suppl 5B):1S–33S, 1990.

65. Remick S, Follansbee S, Olson R, et al. The efficacy of zalcitabine (ddC, HIVID) versus zidovudine (ZDV) as monotherapy in ZDV naive patients with advanced HIV disease: A randomized, double-blind comparative trial (ACTG 114; N3300) (abstract). Ninth International Conference on AIDS, Berlin, June, 1993.

66. Fischl MA, Olson RM, Follansbee SE, et al. Zalcitabine compared with zidovudine in patients with advanced HIV-1 infection who received previous zidovudine therapy. *Ann Intern Med* 118:762–769, 1993.

67. Fischl MA, Stanley K, Collier AC, et al. Combination and monotherapy with zidovudine and zalcitabine in patients with advanced HIV disease. *Ann Intern Med* 122:24–32, 1995.

68. Abrams DI, Golman AI, Launer C, et al. A comparative trial of didanosine and zalcitabine after treatment with zidovudine in patients with human immunodeficiency virus infection. *N Engl J Med* 330:657–662, 1994.

69. Saag MS. What to do when zidovudine fails? *N Engl J Med* 330:706–707, 1994.

70. Meng TC, Fischl MA, Boota AM, et al. Combination therapy with zidovudine and dideoxycytidine in patients with advanced human immunodeficiency virus infection. *Ann Intern Med* 116:85–86, 1992.

71. Collier AC, Coombs RW, Fischl MA, et al. Combination therapy with zidovudine and didanosine compared to zidovudine alone in HIV-1 infection. *Ann Intern Med* 119:786–793, 1993.

72. Yarchoan R, Lietzau JA, Nguyen BY, et al. A randomized study of alternating or simultaneous zidovudine and didanosine therapy in patients with symptomatic human immunodeficiency virus infection. *J Infect Dis* 169:9–17, 1994.

73. Browne MJ, Mayer KH, Chafee SBD, et al. 2'3'-Didehydro-3'-deoxythymidine (d4T) in patients with AIDS or AIDS-related complex: A phase I trial. *J Infect Dis* 167:21–29, 1993.

74. Package insert. Zerit (stavudine). Wallingford, CT: Bristol-Myers Squibb, 1994.

75. Lin PF, et al. Genotypic and phenotypic analysis of HIV type I isolates from patients on prolonged stavudine therapy. *J Infect Dis* 170:1157–1164, 1994.

76. Pluda J, Cooley T, Montaner J, et al. Phase I/II study of 3TC (GR109714X) in adults with ARC or AIDS. Ninth International Conference on AIDS, Berlin, June, 1993.

77. van Leeuwen R, et al. Evaluation of safety and efficacy of 3TC (lamivudine) in patients with asymptomatic or mildly symptomatic human immunodeficiency virus infection: a phase I/II study. *J Infect Dis* 171:1166–1171, 1995.

78. Pluda JM, et al. Phase I/II study of 2'-deoxy-3'-thiacytidine (lamivudine) in patients with advanced human immunodeficiency virus infection. *J Infect Dis* 171:1438–1447, 1995.

79. Reports from the Second National Conference on Human Retroviruses and Related Infections. Washington, DC: January, 1995.
80. Delfraissy JF, Serini D, Brun-Veziniet F, et al. A phase I–II dose ranging study of the safety and activity of Ro 31-8959 (HIV proteinase inhibitor) in previously zidovudine (ZDV) treated HIV-infected individuals (abstract). Ninth International Conference on AIDS, Berlin, June 1993.
81. Schooley RT, et al. Recombinant soluble CD4 therapy in patients with the acquired immunodeficiency syndrome (AIDS) and AIDS-related complex: A phase I–II escalating dosage trial. *Ann Intern Med* 112:247–253, 1990.
82. Finberg RW, Wahl SM, Allen JB, et al. Selective elimination of HIV-1 infected cells with an interleukin-2 receptor specific cytotoxin. *Science* 252:1703–1705, 1991.
83. Lane HC, Davey V, Kovacs JA, et al. Interferon-alpha in patients with asymptomatic human immunodeficiency virus (HIV) infection. *Ann Intern Med* 112:805–810, 1990.
84. Kovacs JA, et al. Increases in CD4 T lymphocytes with intermittent courses of interleukin-2 in patients with human immunodeficiency virus infection: A preliminary study. *N Engl J Med* 332:567–575, 1995.
85. Pedersen C, Sandstrom E, Petersen CS, et al. The efficacy of inosine pranobex in preventing the acquired immunodeficiency syndrome in patients with human immunodeficiency virus infection. *N Engl J Med* 322:1757–1763, 1990.
86. Kweder SL, Schnur RA, Cooper EC. Inosine pranobex: Is a single positive trial enough? (editorial). *N Engl J Med* 322:1807–1809, 1990.
87. Caliendo A, Hirsch M. Combination therapy for infection due to HIV. *Clin Infect Dis* 18:516–524, 1994.
88. Hartshorn KL, Vogt MW, Neumeyer D, et al. Synergistic inhibition of HIV replication in vitro by AZT and recombinant interferon alpha. *Antimicrob Agents Chemother* 31:168–172, 1987.
89. Kovacs JA, Deyton L, Davey R, et al. Combined zidovudine and interferon-alpha therapy in patients with Kaposi sarcoma and the acquired immunodeficiency syndrome (AIDS). *Ann Intern Med* 111:280–287, 1989.
90. Krown JA, Gold JWM, Niedzwiecki D, et al. Interferon-alpha with zidovudine: Safety, tolerance, and clinical and virologic effects in patients with Kaposi sarcoma associated with the acquired immunodeficiency syndrome (AIDS). *Ann Intern Med* 112:280–287, 1990.
91. Fischl MA, Uttamchandani RB, Resnick L, et al. A phase I study of recombinant human interferon-alpha-2a or human lymphoblastoid interferon-alpha-n1 and concomitant zidovudine in patients with AIDS-related Kaposi's sarcoma. *J Acquir Immune Defic Syndr* 4:1–10, 1991.
92. Surbone A, Yarchoan R, McAtee N, et al. Treatment of the acquired immunodeficiency syndrome (AIDS) and AIDS-related complex with a regimen of 3'-azido-2',3'-dideoxythymidine (azidothymidine or zidovudine) and acyclovir. *Ann Intern Med* 108:534–540, 1988.
93. Hollander H, Lifson AR, Maha M, et al. Phase I study of low-dose zidovudine and acyclovir in asymptomatic human immunodeficiency virus seropositive individuals. *Am J Med* 87:628–632, 1989.
94. de Wolf F, Lange JM, Goudsmit J, et al. Effect of zidovudine on serum

human immunodeficiency virus antigen levels in symptom-free subjects. *Lancet* 1:373–376, 1988.

95. Collier AC, Bozette S, Coombs RW, et al. A pilot study of low dose zidovudine in human immunodeficiency virus infection. *N Engl J Med* 323:1015–1021, 1990.

96. Cooper DA, Pedersen C, Aiuti F, et al. The efficacy and safety of zidovudine with or without acyclovir in the treatment of patients with AIDS-related complex. *AIDS* 5:933–943, 1991.

97. Cooper DA, Pehrson PO, Pedersen C, et al. The efficacy and safety of zidovudine alone or as cotherapy with acyclovir for the treatment of patients with AIDS or AIDS-related complex: A double-blind randomized trial. European-Australian Collaborative Group. *AIDS* 7:197–207, 1993.

98. Stein DS, et al. The effect of the interaction of acyclovir with zidovudine on progression to AIDS and survival. *Ann Intern Med* 121:100–108, 1994.

99. Youle MS, et al. Effects of high-dose oral acyclovir on herpesvirus disease and survival in patients with advanced HIV disease: A double-blind, placebo-controlled study. *AIDS* 5:641–650, 1994.

100. Holodniy M, Katzenstein D, Winters M, et al. Measurement of HIV virus load and genotypic resistance by gene amplification in asymptomatic subjects treated with combination therapy. *J Acquir Immune Defic Syndr* 6:366–369, 1993.

101. DeClerq E. HIV-1-specific RT inhibitors: Highly selective inhibitors of human immunodeficiency virus type 1 that are specifically targeted at the viral reverse transcriptase. *Med Res Rev* 13:229–258, 1993.

102. Larder BA, Kellam P, Kemp SD. Convergent combination therapy can select viable multi-drug resistant HIV-1 in vitro. *Nature* 365:451–453, 1993.

103. Chow Y-K, Hirsch MS, Merrill DP, et al. Use of evolutionary limitations of HIV-1 multi-drug resistance to optimize therapy. *Nature* 361:650–654, 1993.

104. Saag MS, Emini EA, Laskin OL, et al. A short-term clinical evaluation of L-697,661, a non-nucleoside inhibitor of HIV-1 reverse transcriptase. *N Engl J Med* 329:1065–1072, 1993.

105. Havir D. Antiviral activity of nevirapine at 400 mg in p24 antigen positive adults. Ninth International Conference on AIDS, Berlin, June, 1993.

106. Reichman M, Fischl M, Para M, et al. Phase I study of atevirdine (ATV), a non-nucleoside reverse transcriptase inhibitor, given in combination with zidovudine (ZDV) (abstract). Ninth International Conference on AIDS, Berlin, June, 1993.

107. Investigator brochure. Delavirdine mesylate (U-90152S). Kalamazoo, MI: The Upjohn Company, 1994.

Ambulatory Management of HIV Infection 32

Jon D. Fuller, Howard Libman

The management of HIV infection in the ambulatory setting begins with the recognition that education about disease prevention should be part of routine health care maintenance. Clinicians who provide an opportunity for patients to ask frank questions about HIV infection will help them to acquire an understanding of behaviors that could place them at risk and aid them in assessing the need for HIV antibody testing. Education about the types of casual contact that do not lead to viral transmission will assist them in learning to live and work comfortably with HIV-infected individuals.

HIV Antibody Testing

Some patients seek HIV antibody testing on their own, often outside the primary care context, such as at a sexually transmitted disease clinic or an anonymous test site. In other cases, the clinician takes the initiative by recommending HIV antibody testing to patients with historical risks for HIV infection or suggestive clinical findings [1–7] (Table 32-1).

Pretest and Post-Test Counseling

The personal benefits of learning that one is HIV antibody positive early in the course of infection include the capacity to receive appropriate medical care and to modify behaviors in order to decrease the risk of transmission to others (Table 32-2). However, testing is also associated with certain risks. Receiving a positive result can have devastating personal and social effects. HIV seropositivity may adversely affect one's

Table 32-1 *Indications and contraindications for HIV antibody testing*

Historical indications
  Men who have sex with men
  Persons with multiple sexual partners
  Current or past injection drug users
  Recipients of blood products between 1978 and 1985
  Persons with current or past sexually transmitted diseases
  Prostitutes and their sexual partners
  Women of childbearing age who are at risk through drug use, prostitution, or unprotected sex
  Children born to HIV-infected mothers
  Sexual partners of those at risk for HIV infection
Clinical indications
  Tuberculosis
  Syphilis
  Recurrent shingles
  Unexplained chronic constitutional symptoms
  Unexplained chronic generalized adenopathy
  Unexplained diarrhea or wasting
  Unexplained encephalopathy
  Unexplained thrombocytopenia
  Unexplained thrush or chronic vaginal candidiasis
Contraindications
  Pretest and post-test counseling unavailable
  Inability to provide informed consent
  Acute psychosis or severe emotional disturbance
  Suicidality
  Lack of adequate personal support system

Table 32-2 *Potential benefits and risks of HIV antibody testing*

Benefits
  Individual health
    Antiretroviral therapy
    Prophylaxis for opportunistic infections
    Screening and prophylaxis for tuberculosis
    Screening for and treatment of syphilis and other sexually transmitted diseases
    Administration of appropriate vaccinations
    Other routine health care maintenance
    Patient education
  Public health
    Reduction of high-risk behaviors
    Monitoring of HIV infection epidemiology

Risks
  False-positive test result
  False-negative test result
  Adverse psychological reactions
  Breach of confidentiality
  Societal discrimination

eligibility for life insurance, health insurance, employment, and housing, and suicide has been reported in asymptomatic persons who have received the news of a positive test result [8–12]. Patients who undergo HIV antibody testing should have a full understanding of its ramifications through pretest and post-test counseling. Antibody testing is contraindicated in patients who cannot provide informed consent; who are unable to understand the implications of test results; who are psychotic, suicidal, or emotionally disturbed; or who lack adequate personal support systems to cope with the stress of receiving a positive test result (see Table 32-1).

Confirmation of Reported Seropositivity

A variety of economic and health care benefits may become available to HIV-infected patients, and several case reports have documented individuals who misrepresent themselves as seropositive in order to take advantage of these. This behavior may also be a manifestation of the Munchausen syndrome, with the desire to repeatedly undergo unnecessary and often invasive diagnostic procedures [13–15]. For these reasons, it is prudent to confirm a verbally reported positive HIV antibody test result in patients without characteristic manifestations of HIV disease [16].

Clinical Evaluation

The initial evaluation of HIV-infected patients includes a careful history and physical examination, appropriate baseline laboratory studies, and attention to their psychosocial and educational needs.

Medical History

While certain disease manifestations may be seen with a higher incidence in particular populations, such as Kaposi's sarcoma (KS) in homosexual men and recurrent bacterial pneumonia in injection drug users (IDUs), the manner in which an individual has acquired HIV infection does not generally have an impact on clinical management. However, for the purposes of epidemiologic reporting, it is important to identify the HIV risk behavior(s) for each individual. This information also guides the clinician in educating the patient about specific changes in behavior necessary to minimize the risk of transmitting HIV to others.

Particular items in the medical history are of significance in managing HIV-infected patients. It is important to establish if the patient has a history of syphilis because of the increased risk of relapse following treatment and central nervous system (CNS) involvement. A history of genital warts or receptive anal intercourse in men and women should be carefully sought; human papillomavirus (HPV) infection in association with HIV-induced immune suppression can predispose to cervical dysplasia and cancer, as well as squamous cell carcinoma of the anus [17–22]. Many common skin conditions, including eczema, seborrhea, psoriasis, warts, molluscum contagiosum, and herpes simplex virus (HSV) infection, may be exacerbated by HIV infection. Patients with a history of hepatitis B virus (HBV) infection may experience viral reactivation, leading to reversion to infectious status or clinical hepatitis [23–25]. Since the immune response to HBV infection causes hepatitis, the condition may not be apparent until therapy with immunorestorative agents such as zidovudine (ZDV) is initiated. A history of tuberculosis (TB) exposure is important to obtain, since the risk of developing active disease is significantly increased in HIV-infected individuals [26].

Review of Systems

Since severe weight loss can accompany many of the infectious or neoplastic complications of HIV infection, significant decrease in weight should prompt an evaluation for opportunistic disease. Weight loss may also be an indication for the use of nutritional supplements, appetite stimulants such as megestrol acetate or dronabinol, or a trial of recombinant human growth hormone [27–33]. The presence of chronic, low-grade fever may be the earliest manifestation of infections, such as *Pneumocystis carinii* pneumonia (PCP), mycobacterial disease, or cryptococcosis, or of neoplasia, especially lymphoma. Chronic sweats may result from cytokines released in response to HIV infection; they can also be an indication of occult opportunistic infection or neoplasia.

Generalized lymphadenopathy is frequently seen in HIV-infected patients and usually represents a benign, reactive process that may regress with more advanced disease [34]. However, individual nodes or groups of nodes that are bulky, matted, or tender may warrant evaluation for infection or tumor, particularly if constitutional symptoms or pancytopenia are present [35, 36].

A history of new, pigmented skin lesions should raise the clinician's suspicion for KS (see Plates 15, 16). However, cat-scratch bacillus can also cause erythematous, nodular lesions that resemble KS, making biopsy preferable to empiric diagnosis [37, 38]. Mucocutaneous ulcers may represent infection with HSV, cytomegalovirus (CMV), *Staphylococcus aureus*, or mycobacteria. Nodular skin lesions may indicate the presence of molluscum contagiosum (see Plate 11) or verruca vulgaris, both of which may grow rapidly in the setting of immune dysfunction.

Human immunodeficiency virus can enter the CNS at the time of primary infection, or subsequently, resulting in a variety of neurologic syndromes, including aseptic meningitis, encephalopathy, and myelitis, as well as peripheral and autonomic neuropathies. Persistent headache, mental status changes, memory loss, and an inability to concentrate may be manifestations of HIV itself or of an opportunistic infection or tumor involving the CNS [39–49]. Peripheral nerve involvement by HIV may manifest as painful paresthesias, numbness, or weakness. Autonomic neuropathy may produce orthostatic hypotension, nocturia, urinary or fecal incontinence, or gastroparesis.

HIV-related oral manifestations include white patches or plaques on the tongue or buccal mucosa (thrush or hairy leukoplakia), gingival inflammation or swelling (necrotizing gingivitis), ulceration (HSV, CMV, or aphthous stomatitis), condylomas, and KS of the palate, gingiva, or pharynx (see Plates 1–6). Bacterial sinusitis, bronchitis, and pneumonia are seen with increased frequency in HIV-infected patients and generally present with typical symptoms [50–52]. Shortness of breath and dyspnea on exertion may be manifestations of PCP, pulmonary KS, lymphoid interstitial pneumonitis (LIP), or HIV-related cardiomyopathy.

Retrosternal chest pain with swallowing (odynophagia) can be seen with esophagitis caused by many infections, including *Candida albicans*, HSV, CMV, and HIV, as well as drugs, including zalcitabine (formerly dideoxycytidine or ddC) [53–56]. Aphthous-like ulcers involving the esophagus are diagnosed by excluding other causes and may respond to therapy with topical or systemic corticosteroids or thalidomide [57–60]. Difficulty in coordinating the movements of swallowing (dysphagia) may be a manifestation of autonomic neuropathy; CNS involvement by infection, neoplasia, or degenerative disease, such as progressive multifocal leukoencephalopathy (PML); or HIV encephalopathy. Diarrhea may result from opportunistic diseases of the gastrointestinal tract or drug toxicity.

Myalgias and arthralgias may represent, respectively, HIV-induced myositis and arthritis, including Reiter's syndrome, psoriatic arthritis, and reactive arthropathy [61–64]. Myalgias may also indicate myopathy associated with chronic ZDV therapy [65, 66]. The fibromyalgia syndrome—the triad of depression, insomnia, and pain at tendon insertions—has also been described with increased frequency among HIV-infected patients [67].

Physical Examination

Skin

Seborrheic dermatitis may present atypically with a papular or nodular appearance in HIV-infected patients [68] (see Plate 14). This condition often involves the mustache, beard, eyebrows, scalp, forehead, retroauricular skin, nipples, and perianal area. Psoriasis may be exacerbated by HIV infection and improve during ZDV therapy [69–72].

An otherwise rare skin condition known as eosinophilic folliculitis (EF) has been described in HIV-infected patients and may be mistaken for one of the atypical presentations of seborrheic dermatitis. EF frequently begins as a pruritic, papular eruption and develops into a weeping, crusting ulcer with a hypertrophic margin and central healing. While the etiology of EF remains obscure, it may represent a nonspecific response to skin saprophytes [73, 74]. The condition is generally responsive to ultraviolet light therapy.

Staphylococcus aureus infection may result in recurrent folliculitis, impetigo (see Plate 12), furuncles, or abscesses. Bacteremia may develop even in patients without intravascular catheters or other predisposing factors [75].

Mycotic infection of the nail bed, onychomycosis, is common and may present as typical "powdery" disintegration or discoloration of the distal nail or as thickening of the nail bed. Patients receiving ZDV frequently develop nail bed dyschromia, which manifests as asymptomatic vertical, and occasionally horizontal, dark striping [76–78].

Herpes simplex virus infection may cause chronic or recurrent ulceration of the oral, labial, buccal, genital, or perirectal tissues (see Plate 9). Relapse is common and may require chronic suppressive antiviral therapy. If HSV infection is present for more than one month in an HIV-infected person, it constitutes an AIDS-defining diagnosis.

Recurrent shingles (reactivation of varicella-zoster virus [VZV]) is increased in frequency and may be seen at any time in the course of HIV disease [79, 80] (see Plate 10). Zoster may present as localized or disseminated disease, and is manifested by a painful or dysesthetic prodrome followed by vesicles that weep and gradually crust. Complications of zoster may include encephalitis, ophthalmitis, and rapidly progressing necrotizing retinitis (acute retinal necrosis syndrome) [81–85]. Although disseminated VZV infection generally responds well to acyclovir, increased morbidity and mortality have been reported in this population [86].

Kaposi's sarcoma of the skin can present as macules, plaques, or nodules, and may wax and wane even without therapy (see Plates 15, 16). While KS lesions are characteristically blue-red or purple, they may become brown with age. Cutaneous KS of the extremities or involvement of regional lymph nodes can lead to lymphatic obstruction and chronic dependent edema. Sites with a particularly high incidence of KS include the lower extremities, tip of the nose, oral cavity (gums, hard palate, posterior pharynx; see Plate 5), and bulbar and palpebral conjunctivae. Kaposi's sarcoma lesions may appear less violaceous on dark-skinned persons and are sometimes mistaken for nevi.

Many localized and disseminated infections may present as nodules, papules, pustules, or plaques; facial involvement may be incorrectly diagnosed as seborrhea [87]. Any skin lesion that is unresponsive to empiric therapy, especially in the presence of systemic symptoms, should be considered for biopsy and culture.

Lymph Nodes

Generalized lymphadenopathy is common, with intermittent symptoms corresponding to nodal enlargement and involution. Involved sites may include the cervical, occipital, axillary, and femoral/inguinal chains. Lymph nodes are typically 1 to 2 cm in diameter, firm, nontender, and nonadherent.

Oropharynx

Thrush or oropharyngeal candidiasis may present in several patterns. In the pseudomembranous form, it is a white, curd-like membrane that can be removed to reveal an erythematous mucosal surface; potassium hydroxide preparation of mucosal scrapings demonstrates budding yeast and pseudohyphae (see Plate 1). Pseudomembranous thrush may interfere with eating, cause a bad taste in the mouth, or be cosmetically unacceptable. Atrophic thrush is slightly tender and appears as an erythematous, smooth, or papular region on mucous membranes, especially the hard palate. Angular cheilitis manifests as fissuring and erythema of the corners of the mouth.

Hairy leukoplakia is a white, vertical, corrugated lesion usually appearing on the sides or dorsum of the tongue or buccal mucosa (see Plate 3). Epstein-Barr virus can be detected in many biopsy specimens, although other viruses, including HSV and HPV, have also been suggested as causative agents [88–90]. Hairy leukoplakia is not dangerous in itself, but it is a marker for immunodeficiency and has been correlated with more rapid HIV disease progression [91]. It may regress spontaneously or during antiviral therapy with ganciclovir, acyclovir, and possibly ZDV [92–95]. Because the condition is asymptomatic, specific treatment is generally not necessary.

Acute necrotizing ulcerative gingivitis (ANUG) manifests as painful, swollen gums associated with an erythematous, horizontal line at the gingivodental border (see Plate 4). ANUG can lead to severe and sometimes rapidly progressive periodontal disease. Patients with significant gingival or periodontal abnormalities should be empirically started on penicillin or clindamycin and promptly referred to a dentist or oral surgeon [96].

Eyes

Since a variety of opportunistic infections may involve the cornea, conjunctiva, or retina of HIV-infected patients, a careful eye examination should be performed regularly. A dilated funduscopic examination is necessary to visualize the peripheral retina. Lesions of the cornea or conjunctiva may occur with KS, or with VZV or *Microsporidia* infection [97, 98]. Retinal lesions may be caused by HIV, CMV, *P. carinii*, *Toxoplasma gondii*, syphilis, *Candida*, or histoplasmosis [99–105].

Cotton-wool spots, a manifestation of retinal ischemia frequently associated with HIV infection, are pale, moderately well-delineated white patches with fluffy or discrete borders (see Plate 7). Usually asymptomatic, they may remain stable over time or disappear in one location as they develop in another. While the etiology of cotton-wool spots is unknown, they may represent a response to HIV itself [106].

Cytomegalovirus retinitis is one of the most serious and frequent ophthalmologic complications of HIV infection, occurring in 15 to 40 percent of persons diagnosed with AIDS and often causing monocular or binocular blindness [107]. Cytomegalovirus infection manifests as perivascular yellow or white lesions, usually associated with areas of hemorrhage (see Plate 8). In contrast to the smooth, homogeneous appearance of cotton-wool patches, CMV retinitis is patchy or "chunky," and has been described as resembling "scrambled eggs and ketchup." Early CMV disease may be limited to the periphery of the retina and be observable only on dilated examination. HIV-infected patients noted to have retinal lesions should be evaluated by an ophthalmologist, as should individuals with new visual symptoms, such as "floaters," decreased acuity, or flashing bright lights.

Cardiopulmonary System
While cardiopulmonary examination is often nonspecific, several HIV-related conditions may result in characteristic physical findings [108]. *Pneumocystis carinii* pneumonia may be accompanied by dry basilar rales and is occasionally associated with malar rash and arthropathy. Pulmonary KS may present with pleural effusion, frequently unilateral, manifested by decreased breath sounds and dullness to percussion. Congestive cardiomyopathy can result from HIV infection, antiretroviral agents, or opportunistic infections such as PCP or toxoplasmosis [109, 110]. Bacteremia from intravascular devices occurs with increased frequency in this population [111, 112]. If valvular disease develops as a complication of bacteremia, signs of endocarditis, including a new regurgitant murmur, peripheral stigmata, or both, are sometimes present.

Abdomen
Hepatic tenderness or enlargement may signify infiltration with opportunistic infection or tumor, or the presence of viral hepatitis. Splenomegaly may be due to tumor, bacterial or mycobacterial abscess, or disseminated *P. carinii* infection. Abdominal masses may result from lymphoma, KS, or involvement of mesenteric nodes with *Mycobacterium avium* complex (MAC) or other opportunistic infections.

Rectum
Genital warts and HSV infection are the most frequently encountered perirectal pathology in HIV-infected patients; KS, candidiasis, or psoriasis may also be seen. Anal squamous cell cancers, which occur in association with HPV infection, are often palpable on digital examination and may be tender and friable.

Genitourinary Tract

Recurrent vulvovaginal candidiasis and HSV infection occur with increased frequency in HIV-infected women, and pelvic inflammatory disease may be more severe and complicated by tuboovarian abscess formation [113–116]. Candidal and herpetic infections are prone to relapse and may require chronic suppressive therapy. Human papillomavirus infection can lead to the development of cervical dysplasia and cancer, which may be more aggressive in this population.

Nervous System

Because screening mental status examination may be insensitive to subtle manifestations of HIV encephalopathy, patients who complain of decreased concentration or memory should undergo formal neuropsychological testing. The Mental Alternation Test of cognition has been reported as a reliable means to identify HIV-infected patients who require further cognitive evaluation [117]. Other neurologic abnormalities on examination may include cranial and peripheral nerve palsies, painful peripheral neuropathy, or focal motor deficits caused by intracranial mass lesions or spinal cord involvement by HIV or CMV.

Laboratory Studies

Baseline laboratory evaluation of the HIV-infected patient is important to screen for occult systemic disease, to identify latent infections that may reactivate, and to monitor for drug toxicity (Table 32-3).

Complete Blood Count

A complete blood and differential count should be performed on all patients. Cytopenias may occur without symptoms and should prompt

Table 32-3 *Baseline laboratory evaluation of the HIV-infected patient*

Complete blood and differential counts
Liver function tests
Hepatitis B and C virus serologies
Syphilis serology
Purified protein derivative (PPD) and anergy panel
Chest x-ray
Urinalysis
Renal function tests
(?) Toxoplasmosis serology
(?) Cytomegalovirus serology
(?) Serum cryptococcal antigen
Glucose 6-phosphate dehydrogenase
CD4 cell count

appropriate evaluation. Anemia, thrombocytopenia, and/or leukopenia may be caused by HIV-induced marrow suppression, antiviral therapy, or infiltration of the marrow by infection or tumor; thrombocytopenia and leukopenia may also be mediated by autoantibody production.

Liver Function Tests and Hepatitis Serologies
Because hepatitis B, C, and D (delta) are known to occur with an increased frequency among HIV-infected patients, liver function tests and serologies for HBV, HCV, and, if HBV-positive, HDV, are recommended as part of the initial evaluation [118–125]. These studies will help in assessing the need for HBV vaccination in susceptible individuals and alert the clinician to the presence of HBV or HCV infection [126, 127]. Liver biopsy and treatment with interferon-alpha should be considered for symptomatic chronic viral hepatitis [128–130]. An isolated increased serum alkaline phosphatase may prompt evaluation for hepatic involvement by TB or MAC.

Syphilis Serology
Syphilis may progress more rapidly, be more resistant to standard therapies, be more prone to reactivation, and be more difficult to detect by standard serologic testing in HIV-infected individuals [131–136]. Baseline screening for syphilis and annual retesting are warranted in all patients, and central nervous system involvement should be considered in anyone with a positive syphilis serology.

Tuberculosis Testing
Since HIV is the most potent known activator of latent TB, baseline and follow-up skin testing with controls is critically important in identifying patients who should receive antimicrobial prophylaxis [137–141]. Because skin testing depends on intact cell-mediated immunity, anergy is more common with advanced immunodeficiency. For this reason, induration of 5 mm or more in response to an inoculum of intermediate-strength purified protein derivative (PPD) is considered positive in HIV-infected patients [142]. Since the risk of developing active tuberculosis in this population is greater than that of isoniazid hepatitis, a positive PPD is an indication for prophylactic therapy in the previously untreated individual regardless of age and timing of PPD conversion. Isoniazid prophylaxis for one year should also be given to anergic HIV-seropositive patients at high risk for TB, including IDUs, the homeless, prisoners, alcoholics, immigrants from endemic countries, and those with recent TB exposure [143].

Chest Roentgenography
A screening chest x-ray may be helpful in detecting the subtle changes of early PCP in the future time. For this reason, it is desirable in the

patient with a history of cigarette smoking or injection drug use to obtain a baseline x-ray. Asymptomatic hilar adenopathy due to MAC, histoplasmosis, TB, cryptococcosis, or lymphoma may also be detected on screening radiographs.

Urinalysis and Renal Function Tests

HIV-related renal disease, including focal and segmental glomerulosclerosis, may be suspected on the basis of baseline urinalysis and renal function tests [144, 145]. These studies are also useful in that many drugs used in the management of HIV disease require dosage adjustment in the presence of renal dysfunction.

Toxoplasma Serology

Some authors have recommended that *Toxoplasma* antibody titers be obtained as part of the baseline evaluation of HIV-infected patients. This information may have value in selecting patients for antimicrobial prophylaxis and in identifying patients at risk for developing active disease.

Cytomegalovirus Serology

Cytomegalovirus serology has been advocated by some authorities as a screening test to determine which patients are at increased risk for developing CMV infection with advanced HIV disease. It may also be useful in patients requiring blood transfusion to identify those individuals who should be given white-blood-cell-poor products [146].

Serum Cryptococcal Antigen

Serum assay for polysaccharide capsule antigens of *Cryptococcus neoformans* has been reported to be 99 percent sensitive in detecting meningitis [147]. However, routine serum antigen screening of asymptomatic individuals is of little clinical utility at present.

Glucose 6-Phosphate Dehydrogenase

Patients who are deficient in glucose 6-phosphate dehydrogenase (G6PD) are at risk for hemolysis should they need to take a sulfone such as dapsone for PCP prophylaxis or therapy. Having baseline information on a patient's G6PD status allows for immediate therapy should it be necessary.

HIV Disease Staging

A number of clinical and laboratory variables are useful in staging HIV infection. Staging guides decisions regarding antiretroviral and prophylactic therapies, provides prognostic information, and helps to focus the differential diagnosis for specific clinical problems.

Clinical Markers

Information from a number of natural history studies suggests that certain clinical features may identify patients at risk for disease progression. Being at either end of the age spectrum appears to confer a negative prognosis, as does the presence of systemic symptoms, hairy leukoplakia, thrush, anemia, or leukopenia. Neither VZV infection nor generalized lymphadenopathy suggests a poor prognosis, although previously swollen nodes that involute may signal a decline in immune function. There are conflicting data regarding the prognostic significance of thrombocytopenia [148–155].

Laboratory Studies

CD4 Cell Count

CD4 cell counts are highly correlated with the progression of HIV disease. While the normal CD4 count ranges between 1,300/mm³ and 430/mm³, it is generally above 800/mm³ in healthy persons [156]. CD4 cell counts have been shown to decrease by 50 to 85 cells/mm³/yr in HIV-infected individuals, although one study suggested that this decline may be as low as 15 cells/mm³/yr in IDUs [157–159]. While opportunistic infections do not usually occur with CD4 counts between 800/mm³ and 500/mm³, HSV, VZV, thrush, and fungal or bacterial infections of the skin may be seen with counts below 500/mm³ (Fig. 32-1). A CD4 count of less than 200/mm³ indicates significant immunodefi-

Figure 32-1. Relationship of CD4 cell count to clinical manifestations of HIV infection.

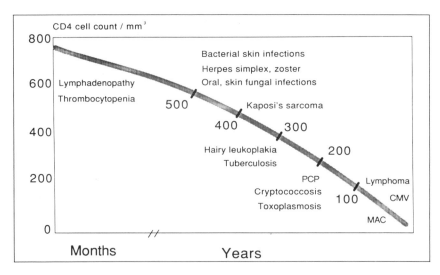
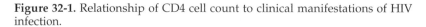

ciency with increased risk for serious opportunistic infections, such as PCP, toxoplasmosis, and cryptococcal meningitis. Patients with counts of less than $100/mm^3$ are also at risk for CMV and MAC infections, and for lymphoma. It is important to remember, however, that some patients with very low CD4 counts may be symptom free for months to a year or more [160].

Some investigators have suggested that the percentage of total lymphocytes that are CD4 cells may provide a more reliable indication of immune function than the absolute CD4 cell count [161]. However, current Centers for Disease Control (CDC) recommendations for instituting PCP prophylaxis do not include a CD4 percentage criterion [162].

CD4 cell count results may not always be reliable [163]. Since CD4 counts have a diurnal variation in most individuals, serial samples should be obtained at approximately the same time of day. Intercurrent illnesses, especially herpesvirus infections, may cause transient CD4 cell count depression. Since inter- and intralaboratory variation in test results may occur, it is wise to confirm the initial CD4 count and any subsequent values that are grossly different from baseline, especially if such results would lead to new therapeutic interventions.

Quantitation of Viral Plasma RNA
Several assays have recently been described for quantifying viral activity by directly measuring plasma HIV RNA. They have been shown to correlate well with disease stage and to predict benefit from antiretroviral treatment better than CD4 count response [164–166]. These assays will likely become more generally available and come into increased clinical use over the next few years.

p24 Antigenemia
The *gag* gene of HIV codes for a nuclear protein of 24 daltons known as the p24 antigen. p24 Antigenemia has been correlated with active viral replication and progression of HIV disease [167].

$ß_2$-Microglobulin
$ß_2$-Microglobulin is a low molecular weight globulin that forms part of the class 1 histocompatibility complex present on most somatic cells. $ß_2$-Microglobulin levels correlate with increased cell death and reflect the general level of lymphoid activation; they are increased in the presence of viral infections and hematologic malignancies. $ß_2$-Microglobulin levels greater than 5 µg/ml are associated with progression of HIV disease [168, 169]. Despite being a relatively inexpensive assay, $ß_2$-microglobulin testing is not available in many clinical settings. $ß_2$-Microglobulin levels may be increased in seronegative IDUs, diminishing the assay's usefulness in HIV-infected drug users [170].

Neopterin

Macrophages increase their production of neopterin, a metabolite of guanosine triphosphate, under the influence of gamma-interferon secreted from activated T cells. Increased serum or urinary neopterin levels in HIV-infected patients have a prognostic value that is independent of CD4 cell count [171–173].

Use of Laboratory Studies for Staging and Management

The CD4 cell count has historically been the principal means for clinical staging of patients and initiation and modification of antiretroviral and prophylactic therapies. p24 Antigen, β_2-microglobulin, and neopterin have proved less useful for staging but do contribute information on the degree of viral activation and may complement the CD4 count in making treatment decisions.

Although the baseline CD4 count has been shown to correlate well with the risk of developing complications of HIV disease, two studies have suggested that an improvement in the CD4 count (or a delay in decline of the CD4 count) associated with antiretroviral therapy does not necessarily indicate slowed clinical progression or improved survival [174, 175]. For this reason, the CD4 count response to therapy may have limited usefulness in judging the benefit of a particular drug regimen. Further studies are necessary to define more clearly the role of viral plasma RNA levels in clinical practice, but these assays carry great promise for staging patients and tailoring antiretroviral treatment.

Therapeutic Interventions

Initiation of Antiretroviral Therapy

The question of when antiretroviral therapy should be started is one of the more controversial treatment decisions at the present time. On the one hand, it is known that (1) an enormous viral load is present in peripheral lymph nodes even in the earliest stages of HIV infection [176]; (2) once a high peripheral viral burden develops, it tends to remain elevated in the absence of antiretroviral treatment [164]; (3) decreased viremia correlates with slowed disease progression; and (4) antiretroviral therapy may delay the onset of opportunistic infections [177]. For all these reasons, there is a theoretical advantage to initiating antiretroviral therapy early in the course of HIV infection.

However, currently available data on clinical outcomes such as progression to AIDS or death do not convincingly show a benefit associated with ZDV monotherapy in patients with a CD4 count of 500/mm^3 or higher. The only studies demonstrating increased survival have been in individuals with an AIDS-defining opportunistic infection or a CD4 count below 200/mm^3. While some patients may put a high priority on decreased symptomatology, even in the absence of a survival benefit, others may prefer to delay initiation of therapy, given its cost and potential toxicity, if they could achieve a similar effect with later treatment. Since most trials to date have focused on beginning antiretroviral monotherapy, it may be that the discrepancy between observed benefits and those predicted from natural history studies suggests that HIV infection should be optimally treated with more than one agent. Indeed, a number of studies looking at the impact of combination therapy on viral burden indicate that such regimens may be appropriate as the first mode of treatment [178–181].

If the utility of plasma RNA measurements is validated, it may be possible to tailor antiretroviral treatment in individual patients [182]. In those patients in whom no virologic improvement is seen, one of several possible changes in therapy could be tried, such as the addition of a second drug or use of another type of antiretroviral agent. This approach might allow the clinician to respond to viral characteristics, such as drug resistance and phenotype (SI vs NSI), without actually having to test for them.

Recommendations for Antiretroviral Therapy

Given that plasma RNA assays are still being validated in clinical practice and that the number of published clinical trials starting with or switching to combination therapy are few, how should the clinician approach the question of when to begin antiretroviral therapy? For patients with prior PCP or HIV-related symptoms and a CD4 count of $200/mm^3$ or less, there is no doubt that initiation of monotherapy with ZDV slows disease progression and improves survival [183, 184]. Combination antiretroviral therapy has also been proposed for patients in this group and is currently being evaluated in clinical trials [185].

For both symptomatic and asymptomatic patients with a CD4 count between $200/mm^3$ and $500/mm^3$, two large studies have shown that ZDV monotherapy leads to a reduction by at least half in progression to AIDS or severe symptoms but does not affect survival [186, 187]. The decision as to whether to initiate antiretroviral therapy for individuals in this group should be based on an assessment of its potential benefits compared to the cost, side effects, and the need for monitoring visits [188]. Because there appears to be a limited (1–3 year) duration of benefit with existing treatments [189] and only one type of agent (nucleoside analogue reverse transcriptase inhibitors) is currently available, theoretical concern could be raised about starting antiretroviral therapy in the absence of significant symptoms, only to be left with no options later in the course of HIV disease. On the other hand, the clinician might try to obtain limited benefit from currently available drugs as soon as the CD4 count drops to $500/mm^3$ in anticipation that new agents may provide greater therapeutic effect in the future [190].

For asymptomatic patients with a CD4 count greater than $500/mm^3$, only one study has shown a delay in HIV disease progression but included such relatively "soft" endpoints as hairy leukoplakia and herpes zoster [191]. Since there was no observed delay in progression to AIDS, antiretroviral therapy is not currently recommended for this group of patients.

Overview of Currently Available Nucleoside Analogues

For initial monotherapy, studies have shown that ZDV is preferable to didanosine (ddI) or ddC [192, 193]. Didanosine, ddC, and stavudine (d4T) can all be considered as alternative agents should the patient experience drug intolerance or clinical or immunologic progression [194–196]. Combinations of ZDV with ddI or ddC can also be attempted if monotherapy fails; using one of these combinations for patients starting antiretroviral therapy who have a CD4 count less than 200/mm³ has also been proposed [181, 197]. While combination treatment may be better than monotherapy in some patients, a retrospective analysis of ACTG 155 demonstrated a slowing of disease for individuals with CD4 counts between 150/mm³ and 300/mm³ who received ZDV and ddC, but possibly a worse outcome for those with CD4 counts less than 50/mm³ [198]. Indeed, if nucleoside analogues have significant toxicity in patients with very low CD4 counts or do not appear to confer benefit, discontinuation of antiretroviral therapy is a reasonable option in this setting [197].

Lamivudine (3TC), a new nucleoside analogue, and saquinavir and indinavir, two protease inhibitor drugs, have recently become available through pharamaceutical company parallel track programs. Their role in clinical practice is as yet undefined (see Chap. 31).

Clinical Use of Nucleoside Analogues

Zidovudine

Zidovudine is given in a total daily dose of 500 to 600 mg, administered either as one 100-mg capsule five times a day or two capsules three times a day. Headache and nausea, which may occur with initiation of therapy, can be minimized by gradually increasing the dose over a week or more and by using analgesics and antiemetics as needed. Chronic toxicities include bone marrow suppression, myositis, and rarely, liver function test abnormalities. Patients in whom anemia or neutropenia develops on ZDV can be treated with colony stimulating factors, such as erythropoietin or granulocyte colony stimulating factor (G-CSF), or switched to another agent. Patients receiving ZDV who have evidence of disease progression manifested by the development of an opportunistic infection or decline in CD4 cell count should be considered for other antiretroviral regimens.

Didanosine

Didanosine dosing is calculated by weight (125 mg bid in patients < 60 kg, and 200 mg bid for those ≥ 60 kg), with patients taking two tablets at each dose in order to receive an adequate amount of incorporated antacid. A powder preparation is also available, but the dosage differs from that of the tablet preparation. Didanosine should be administered 1 hour before or 2 hours after eating to maximize absorption. Tablets must be chewed or predissolved in water but should not be swallowed whole. Didanosine may interfere with absorption of dapsone if the two drugs are taken simultaneously. The principal toxicities of ddI are peripheral neuropathy and pancreatitis, and therapy should be discontinued if either develops. Neuropathy is generally reversible once the agent is stopped and may not recur if it is resumed at a lower dose. Serum amylase or lipase levels should be evaluated periodically to detect asymptomatic pancreatitis.

Zalcitabine

Zalcitabine in combination with ZDV is an option for patients who have progressed on ZDV monotherapy. Zalcitabine can also be used as monotherapy for patients with advanced HIV disease who are intolerant of ZDV or who have evidence of disease progression on therapy [195]. Zalcitabine is administered as one 0.75-mg tablet three times a day, both for monotherapy or in combination with other agents. The most frequently encountered side effects include peripheral neuropathy, oral ulcerations, and pancreatitis. Fatal cases of hepatomegaly with steatosis and lactic acidosis have also been reported [199]. Patients receiving ZDV and ddC who experience anemia or neutropenia should be treated with colony stimulating factors or have their ZDV dose reduced or the drug discontinued; those in whom gastrointestinal dysfunction or peripheral neuropathy develops should have their ddC therapy stopped and reintroduced at a lower dose after symptoms have resolved.

Stavudine

Like ZDV, d4T is a nucleoside analogue of thymidine. Stavudine has been approved as monotherapy for HIV-infected patients who are intolerant of ZDV or who have experienced toxicity to other agents. This is based on a study showing improvement in CD4 counts in patients switched to d4T after at least 24 weeks of prior ZDV therapy compared with those who continued on ZDV [196]. Peripheral neuropathy is the side effect most frequently described, followed by transiently increased hepatic transaminase levels. Insomnia, anxiety, and acute panic were also observed in one retrospective study of 96 patients being treated in the d4T parallel track program [200]. Stavudine is administered by weight, with patients of 60 kg or greater receiving 40 mg twice a day

Table 32-4 *Prophylactic antimicrobial therapies in HIV disease*[a]

	CD4 cell count		
Infection	*> 500/mm³*	*500–200/mm³*	*< 200/mm³*
PCP	None	None	TMP-SMX
MAC	None	None	Rifabutin[b]
Tuberculosis	Isoniazid	Same	Same
Fungal infections	None	None	Fluconazole
Toxoplasmosis	None	None	TMP-SMX
HSV	None	Acyclovir	Same
CMV	None	None	(?) Oral ganciclovir

PCP = *Pneumocystis carinii* pneumonia; TMP-SMX = trimethoprim-sulfamethoxazole; MAC = *Mycobacterium avium* complex; HSV = herpes simplex virus; CMV = cytomegalovirus.
[a]See text for discussion. USPHS recommendations are summarized in reference [215].
[b]Recommended for patients with CD4 cell count < 75/mm³.

and those under 60 kg receiving 30 mg twice a day. A reduced dosage should be used for individuals with hepatic dysfunction [196]. Zidovudine should not be administered concurrently with d4T.

Prophylaxis Against Opportunistic Infections

Preventive antimicrobial therapies used in HIV disease can be stratified by CD4 cell count (Table 32-4). The effectiveness of primary prophylaxis for PCP and MAC infection has been well documented (see below). Patients who have a history of a positive PPD or who are anergic and at risk for TB should receive one year of isoniazid therapy. Recent studies suggest that fluconazole is effective in preventing candidiasis and cryptococcosis in patients with advanced HIV disease [201, 202]. Trimethoprim-sulfamethoxazole confers some protection against toxoplasmosis, and dapsone alone or in combination with pyrimethamine appears to do so as well. Acyclovir is useful in preventing relapse of HSV infection, but its role in primary prophylaxis has not been established. However, it may be associated with a survival advantage in advanced HIV disease (see Clinical Use of Acyclovir). Oral ganciclovir is currently being evaluated for the prevention of CMV infection.

Pneumocystis carinii Pneumonia

Data continue to accrue regarding the relative efficacy of various prophylactic regimens in different patient populations. Based on the results of a trial comparing trimethoprim-sulfamethoxazole (TMP-SMX) with aerosol pentamidine (AP) as secondary prophylaxis, the CDC has recommended oral TMP-SMX as the drug of choice to prevent PCP [162] (see Fig. 19-3). While TMP-SMX, one double-strength tablet daily, is suggested, one published series of patients with CD4 counts less than 200/mm³ experienced no breakthrough infections using one double-strength tablet three times a week [203]. Patients can be rechallenged with TMP-SMX if a mild reaction develops, but those with major toxicity should either be treated with another regimen or desensitized using gradually increasing doses of TMP-SMX [204–206] (see Table 19-4). For those patients intolerant of TMP-SMX who cannot be desensitized, a number of alternative strategies are available. Dapsone has been used in treatment regimens including 50 mg per day and 100 mg three times a week [207]. Patients who experience an allergic reaction to dapsone may also benefit from desensitization [208]. Aerosol pentamidine is effective for prophylaxis against PCP, although less so than TMP-SMX and probably dapsone [209, 210]. For patients who cannot tolerate any of these regimens, other agents should be considered, including intravenous pentamidine, atovaquone, or pyrimethamine-sulfadoxine.

Mycobacterium avium Complex

Mycobacterium avium complex bacteremia has been shown to occur in up to 43 percent of patients within 2 years of an AIDS diagnosis. This incidence rises as the CD4 count declines and appears to be especially high in patients with a positive MAC culture of sputum or stool [211, 212]. Since untreated MAC bacteremia significantly decreases survival and treatment is only partially effective, antibiotic prophylaxis could potentially improve both quality of life and prognosis [213].

Two controlled trials evaluating rifabutin for prevention of MAC have been conducted involving a total of 590 patients with CD4 counts less than $200/mm^3$. Bacteremia was reduced from 18 percent in those receiving placebo to 9 percent in the treatment group [214]. In addition, rifabutin prophylaxis significantly delayed constitutional symptoms, laboratory abnormalities, and frequency of hospitalization, although no improvement in survival was seen. As a result of these studies, the United States Public Health Service has recommended that patients with HIV infection and CD4 count less than $75/mm^3$ receive lifetime preventive therapy for MAC with rifabutin 300 mg by mouth daily after excluding the presence of active mycobacterial disease [215]. However, in making a decision about rifabutin prophylaxis, its potential benefits should be weighed against its cost, toxicity, potential interaction with other drugs, and theoretical concerns about increased MAC and *M. tuberculosis* resistance [216–220].

Several recent preliminary studies have suggested that clarithromycin may also be effective for the primary prophylaxis of MAC infection [221–223]. The recommended preventive dose of clarithromycin is 500 mg by mouth twice a day.

Clinical Use of Acyclovir

Considerable interest has been generated regarding the potential use of acyclovir, with or without antiretroviral agents, in HIV-infected patients. An early trial randomized 130 patients with a diagnosis of

AIDS to receive ZDV alone (250 mg qid) or in combination with acyclovir (800 mg qid). At the end of a 24-week observation period, the combination treatment group had a survival rate of 85 percent compared with 66 percent for the monotherapy group [224]. Another study prospectively evaluated 302 HIV-infected patients with CD4 counts less than 150/mm³ who were randomized to receive placebo or 3,200 mg acyclovir per day for up to 48 weeks. Although suppression of clinical CMV infection was not observed, a survival benefit of 50 percent was reported in those treated with acyclovir [225]. On the other hand, a trial comparing no treatment to ZDV alone (2 gm/day for 1 month, followed by 1 gm/day) to the same dose of ZDV plus acyclovir (800 mg 5 times/day) in 199 patients with AIDS-related complex (ARC) found no advantage with combination therapy over a 6-month observation period [226]. Another study compared ZDV monotherapy to ZDV in combination with acyclovir (in the same doses as the aforementioned trial) in 302 patients with ARC and AIDS for a period of 12 months [227]. Initial analysis suggested as much as a 50 percent decreased mortality in the combination therapy group, especially in patients with AIDS. However, after adjusting for entry CD4 counts and severity of illness, only a statistically insignificant trend toward improved survival remained. More recently, retrospective analysis of data from the Multicenter AIDS Cohort Study demonstrated as much as a 36 percent reduction in the risk for death in patients with AIDS who had received a median of 600 to 800 mg per day of acyclovir in addition to ZDV, increasing survival by as much as 6 months [228]. Although no decrease in herpesvirus manifestations was noted in any of these trials, it is postulated that acyclovir may inhibit the stimulatory activity of these viruses on HIV replication [229–231].

Taken together, these reports suggest that acyclovir, alone or in combination with ZDV, may prolong survival in AIDS patients. While the data are encouraging, it is important to realize that only one prospective trial has thus far demonstrated a statistically significant benefit [225].

Overview of Stratified Management

CD4 Cell Count Greater Than 500/mm³
As a general rule, clinical studies do not support antiretroviral therapy for patients in this group, although those with HIV-related thrombocytopenia, constitutional symptoms, or encephalopathy may benefit from initiation of ZDV [232–236] (Table 32-5). While there are few specific therapeutic interventions to offer, patients should be provided education about their disease, emotional support, and routine health care maintenance. Medical follow-up for this group should be scheduled every 3 to 6 months.

Table 32-5 *Stratified management of HIV infection*

CD4 cell count > 500/mm^3
    No specific therapy (in absence of thrombocytopenia, dementia, or other
       HIV-related symptoms)
    Focus on patient education and health care maintenance issues
    Follow-up visits q3–6 mo
    Repeat CD4 counts q6 mo
CD4 cell count of 500–200/mm^3
    Discuss initiation of antiretroviral therapy (see text)
    Follow-up visits q1–3 mo
    Repeat CD4 counts q3 mo
CD4 cell count of 200–100/mm^3
    Initiate *Pneumocystis carinii* prophylaxis
    Encourage antiretroviral therapy if not previously initiated
    Consider switching patients receiving ZDV to another antiretroviral agent or
       adding a second agent
    Consider addition of acyclovir therapy
    Close surveillance for opportunistic infections
    Follow-up visits q4–6 wk
    Repeat CD4 counts q3 mo
CD4 cell count < 100/mm^3
    Consider initiating MAC prophylaxis
    Consider further modification of antiretroviral regimen, including
       discontinuation of drug(s)
    Close surveillance for CMV, MAC, and lymphoma
    Follow-up visits q1–4 wk
    Repeat CD4 counts unnecessary when CD4 count < 50/mm^3

CD4 Cell Count Between 500/mm^3 and 200/mm^3

As previously noted, initiation of antiretroviral treatment should
be individualized in this group based on its potential benefits and
toxicities and taking into account patient preference. In asymptomatic
or mildly symptomatic persons, monitoring without therapy is a reasonable option. Follow-up visits should be scheduled at 1- to 3-month
intervals, with attention focused on surveillance for HIV-related symptoms and monitoring for toxicity in those receiving antiretroviral
therapy.

CD4 Cell Count Less Than 200/mm^3

Prophylaxis for PCP should be initiated once the CD4 count falls below
200/mm^3; it is also indicated in patients with a prior history of PCP and
in those with counts above 200/mm^3 who have thrush or persistent,
unexplained fever [163]. This group is at greatest risk for serious opportunistic infections and neoplasms and should be seen in follow-up
at 4- to 6-week intervals. Patients should be encouraged to begin
antiretroviral therapy if they have not previously done so; modification of their regimen, with addition of a second agent or switching to

another drug, should be considered for those with evidence of disease progression. Clinicians may also want to consider adding acyclovir in a dose of 400 to 800 mg twice a day, based on the data suggesting a survival advantage.

CD4 Cell Count Less Than 100/mm³

Rifabutin prophylaxis should be considered for all patients in this group. Individuals whose CD4 count is less than 50/mm³ are at increased risk for death and should be monitored carefully for CMV and MAC infections as well as lymphoma [237, 238]. As previously noted, further modification or discontinuation of antiretroviral therapy should be considered if the CD4 count continues to decline.

Other Considerations in Clinical Management

Alternative Medical Therapies

Alternative medical therapies are commonly used by HIV-infected patients, often in conjunction with conventional treatments, but individuals may not volunteer such information unless it is specifically requested [239]. The rationale, safety, and efficacy of alternative medical therapies for HIV disease are summarized in Appendix B.

Clinical Trials

Participation in clinical trials should be encouraged for HIV-infected patients in therapeutic areas where optimal management is not known (see Chap. 33). Good communication between research staff and the primary care provider is important to ensure coordination of care.

Substance Abuse Issues

Many HIV-infected patients have a history of substance abuse involving alcohol, cocaine, crack, or opiates. Clinicians should recognize that the stress of being seropositive or developing symptomatic disease may lead to substance abuse relapse. Maintenance of sobriety is a key component of comprehensive care, and, in some situations, substance abuse treatment may be a higher priority than treatment for HIV infection, since the latter may be impossible or ineffective in the context of active drug use.

Psychosocial Support

Informing patients about support groups and AIDS service organizations available within the community is another important aspect of primary care. "Buddies" available through service organizations can provide long-term emotional support that may otherwise be unavailable to patients who have been estranged from family or the community at large.

Personal Finances

Assessment of the patient's financial situation and insurance status should also be part of the intake process, with attention given to ascertaining eligibility for entitlement programs for health care, general relief, disability, and housing.

Legal Issues

A variety of legal issues can take on dramatic significance for those with life-threatening HIV disease, especially if the patient is a single parent or involved in a nontraditional relationship such as a long-term homosexual union. Patients may need to anticipate transfer of custody for their children and should also be encouraged to arrange for others to make medical judgments on their behalf in case of severe illness by executing an advance directive for health care, a durable power of attorney, or both. Many AIDS service organizations provide legal services to help patients draw up legal instruments and deal with custody issues.

Food Safety

Caution in food preparation and handling is important given the vulnerability to infections that accompanies immunodeficiency. Using a plastic or glass instead of wooden cutting board may decrease the chance of bacterial contamination. Microwaved foods, especially poultry, should be allowed to stand for a few minutes after cooking to ensure that heat is evenly distributed. Because of the risk of salmonellosis, raw egg products should not be consumed. Raw seafood (sashimi, sushi, oysters) or meat (steak tartare) should also be avoided because of potential transmission of bacterial and protozoal pathogens.

Pet Safety

Pets can be an important source of companionship, affection, and comfort for HIV-infected patients [240]. While a few animals may present a risk for acquiring particular infections, most domestic pets can be cared for safely if common sense guidelines are followed [241, 242] (Table 32-6).

Health Care Maintenance

The provision of primary care to HIV-infected patients includes routine health care maintenance, as well as vaccination and screening

Table 32-6 *Pet care guidelines*

General pet hygiene
    Wash hands frequently after animal contact
    Use gloves when changing litter box or cleaning aquarium
    Keep the pet's living and feeding area clean, and control fleas
    Avoid contact with a pet's body fluids
Cats
    Cats can carry toxoplasmosis and transmit it through contact with feces or
      cat litter
    Keep cat litter boxes away from kitchen and eating areas and change the
      litter box daily, using care to avoid inhalation of dust particles
    Disinfect the litter box at least once a month
    Keep fleas under control to decrease the risk of transmitting
      Rochalimaea henselae (cat-scratch disease)
Preventive veterinary medicine
    Keep vaccinations current
    Take pet in for a routine examination at least once a year
    Contact a veterinarian if animal shows signs of possible illness
    Have new pets examined by a veterinarian to screen for diseases and
      parasites
Animal bites
    Tend to any animal bites immediately to help prevent infection by rinsing
      with cold running water
    Disinfect with a preparation such as povidone-iodine (Betadine) solution
    After first aid, always contact your physician

Source: Modified from Pets Are Wonderful Support (PAWS). *Safe Pet Guidelines.* Education Department, PO Box 460489, San Francisco, CA 94146-0489 (telephone: 415-824-4040).

examination protocols adapted to this population. A recommended health care maintenance schedule is presented in Table 32-7.

Periodic Physical Examination

Pelvic Examination

As previously noted, HIV-infected women with HPV infection may be at increased risk for cervical cancer. Although an early report suggested that a relative insensitivity of the Papanicolaou (Pap) smear might necessitate colposcopy to screen for cervical neoplasia in HIV-infected women, several subsequent studies have indicated that the standard screening test appears to be adequate [243–245]. While the CDC currently recommends only annual Pap smears [246], Pap smears twice each year are suggested to HIV-infected women at our institutions, with colposcopic evaluation of any suspicious lesions.

Rectal Examination

Patients with a history of receptive anal intercourse or anogenital condylomas should have surveillance rectal examinations performed annually.

Table 32-7 *HIV infection health care maintenance schedule*

Issue	Intake	Semiannually	Annually
Pneumococcal vaccine	X		
Hepatitis B vaccine	X[a]		
Influenza vaccine			X
Haemophilus vaccine	X		
Rectal examination	X		X[b]
Breast examination	X[c]		X[c]
Syphilis serology	X		X
Chlamydia/gonorrhea	X		X[c]
Pap smear	X[c]	X[c]	
Mammography	X[c,d]		X[c,d]
PPD, controls	X		X[e]
Patient education	X[f]		
Mental health assessment	X[f]		
Addiction assessment	X[f]		

[a]HBV-seronegative patients.
[b]Patients with a history of receptive anal intercourse and/or HPV infection.
[c]Women only.
[d]Baseline at age 35–40; annually after the age of 40 or 50.
[e]PPD-negative or previously anergic patients with improved CD4 cell counts.
[f]As needed thereafter based on patient characteristics.

Immunizations

Overview
Administration of appropriate immunizations constitutes an important part of routine health care for HIV-infected patients but appears to be underutilized [247] (Table 32-8; see also Table 32-7). Because diminished antibody production in response to vaccination is associated with profound immunodeficiency, immunizations should be administered as early in the course of HIV disease as possible.

Questions regarding safety of live-virus vaccines in HIV-infected persons were raised in 1987, when disseminated vaccinia developed in an asymptomatic, seropositive military recruit after the administration of smallpox vaccine [248, 249]. Disseminated mycobacterial disease was also reported following bacillus Calmette-Guérin (BCG) vaccination in two symptomatic HIV-infected adults [250, 251]. However, these cases represent the only serious morbidity from live viral vaccination of HIV-infected patients reported to date.

Influenza Vaccine
Although annual immunization with influenza vaccine has been recommended for HIV-infected persons, diminished antibody response has been associated with advanced immunodeficiency [252]. In one

Table 32-8 *Use of immunizations in HIV-infected patients**

Vaccine	Children	Adults
DPT	Yes	Td preparation
OPV	No	No
e-IPV	Yes	No
MMR	Yes	Yes
Hib	Yes	Yes
Hepatitis B	Yes	Yes
Influenza	Yes	Yes
Pneumococcal	Yes	Yes

DPT = diphtheria-pertussis-tetanus; Td = diphtheria-tetanus; OPV = oral poliovirus vaccine; e-IPV = enhanced inactivated polio vaccine; MMR = measles-mumps-rubella; Hib = *Haemophilus influenzae* type b conjugate vaccine.
*See text for discussion.
Source: Adapted from DE Craven et al. Immunization of adults and children infected with human immunodeficiency virus. *Infect Dis Clin Prac* 1:330–338, 411–423, 1992; American College of Physicians Task Force on Adult Immunization and Infectious Disease Society of America. *Guide for Adult Immunization* (2nd ed), 1990; Centers for Disease Control. Update of adult immunization: Recommendations of the Immunization Practices Advisory Committee. *MMWR* 40:1–94, 1991; and American Academy of Pediatrics. *Report of the Committee on Infectious Diseases* (22nd ed), 1991.

study, 94 to 100 percent of seronegative control subjects had an adequate antibody response, compared to 52 to 89 percent of asymptomatic seropositive individuals and 13 to 50 percent of those with advanced HIV disease [253].

Pneumococcal Vaccine
Pneumococcal pneumonia and bacteremia have been shown to occur with increased frequency in HIV-infected patients [254, 255]. Pneumococcal vaccine is recommended for persons who are predisposed to bacteremic pneumococcal disease if they are capable of producing an antibody response [256]. Although some studies have described impaired responsiveness to pneumococcal vaccine in patients with symptomatic HIV disease, others have suggested that adequate antibody response is achievable in asymptomatic seropositive individuals and those with mild HIV-related symptoms [257–259].

Haemophilus influenzae, Type B, Vaccine
Because patients with HIV infection are at increased risk for bacteremic hemophilus infection, routine use of *H. influenzae* vaccine has been advocated for this population, although its efficacy has not been demonstrated [260].

Measles-Mumps-Rubella Vaccine (MMR)
Six fatal cases of measles in unvaccinated HIV-infected children have been reported to the CDC, suggesting that the risk of life-threatening

measles in unvaccinated HIV-infected children appears to be greater than the risk of developing disease as a result of vaccination [261]. MMR is given at the usual ages for all asymptomatic HIV-infected children and should also be considered in those who are symptomatic. Severe immunodeficiency from HIV infection has not been associated with decreased immunity to measles in previously vaccinated adults. It has been suggested that the measles antibody status of HIV-infected adults without proof of prior immunization should be ascertained and that live measles vaccine be administered to susceptible individuals [262, 263].

Polio Vaccine

Oral poliovirus vaccine (OPV) results in shedding of live virus. Although vaccination-related paralytic poliomyelitis is rare (1 in 2.6-4.3 million doses), most recent cases of polio in the United States have resulted from vaccination [264, 265]. Despite this risk, administration of OPV to many HIV-infected children in Europe and the United States has not resulted in adverse reactions [266]. Nevertheless, to minimize the possibility of active disease, enhanced inactivated polio vaccine (e-IPV) should be used instead of OPV to immunize HIV-infected children and their household contacts [267]. Enhanced inactivated polio vaccine should also be administered to HIV-seronegative children residing in the same household with HIV-infected adults or children. Adults who were not vaccinated as children do not need to be immunized.

Hepatitis B Vaccine

Some decreased responsiveness to antibody production following vaccination with hepatitis B vaccine has been noted in the HIV-infected population [268, 269]. Nevertheless, patients who are hepatitis B surface antigen and antibody negative and remain at risk for acquiring HBV should be considered for vaccination.

Tetanus Toxoid

No adverse reactions to the administration of tetanus toxoid have been reported among HIV-infected children or adults. Current recommendations are for children to receive the usual sequence of diphtheria-pertussis-tetanus (DPT) injections and for adults to receive a booster dose (Td) every 10 years.

References

1. Gabel RH, Barnard N, Norko M, O'Connel RA. AIDS presenting as mania. *Compr Psychiatry* 27:251–254, 1986.
2. Jones GH, Kelly CL, Davies JA. HIV and onset of schizophrenia. *Lancet* 1:982, 1987.

3. Perry S, Jacobsen P. Neuropsychiatric manifestations of AIDS-spectrum disorders. *Hosp Community Psychiatry* 37:135–142, 1986.

4. Maccario M, Scharre DW. HIV and acute onset of psychosis. *Lancet* 2:342, 1987.

5. Berman A, Espinoza LR, Diax JD, et al. Rheumatic manifestations of human immunodeficiency virus infection. *Am J Med* 85:59–64, 1988.

6. Buskila D, Gladman D. Musculoskeletal manifestations of infection with human immunodeficiency virus. *Rev Infect Dis* 12:223–235, 1990.

7. Fuente C, Velez A, Martin N, et al. Reiter's syndrome and human immunodeficiency virus infection: Case report and review of the literature. *Cutis* 47:181–185, 1991.

8. Foreman J. Suicides raise question on AIDS testing. *The Boston Globe* February 2, 1987.

9. Glass RM. AIDS and suicide. *JAMA* 259:1369–1370, 1988.

10. Goldblum P, Moulton J. AIDS-related suicide: A dilemma for health care providers. *Focus* 2:1–2, 1986.

11. Marzuk PM, Tierney H, Tardiff K, et al. Increased risk of suicide in persons with AIDS. *JAMA* 259:1333–1337, 1989.

12. Pierce C. Suicides underscore urgency of HIV test counseling. *Fam Pract News* 17:16, 1987.

13. Tyson E, Fortenberry JD. Fraudulent AIDS: A variant of Munchausen's syndrome. *JAMA* 258:1889–1890, 1987.

14. Evans GA, Gill MJ, Gerhart S. Factitious AIDS. *N Engl J Med* 319:1605–1606, 1988.

15. Levine SS. An AIDS diagnosis used as focus of malingering. *West J Med* 148:337–338, 1988.

16. Craven DE, et al. Factitious HIV infection: The importance of documenting infection. *Ann Intern Med* 121:763–766, 1994.

17. Daling JR, Weiss NS, Hislop G, et al. Sexual practices, sexually transmitted diseases, and the incidence of anal cancer. *N Engl J Med* 317:973–977, 1987.

18. Enck RE. Squamous cell cancers and the acquired immunodeficiency syndrome. *Ann Intern Med* 106:773, 1987.

19. Overly WL, Jakubek DJ. Multiple squamous cell carcinomas and human immunodeficiency virus infection. *Ann Intern Med* 102:334, 1987.

20. Sonnex C, Mindel A. Sexual practices, sexually transmitted diseases, and the incidence of anal cancer. *N Engl J Med* 318:990, 1988.

21. Centers for Disease Control. Risk for cervical disease in HIV-infected women—New York City. *MMWR* 39:846–849, 1990.

22. Melbye M, Cote TR, Kessler L, et al. High incidence of anal cancer among AIDS patients. *Lancet* 343:636–639, 1994.

23. Bodsworth N, Donovan B, Nightingale BN. The effect of concurrent human immunodeficiency virus infection on chronic hepatitis B: A study of 150 homosexual men. *J Infect Dis* 160:577–582, 1989.

24. Bodsworth NJ, Cooper DA, Donovan B. The influence of human immunodeficiency virus type 1 infection on the development of the hepatitis B virus carrier state. *J Infect Dis* 163:1138–1140, 1991.

25. Vento S, Di Perri G, Luzzati R, et al. Clinical reactivation of hepatitis B in anti-HBs-positive patients with AIDS. *Lancet* 1:332–333, 1989.

26. Selwyn PA, Hartel D, Lewis VA, et al. A prospective study of the risk of tuberculosis among intravenous drug users with human immunodeficiency virus infection. *N Engl J Med* 320:545–550, 1989.
27. Furth PA. Megestrol acetate and cachexia associated with human immunodeficiency virus (HIV) infection. *Ann Intern Med* 110:667, 1989.
28. Von Roenn JH, Murphy RL, Weber KM, et al. Megestrol acetate for treatment of cachexia associated with human immunodeficiency virus (HIV) infection. *Ann Intern Med* 109:840–841, 1988.
29. Von Roenn JH, Armstrong D, Kotler DP, et al. Megestrol acetate in patients with AIDS-related cachexia. *Ann Intern Med* 121:393–399, 1994.
30. Oster MH, Enders SR, Samuels SJ, et al. Megestrol acetate in patients with AIDS and cachexia. *Ann Intern Med* 121:400–408, 1994.
31. Haller DG. Weight gain in patients with AIDS-related cachexia: Is bigger better? *Ann Intern Med* 121:462–463, 1994.
32. Gorter R, Seefried M, Volberding P. Dronabinol effects on weight in patients with HIV infection. *AIDS* 6:127, 1992.
33. Schambelan M, LaMarca A, Mulligan K, et al. Growth hormone therapy of AIDS wasting. Tenth International Conference on AIDS, Yokohama, August 1994.
34. Gold JWM, Weikel CS, Godbold J, et al. Unexplained persistent lymphadenopathy in homosexual men and the acquired immune deficiency syndrome. *Medicine (Baltimore)* 64:203–213, 1985.
35. Abrams DI. AIDS-related lymphadenopathy: The role of biopsy. *J Clin Oncol* 4:126–127, 1986.
36. Libman H. Generalized lymphadenopathy. *J Gen Intern Med* 2:48–58, 1987.
37. Koehler JE, LeBoit PE, Egbert BM, Berger TG. Cutaneous vascular lesions and disseminated cat-scratch disease in patients with the acquired immunodeficiency syndrome (AIDS) and AIDS-related complex. *Ann Intern Med* 109:449–455, 1988.
38. Koehler JE, Tappero JW. Bacillary angiomatosis and bacillary peliosis in patients infected with human immunodeficiency virus. *Clin Infect Dis* 17:612–624, 1993.
39. Denning DW, Anderson J, Rudge P, Smith H. Acute myelopathy associated with primary infection with human immunodeficiency virus. *Br Med J* 143–144, 1987.
40. Goudsmit J, De Wolf F, Paul DA, et al. Expression of human immunodeficiency virus antigen (HIV-Ag) in serum and cerebrospinal fluid during acute and chronic infection. *Lancet* 2:177–180, 1986.
41. So YT, Holtzman DM, Abrams DI, Olney RK. Peripheral neuropathy associated with acquired immunodeficiency syndrome: Prevalence and clinical features from a population-based survey. *Arch Neurol* 45:945–948, 1988.
42. de la Monte SM, Gabuzda DH, Ho DD, et al. Peripheral neuropathy in the acquired immunodeficiency syndrome. *Ann Neurol* 23:485–492, 1988.
43. Husstedt IW, Grotemeyer KH, Busch H, Zidek W. Progression of distal-symmetric polyneuropathy in HIV infection: A prospective study. *AIDS* 7:1069–1073, 1993.
44. Villa A, Foresti V, Confalonieri F. Autonomic neuropathy and HIV infection. *Lancet* 2:915, 1987.

45. Craddock C, Pasvol G, Bull R, et al. Cardiorespiratory arrest and autonomic neuropathy in AIDS. *Lancet* 2:16–18, 1987.

46. Carne CA, Tedder RS, Smith A, et al. Acute encephalopathy coincident with seroconversion for anti-HTLV-III. *Lancet* 2:1206–1208, 1985.

47. Navia BA, Jordan BD, Price RW. The AIDS dementia complex: I. Clinical features. *Ann Neurol* 19:517–524, 1986.

48. Petito CK, Navia BA, Cho ES, et al. Vacuolar myelopathy pathologically resembling subacute combined degeneration in patients with the acquired immunodeficiency syndrome. *N Engl J Med* 312:874–879, 1985.

49. Singh BM, Levine S, Yarrish RL, et al. Spinal cord syndromes in the acquired immune deficiency syndrome. *Acta Neurol Scand* 73:590–598, 1986.

50. Godofsky EW, Zinreich J, Armstrong M, et al. Sinusitis in HIV-infected patients: A clinical and radiographic review. *Am J Med* 93:163–170, 1992.

51. Small CB, Kaufman A, Armenaka M, Rosenstreich DL. Sinusitis and atopy in human immunodeficiency virus infection. *J Infect Dis* 167:283–290, 1993.

52. Zurlo JJ, Feuerstein IM, Lebovics R, Lane CH. Sinusitis in HIV-1 infection. *Am J Med* 93:157–162, 1992.

53. Rabeneck L, Popovic M, Gartner S, et al. Acute HIV infection presenting with painful swallowing and esophageal ulcers. *JAMA* 263:2318–2322, 1990.

54. Edwards P, Turner J, Gold J, Cooper DA. Esophageal ulceration induced by zidovudine. *Ann Intern Med* 112:65–66, 1990.

55. Indorf AS, Pegram PS. Esophageal ulceration related to zalcitabine (ddC). *Ann Intern Med* 117:133–134, 1992.

56. Wilcox CM. Esophageal disease in the acquired immunodeficiency syndrome: Etiology, diagnosis and management. *Am J Med* 92:412–421, 1992.

57. Slomianski A, Snyder M, Goldmeier P. Concomitant esophageal and penile ulcerations healed with steroid therapy in a patient with AIDS: A case report. *Clin Infect Dis* 15:861–862, 1992.

58. Bach MC, Howell DA, Valenti AJ, et al. Aphthous ulceration of the gastrointestinal tract in patients with acquired immunodeficiency syndrome (AIDS). *Ann Intern Med* 112:465–467, 1990.

59. Wilcox CM, Schwartz DA. A pilot study of oral corticosteroid therapy for idiopathic esophageal ulcerations associated with human immunodeficiency virus infection. *Am J Med* 93:131–134, 1992.

60. Youle M, Clarbour J, Farthing C, et al. Treatment of resistant aphthous ulceration with thalidomide in patients positive for HIV antibody. *Br Med J* 298:432, 1989.

61. Winchester R, Bernstein DH, Fischer HD, et al. The co-occurrence of Reiter's syndrome and acquired immunodeficiency. *Ann Intern Med* 106:19–26, 1987.

62. Fuente C, Velez A, Martin N, et al. Reiter's syndrome and human immunodeficiency virus infection: Case report and review of the literature. *Cutis* 47:181–185, 1991.

63. Buskila D, Gladman D. Musculoskeletal manifestations of infection with human immunodeficiency virus. *Rev Infect Dis* 12:223–235, 1990.

64. Forster SM, Seifert MH, Keat AC, et al. Inflammatory joint disease and human immunodeficiency virus infection. *Br Med J* 296:1625–1627, 1988.

65. Dalakas MC, Illa I, Pezeshkpour GH, et al. Mitochondrial myopathy caused by long-term zidovudine therapy. *N Engl J Med* 322:1098–1105, 1990.
66. Arnaudo E, Dalakas M, Shanske S, et al. Depletion of muscle mitochondrial DNA in AIDS patients with zidovudine-induced myopathy. *Lancet* 337:508–510, 1991.
67. Simms RW, Zerbini CAF, Ferrante N, et al. Fibromyalgia syndrome in patients infected with human immunodeficiency virus. *Am J Med* 92:368–374, 1992.
68. Eisenstat BA, Wormser GP. Seborrheic dermatitis and butterfly rash in AIDS. *N Engl J Med* 311:189, 1984.
69. Johnson TM, Duvic M, Rapini RP, et al. AIDS exacerbates psoriasis. *N Engl J Med* 313:1415, 1985.
70. Fuchs D, Hausen A, Reibnegger G, et al. Psoriasis, gamma-interferon, and the acquired immunodeficiency syndrome. *Ann Intern Med* 106:165, 1987.
71. Duvic M, Rios A, Brewton GW. Remission of AIDS-associated psoriasis with zidovudine. *Lancet* 2:627, 1987.
72. Ruzicka T, Froschl M, Hohenleutner U. Treatment of HIV-induced retinoid-resistant psoriasis with zidovudine. *Lancet* 2:1469–1470, 1987.
73. Soeprono FF, Schinella RA. Eosinophilic pustular folliculitis in patients with acquired immunodeficiency syndrome. *J Am Acad Dermatol* 14:1020–1022, 1986.
74. Buchness MR, Lim HW, Hatcher VA, et al. Eosinophilic pustular folliculitis in the acquired immunodeficiency syndrome: Treatment with ultraviolet B phototherapy. *N Engl J Med* 318:1183–1186, 1988.
75. Jacobson MA, Gellermann H, Chambers H. *Staphylococcus aureus* bacteremia and recurrent staphylococcal infection in patients with acquired immunodeficiency syndrome and AIDS-related complex. *Am J Med* 85:172–176, 1988.
76. Furth PA, Kazakis AM. Nail pigmentation changes associated with azidothymidine (zidovudine). *Ann Intern Med* 107:350, 1987.
77. Panwalker AP. Nail pigmentation in the acquired immunodeficiency syndrome (AIDS). *Ann Intern Med* 107:943–944, 1987.
78. Vaiopoulos G, Mangakis J, Karabinis A, et al. Nail pigmentation and azidothymidine. *Ann Intern Med* 108:777, 1988.
79. Buchbinder SP, Katz MH, Hessol NA, et al. Herpes zoster and human immunodeficiency virus infection. *J Infect Dis* 166:1143–1156, 1992.
80. Rogues AM, Dupon M, Ladner J, et al. Herpes zoster and human immunodeficiency virus infection: A cohort study of 101 coinfected patients. *J Infect Dis* 168:245, 1993.
81. Sandor EV, Millman A, Croxson TS, et al. Herpes zoster ophthalmicus in patients at risk for the acquired immunodeficiency syndrome (AIDS). *Am J Ophthalmol* 101:153–155, 1986.
82. Ryder JW, Croen K, Kleinschmidt-DeMaster K. Progressive encephalitis three months after resolution of cutaneous zoster in a patient with AIDS. *Ann Neurol* 19:182–188, 1986.
83. Forster DJ, Dugel PU, Frangieh GT, et al. Rapidly progressive outer retinal necrosis in the acquired immunodeficiency syndrome. *Am J Ophthalmol* 110:341–348, 1990.

84. Margolis TP, Lowder CY, Holland GN, et al. Varicella-zoster virus retinitis in patients with the acquired immunodeficiency syndrome. *Am J Ophthalmol* 112:119–131, 1991.

85. Hellinger WC, Bolling JP, Smith TF, Campbell RJ. Varicella-zoster virus retinitis in a patient with AIDS-related complex: Case report and brief review of the acute retinal necrosis syndrome. *Clin Infect Dis* 16:208–212, 1993.

86. Cohen PR, Beltrani VP, Grossman ME. Disseminated herpes zoster in patients with human immunodeficiency virus infection. *Am J Med* 84:1076–1080, 1988.

87. Perniciaro C, Peters MS. Tinea faciale mimicking seborrheic dermatitis in a patient with AIDS. *N Engl J Med* 314:315–316, 1986.

88. Oral viral lesion (hairy leukoplakia) associated with acquired immunodeficiency syndrome. *MMWR* 34:549–550, 1985.

89. Greenspan JS, Greenspan D, Lennette ET, et al. Replication of Epstein-Barr virus within the epithelial cells of oral "hairy" leukoplakia, an AIDS-associated lesion. *N Engl J Med* 313:1564–1571, 1985.

90. Friedman-Kien AE. Viral origin of hairy leukoplakia. *Lancet* 2:694, 1986.

91. Greenspan D, Greenspan JS, Hearts NG, et al. Relation of oral hairy leukoplakia to infection with the human immunodeficiency virus and the risk of developing AIDS. *J Infect Dis* 155:475–481, 1987.

92. Newman C, Polk F. Resolution of oral hairy leukoplakia during therapy with 9-(1,3-dihydroxy-2-propoxymethyl) guanine (DHPG). *Ann Intern Med* 107:348–350, 1987.

93. Friedman-Kien AE. Viral origin of hairy leukoplakia. *Lancet* 2:694, 1986.

94. Katz MH, Greenspan D, Heinic GS, et al. Resolution of hairy leukoplakia: An observational trial of zidovudine versus no treatment. *J Infect Dis* 164:1240–1241, 1991.

95. Resnick L. Herbst JS, Ablashi DV, et al. Regression of oral hairy leukoplakia after orally administered acyclovir therapy. *JAMA* 259:384–388, 1988.

96. Greenspan JS, Greenspan D, Winkler JR. Diagnosis and Management of the Oral Manifestations of HIV Infection and AIDS. In MA Sande, PA Volberding (eds), *The Medical Management of AIDS*. Philadelphia: Saunders, 1988. P 131.

97. Krause PR, Straus SE. Zoster and its complications. *Hosp Pract* 25:61–76, 1990.

98. Centers for Disease Control. Microsporidian keratoconjunctivitis in patients with AIDS. *MMWR* 39:188–189, 1990.

99. Sneed SR, Blodi CF, Berger BB, et al. *Pneumocystis carinii* choroiditis in patients receiving inhaled pentamidine. *N Engl J Med* 322:936–937, 1990.

100. Cantrill HL, Henry K, Sannerud K, Balfour HH. HIV infection of the retina. *N Engl J Med* 318:1539, 1988.

101. Pomerantz RJ, Kuritzkes DR, De la Monte SM, et al. Infection of the retina by human immunodeficiency virus type 1. *N Engl J Med* 317:1643–1647, 1987.

102. Holland GN, Pepose JS, Pettit TH, et al. Acquired immune deficiency syndrome: Ocular manifestations. *Ophthalmology* 90:859–873, 1983.

103. Mines JA, Kaplan HJ. Acquired immunodeficiency syndrome (AIDS): The disease and its ocular manifestations. *Int Ophthalmol Clin* 26:73–115, 1986.

104. deSmet MD, Nussenbatt RB. Ocular manifestations of AIDS. *JAMA* 266:3019–3022, 1991.
105. deSmet MD. Differential diagnosis of retinitis and choroiditis in patients with acquired immunodeficiency syndrome. *Am J Med* 92 (suppl 2A):17S–21S, 1992.
106. Freeman WR, Chen A, Henderly DE, et al. Prevalence and significance of acquired immunodeficiency syndrome-related microvasculopathy. *Am J Ophthalmol* 107:229–235, 1990.
107. Bloom JN, Palestine AG. The diagnosis of cytomegalovirus retinitis. *Ann Intern Med* 109:963–969, 1988.
108. Acierno LJ. Cardiac complications in acquired immunodeficiency syndrome (AIDS): A review. *J Am Coll Cardiol* 13:1144–1154, 1989.
109. Herskowitz A, et al. Cardiomyopathy associated with antiretroviral therapy in patients with HIV infection: A report of six cases. *Ann Intern Med* 116:311–313, 1992.
110. Calabrese LH, Proffitt MR, Yen-Lieberman B, et al. Congestive cardiomyopathy and illness related to the acquired immunodeficiency syndrome (AIDS) associated with isolation of retrovirus from myocardium. *Ann Intern Med* 107:691–692, 1987.
111. Raviglione MC, Battan R, Pablos-Mendez A, et al. Infections associated with Hickman catheters in patients with acquired immunodeficiency syndrome. *Am J Med* 86:780–786, 1989.
112. Skoutelis AT, Murphy RL, MacDonell KB, et al. Indwelling central venous catheter infections in patients with acquired immune deficiency syndrome. *J Acquir Immune Defic Syndr* 3:335–342, 1990.
113. Biggers SD, Laguardia KD. The effect of human immunodeficiency virus infection on the course of pelvic inflammatory disease. Tenth International Conference on AIDS, Yokohama, August 1994.
114. Hankins CA. Issues involving women, children, and AIDS primarily in the developed world. *J Acquir Immune Defic Syndr* 3:443–448, 1990.
115. Imam N, Carpenter CCJ, Mayer KH, et al. Hierarchical pattern of mucosal *Candida* infections in HIV-seropositive women. *Am J Med* 89:142–146, 1990.
116. Rhoads JL, Wright DC, Redfield RR, Burke DS. Chronic vaginal candidiasis in women with human immunodeficiency virus infection. *JAMA* 257:3105–3107, 1987.
117. Jones BN, Teng EL, Folstein MF, Harrison KS. A new bedside test of cognition for patients with HIV infection. *Ann Intern Med* 119:1001–1004, 1993.
118. Sherman KE, Freeman S, Harrison S, Andron L. Prevalence of antibody to hepatitis C virus in patients infected with the human immunodeficiency virus. *J Infect Dis* 163:414, 1991.
119. Eyster ME, Alter HJ, Aledort LM, et al. Heterosexual co-transmission of hepatitis C virus (HCV) and human immunodeficiency virus (HIV). *Ann Intern Med* 115:764–768, 1991.
120. Gordin FM, Gibert C, Hawley HP, Willoughby A. Prevalence of human immunodeficiency virus and hepatitis B virus in unselected hospital admissions: Implications for mandatory testing and universal precautions. *J Infect Dis* 161:14–17, 1990.
121. Kingsley LA, Rinaldo CR, Lyter DW, et al. Sexual transmission efficiency

of hepatitis B virus and human immunodeficiency virus among homosexual men. *JAMA* 264:230–234, 1990.

122. Thomas DL, Cannon RO, Shapiro CN, et al. Hepatitis C, hepatitis B, and human immunodeficiency virus infections among non-intravenous drug-using patients attending clinics for sexually transmitted diseases. *J Infect Dis* 169:990–995, 1994.

123. Kreek MJ, Des Jarlais DC, Trepo CL, et al. Contrasting prevalence of delta hepatitis markers in parenteral drug abusers with and without AIDS. *J Infect Dis* 162:538–541, 1990.

124. Buti M, Esteban R, Espanol MT, et al. Influence of human immunodeficiency virus infection on cell-mediated immunity on chronic D hepatitis. *J Infect Dis* 163:1351–1353, 1991.

125. Solomon RE, Kaslow RA, Phair JP, et al. Human immunodeficiency virus and hepatitis delta virus in homosexual men: A study of four cohorts. *Ann Intern Med* 108:51–54, 1988.

126. Centers for Disease Control. Update on adult immunization: Recommendations of the Immunization Practices Advisory Committee (ACIP). *MMWR* 40(RR–12):8–9, 1991.

127. Centers for Disease Control and Prevention. Recommendations of the Advisory Committee on Immunization Practices (ACIP): Use of vaccines and immune globulins in persons with altered immunocompetence. *MMWR* 42(RR–5):1–18, 1993.

128. Boyer N, Marcellin P, Degott C, et al. Recombinant interferon-alpha for chronic hepatitis C in patients positive for antibody to human immunodeficiency virus. *J Infect Dis* 165:723–726, 1992.

129. Wong DKH, Cheung AM, O'Rourke K, et al. Effect of alpha-interferon treatment in patients with hepatitis B e antigen–positive chronic hepatitis B: A meta-analysis. *Ann Intern Med* 119:312–323, 1993.

130. Cital JL, Villarreal C, Robles M, et al. Interferon alpha 2-b in 20 patients with HIV+ and concomitant chronic hepatitis B or C. Ninth International Conference on AIDS, Berlin, June 1993.

131. Tramont EC. Syphilis in the AIDS era. *N Engl J Med* 316:1600–1601, 1987.

132. Berry CD, Hooton TM, Collier AC, et al. Neurologic relapse after benzathine penicillin therapy for secondary syphilis in a patient with HIV infection. *N Engl J Med* 316:1587–1589, 1987.

133. Johns DR, Tierney M, Felsenstein D. Alteration in the natural history of neurosyphilis by concurrent infection with the human immunodeficiency virus. *N Engl J Med* 316:1569–1572, 1987.

134. Hicks CB, Benson PM, Luptom GP, et al. Seronegative secondary syphilis in a patient infected with the human immunodeficiency virus (HIV) with Kaposi's sarcoma: A diagnostic dilemma. *Ann Intern Med* 107:492–495, 1987.

135. Centers for Disease Control. Continuing increase in infectious syphilis—United States. *MMWR* 37:35–38, 1988.

136. Spence MR, Abrutyn E. Syphilis and infection with the human immunodeficiency virus. *Ann Intern Med* 107:587, 1987.

137. Centers for Disease Control. Tuberculosis and human immunodeficiency virus infection: Recommendations of the Advisory Committee for the Elimination of Tuberculosis (ACET). *MMWR* 38:236–250, 1989.

138. Hopewell PC. Impact of human immunodeficiency virus infection on the epidemiology, clinical features, management, and control of tuberculosis. *Clin Infect Dis* 15:540–547, 1992.

139. Markowitz N, Hansen NI, Wilcosky TC, et al. Tuberculin and anergy testing in HIV-seropositive and HIV-seronegative persons. *Ann Intern Med* 119:185–193, 1993.

140. Sunderam G, McDonald RJ, Maniatis T, et al. Tuberculosis as a manifestation of the acquired immunodeficiency syndrome (AIDS). *JAMA* 265:362–366, 1986.

141. Chaisson RE, Schecter GF, Theuer CP, et al. Tuberculosis in patients with the acquired immunodeficiency syndrome: Clinical features, response to therapy, and survival. *Am Rev Respir Dis* 136:570–574, 1987.

142. Centers for Disease Control. Purified protein derivative (PPD)-tuberculin anergy and HIV infection: Guidelines for anergy testing and management of anergic persons at risk of tuberculosis. *MMWR* 40:27–33, 1991.

143. Centers for Disease Control. Tuberculosis and human immunodeficiency virus infection: Recommendations of the Advisory Committee for the Elimination of Tuberculosis (ACET). *MMWR* 38:237–238, 243–250, 1989.

144. Sreepada TK, Filippone EJ, Nicastri AD, et al. Associated focal and segmental glomerulosclerosis in the acquired immunodeficiency syndrome. *N Engl J Med* 310:669–673, 1984.

145. Carbone L, D'Agati V, Chent JT, Appel GB. Course and prognosis of human immunodeficiency virus-associated nephropathy. *Am J Med* 87:389–395, 1989.

146. Rabkin CS, et al. Cytomegalovirus infection and the risk of AIDS in human immunodeficiency virus-infected hemophilia patients. *J Infect Dis* 168:1260–1263, 1993.

147. Chuck SL, Sande MA. Infections with *Cryptococcus neoformans* in the acquired immunodeficiency syndrome. *N Engl J Med* 321:794–799, 1989.

148. Eyster ME, Gail MH, Ballard JO, et al. Natural history of human immunodeficiency virus infections in hemophiliacs: Effects of T-cell subsets, platelet counts, and age. *Ann Intern Med* 107:1–6, 1987.

149. Moss AR. Predicting who will progress to AIDS. *Br Med J* 197:1067–1068, 1988.

150. Polk BF, Fox R, Brookmeyer R, et al. Predictors of the acquired immunodeficiency syndrome developing in a cohort of seropositive homosexual men. *N Engl J Med* 316:61–66, 1987.

151. Lefrere JJ, Salmon D, Courouce AM. Evolution towards AIDS in HIV-infected individuals. *Lancet* 1:1220–1221, 1988.

152. Kaplan JE, Spira TJ, Fishbein DB, et al. A six-year follow-up of HIV-infected homosexual men with lymphadenopathy: Evidence for an increased risk of developing AIDS after the third year of lymphadenopathy. *JAMA* 260:2694–2697, 1988.

153. Holzman RS, Walsh CM, Karpatkin S. Risk for the acquired immunodeficiency syndrome among homosexual men seropositive for the human immunodeficiency virus. *Ann Intern Med* 106:383–386, 1987.

154. Kaslow RA, Phair JP, Friedman HB, et al. Infection with the human immunodeficiency virus: Clinical manifestations and their relationship to immune deficiency. *Ann Intern Med* 107:474–480, 1987.

155. Fuchs D, Reibnegger G, Wachter H. Neopterin levels correlating with the Walter Reed staging classification in human immunodeficiency virus (HIV) infection. *Ann Intern Med* 107:784–785, 1987.

156. Macy EM, Adelman DC. Abnormal T-cell subsets in normal persons. *N Engl J Med* 319:1608–1609, 1988.

157. Moss AR, Bacchetti P, Osmond D, et al. Seropositivity for HIV and the development of AIDS or AIDS related condition: Three year follow-up of the San Francisco General Hospital cohort. *Br Med J* 296:745–750, 1988.

158. Munoz A, Carey V, Saah AJ, et al. Predictors of decline in CD4 lymphocytes in a cohort of homosexual men infected with human immunodeficiency virus. *J Acquir Immune Defic Syndr* 1:396–404, 1988.

159. Margolick JB, Munoz A, Vlahov D, et al. Changes in T-lymphocyte subsets in intravenous drug users with HIV-1 infection. *JAMA* 267:1631–1636, 1992.

160. Phillips AN, Lee CA, Elford J, et al. Serial CD4 lymphocyte counts and development of AIDS. *Lancet* 337:389–392, 1991.

161. Kessler HA, Landay A, Pottage JC, Benson CA. Absolute number versus percentage of T-helper lymphocytes in human immunodeficiency virus infection. *J Infect Dis* 161:356–357, 1990.

162. Centers for Disease Control. Recommendations for prophylaxis against *Pneumocystis carinii* pneumonia for adults and adolescents infected with human immunodeficiency virus. *MMWR* 41(RR-4):1–11, 1992.

163. Hoover DR, et al. Effect of CD4 cell count measurement variability on staging HIV-1 infection. *J Acquir Immune Defic Syndr* 5:794–802, 1992.

164. Coombs RW, Collier AC, Allain JP, et al. Plasma viremia in human immunodeficiency virus infection. *N Engl J Med* 321:1626–1631, 1989.

165. Vahey MT, Mayers DL, Wagner KF, et al. Plasma HIV RNA predicts clinical outcome on AZT therapy. Tenth International Conference on AIDS, Yokohama, August 1994.

166. Yerly S, et al. Response of HIV RNA to didanosine as a predictive marker of survival. *AIDS* 9:159–163, 1995.

167. MacDonnell KB, Chmiel JS, Poggensee L, et al. Predicting progression to AIDS: Combined usefulness of CD4 lymphocyte counts and p24 antigenemia. *Am J Med* 89:706–712, 1990.

168. Heering P, Arning M. Neopterin and ß2-microglobulin as markers for AIDS. *Lancet* 1:281, 1987.

169. Zolla-Pazner S, William D, El-Sadr W, et al. Quantitation of ß2-microglobulin and other immune characteristics in a prospective study of men at risk for acquired immune deficiency syndrome. *JAMA* 251:2951–2955, 1984.

170. Davenny K, Buono D, Schoenbaum E, et al. Baseline health status of intravenous drug users with and without HIV infection. Seventh International Conference on AIDS, Florence, June 1991.

171. Davey RT, Lane HC. Laboratory methods in the diagnosis and prognostic staging of infection with human immunodeficiency virus type 1. *Rev Infect Dis* 12:912–930, 1990.

172. Fahey JL, Taylor JMG, Detels R, et al. The prognostic value of cellular and serologic markers in infection with human immunodeficiency virus type 1. *N Engl J Med* 322:166–172, 1989.

173. Polis MA, Masur H. Predicting the progression to AIDS. *Am J Med* 89:701–705, 1990.
174. Volberding PA, et al. A comparison of immediate with deferred zidovudine therapy for asymptomatic HIV-infected adults with CD4 cell counts of 500 or more per cubic millimeter. *N Engl J Med* 333:401–407, 1995.
175. Seligman M, Warrell DA, Aboulker JP, et al. Concorde: MRC/ANRS randomised double-blind controlled trial of immediate and deferred zidovudine in symptom-free HIV infection. *Lancet* 343:871–881, 1994.
176. Haase AT. New molecular technology in HIV research. Tenth International Conference on AIDS, Yokohama, August 1994.
177. Kinloch-de Loës S, et al. A controlled trial of zidovudine in primary human immunodeficiency virus infection. *N Engl J Med* 333:408–413, 1995.
178. Thompson M, Creagh T, Rimland D, et al. Impact of AZT monotherapy versus sequential or combination antiretroviral therapy on survival. Tenth International Conference on AIDS, Yokohama, August 1994.
179. Collier AC, Coombs RW, Fischl MA, et al. Combination therapy with zidovudine and didanosine compared with zidovudine alone in HIV-1 infection. *Ann Intern Med* 119:786–793, 1993.
180. Collier AC, Coombs RW, Timpone J, et al. Comparative study of Ro 31-8959 and zidovudine (ZDV) vs. ZDV and zalcitabine (ddC) vs. Ro 31-8959, ZDV, and ddC. Tenth International Conference on AIDS, Yokohama, August 1994.
181. Meng TC, Fischl MA, Boota AM, et al. Combination therapy with zidovudine and dideoxycytidine in patients with advanced human immunodeficiency virus infection: A phase I/II study. *J Infect Dis* 116:13–20, 1992.
182. Mayers DL, Wagner KF, Chung RCY, et al. Virologic response to ddI following prolonged AZT Rx. Tenth International Conference on AIDS, Yokohama, August 1994.
183. Fischl MA, Richman DD, Grieco MH, et al. The efficacy of azidothymidine (AZT) in the treatment of patients with AIDS and AIDS-related complex: A double-blind, placebo-controlled trial. *N Engl J Med* 317:185–191, 1987.
184. Creagh-Kirk T, Doi P, Andrews E, et al. Survival experience among patients with AIDS receiving zidovudine: Follow-up of patients in a compassionate plea program. *JAMA* 260:3009–3015, 1988.
185. Caliendo AM, Hirsch MS. Combination therapy for infection due to human immunodeficiency virus type 1. *Clin Infect Dis* 18:516–524, 1994.
186. Fischl MA, Richman DD, Hansen N. The safety and efficacy of zidovudine (AZT) in the treatment of subjects with mildly symptomatic human immunodeficiency virus type 1 (HIV) infection: A double-blind, placebo-controlled trial. *Ann Intern Med* 112:720–737, 1990.
187. Volberding PA, Lagakos SW, Koch MA, et al. Zidovudine in asymptomatic human immunodeficiency virus infection: A controlled trial in persons with fewer than 500 CD4-positive cells per cubic millimeter. *N Engl J Med* 322:941–949, 1990.
188. Lenderking WR, Gelber RD, Cotton DJ, et al. Evaluation of the quality of

life associated with zidovudine treatment in asymptomatic human immunodeficiency virus infection. *N Engl J Med* 330:738–743, 1994.

189. Volberding PA, Lagakos SW, Grimes JM, et al. The duration of zidovudine benefit in persons with asymptomatic HIV infection: Prolonged evaluation of protocol 019 of the AIDS Clinical Trials Group. 272:437–442, 1994.

190. Saag MS. What to do when zidovudine fails. *N Engl J Med* 330:706–707, 1994.

191. Cooper DA, Gatell JM, Kroon S, et al. Zidovudine in persons with asymptomatic HIV infection and CD4+ cell counts greater than 400 per cubic millimeter. *N Engl J Med* 329:297–303, 1993.

192. Bozzette SA, Kanouse D, Berry S, et al. Relative effects of ddC or ddI versus ZDV on health status, function and disability in N3300 (ACTG 114) and ACTG 116b/117. Eighth International Conference on AIDS, Amsterdam, July 1992.

193. National Institute of Allergy and Infectious Diseases Press Release, Washington, DC: December 1992.

194. Kahn JO, Lagakos SW, Richman DD, et al. A controlled trial comparing continued zidovudine with didanosine in human immunodeficiency virus infection. *N Engl J Med* 327:581–587, 1992.

195. Abrams DI, Goldman AI, Launer C, et al. A comparative trial of didanosine or zalcitabine after treatment with zidovudine in patients with human immunodeficiency virus infection. *N Engl J Med* 330:657–662, 1994.

196. Bristol-Myers Squibb (Princeton, NJ). Zerit (stavudine) package insert. June 1994.

197. Sande MA, Carpenter CCJ, Cobbs CG, et al. Antiretroviral therapy for adult HIV-infected patients: Recommendations from a state-of-the-art conference. *JAMA* 270:2583–2589, 1993.

198. Fischl M, Collier A, Stanley K, et al. The safety and efficacy of zidovudine (ZDV) and zalcitabine (ddC) or ddC alone versus ZDV. Ninth International Conference on AIDS, Berlin, June 1993.

199. Roche Laboratories. Stavudine package insert, June 1994.

200. Conant M, Mitsunori O, Slaton A, et al. d4T (stavudine) therapy: One large clinic's experience. Tenth International Conference on AIDS, Yokohama, August 1994.

201. Powderly WG, et al. A randomized trial comparing fluconazole with clotrimazole troches for the prevention of fungal infections in patients with advanced human immunodeficiency virus infection. *N Engl J Med* 332:700–705, 1995.

202. Quagliarello VJ, et al. Primary prevention of cryptococcal meningitis by fluconazole in HIV-infected persons. *Lancet* 345:548–552, 1995.

203. Ruskin J, LaRiviere M. Low-dose co-trimoxazole for prevention of *Pneumocystis carinii* pneumonia in human immunodeficiency virus disease. *Lancet* 337:468–471, 1991.

204. Torgovnick J, Arsura E. Desensitization to sulfonamides in patients with HIV infection. *Am J Med* 88:458–459, 1990.

205. Saavedra S, Rivera VC, Buonomo L, Ramirez-Ronda C. It is safe to desensitize the HIV patient allergic to TMP-SMX. Tenth International Conference on AIDS, Yokohama, August 1994.

206. Guerin C, Bachmeyer C, Salmon D, et al. Trimethoprim-sulfamethoxazole

desensitization in HIV patients. Tenth International Conference on AIDS, Yokohama, August 1994.

207. Torres R, Thorn M, Barr M, Britton DJ. Dapsone prophylaxis for toxoplasmosis and *Pneumocystis carinii* pneumonia. Seventh International Conference on AIDS, Florence, 1991.

208. Metroka CE, Lewis NJ, Jacobus DP. Desensitization to dapsone in HIV-positive patients. *JAMA* 267:512, 1992.

209. Hirschel B, Lazzarin A, Chopard P, et al. A controlled study of inhaled pentamidine for primary prevention of *Pneumocystis carinii* pneumonia. *N Engl J Med* 324:1079–1083, 1991.

210. Montaner JSG, Lawson LM, Gervais A, et al. Aerosol pentamidine for secondary prophylaxis of AIDS-related *Pneumocystis carinii* pneumonia: A randomized, placebo-controlled study. *Ann Intern Med* 114:948–953, 1991.

211. Nightingale SD, Byrd LT, Southern PM, et al. Incidence of *Mycobacterium avium-intracellulare* complex bacteremia in human immunodeficiency virus–positive patients. *J Infect Dis* 165:1082–1085, 1992.

212. Chin DP, Hopewell PC, Yajko DM, et al. *Mycobacterium avium* complex in the respiratory or gastrointestinal tract and the risk of *M. avium* complex bacteremia in patients with human immunodeficiency virus infection. *J Infect Dis* 169:289–295, 1994.

213. Horsburgh CR, Havlik JA, Ellis DA, et al. Survival of patients with acquired immunodeficiency syndrome and disseminated *Mycobacterium avium* complex infection with and without antimycobacterial chemotherapy. *Am Rev Respir Dis* 144:557–559, 1991.

214. Nightingale SD, Cameron DW, Gordin FM, et al. Two controlled trials of rifabutin prophylaxis against *Mycobacterium avium* complex infection in AIDS. *N Engl J Med* 329:828–833, 1993.

215. Centers for Disease Control. USPHS/IDSA guidelines for the prevention of opportunistic infections in persons infected with human immunodeficiency virus: A summary. *MMWR* 44(RR-8):1–34, 1995.

216. Fuller JD, Stanfield LED, Craven DE. Rifabutin prophylaxis and uveitis. *N Engl J Med* 330:1315–1316, 1994.

217. Narang PK, Trapnell CB, Schoenfelder JR, et al. Fluconazole and enhanced effect of rifabutin prophylaxis. *N Engl J Med* 330:1316–1317, 1994.

218. Gordin F, Masur H. Prophylaxis of *Mycobacterium avium* complex bacteremia in patients with AIDS. *Clin Infect Dis* 18 (suppl 3):S223–S226, 1994.

219. von Reyn CF, Brown ST, Arbeit RD. Rifabutin prophylaxis against *Mycobacterium avium* complex infection. *N Engl J Med* 330:437, 1994.

220. Reichman LB, McDonald RJ, Mangura BT. Rifabutin prophylaxis against *Mycobacterium avium* complex infection. *N Engl J Med* 330:437–438, 1994.

221. Pierce M, Heifets L, Crampton S. Clarithromycin for the prevention of *Mycobacterium avium* complex in AIDS. Tenth International Conference on AIDS, Yokohama, August 1994.

222. Oualls J, Salvato P, Thompson C. *Mycobacterium avium* complex prevention: Clarithromycin versus rifabutin. Tenth International Conference on AIDS, Yokohama, August 1994.

223. Hellinger JA, Cohen CJ, Mazzullo J. Clarithromycin for the prevention of

Mycobacterium avium complex in AIDS. Tenth International Conference on AIDS. Yokohama, August 1994.

224. Fiddian AP, Collaborative European/Australian Study Group. Preliminary report of a multicentre study of zidovudine plus or minus acyclovir in patients with acquired immune deficiency syndrome or acquired immunodeficiency syndrome–related complex. *J Infect Dis* 18 (suppl 1):79–80, 1989.

225. Youle M, European-Australian Acyclovir Study Group. Double blind, placebo controlled trial of high dose acyclovir for the prevention of cytomegalovirus (CMV) disease in late stage HIV disease. Eighth International Conference on AIDS, Amsterdam, July 1992.

226. Cooper DA, Pederson C, Aiuti F, et al. The efficacy and safety of zidovudine with or without acyclovir in the treatment of patients with AIDS-related complex. *AIDS* 5:933–943, 1991.

227. Cooper DA, Pehrson PO, Pedersen C, et al. The efficacy and safety of zidovudine alone or as cotherapy with acyclovir for the treatment of patients with AIDS and AIDS-related complex: A double-blind, randomized trial. *AIDS* 7:197–207, 1993.

228. Stein DS, Graham NMH, Park LP, et al. The effect of the interaction of acyclovir with zidovudine on progression to AIDS and survival: Analysis of data in the Multicenter AIDS Cohort Study. *Ann Intern Med* 121:100–108, 1994.

229. Golden MP, Kim S, Hammer SM. Activation of human immunodeficiency virus by herpes simplex virus. *J Infect Dis* 166:494–499, 1992.

230. Laurence J. Molecular interactions among herpesviruses and human immunodeficiency viruses. *J Infect Dis* 162:338–346, 1990.

231. Rosenthal L, Sadaie MR, Kashanchi F. HHV-6 Sal/I-L ORF-1 reactivates HIV-1 provirus. Tenth International Conference on AIDS, Yokohama, August 1994.

232. Pottage JC, Benson CA, Spear JB, et al. Treatment of human immunodeficiency virus–related thrombocytopenia with zidovudine. *JAMA* 260:3045–3048, 1988.

233. Oksenhendler E, Bierling P, Ferchal F, et al. Zidovudine for thrombocytopenic purpura related to human immunodeficiency virus (HIV) infection. *Ann Intern Med* 110:365–368, 1989.

234. Swiss Group for Clinical Studies on the Acquired Immunodeficiency Syndrome (AIDS). Zidovudine for the treatment of thrombocytopenia associated with human immunodeficiency virus: A prospective study. *Ann Intern Med* 109:718–721, 1988.

235. Yarchoan R, Berg G, Brouwers P, et al. Response of human-immunodeficiency-virus–associated neurological disease to 3'-azido-3'-deoxythymidine. *Lancet* 1:132–135, 1987.

236. Schmitt FA, Bigley JW, McKinnis R, et al. Neuropsychological outcome of zidovudine (AZT) treatment of patients with AIDS and AIDS-related complex. *N Engl J Med* 319:1573–1578, 1988.

237. Yarchoan R, Venzon DJ, Pluda JM, et al. CD4 count and the risk for death in patients infected with HIV receiving antiretroviral therapy. *Ann Intern Med* 115:184–189, 1991.

238. Phillips AN, Elford J, Sabin C, et al. Immunodeficiency and the risk of death in HIV infection. *JAMA* 268:2662–2666, 1992.
239. Dwyer JT, Salvato-Schille AM, Coulston A, et al. The use of unconventional remedies among HIV-positive men living in California. *J Assoc Nurses AIDS Care* 6:17, 1995.
240. Haladay J. Animal assisted therapy for PWAs: Bringing a sense of connection. *AIDS Patient Care* 3:38–39, February 1989.
241. Glaser CA, Angulo FJ, Rooney JA. Animal-associated opportunistic infections among persons infected with the human immunodeficiency virus. *J Infect Dis* 18:14–24, 1994.
242. Koehler JE, Glaser CA, Tappero JW. *Rochalimaea henselae* infection: A new zoonosis with the domestic cat as reservoir. *JAMA* 271:531–535, 1994.
243. Tarricone NJ, Maiman M, Vieira J. Colposcopic evaluation of HIV seropositive women. Sixth International Conference on AIDS, San Francisco, June 1990.
244. Norton D, Brosgart C, Barkin M, et al. Papanicolaou (PAP) smears versus colposcopy as screening tests for cervical intraepithelial neoplasia (CIN) in HIV seropositive women. Tenth International Conference on AIDS, Yokohama, August 1994.
245. Gagnon S, Cohn J, Spence M, et al. Comparison of cervical cytology with colposcopic biopsies in U.S. HIV-infected women. Tenth International Conference on AIDS, Yokohama, August 1994.
246. Centers for Disease Control. AIDS in women—United States. *MMWR* 39:845–846, 1990.
247. Wortley PM, et al. Pneumococcal and influenza vaccination levels among HIV-infected adolescents and adults receiving medical care in the United States. *AIDS* 8:941–944, 1994.
248. Immunization Practices Advisory Committee, Centers for Disease Control. General Recommendations on Immunization. *Ann Intern Med* 98:615–622, 1983.
249. Redfield RR, Wright DC, James WD, et al. Disseminated vaccinia in a military recruit with human immunodeficiency virus (HIV) disease. *N Engl J Med* 316:673–676, 1987.
250. Centers for Disease Control. Disseminated *M. bovis* infection from BCG vaccination of a patient with acquired immunodeficiency syndrome. *MMWR* 34:227–228, 1986.
251. Tardieu M, Truffot-Pernot C, Carrire JP, et al. Tuberculous meningitis due to BCG in two previously healthy children. *Lancet* 1:440–441, 1988.
252. Immunization Practices Advisory Committee: Prevention and control of influenza. *MMWR* 36:373–387, 1987.
253. Nelson KE, Clements ML, Miotti P, et al. The influence of human immunodeficiency virus (HIV) infection on antibody responses to influenza vaccines. *Ann Intern Med* 109:383–388, 1988.
254. Whimbey E, Gold JWM, Polsky B. Bacteremia and fungemia in patients with the acquired immunodeficiency syndrome. *Ann Intern Med* 104:511–514, 1986.
255. Simberkoff MS, Sadr WE, Schiffman G, Rahal JJ. *Streptococcus pneumoniae* infections and bacteremia in patients with acquired immunodeficiency

syndrome, with report of a pneumococcal vaccine failure. *Am Rev Respir Dis* 130:1174–1176, 1984.

256. Health and Public Policy Committee, American College of Physicians. Pneumococcal vaccine. *Ann Intern Med* 104:118–120, 1986.
257. Amman AJ, Schiffman G, Abrams D, et al. B-cell immunodeficiency in acquired immunodeficiency syndrome. *JAMA* 251:1447–1449, 1984.
258. Huang KL, Ruben FL, Rinaldo CR, et al. Antibody responses after influenza and pneumococcal immunization in HIV-infected homosexual men. *JAMA* 257:2047–2050, 1987.
259. Masur H, Michelis MA, Greene JB, et al. An outbreak of community-acquired *Pneumocystis carinii* pneumonia: Initial manifestation of cellular immune dysfunction. *N Engl J Med* 305:1431–1438, 1981.
260. Casadevall A, et al. *Haemophilus influenzae* type b bacteremia in adults with AIDS and at risk for AIDS. *Am J Med* 92:587–590, 1992.
261. Centers for Disease Control. Measles in HIV-infected children, United States. *MMWR* 37:183–186, 1988.
262. Zolopa AR, Kemper CA, Shiboski S, et al. Progressive immunodeficiency due to infection with human immunodeficiency virus does not lead to waning immunity to measles in a cohort of homosexual men. *Clin Infect Dis* 18:636–638, 1994.
263. Glaser JB, Greifinger R. Measles antibodies in human immunodeficiency virus–infected adults. *J Infect Dis* 165:589, 1992.
264. Schonberger LB, McGowan JE, Gregg MB. Vaccine-associated poliomyelitis in the United States: 1961–1972. *Am J Epidemiol* 104:202–211, 1976.
265. Immunization Practices Advisory Committee. Poliomyelitis prevention. *MMWR* 31:106, 1982.
266. von Reyn CF, Clements CJ, Mann JM. Human immunodeficiency virus infection and routine childhood immunisation. *Lancet* 2:669–672, 1987.
267. Immunization Practices Advisory Committee. Poliomyelitis prevention: Enhanced-potency inactivated poliomyelitis vaccine—supplementary statement. *MMWR* 36:795–799, 1987.
268. Odaka N, Eldred L, Cohn S. Comparative immunogenicity of plasma and recombinant hepatitis B virus vaccines in homosexual men. *JAMA* 260:3635–3637, 1988.
269. Collier AC, Corey L, Murphy VL, Handsfield HH. Antibody to human immunodeficiency virus (HIV) and suboptimal response to hepatitis B vaccination. *Ann Intern Med* 109:101–105, 1988.

Understanding Clinical Trials *33*

Kenneth A. Freedberg, Calvin J. Cohen

With the evolution of the HIV epidemic has come the rapid development of clinical information regarding therapies directed at the virus and associated opportunistic diseases. Because of these therapeutic interventions, the expected life span of a person diagnosed with AIDS manifested by *Pneumocystis carinii* pneumonia (PCP) has increased by about one year over the past decade [1]. Pneumocystis prophylaxis has been an important advance in patient care. While the impact of antiretroviral drugs on survival remains controversial, these agents do slow the rate of decline in immune function in some individuals [2, 3].

Such improvements in standard of care have been the result of many well-designed, controlled clinical trials documenting the impact of specific pharmacologic interventions. This chapter provides an overview of clinical trials and describes the roles that patients and health care providers play in the process.

The Drug Development Process

In general, the purpose of any trial is to answer an important question about the clinical impact of a specific treatment, for which there exists some rationale but insufficient data [4]. This principle holds true at each phase of drug testing, although, as the amount of knowledge increases, the nature of the question evolves.

A chemical compound is generally identified as promising for development as a result of preclinical work including both in vitro and animal studies. In the case of antiretroviral drugs, the focus has been on finding agents that interfere with one or more steps in the viral life cycle but leave the human cell intact. As an example, zidovudine (ZDV) had

523

been described in 1964 as a potential drug for cancer treatment. While it was proved ineffective for that purpose, it was later rescreened for anti-HIV effect, which ultimately led to human trials [5]. Unfortunately, it is the minority of compounds with in vitro activity that proceed in this fashion because many are either too toxic or expensive to produce commercially [6]. It is also worth noting that compounds traditionally used for other purposes are sometimes identified as having promise through clinical observation. For example, a recent report noted increased CD4 cell counts in HIV-infected patients taking sulfasalazine for Reiter's syndrome [7].

If preclinical data are favorably reviewed by the Food and Drug Administration (FDA), the compound enters phase I testing (Table 33-1). Since this may be the first time the compound has been given to human subjects, such testing generally involves a small number of people, often fewer than 100. The major focus at this stage of drug development is to define short-term safety. Phase I study design usually involves dose escalation, that is, administration of the study drug starting at a dose below which toxicity would be anticipated and increasing it incrementally. The target for dose escalation is often based on serum levels of the drug that, from in vitro data, would be expected to result in clinical benefit.

If doses are identified in phase I that are reasonably well tolerated and could be expected to have therapeutic effect, the drug enters phase II testing. In this phase, more subjects are studied using the doses identified as safe in phase I testing, with the goal to look for evidence of clinical benefit. By definition, this phase of research must be performed in subjects who have the disease requiring treatment, whereas phase I testing can be done in either persons with the disease or healthy individuals.

If phase II shows evidence of potential clinical benefit, the drug en-

Table 33-1 *Traditional stages of new drug development and testing*

Study stage	Objective(s)	Length of stage
Preclinical	Drug development, in vitro and animal testing	Months to years
IND application	FDA review	30 days, if no objections
Phase I	Toxicity, dose ranging	6 mo–1 yr
Phase II	Efficacy, toxicity	6 mo–2 yr
Phase III	Efficacy, safety, dosage, comparison	1–4 yr
NDA	FDA drug approval	2–3 yr
Phase IV	Postmarketing studies	Variable

IND = investigational new drug; NDA = new drug application.

ters phase III testing, where it is compared in a randomized fashion against conventional treatment for the disorder. If there is no established standard of care, the drug is compared with placebo, usually in a double-blinded study. FDA drug approval occurs if the results of all three phases demonstrate acceptable safety and clinical efficacy. Following approval, further studies of the drug, called phase IV, are sometimes performed, in which refinements of drug dosage or indication are examined.

The History of Clinical Trials in HIV Disease

In HIV disease, the traditional process of drug testing has been accelerated considerably. The objectives of phases I and II have been combined, so that early testing looks for evidence of both safety and clinical benefit, the latter assessed on the basis of surrogate disease markers [8]. For antiretroviral agents, these may include measures of viral activity, such as p24 antigen or quantitative polymerase chain reaction (PCR); immune function, such as CD4 count or $ß_2$-microglobulin; or short-term clinical effect, such as weight gain or improvement in quality of life. If there is sufficient evidence of benefit at a dose that has acceptable toxicity, the drug then proceeds to phase II/III testing, which is designed to enroll an adequate number of subjects to provide meaningful information about clinical efficacy.

However, given the large number of subjects required for such trials and the length of time needed to demonstrate benefit, the FDA has also introduced an "accelerated approval" process for HIV drugs, in order to provide earlier access to potentially promising agents [9]. It is important to note that these new drugs are not required to be superior or even as effective as currently available medications but only clinically effective for the specific indication [10]. The FDA regulations permit approval after phase I/II testing is completed, if such studies show some evidence of activity that can be reasonably expected to produce clinical benefit. They also allow the agency to grant drug approval on the basis of surrogate marker changes alone, before its clinical impact is known. While there is a general expectation that clinical effectiveness will be defined in postmarketing studies, this is not required.

In addition, the FDA has provided a mechanism for access to a drug before its approval for prescription use, called the "treatment IND" (investigational new drug). While technically available for many years, the procedures are not well known to most practitioners. Before the HIV epidemic, a treatment IND was usually activated after successful phase III testing was completed but before drug approval and commercial availability [11]. However, input from patient advocates changed this policy when data from phase I/II studies of didanosine (ddI) became available [12]. It was argued successfully that surrogate marker data provided sufficient evidence that ddI might reasonably be expected to provide clinical benefit at an acceptable level of risk. In response to this, Dr. Anthony Fauci, then director of the National Institute of Allergy and Infectious Diseases, announced the beginning of the "parallel track" program, which would release a drug simultaneously with ongoing clinical trials [13].

The first pharmaceutical company to use this mechanism, Bristol-Myers Squibb, created a drug distribution system that allowed physicians to apply for access to ddI even as it was entering phase II/III testing. This initially created tension in the medical community because of concern that such general availability might seriously threaten enrollment in trials that were essential to defining its clinical utility [14]. However, even though over 20,000 people participated in the parallel track, all of the clinical trials evaluating ddI were fully enrolled and completed [15].

Since then, other antiretroviral agents have entered the parallel track: zalcitabine (formerly dideoxycytidine or ddC), stavudine (d4T), lamivudine (3TC), and protease inhibitor drugs. This pattern has led some to make the assumption that once a drug enters the parallel track, it is likely to be proved clinically effective. This is consistent with the drug approval process in cancer research, in which over 90 percent of the agents found useful based on phase II data have been confirmed as effective in phase III studies [16].

The parallel track has been changed recently in a small but important way, allowing researchers to learn more about the drug. For example, parallel track access to d4T included two doses given in a randomized double-blinded design. As a result, it became evident that a lower dose of the drug was associated with a decreased incidence of peripheral neuropathy but a similar survival rate compared to a higher dose [17].

Why Participate in Clinical Trials?

People with HIV infection, as well as their primary care providers, may want to participate in clinical trials for many reasons. From the patient perspective, involvement in trials might allow them to be on the "cutting edge" of care, with access to new, experimental therapies which might provide clinical benefit. It may also permit access, at no cost, to other medications, as well as laboratory testing, including experimental surrogate markers of HIV disease. Involvement generally offers participants regular contact with study nurses and physicians, which may complement relationships with their primary providers. Lastly, many patients feel good knowing that they are playing an important role in advancing knowledge related to the AIDS epidemic. By facilitating enrollment of their patients in clinical trials, primary care providers gain access to the newest therapeutic interventions and to a team of experts for consultation.

It is equally important to understand why some patients may not want to participate in clinical trials. Fear of unknown drug toxicities, the potential of receiving an ineffective agent, and the need for additional visits are important considerations. In addition, enrollment in one study may exclude participation in potentially more attractive trials at a future date. Furthermore, difficulties with transportation, child care, and release time from work may make trial participation problematic for some patients.

Recent evidence suggests that patient involvement in clinical trials may also be influenced by ethnicity and gender. For example, a major reason that some African-Americans do not participate in trials is continued concern about the ethics of researchers, as exemplified by the notorious Tuskegee syphilis study [18]. Stone and associates [19] found that the primary reason for lack of study participation differed according to ethnicity: Non-Hispanic whites identified ineligibility, African-Americans noted concern about being a "guinea pig," and Latinos stated that they were not offered enrollment. In addition, problems with language may often make participation more difficult for non–English-speaking populations. Traditionally, women have been underrepresented in clinical trials for a variety of reasons, including study designs that exclude women of childbearing age [20].

The Importance of Clinical Trials in HIV Care

Progress in the management of HIV disease has been the direct result of information from clinical trials. A review of the steps that have led to the use of PCP prophylaxis and antiretroviral therapy demonstrates this point.

Initially, it was through a large natural history study, the Multicenter AIDS Cohort Study (MACS), that the stages of HIV infection were defined. These data showed that there was differential risk of opportunistic infections on the basis of CD4 count and that this marker was better than any other laboratory test [21]. Based on this information, prophylactic interventions were targeted to patients at highest risk of developing PCP, the most prevalent opportunistic infection.

Using a dose comparison design with aerosol pentamidine (AP), community-based researchers in San Francisco and New York enrolled individuals at high risk for PCP. The most effective of the three doses studied was subsequently approved by the FDA for PCP prophylaxis [22]. At about the same time, trimethoprim-sulfamethoxazole (TMP-SMX) was also documented as an effective preventive agent [23]. Since there were no comparative data, clinicians used their own judgment in choosing therapy, generally basing this decision on cost and anticipated side effects [24, 25]. Subsequently, a follow-up trial in persons who had recovered from PCP compared AP with TMP-SMX and documented the superiority of the latter drug for this indication [26]. Other data from trials using dapsone, either alone or in combination with pyrimethamine, showed that it, too, was effective for PCP prophylaxis, with a success rate similar to that for AP [27]. Some patients are unable to tolerate any of these medications, and others have recurrent disease despite their use. Therefore, trials are ongoing to evaluate alternative agents, such as atovaquone, for PCP prophylaxis [28].

More controversial are the clinical trials that have guided the use of antiretroviral agents. The earliest studies focused on ZDV, targeting patients at highest risk for disease progression, including those who had recovered from PCP or had CD4 counts less than $200/mm^3$ and other HIV-related symptoms. The first phase II/III trial documented a clear clinical benefit from ZDV and was stopped earlier than originally planned because of decreased mortality in individuals receiving the drug compared to placebo [29]. The results of this single trial, along with the phase I data available, provided evidence that the FDA considered sufficient to warrant drug approval. Follow-up studies, which included asymptomatic patients and symptomatic individuals without AIDS, were performed to define the effectiveness of ZDV at other stages of HIV disease. Because both groups demonstrated a reduction in the rate of progression to an AIDS-defining opportunistic infection or death, they led to what became the standard of care in the United States: to offer ZDV to all patients with CD4 counts less than $500/mm^3$, whether or not they were symptomatic [30]. A limitation of these trials was that the average duration of follow-up was about one year, and it was unclear whether clinical effectiveness would be maintained over longer periods of time.

Several years later, two European studies addressed the question of long-term benefit from ZDV but provided contrasting conclusions. One study documented that ZDV remained effective over 3 years in slowing the rate of progression to symptomatic HIV disease [31]. However, an even larger trial, known as the Concorde study, compared the strategy of starting ZDV when the patient was asymptomatic to delaying it until the development of symptoms [2]. This study demonstrated similar benefits to starting ZDV early as were seen in the United States trials, but, by year three, no differences were evident for any clinical outcome. Also of note was that the CD4 count remained increased in those who started on ZDV but that the change in this surrogate marker did not correlate with clinical benefit. These data have led to uncertainty regarding the strategy of using ZDV for asymptomatic patients, suggesting instead that therapy could be postponed until symptoms appear [32].

Several studies regarding the use of other antiretroviral drugs have also been published, noting that there is improved short-term clinical outcome for patients who switch to alternative agents after receiving

ZDV for a period of time [15]. There are also data showing that the concurrent use of two drugs has a greater impact on the CD4 count compared with an alternating regimen of the same agents [33]. However, so far, studies have not yielded clinical outcome results that justify widespread use of combination drug treatment [34].

All of the above trials have contributed to the development of guidelines for antiretroviral therapy [32]. It is clear that each study has yielded information that has an incremental effect on medical care. While physicians may differ on what constitutes the correct clinical decision in a given situation, it is only possible to come to an informed opinion based on the results of clinical trials.

Academic-Based and Community-Based Trials

There are several different ways in which clinical trials can be performed. While phase I studies are usually small enough to be done at one institution, phase II/III studies generally require multiple sites. These are often linked to constitute networks, with the goal of streamlining enrollment procedures and data management. Such networks also have the advantage of pooling the expertise of researchers and clinicians from several institutions.

The first national network was the AIDS Clinical Trials Group (ACTG). This National Institutes of Health (NIH)–funded group consists of sites in academic institutions across the United States. The ACTG has been responsible for many important clinical trials. However, concerns have been raised about relying solely on the ACTG for trials development, in that many potential study participants receive their primary care outside of academic institutions and may not feel comfortable accessing these sites for research studies [18].

Other networks have evolved as well in recent years, some of which have been designed to build on the established relationships between clinicians and their patients. One, the Community Program for Clinical Research on AIDS (CPCRA), is also funded by the NIH [18]. This network has 17 sites, chosen in part to maximize the ability to recruit underrepresented racial minorities with HIV infection. Another, the Community Based Clinical Trials Network (CBCTN), has been funded by the American Foundation for AIDS Research (AmFAR) [35]. Both networks rely primarily on the expertise of primary care providers, in concert with their patients, to design trials that address issues of clinical importance. These networks have a track record of producing useful results, as evidenced by the original PCP AP prophylaxis study and evaluation of the utility of rifabutin for *Mycobacterium avium* complex (MAC) prevention [22, 36]. In addition to these two networks, researchers may contract directly with a pharmaceutical sponsor, providing an additional mechanism for accessing investigational treatments. Thus, between the ACTG, the two community-based networks, and other freestanding sites, patients and health care providers have numerous opportunities to participate in clinical trials.

Non–Trial-Based Experimental Therapy

It has been noted in several surveys of HIV-seropositive persons that there is widespread use of treatments for which only limited information is available to justify their use [37] (see Appendix B). What has generally been found, however, is that the choice of therapy is often based on extrapolating from early-phase scientific data [38]. For example, high-dose vitamin C has been advocated by some for the treatment of HIV disease. Initial interest was sparked by published reports of in vitro activity of vitamin C against a human retrovirus [39]. After many years of research into the potential clinical use of antioxidants, the NIH is actively reviewing a protocol that will evaluate the impact of vitamin C on a variety of HIV surrogate markers (Richard Elion, MD, personal communication, 1994).

The scientific method is not inherently limited to studying drugs produced by the pharmaceutical industry. Any substance, including naturally occurring substances, can be studied using clinical trial methodology. There are currently a few examples of plant products that have been identified by in vitro testing as having activity against HIV and for which phase I/II testing is ongoing or planned. These include hypericin, an extract from St. Johnswort, and curcumin, an extract of turmeric [7].

Several newsletters are published that review information about current and experimental treatment options (Table 33-2). Each of these serves to inform the HIV-infected community of recent data presented in a variety of journals, including some that may not be known to primary care providers. These newsletters have an important impact on many patients and, for some, are the most influential resource guiding treatment decisions [40].

Conclusions

There remain many unanswered questions about the optimal management of HIV disease. Most clinical advances to date have come from a combination of preclinical research, clinical trials, and observation. Although a single trial can only answer a specific question at one moment in time, the sum of knowledge for managing HIV infection continues to advance in stepwise fashion based in large measure on the efforts of study participants.

Table 33-2 *Selected treatment directories and newsletters*

AIDS Treatment News. Published by John S. James. Issued semiweekly. 1-800-TREAT-12.

AIDS/HIV Treatment Directory. Published by the American Foundation for AIDS Research (AmFAR). Updated quarterly. 1-212-682-7440. Also contains complete listing of other publications and treatment directories, including currently available clinical trials.

Bulletin of Experimental Treatments for AIDS (BETA). Published by the San Francisco AIDS Foundation. Issued quarterly. 1-800-327-9893.

National AIDS Treatment Information Project. Funded by the Kaiser Family Foundation. Treatment information for patients and community organizations. 1-617-667-5520.

P.I. Perspective. Published by Project Inform. Issued approximately every 4 months. 1-800-334-7422.

Treatment Issues. Published by Gay Men's Health Crisis (GMHC). Issued 10 times per year. 1-212-337-3613.

References

1. Osmond D, Charlebois E, Lang W, et al. Changes in AIDS survival time in two San Francisco cohorts of homosexual men, 1983 to 1993. *JAMA* 271:1083–1087, 1994.
2. Concorde Coordinating Committee. Concorde: MRC/ANRS randomized double-blind controlled trial of immediate and deferred zidovudine in symptom-free HIV infection. *Lancet* 343:871–878, 1994.
3. Graham NMH, Zeger SL, Park LP, et al. The effects of early treatment on survival in the Multi-Center AIDS Cohort Study. *N Engl J Med* 326:1737–1742, 1992.
4. Passamani E. Clinical Trials—are they ethical? *N Engl J Med* 324:1589–1592, 1991.
5. Yarchoan R, Klecker RW, Weinhold KJ, et al. Administration of 3'-azido 3'deoxythymidine, an inhibitor of HTLV-III/LAV replication, to patients with AIDS or AIDS-related complex. *Lancet* 1:575–580, 1986.
6. Young FE. The reality behind the headlines. *FDA Consumer* 4–5, 1988.
7. Abrams D, Cotton D, Mayer K. *AmFAR AIDS/HIV Treatment Directory* 7:57, 1994.
8. Byar DP, Schoenfeld DA, Green SB, et al. Design considerations for AIDS trials. *N Engl J Med* 323:1343–1348, 1990.
9. Cotton P. FDA "pushing envelope" on AIDS drug. *JAMA* 266:757–758, 1991.
10. Lasagna L (Chair). *Final Report of the National Committee to Review Current Procedures for Approval of New Drugs for Cancer and AIDS.* Washington DC: National Cancer Institute, August 15, 1990.
11. Young FE, Norris JA, Levitt JA, et al. The FDA's new procedures for the use of investigational drugs in treatment. *JAMA* 259:2267–2270, 1988.

12. Cooley TP, Kunches LM, Saunders CA, et al. Once daily administration of 2'3'-dideoxyinosine (ddI) in patients with the acquired immunodeficiency syndrome or AIDS-related complex: Results of a phase I trial. *N Engl J Med* 322:1340–1345, 1990.

13. US Public Health Service, Food and Drug Administration. Expanded availability of investigational new drugs through a parallel track mechanism for people with AIDS and other HIV-related disease. *Federal Register* 57:13244–13259, 1992.

14. Volberding P, Dobson J, Thorne B. Expanded access to AIDS treatments would benefit all. *AmFAR AIDS/HIV Experimental Treatment Directory* 3:51, 1990.

15. Kahn JO, Lagakos SW, Richman DD, et al. A controlled trial comparing continued zidovudine with didanosine in human immunodeficiency virus infection. *N Engl J Med* 327:581–587, 1992.

16. Lasagna L (Chair). *Final Report of the National Committee to Review Current Procedures for Approval of New Drugs for Cancer and AIDS.* Washington DC: National Cancer Institute, August 15, 1990. P 50.

17. Stavudine. *Physicians Desk Reference.* Montvale NJ: Medical Economics, 1995. Pp. 697–700.

18. El-Sadr W, Capps L. The challenge of minority recruitment in clinical trials for AIDS. *JAMA* 267:954–957, 1992.

19. Stone VE, Mauch MY, Steger K, Craven DE. Participation of women and persons of color in AIDS clinical trials (abstract). *J Gen Intern Med* 9:108, 1994.

20. Cotton DJ, Finkelstein DM, He W, Feinberg J. Determinants of accrual of women to a large, multicenter clinical trials program of human immunodeficiency virus infection: The AIDS Clinical Trials Group. *J Acquir Immune Defic Syndr* 6:1322–1328, 1993.

21. Masur H, Ognibene FP, Yarchoan R, et al. CD4 counts as predictors of opportunistic pneumonias in human immunodeficiency virus (HIV) infection. *Ann Intern Med* 111:223–231, 1989.

22. Leoung GS, Feigal DW, Montgomery AB, et al. Aerosolized pentamidine for prophylaxis against *Pneumocystis carinii* pneumonia: The San Francisco Community Prophylaxis Trial. *N Engl J Med* 323:769–775, 1990.

23. Fischl MA, Dickinson GM, La Voie L, et al. Safety and efficacy of sulfamethoxazole and trimethoprim chemoprophylaxis for *Pneumocystis carinii* pneumonia. *JAMA* 259:1185–1189, 1988.

24. Freedberg KA, Tosteson ANA, Cohen CJ, et al. Primary prophylaxis for *Pneumocystis carinii* pneumonia in HIV-infected people with CD4 counts below 200/mm³: A cost-effectiveness analysis. *J Acquir Immune Defic Syndr* 4:521–531, 1991.

25. Mayer KH. A new decade. *AmFAR AIDS/HIV Experimental Treatment Directory* 3:46–50, 1990.

26. Hardy WD, Feinberg J, Finkelstein DM, et al. A controlled trial of trimethoprim-sulfamethoxazole or aerosolized pentamidine for secondary prophylaxis of *Pneumocystis carinii* pneumonia in patients with acquired immunodeficiency syndrome. *N Engl J Med* 327:1842–1848, 1992.

27. Girard PM, Landman R, Gandebout C, et al. Dapsone-pyrimethamine compared with aerosolized pentamidine as primary prophylaxis against

Pneumocystis carinii pneumonia and toxoplasmosis in HIV infection. *N Engl J Med* 328:1514–1520, 1993.

28. Abrams D, Cotton D, Mayer K (eds). *AmFAR AIDS/HIV Treatment Directory* 7:197–198, 1994.
29. Fischl MA, Richman DD, Grieco MH, et al. The efficacy of azidothymidine in patients with AIDS or AIDS related complex: A double blind, placebo-controlled trial. *N Engl J Med* 317:185–191, 1987.
30. NIH state-of-the-art conference on azidothymidine therapy for early HIV infection. *Am J Med* 89:335–344, 1990.
31. Cooper DA, Gatell JM, Kroon S, et al. Zidovudine in persons with asymptomatic HIV infection and CD4 cell counts greater than 400 per cubic millimeter. *N Engl J Med* 329:297–303, 1993.
32. Sande MA, Carpenter CCM, Cobbs CG, et al. Antiretroviral therapy for adult HIV-infected patients. *JAMA* 270:2583–2589, 1993.
33. Yarchoan R, Lietzau JA, Nguyen B, et al. A randomized pilot study of alternating or simultaneous zidovudine and didanosine therapy in patients with symptomatic human immunodeficiency virus infection. *J Infect Dis* 169:9–17, 1994.
34. Fischl MA, et al. The safety and efficacy of zidovudine (ZDV) and zalcitabine (ddC) or ddC alone versus ZDV. Ninth International Conference on AIDS, Berlin, June 1993.
35. Cohen CJ, Shevitz A, Mayer KH. Expanding access to investigational new therapies. *Primary Care* 19:87–96, 1992.
36. Nightingale SD, et al. Two controlled trials of rifabutin prophylaxis against *Mycobacterium avium* complex infection in AIDS. *N Engl J Med* 329:828–833, 1993.
37. Cohen CJ, Mayer KH, Eisenberg DM, et al. Prevalence of nonconventional medical treatments in HIV-infected patients: Implications for primary care. *Clin Research* 38:692A, 1990.
38. Abrams DI. Alternative therapies in HIV infection. *AIDS* 4:1179–1187, 1990.
39. Harakeh S, Jariwalla RJ, Pauling L. Suppression of human immunodeficiency virus replication by ascorbate in chronically and acutely infected cells. *Proc Natl Acad Sci USA* 87:7245–7249, 1990.
40. Cohen CJ, Mayer KH, Eisenberg DM, et al. Determinants of nonconventional treatment use among HIV infected individuals. Sixth International Conference on AIDS, San Francisco, July 1990.

Management of Advanced HIV Disease

34

Thomas W. Barber

> AIDS is progressive, a disease of time. Once a certain density of symptoms is attained, the course of illness can be swift, and brings atrocious suffering. . . . [A] plethora of disabling, disfiguring, and humiliating symptoms make the AIDS patient steadily more infirm, helpless, and unable to control or take care of basic functions and needs.
>
> Susan Sontag, *AIDS and Its Metaphors*

Our understanding of the natural history of HIV infection is in a state of continual evolution, changing as we gain new insights about disease pathogenesis and treatment and as the epidemic extends into new populations. The prognosis for survival for patients with HIV infection has improved significantly in recent years, attributable largely to effective strategies for prevention of *Pneumocystis carinii* pneumonia (PCP), the treatment of opportunistic infections, and the use of antiretroviral drugs such as zidovudine (ZDV).

The clinical course of HIV infection is extremely variable. Some patients develop one opportunistic infection after another and rapidly progress to death, despite aggressive medical management. There are also many patients who survive for years, despite profoundly low CD4 cell counts and an increasing number of HIV-related complications. This latter group is the subject of this chapter.

The terms *AIDS* (acquired immunodeficiency syndrome) and *ARC* (AIDS-related complex) have begun to lose their usefulness as prophylactic and therapeutic regimens influence the course of the disease. Both of the patients described below have AIDS, yet an enormous gulf separates the two in terms of prognosis, functional status, and quality of life.

Mr. A was diagnosed with HIV infection after presenting with a mild case of PCP. He is followed regularly by a primary care physician and is now receiving secondary PCP prophylaxis and antiretroviral therapy. His CD4 count is 180 cells/mm³, and he feels good physically. He is able to work and looks to the future with hope.

Ms. B was diagnosed with HIV infection 6 years ago. She has had many complications, including several AIDS-defining opportunistic infections. Her CD4 count is 10 cells/mm³. She has a permanent central line through which she receives daily infusions of antibiotics and parenteral nutrition. She receives two different hematopoietic growth factors by injection every day. She has chronic fever, pain and nausea, markedly impaired vision, progressive dementia, wasting syndrome, urinary and fecal incontinence, sacral and hip pressure ulcers, and a number of iatrogenic complications related to her central line and medication regimen. She has been hospitalized frequently in recent months.

Ms. B has been unemployed for several years. She has lived in numerous residences since losing her job because of financial problems. She is depressed and suicidal, and she is worried about the impact of her death on her children.

Advanced HIV Infection

How can we conceptualize the stage of disease exemplified by Ms. B? In seeking terminology that is descriptive yet does not carry pejorative connotations, many clinicians use the term *advanced HIV infection* to describe their patients with severe immunodeficiency who have multiple medical, social, and psychological complications. While such terminology is difficult to define precisely, its most important characteristics include chronicity, complexity, severity, unpredictability, and poor quality of life.

Chronicity

Most patients described as having advanced HIV infection have CD4 cell counts below 100/mm³ and have been symptomatic for a considerable period of time. They have much in common with persons living with other chronic diseases, such as cancer, systemic lupus erythematosus, or multiple sclerosis. Their illness becomes a central feature of daily life, profoundly influencing their goals and expectations, interpersonal relationships, and ability to work.

Complexity

As HIV disease progresses, patients typically experience a series of medical complications, many of which require long-term therapy to prevent relapse. Individuals are placed on increasingly complex medical regimens designed to ameliorate or stabilize their condition. Many of these medications are new or experimental, have significant side effects, and are expensive. Adverse drug reactions and interactions may become as difficult to manage as the disease itself.

Severity

Severity can be measured both in terms of the intensity of the disease and its overall impact on the lives of patients. Each HIV-related opportunistic infection, malignancy, and degenerative disorder may cause substantial morbidity and mortality. Earlier diagnosis and better treatment have helped to reduce the severity of many of these complications. However, greater longevity has resulted in an increasing number of illnesses for many patients and the emergence of new opportunistic diseases.

Unpredictability

Despite the progressive damage to the immune system inflicted by HIV infection, the course of disease for a given patient is remarkably unpredictable. Some patients who have experienced severe complications go on to have prolonged asymptomatic periods. One individual may experience a sudden deterioration in functional status, while another will undergo gradual decline. Some patients have localized disease manifestations, whereas in others debilitating multiorgan system involvement develops.

Quality of Life

The concepts of chronicity, complexity, severity, and unpredictability are directly related to the issue of quality of life. Patients are acutely aware, as clinicians should be, that optimizing and preserving the quality of life are at least as important as prolonging its duration. While each of the features of advanced HIV infection described above represents a subjective concept, the idea of quality of life is a uniquely personal notion. Recent studies have attempted to assess the impact of various diseases and treatments on the quality of life of HIV-infected patients [2].

Practical Approach to Care

Geriatricians have distinguished between the "young old" and the "old old." The young old are elderly but enjoy relatively good health and maintain the ability to live independently. The old old, in contrast, are identified primarily by the impact that disease and disability have had on their functional status and independence. Patients with advanced HIV infection often deal with problems that affect their lives in similar ways to the "old old" population, but they are a distinct group with special medical and psychosocial needs.

High-quality care for patients with advanced HIV infection requires an appreciation of the interrelatedness of its medical, psychological, social, economic, and spiritual consequences (Table 34-1). This, in turn, demands a blend of comprehensiveness and flexibility: Clinicians must be able to apply medical knowledge and technology in a way that is consistent with the patient's personal goals and beliefs and is responsive to rapid changes in functional status. As with any successful patient-clinician interaction, the relationship must be based on mutual trust and understanding.

Successful programs for patients with advanced HIV infection generally employ a multidisciplinary team approach (Table 34-2). This collaboration takes advantage of the complementary skills and perspectives of a variety of health providers and facilitates the accomplishment of the goals described below.

History, Physical Examination, and Laboratory Screening

The medical history for the patient with advanced HIV infection is similar to that elicited at other stages of disease (Table 34-3). This list is very comprehensive and beyond the scope of a single visit. Instead, the information should be gathered over a series of interactions with the patient, with the more concrete issues discussed initially and the more complex and emotionally laden ones addressed later.

The clinician collects data regarding active symptoms, past complications and treatment of HIV infection, and mode of HIV acquisition. A careful review of systems is performed, given the multiplicity of problems to which the patient is prone. There should be open discussion of

---

Table 34-1 *Goals for care of patients with advanced HIV infection*

Establish and maintain relationship based on trust, understanding, and knowledge
Use multidisciplinary team approach
Screening: history, physical examination, laboratory evaluation
Prevention: behavioral, environmental, immunologic, pharmacologic
Treatment: medical, psychiatric, addiction, nutrition
Surveillance: anticipatory monitoring
Support to patient and significant others
Individualize approach, within context of guidelines; recognize and respect competing priorities (housing, addiction, finances, family, independence)
Plan for terminal care
Maintain involvement through stages of dying and death

Table 34-2 *The multidisciplinary team*

Essential elements
  Primary care physician and physician assistant or nurse practitioner
  Registered nurse, institution-based or home-based
  Social worker
  Mental health provider
  Physical therapist
  Clergy member
  Case manager
Optional elements (included as applicable)
  Medical subspecialty consultants
  Expert in substance abuse/addiction
  Advocates for special groups
  Hospice provider

past and present sexual practices, as well as patterns of drug and alcohol use. Equally important is evaluation of the patient's mental health. Psychiatric disease, ranging from transient situational anxiety and depression to suicidality and psychosis, is extremely common in this population. The patient's social situation, significant others and support networks, and the status and stability of finances and housing should also be assessed.

Having collected this information, the clinician can begin to learn more about the patient's goals regarding health care. These goals typically evolve over time, and it can be helpful to reassess them periodi-

Table 34-3 *Components of the medical history in advanced HIV infection*

Present symptoms
Mode(s) of HIV acquisition
Date of and reason for original HIV testing
Review of systems
History
  Past medical/surgical/gynecologic
  Sexual, past and present
  Drug and alcohol use, past and present
  Psychiatric
Medications
  Past and present
  Adverse reactions with details
Use of alternative therapies and underground drug networks
Assessment
  Social situation, support network, financial resources, housing
  Goals for medical care
  Health beliefs
  Quality of life
  Functional status
  Wishes for treatment and/or support in terminal stages of disease

cally. It is also valuable to elicit from the patient a description of his or her health beliefs and practices. People of all socioeconomic and ethnic groups participate in systems of healing outside of allopathic or mainstream Western medicine [3]. These may include health practices from Eastern, Native American, African, Caribbean, Latino, and other traditions, and may embrace religious or New Age philosophies. Patients may have unusual dietary habits or use "natural" products as remedies. Some individuals participate in underground "buyer's clubs" of drugs not fully tested for use in HIV infection. Few will volunteer information about such health beliefs and practices unless they are specifically asked about them.

Questions to be addressed include the following: What impact has HIV infection had on the patient's life? What is the patient's view of the quality of his or her life now, and what might be done to improve it? Are there any limitations on the patient's ability to carry out the basic activities of daily living (ADLs) [4] required to maintain independence? The answers to these questions form the basis for the management plan for the patient with advanced HIV infection [5]. Once limitations of functional status have been identified [6], an appropriate rehabilitation program can be designed [7, 8].

Discussions of limitations on quality of life and independence flow naturally to dialogue about dying and death, as well as planning for terminal care. Although these discussions are sometimes difficult, it is well recognized that most patients want to address such issues, including their ideas, fears, and wishes, with their physician. It is only with this information that the clinician can offer reasonable guidance about what types of treatment and level of care may be most appropriate.

The physical examination should be comprehensive, with particular attention paid to the skin, ocular fundi, mouth, lymph nodes, lungs, abdomen, rectum, and central nervous system. Baseline laboratory testing should include a complete blood count with white blood cell differential, CD4 cell count, liver and renal function tests, syphilis and hepatitis B and C serologies, skin testing for tuberculosis along with control antigens, and a Papanicolaou smear in women.

Medical Management

Once the above information has been collected, the clinician can make rational recommendations to the patient with advanced HIV infection about how to optimize his or her health status and prevent intercurrent illness in a manner consistent with personal goals and expectations (Table 34-4).

As detailed elsewhere in this text, there is strong evidence that prophylaxis against PCP with trimethoprim-sulfamethoxazole, or alternatively with dapsone or aerosol pentamidine, reduces morbidity and mortality. All patients with advanced HIV infection should be provided PCP prophylaxis. Likewise, patients previously diagnosed with an op-

Table 34-4 *Hierarchy of interventions in advanced HIV infection*

1. Primary or secondary prophylaxis of *Pneumocystis carinii* pneumonia
2. Maintenance treatment for opportunistic infections
3. Screening for and appropriate prophylaxis of latent tuberculosis or treatment of active tuberculosis
4. Screening for and appropriate treatment of syphilis and other sexually transmitted diseases
5. Prophylaxis against *Mycobacterium avium* complex infection
6. Antiretroviral therapy
7. Immunizations
8. Patient education and risk reduction: sexual practices, alcohol and illicit drugs, nutrition, exercise

portunistic infection for which maintenance therapy prevents relapse should continue to receive the appropriate pharmacologic agent(s).

Patients with advanced HIV infection should be screened for tuberculosis and for treatable sexually transmitted diseases such as syphilis. While testing for tuberculosis with purified protein derivative (PPD) should be performed routinely in all patients, its diagnostic usefulness is limited because of the high prevalence of anergy to skin tests in this population. Therefore, special attention should be paid to any symptoms or signs suggestive of tuberculosis, especially in patients with possible exposure to the disease.

Patients with advanced HIV infection and CD4 cell counts less than $75/mm^3$ may benefit from prophylaxis against *Mycobacterium avium* complex (MAC) infection with rifabutin. Published reports have demonstrated that daily administration of rifabutin can reduce the likelihood of MAC bacteremia by 50 percent [9], although no improvement in survival has been shown. Some clinicians have raised concerns about the drug's potential toxicity, interactions with other agents, cost, and effects on antibiotic resistance patterns of other bacteria including *Mycobacterium tuberculosis*. There is preliminary information that clarithromycin may also be effective in preventing MAC infection.

Whenever possible, patients with advanced HIV infection should be offered antiretroviral therapy. Zidovudine and didanosine have been used extensively in this population, and, while their effectiveness is uncertain, they may confer therapeutic benefit for some patients. Interested persons should be considered for participation in clinical trials evaluating new approaches to antiretroviral therapy.

Although patients with advanced HIV infection usually have markedly impaired antibody responses to vaccines, efforts should be made to immunize them as early as possible in the course of their disease against pneumococcus; *Haemophilus influenzae*, type B; and tetanus; and measles, mumps, and rubella, if indicated. If the patient is seronegative for hepatitis B and at continued risk for this infection, hepatitis B vaccine should be considered as well [10]. Patients should also be offered annual immunization against influenza virus.

HIV-infected patients should be educated about modifying behaviors that increase the risk of disease transmission, progression, or complication. For example, the clinician should discuss "safer sex" practices to prevent HIV transmission and the acquisition of other sexually transmitted diseases. Efforts should be made to treat ongoing alcohol or substance abuse. HIV disease progression may also be reduced and quality of life enhanced by fostering good nutritional and exercise habits.

Monitoring for Complications

Once appropriate management strategies have been implemented, the patient with advanced HIV infection enters a period of anticipatory monitoring or surveillance (Table 34-5). Periodic follow-up visits are arranged at regular intervals, and the patient is encouraged to contact the clinician whenever any changes in health status occur. During these visits, there is a brief review of new symptoms and drug toxicities, confirmation of medications, and an update on the psychosocial and functional status of the patient. Physical examination should focus on evaluation of new symptoms and those organ systems most frequently affected by HIV disease.

Laboratory testing should be guided by symptoms, although it may be helpful to follow complete blood counts and liver function tests looking for early evidence of medication toxicity or new complications. Periodic screening for syphilis and viral hepatitis may be helpful in patients who remain sexually active or continue to use injection drugs and have had negative tests in the past. Likewise, the PPD should be repeated periodically if prior tests have been negative and the patient is not anergic. It is probably not useful to monitor the CD4 cell count if it has been persistently below $50/mm^3$, as results are not likely to affect management. Blood culture surveillance for MAC may be useful in establishing early diagnosis of disseminated infection.

Throughout this period of surveillance, the patient's needs should be continually reassessed, and services adjusted accordingly. The patient and clinician should seek a balance between suppression of HIV complications and the potential adverse impact of treatment on the patient's quality of life. The clinician should address limitations of treatment periodically and provide support to the patient who appropriately chooses to defer evaluations or treatments.

Whenever possible, patients with end-stage HIV disease should be offered treatment at home. A wide range of home services, including nursing care, home infusion, physical therapy, diagnostic testing, and hospice care, are now available to HIV-infected patients. For patients who have unstable home situations, who are homeless, or who cannot manage at home, a variety of alternative care sites may be available [11–13]. These include an acute care hospital, rehabilitation or chronic care hospital, nursing home [14], day care center, and hospice. Specialized services or units are now available in many settings for patients

Table 34-5 *Anticipatory monitoring in advanced HIV infection*

History
    Identification of new symptoms and drug toxicities
    Review of old problems
    Confirmation of medications
    Update on psychological status, social situation
    Update of functional status assessment
Physical examination
    Vital signs
    Evaluation of new symptoms
    Periodic reassessment of organ systems at risk: skin, ocular fundi, mouth,
       lymph nodes, lungs, abdomen, rectum, and central nervous system
Laboratory evaluation
    Complete blood count with white cell differential, liver function tests, Pap
       smear, syphilis serology if patient is sexually active, PPD if negative in
       past and patient not anergic
    (?) Isolator blood cultures for *Mycobacterium avium* complex
Patient education/risk reduction
Reassess needs/reorganize support services

with HIV infection, drawing together health care professionals with special expertise.

Terminal Illness

Perhaps to a greater degree than in other chronic diseases, it can be difficult to recognize the terminal stage of HIV infection. Its clinical manifestations are so variable, and their impact on the individual's quality of life so unpredictable, that patients, families, partners, and clinicians are sometimes taken by surprise when death finally occurs. Of all the complications of advanced HIV infection, perhaps the neuropsychiatric effects cause the most disability and social isolation.

Whenever possible the patient and clinician should anticipate the dilemmas of end-of-life decision making, establishing mutual goals and priorities, ranking options for late-stage care, and negotiating the limitation or withdrawal of treatments that no longer provide significant benefit. Living wills may help to delineate the patient's wishes, and health care proxies can assist in making decisions, but they are not a substitute for honest discussion about these issues.

References

1. Sontag S. *AIDS and Its Metaphors*. New York: Farrar, Straus and Giroux, 1989. P 21.
2. Wu AW, Rubin HR, Mathews WC, et al. Functional status and well-being

in a placebo-controlled trial of zidovudine in early symptomatic HIV infection. *J Acquir Immune Defic Syndr* 6:452–458, 1993.

3. Eisenberg DM, Kessler RC, Foster C, et al. Unconventional medicine in the United States. Prevalence, costs and patterns of use. *N Engl J Med* 328:246–252, 1993.

4. Katz S, Ford AB, Moskowitz RW, et al. Studies of illness in the aged: The index of ADL, a standardized measure of the biological and psychosocial function. *JAMA* 185:914–919, 1963.

5. Weinstein BD. Assessing the impact of HIV disease. *Am J Occup Ther* 44:220–226, 1990.

6. Stewart AL, Greenfield S, Hays RD, et al. Functional status and well-being of patients with chronic conditions: Results from the medical outcomes study. *JAMA* 262:907–913, 1989.

7. O'Connell PG, Levinson SF. Experience with rehabilitation in the acquired immunodeficiency syndrome. *Am J Phys Med Rehabil* 70:195–200, 1991.

8. Sliwa JA, Smith JC. Rehabilitation of neurologic disability related to human immunodeficiency virus. *Arch Phys Med Rehabil* 72:759–762, 1991.

9. Nightingale S, Cameron DW, Gordin FM, et al. Two controlled trials of rifabutin prophylaxis against *Mycobacterium avium* complex infection in AIDS. *N Engl J Med* 329:828–833, 1993.

10. Craven DE, Fuller JD, Barber TW, Pelton SI. Immunization of adults and children infected with human immunodeficiency virus. *Infect Dis Clin Pract* 1:330–338, 411–423, 1992.

11. Lynn DJ. Allocation and the physician: The impacts of aging and AIDS. *J Gen Intern Med* 4:173–174, 1989.

12. Weinberg DS, Murray HW. Coping with AIDS: The special problems of New York City. *N Engl J Med* 317:1469–1473, 1987.

13. Boccellari AA, Dilley JW. Management and residential placement problems of patients with HIV-related cognitive impairment. *Hosp Community Psychiatry* 43:32–37, 1992.

14. Swan JH, Benjamin AE, Brown A. Skilled nursing facility care for persons with AIDS: Comparison with other patients. *Am J Public Health* 82:453–455, 1992.

HIV Prevention in Clinical Practice

35

Christopher W. Shanahan, Harvey J. Makadon

More than a decade after it was first described, the AIDS epidemic continues virtually unchecked. It is estimated that 40,000 to 80,000 persons are infected annually with HIV in the United States [1]. The absence of a curative treatment or vaccine makes prevention of HIV transmission essential to controlling the epidemic.

Epidemiologic and ethnographic studies indicate that most cases of HIV transmission are causally linked to specific human behaviors and have confirmed the effectiveness of population-based prevention programs [2]. For example, widespread modification of sexual behaviors of gay men in San Francisco and New York has lead to a substantial decrease in HIV transmission [3]. In addition, needle exchange programs appear to be effective in preventing the spread of HIV infection among injection drug users (IDUs) [4].

It is also clear, however, that the overall effectiveness of prevention programs has been quite variable and inconsistent over time [2, 5–9]. In addition, there is recent evidence of increasing HIV transmission in young homosexual men in San Francisco, members of a population that had previously demonstrated significant reduction in high-risk behaviors [10]. This "recidivism" is thought to be the result of several factors, including inadequate patient education, lack of access to drug treatment and harm reduction programs, and the inherent difficulty associated with changing complex personal behaviors [11–14].

As the AIDS epidemic grows, its characteristics are gradually changing [15]. HIV continues disproportionately to affect urban men who have sex with men, who use injection drugs, or both [16]. However, adolescents [17], middle-class adults [18], and homosexual men in smaller cities have also become infected in increasing numbers in recent years [19, 20]. Heterosexuals now compose 7 to 9 percent of the total US AIDS population [21, 22]. Nearly 40 percent of women diag-

545

nosed with AIDS between 1991 and 1993 identified heterosexual contact as their only risk factor for HIV transmission [21]. In some high-prevalence US communities, increasing HIV seroconversion has been reported in persons who lack all risk behaviors except unprotected heterosexual contact. This pattern replicates the predominant mode of HIV transmission observed in much of Africa and Asia [23–26], and appears related to unprotected vaginal and anal intercourse with high-risk individuals [27–31].

A Role for Clinicians in HIV Prevention

HIV infection is now the second most common cause of death in men aged 25 to 44, and the fifth leading cause of death in women of the same age group [32]. Public health authorities had high expectations for prevention campaigns during the first decade of the AIDS epidemic. However, it is now clear that the strategies used have not resulted in durable behavioral changes.

The impact that health care providers have in the area of HIV prevention is only beginning to be explored. Clinicians have been shown to play an important role in the prevention of other public health problems, such as cigarette smoking [33–35], and are in a unique position to provide patient education and counseling [36]. One study found that 59 percent of patients would be glad to have the opportunity to talk about sex with their physician, and 67 percent stated that they would be very comfortable discussing AIDS. However, only 15 percent of patients reported ever having discussed AIDS with their physician during the previous 5 years [37].

Despite patient interest in the subject, physicians have not routinely incorporated discussion of sexuality and drug use into their clinical practices. One national survey of physicians reported that 97 percent "usually" and 84 percent "always" addressed smoking cessation and alcohol use during new patient visits with adults [38]. However, these same physicians said that they discussed sexual orientation, number of sex partners, and condom use at rates of only 27, 22, and 31 percent, respectively. Rabin and associates [39] recently demonstrated that prevention practices by physicians for sexually transmitted diseases can be significantly improved with skills-based education.

The Process of Prevention

Many factors affect the extent of prevention efforts in the primary care setting. Certainly, the ability of a clinician to engage a patient in sensitive discussion is often determined by the availability of adequate time and privacy. In addition, the skills to conduct culturally sensitive sexual and drug use histories and to provide meaningful information for behavioral change vary widely among professionals [40].

Another factor that affects preventive care involves the terms used by health professionals to characterize persons at risk for HIV infection. For example, some men engage in unsafe sex with other men but do not consider themselves to be bisexual, homosexual, or gay [41–43]. Using a label rather than inquiring about specific behaviors may provide inaccurate information and lead to confusion regarding risk for HIV exposure and transmission.

The success of preventive health education in clinical practice may also be influenced by a patient's perception of his or her own vulnerability [44]. For example, individuals in communities with low reported HIV prevalence rates predictably exhibit a low sense of personal risk. This perception may make it more difficult for clinicians to engage such patients in discussion of behavioral change and may place them at higher risk for HIV infection as the seroprevalence rate rises within their community [19]. Since there is no simple way to know the HIV risk or serostatus of another person with certainty, behavioral norms for sexually active and drug-using individuals may need to shift toward mutual self-disclosure to reduce harm [45].

Prevention in the Clinical Encounter

What is HIV Prevention?

Clinical prevention involves providing information to patients in order to help them modify behaviors that place them at risk for HIV infection. The health care provider may be able to effect behavioral changes by

1. Reinforcing the importance of condom use and a mutually monogamous relationship.
2. Identifying and treating drug use.
3. Using appropriate and sensitive patient interviewing techniques.
4. Highlighting the patient's personal investment in change.
5. Supporting the patient's efforts to discuss high-risk behaviors with partners.

Goals for Clinical HIV Prevention

The clinician can assist the patient in evaluating his or her risk for HIV infection by methodically reviewing sexual and drug use histories. Goals for this encounter include reinforcement of prevention practices that the patient has already adopted and eliciting ideas on how to maintain compliance with safer behaviors. Information obtained from the patient should be used to structure interventions; interested individuals can be referred to HIV health educators, counselors, or local AIDS prevention groups for further information.

When discussing HIV transmission, the clinician should tailor topics to the patient's lifestyle and risk behaviors (Tables 35-1, 35-2). The goal for risk reduction should be to create the impetus for behavioral change by discussing self-care as well as protection of others. Drug users have special informational needs. "Crack cocaine" has been associated with an increased risk of HIV infection from sexual behaviors related to drug procurement, including trading sex for drugs, money, or other inducements [46]. When a clinician discusses risk reduction with IDUs, it is insufficient to advise them only "not to share needles." Many drug users do not share injection equipment per se but rather rent it in a "shooting gallery." It is common in this setting for unsterile drug paraphernalia to be used sequentially by multiple clients who never actually see each other [5].

When Should Risk Assessment Begin?

A discussion of HIV prevention during a clinical encounter is generally initiated by the health care provider [37, 47]. Because clinicians see patients in a wide range of situations, the setting often dictates the scope and type of issues that can be addressed. In general, the provider should initiate the discussion, presenting the topic of HIV prevention as part of routine health care maintenance for both new and established patients.

Table 35-1 *Sexual risk reduction topics for discussion with patients*

The importance of taking care of oneself and others by reducing risk for HIV transmission

The role of "safer sex" in the patient's life with all relevant partners—whether regular, occasional, and/or paid

The importance of limiting number of sexual partners

The importance of knowing the serostatus of sexual partners and frankly discussing risk behaviors with them

The risk of unplanned or unprotected sexual contact when using drugs, including alcohol

The risk of HIV transmission during pregnancy

The use of condoms in male-female and male-male sexual activity, including obstacles and strategies to overcome them

The feasibility of unilateral initiation of risk reduction behaviors in their sexual interactions

Table 35-2 *Drug use risk reduction topics for discussion with patients*

The importance of dilute bleach to clean drug paraphernalia
The avoidance of "shooting galleries" or trading sex for drugs or money
The importance of drug treatment and rehabilitation
The opportunity to discuss harm reduction topics and/or offer referral to
  community-based educational services when indicated

Risk Assessment: What Questions Should Be Asked?

While there is no consensus concerning the optimal means of incorporating HIV risk assessment into the visit, certain questions appear to be reasonable (Table 35-3). Who to screen and when to screen are influenced by many factors, including the seroprevalence of HIV in the community and the probability of high-risk sexual and drug use behaviors in the patient being interviewed.

Should Everyone Be Assessed for Risk of HIV Infection?
Yes. A patient's risk cannot be accurately estimated solely by his or her personal appearance or self-reported behaviors.

Should the Assessment Be the Same for All Patients?
Probably not. Detailed sexual and drug use histories can be time-consuming, and easily administered screening instruments may conserve effort and minimize patient anxiety [48]. Evidence of high-risk patient

Table 35-3 *Sample HIV risk assessment instrument for men and women*

Men	Women
Did you receive a transfusion of blood or blood products between 1978 and 1985?	Did you receive a transfusion of blood or blood products between 1978 and 1985?
Have you ever, even once, used any kind of injected drug?	Have you ever, even once, used any kind of injected drug?
Have you ever had a disease that you contracted through sexual contact?	Have you ever had a disease that you contracted through sexual contact?
Have you ever, even once, had sex with a man?	Are you sexually active with men?
Have you ever, even once, had sex with a prostitute or with someone who has used injected drugs?	Have you ever, even once, had sex with a bisexual man or one who has used injected drugs?
Do you have any other reason to suspect you might be at risk for AIDS or the HIV virus?	Do you have any other reason to suspect you might be at risk for AIDS or the HIV virus?

Source: Adapted from N Hearst. AIDS risk assessment in primary care. *J Am Board Fam Pract* 1:44–48, 1994.

behaviors should prompt more detailed inquiry. If there is inadequate time for discussion, the patient should be scheduled for a follow-up visit or be referred to an appropriate professional for continuation of risk assessment.

Who Should be Considered at High Risk for HIV Infection?

Any person who answers yes to screening questions (see Table 35-3) should be considered at high risk and undergo more specific discussion about his or her behaviors and the need for HIV antibody testing [49]. HIV antibody testing should be performed only in the context of appropriate counseling, and discussions should include a thorough explanation of the meaning of the term "confidentiality" [49]. *Confidential testing* implies a level of protection similar to that associated with medical records; that is, information cannot be released to an outside party without the patient's consent. In *anonymous testing*, the patient and his or her blood sample are identified by a number only and cannot be traced. While home HIV antibody testing may soon become a reality, its effect on the behavior of persons engaging in high-risk behaviors is unclear [50].

Prevention in HIV-Seropositive Patients

Prevention efforts in HIV-infected individuals have an important role in clinical care and should focus on how to reduce behaviors that could potentially expose others to the virus. The patient should be counseled on several important issues, including (1) the vital importance of informing sexual and drug-using partners of his or her serostatus; (2) the significance of avoiding high-risk sexual and drug-using behaviors; and (3) the fact that progression of HIV disease is associated with increased risk of viral transmission to sexual partners [51].

Education as Intervention

HIV education is important for all patients regardless of their history, since behavior varies over the course of a lifetime [52, 53]. Persons involved in high-risk behaviors in traditionally "low-risk" settings should be informed of the changing characteristics of the epidemic that may place them at increased risk [19, 20]. It should also be remembered that patients are part of a larger community, and word-of-mouth information may help persons at high risk for HIV infection who do not make regular use of the health care system. For example, investigators have shown that IDUs may reduce their risk by utilizing information obtained solely through talking to others [54].

How questions are asked is just as important as what questions are asked (Tables 35-4, 35-5). A well-conducted medical interview provides reliable data for risk estimation and clinical decision making [55]. Questions should be presented in both an open-ended and close-ended

Table 35-4 *Principles for interviewing patients*

Facilitate discussion
Clarify for patients that increased risk results from intimate behaviors with HIV-
infected individuals whose serostatus may not be known at the time
Educate by giving information about relative risk associated with specific sexual
behaviors (see Table 35-6)
Advise harm reduction strategies when indicated
Use language that is relevant and appropriate for the patient's educational level and
vocabulary
Set goals for behavioral change that are realistic and obtainable

Table 35-5 *Examples of effective and ineffective questions*

Effective	Ineffective
Now I would like to ask you some questions about sexual activity and drug use. I ask all of my patients these questions because doctors now believe that it is extremely important to do so since so many people are affected by HIV, the AIDS virus. I realize that some of the questions may seem awkward to both of us but that is understandable.	No introduction—immediately start asking questions without preparing patient. (**Reason:** *Abrupt introduction of this topic will place both parties ill at ease, providing strong incentive to get it "over with" rather than explore details of risk behaviors in the patient's life.*)
Have you had sex with a man, even once?	Are you gay or bisexual? (**Reason:** *Not all men who engage in anal intercourse consider themselves gay or homosexual; avoid labels that may be misleading.*)
Sometimes when people drink or take drugs, they do things that they typically might not do, like have sex without a condom, or have sex with someone they did not know, or perhaps engage in a sexual act like anal intercourse. Has anything like that ever happened to you? Have you ever not remembered what happened but were worried that you may have done something you would usually not do?	Do you ever have sex under the influence of drugs or alcohol? (**Reason:** *Being considered out of control or sexually promiscuous is socially unacceptable in our society; patients may not tell the truth if they sense that the clinician may view them unfavorably because of their conduct. Normalizing the behavior to a certain extent may permit the patient to talk more freely.*)
Have you ever caught an infection from having sex with someone?	Have you ever had any sexually transmitted diseases? (**Reason:** *Anticipate the need to avoid medical jargon; some patients may deny things they do not understand.*)
People who always use condoms with their sexual partners sometimes don't if the sex is with the person they love or are going out with; do you use a condom every time with your boyfriend/girlfriend/lover?	You always use a condom when you have sex, right? (**Reason:** *Avoid judgmental and insinuating statements. It inhibits the ability to talk freely without fear of scorn or ridicule. Additionally, it inadvertently informs the patient about what the provider probably wants to hear.*)

manner. HIV risk assessment should be introduced by stressing to the patient the importance of discussing the topic and that, while such discussions should be considered routine, they are also sometimes awkward for both parties.

The health care provider should attempt to educate and advise the patient during the interview and use any information obtained to tailor the message, while acknowledging gaps in our knowledge of the relative risks of specific sexual acts (Table 35-6).

HIV Counseling and Testing

Pretest Counseling

HIV antibody testing continues to be an important tool for HIV prevention and treatment. If HIV testing is requested by the patient, the clinician should assess the individual's risk behaviors and motivation. When the physician advises testing, it should only be performed in the context of a detailed risk assessment.

The purpose of pretest counseling is to inform the patient of the nature of the test, as well as the indications and contraindications for testing (Tables 35-7, 35-8; see also Table 32-1). In addition to understanding the meaning of both positive and negative results, the patient should also be informed that, although rare, false-positive and false-negative results sometimes occur. The clinician should explain to the patient that, in the case of recent known high-risk exposure, retesting should be performed in about 6 months. For persons who continue high-risk behaviors, repeat testing may help in the early identification of a new seroconversion [49].

Post-Test Counseling

The time required to report and discuss the results of an HIV antibody test may be quite variable. In general, the clinician should allocate no less than 15 minutes for discussion of a negative test result and at least 30 minutes for a positive result (Table 35-9). Post-test counseling is a complex process influenced by the setting, the experience of the clinician, and the resources available. It may be advisable to employ an HIV counselor or utilize outside testing and counseling services when adequate support is not available in a practice setting. The Centers for Disease Control [56] has published specific standards and guidelines for the notification process, describing the primary public health purposes of counseling during serostatus notification as follows:

1. To reinforce perception of risk for those who are unaware or uninformed.

Table 35-6 *Relative risk of HIV transmission associated with specific sexual practices*

Risk	Sexual practice
Highest risk	Unprotected peno-vaginal intercourse
	Unprotected peno-anal intercourse
Uncertain risk	Oral-genital sex with or without a condom or dental dam
	Peno-anal or peno-vaginal intercourse with a latex condom
	Anal-manual intercourse ("fist fucking")
	Oral-anal sex ("rimming")
	Deep kissing ("French," "wet")
	Sharing of insertive sex toys (e.g., dildos, vibrators)
No risk	Dry kissing
	Hugging
	Mutual masturbation
	Coprolalia ("talking dirty")
	Phone sex
	Exhibitionism/transvestitism/voyeurism
	Holding hands
	Massage

Source: Adapted from *The Complete Guide to Safe Sex*. The Institute for Advanced Study of Human Sexuality. Beverly Hills, CA: The Prevent Group, 1987.

Table 35-7 *Topics for pretest counseling*

A person can be completely healthy and still be infected with HIV
One cannot tell if a person is HIV-positive by just looking at him or her
Persons who are HIV-positive are infectious to others who engage in high-risk behavior with them
A person can be infected with HIV, infectious to others through high-risk behavior, but not have AIDS
Most persons who test HIV-positive develop AIDS within 8 to 10 years, but sometimes it takes longer
Tests for HIV infection are very accurate, but incorrect results do occur. The patient should be retested in 6 months, regardless of the results of the first test, if he or she has engaged in recent high-risk behaviors.

Table 35-8 *Information to obtain from the patient during pretest counseling*

Does anyone else know that the patient plans on being tested?
Does the patient have someone who can accompany him or her to the next visit to receive the test results?
Does the patient have someone to talk to while waiting for the test results?
Does the patient have any current organized supports, such as Alcoholics Anonymous (AA) or Narcotics Anonymous (NA)? If so, the patient should be encouraged to use them.
If necessary, would the patient accept referral for additional support?

Table 35-9 *Topics for post-test counseling*

Allow adequate time for thorough discussion of the test results and their
  implications

Consider using ancillary services if necessary

Assess the patient's capacity to assimilate and cope with test results

If the test results are **POSITIVE:**
  1. Clearly state the results and their proper interpretation
  2. Anticipate the need for extra support
  3. Review the patient's plan for the next 48 hours
  4. Assess the potential for suicide
  5. Arrange for follow-up within 2 to 3 weeks to review test results,
     monitor coping mechanisms, initiate medical evaluation, and continue
     education

If the test results are **NEGATIVE:**
  1. Clearly state the results and their proper interpretation
  2. Emphasize the need for repeat testing in 6 months
  3. Restate the possibility of later seroconversion if recently exposed
  4. Dispel any belief that continuation of high risk behavior is now permis-
     sible because of invulnerability or immunity

---

2. To help uninfected persons initiate and sustain behavioral
   changes that reduce their risk of becoming infected.
3. To arrange access to necessary medical, prevention, and case
   management services for persons with a positive result.
4. To assist those who may be infected to avoid infecting others
   and remain healthy.
5. To support and/or assist infected persons in the referral of sex
   or needle-sharing partners.

If the HIV Test Result Is Positive

Once a patient is told he or she is HIV positive, it is unlikely that the
ensuing discussion will be remembered or fully understood. The clinician must be prepared for a range of reactions, including denial, depressed acceptance, anger directed at self or others, or even frank hys-
teria [57]. Mental health services should be readily available, and the
clinician should inquire about the patient's planned activities for the
next 24 to 48 hours, assessing the potential for depression and suicide
(see Table 35-9). The patient should be referred for initiation of primary
medical care as soon as reasonably possible after being informed about
a positive test result.

In addition to helping patients deal with their emotional response, it
is important to begin the educational process about what it means to
have HIV infection. The clinician should review the natural history of
HIV disease, methods for monitoring the progression of immunodeficiency, and strategies for early intervention [58].

If the HIV Test Result Is Negative

If the HIV test result is negative, the clinician should emphasize some important points. The patient should be reminded that the risk for infection remains if high-risk behaviors are continued and that a negative test result is not a justification for unsafe behavior or indication of "immunity" to HIV infection [58] (see Table 35-9).

Incorporating HIV Prevention in Clinical Practice

How practitioners incorporate primary HIV prevention into their clinical practice will vary based on many factors, including setting, the circumstances, and their level of experience [59].

Time management will become increasingly important for clinicians who screen and educate patients. Given pressures to shorten visits, it may be difficult for some practitioners to take on the responsibilities of HIV risk assessment without appropriate resources. For example, a primary care physician in community practice may have to offer all of the individual components of prevention, including risk assessment, patient education, and, pretest and post-test counseling. On the other hand, a clinician in a practice organized to provide HIV services may only need to address risk assessment and patient education and then refer the patient to another professional for counseling and testing.

It is important for each practitioner to regard his or her role as part of a larger public health strategy for primary HIV prevention. Most regions of the United States have local HIV prevention projects. In addition, several programs may target different specific subpopulations within a geographic area. A single metropolitan area may have a gay men's AIDS prevention group, a needle exchange program for IDUs, and a high school HIV prevention program.

Ultimately, clinical prevention may be facilitated through collaboration with public health organizations. This strategy would recognize the strengths of each of these approaches, while considering the time limitations of clinical practice and acknowledging that specific resources need to be devoted to prevention projects. Health care professionals can assist in these efforts by promoting AIDS prevention activities in their communities.

References

1. Centers for Disease Control. Projections of the number of persons diagnosed with AIDS and the number of immunosuppressed HIV-infected persons—United States, 1992–94. *MMWR* 42:17–18, 1993.

2. Choi K-H, Coates T. *Preventing HIV Infection: What Does the Empirical Literature Say About Programs, Outcomes, Implications and Research Directions?* Unpublished manuscript. Available from Center for AIDS Prevention Studies (CAPS), 74 New Montgomery St, Suite 600, San Francisco CA 64105.

3. Coates TJ. Prevention of HIV-1 infection: Accomplishments and priorities. *J NIH Research* 5:73–76, 1993.

4. Turner CF, Miller HG, Moses LE. *AIDS: Sexual Behavior and Intravenous Drug Use*. Washington DC: National Research Council, National Academy Press, 1989. Pp 202–209.

5. Page JB, Smith PC, Kane N. Shooting Galleries, Their Properties and Implications for Prevention of AIDS. In DG Fisher (ed), *AIDS and Alcohol/Drug Abuse: Psychological Research*. New York: Hawthorn Press, 1992. Pp 69–85.

6. Des Jarlais DC, et al. HIV-1 infection among intravenous drug users in Manhattan, New York City from 1977 through 1987. *JAMA* 261:1008–1012, 1989.

7. Ickovics JR, et al. Limited effects of HIV counseling and testing for women: A prospective study of behavioral and psychological consequences. *JAMA* 272:443–448, 1994.

8. Centers for Disease Control. Antibody to human immunodeficiency virus in female prostitutes. *MMWR* 36:157–161, 1987.

9. Novick DM, et al. Absence of antibody to human immunodeficiency virus in long-term socially rehabilitated methadone maintenance patients. *Arch Intern Med* 150:97–99, 1990.

10. Lemp GF, et al. Seroprevalence of HIV and risk behaviors among young homosexual and bisexual men: The San Francisco/Berkeley Young Men's Survey. *JAMA* 272:449–454, 1994.

11. Dalton HL. AIDS in blackface. *Daedalus* Summer 1989, Pp 205–227.

12. Nelson KE, et al. Human immunodeficiency virus infection in diabetic intravenous drug users. *JAMA* 266:2259–2261, 1991.

13. Des Jarlais DC, Case P. Shaping the Response: Increasing Access to Injection Equipment: Syringe Exchange and Other Examples of Harm Reduction Strategies. In J Mann, D Tarantola, T Netter (eds), *AIDS in the World*. Cambridge MA: Harvard University Press, 1992. Pp 685–990.

14. Peterson JL, et al. High-risk sexual behavior and condom use among gay and bisexual African-American men. *Am J Public Health* 82:1490–1494, 1992.

15. Hu DJ, Fleming PL, Mays MA, Ward JW. The expanding regional diversity of the acquired immunodeficiency syndrome epidemic in the United States. *Arch Intern Med* 154:654–659, 1994.

16. Centers for Disease Control. *HIV/AIDS Surveillance Report* 5:1–33, 1994.

17. Centers for Disease Control. Update: Impact of the expanded AIDS surveillance case definition for adolescents and adults on case reporting—United States, 1993. *MMWR* 43:160–161, 167–170, 1994.

18. Glaser JB, Strange TJ, Rosati D. Heterosexual human immunodeficiency virus transmission among the middle class. *Arch Intern Med* 149:645–649, 1989.

19. Kelly JA, et al. Acquired immunodeficiency syndrome/human immuno-

deficiency virus risk behavior among gay men in small cities: Findings of a 16-city national sample. *Arch Intern Med* 152:2293–2297, 1992.

20. Smucny J, et al. Risk factors for HIV infection in homosexual men: The Cleveland men's study of risks in a low-prevalence area. *Cleve Clin J Med* 59:573–580, 1992.

21. Centers for Disease Control. United States AIDS cases. *AIDS* 8:399–401, 1994.

22. Centers for Disease Control. Heterosexually acquired AIDS—United States, 1993. *MMWR* 43:155–160, 1994.

23. Drucker E. Epidemic in the war zone: AIDS and community survival in New York City. *Int J Health Serv* 20:601–615, 1990.

24. The Collaborative Study Group of AIDS in Haitian Americans. Risk factors for AIDS among Haitians residing in the United States. *JAMA* 257:635–639, 1987.

25. Del Tempelis C, et al. Human immunodeficiency virus infection in women in San Francisco Bay area (letter). *JAMA* 258:474–475, 1987.

26. Zell SC. The AIDS Epidemic in Thailand: Past, present, and future prospects. *J Physicians Assoc for AIDS Care* 1:19–31, 1994.

27. Lazzarin A, et al. Man-to-women sexual transmission of the human immunodeficiency virus: Risk factors related to sexual behavior, man's infectiousness and woman's susceptibility. *Arch Intern Med* 151:2411–2416, 1991.

28. Cameron DW, et al. Female to male transmission of human immunodeficiency virus type-1: Risk factors for seroconversion in men. *Lancet* 2:403–407, 1989.

29. Padian NS, Shiboski SC, Jewell NP. Female-to-male transmission of human immunodeficiency virus. *JAMA* 266:1664–1667, 1991.

30. Padian NS, Shiboski SC, Jewell NP. The effect of number of exposures on the risk of heterosexual HIV transmission. *J Infect Dis* 161:883–887, 1990.

31. de Vinzenzi I, for the European Study Group on Heterosexual Transmission of HIV. A longitudinal study of human immunodeficiency virus transmission by heterosexual partners. *N Engl J Med* 331:341–346, 1994.

32. Centers for Disease Control/National Center for Health Statistics. Advance report of final mortality statistics, 1991. *Monthly Vital Statistics Report* 42: 2 (suppl):22–24, 1993.

33. Russell M, Wilson C, Taylor C, Baker C. Effect of general practitioners' advice against smoking. *Br Med J* 2:31–35, 1979.

34. Cummings SR, et al. Training physicians in counseling about smoking cessation: A randomized trial of the "Quit for Life" program. *Ann Intern Med* 110:640–647, 1989.

35. Cohen SJ, et al. Encouraging primary care physicians to help smokers quit: A randomized, controlled trial. *Ann Intern Med* 110:648–652, 1989.

36. Adams PF, Benson V. Current estimates from the National Health Interview survey, 1990. *Vital Health Stat* 10:1–212, 1991.

37. Gerbert B, Maguire BT, Coates T. Are patients talking to their physicians about AIDS? *Am J Public Health* 80:467–469, 1990.

38. Loft J, et al. HIV prevention practices of primary-care physicians—United States, 1992. *MMWR* 42:988–992, 1994.

39. Rabin DL, et al. Improving office-based physicians' prevention practices for sexually transmitted diseases. *Ann Intern Med* 121:513–519, 1994.
40. Rottello G. "Watch your mouth." *OUT Magazine* June 1994. Pp 148–168.
41. Gonsiorek JC, Weinrich JD. The Definition and Scope of Sexual Orientation. In JC Gonsiorek, JD Weinrich (eds), *Homosexuality: Research Implications for Public Policy*. London: Sage Publications, 1991. Pp 1–12.
42. Carrier JM. Cultural factors affecting urban Mexican male homosexual behavior. *Arch Sex Behav* 5:103–124, 1976.
43. Hernandez M, et al. Sexual behavior and status for human immunodeficiency virus type 1 among homosexual and bisexual males in Mexico City. *Ann J Epidemiol* 135:883–894, 1992.
44. Turner CF, Miller HG, Moses LE. *AIDS: Sexual Behavior and Intravenous Drug Use*. Washington, DC: National Research Council, National Academy Press, 1989. Pp 271–273.
45. Hearst N, Hulley SB. Preventing the heterosexual spread of AIDS: Are we giving our patients the best advice? *JAMA* 259:2428–2432, 1988.
46. Chaisson RE, et al. Cocaine use and HIV infection in intravenous drug users in San Francisco. *JAMA* 261:561–565, 1989.
47. Lewis CE. Sexual practices: Are physicians addressing the issues? *J Gen Int Med* 5 (suppl):S78–S81, 1990.
48. Hearst N. AIDS risk assessment in primary care. *J Am Board Fam Pract* 1:44–48, 1994.
49. Report of the US Preventive Services Task Force. *Screening for Infection with Human Immunodeficiency Virus. Guide to Clinical Preventive Services: An Assessment of the Effectiveness of 169 Interventions*. Williams & Wilkins, Baltimore: 1989. Pp 139–146.
50. Cimons M. Debate revived over home collection HIV tests. *J Physicians Assoc for AIDS Care*. Jul 1:6–7, 31, 1994.
51. Musicco M, et al. Antiretroviral treatment of men infected with human immunodeficiency virus type 1 reduces the incidence of heterosexual transmission. *Arch Intern Med* 154:1971–1976, 1994.
52. Division of Reproductive Health and Division of Adolescent and School Health, Centers for Disease Control. Sexual behavior among high school students. *MMWR* 40:885–888, 1992.
53. Centers for Disease Control. Selected behaviors that increase risk for HIV infection, other sexually transmitted diseases and unintended pregnancy among high school students—United States, 1991. *MMWR* 41:945–950, 1992.
54. Friedman SR, Des Jarlais DC, Sothevan JL. AIDS health education for intravenous drug users. *Health Educ Q* 13:383–393, 1986.
55. Nardone DA, et al. A model for the diagnostic medical interview: Nonverbal, verbal and cognitive assessments. *J Gen Int Med* 7:437–442, 1992.
56. US Department of Health and Human Services/Centers for Disease Control. *HIV Counseling, Testing and Referral; Standards and Guidelines*. Washington DC: Public Health Service, May 1994.
57. National Institutes of Mental Health. *Coping with AIDS: Psychological and Social Considerations in Helping People with HTLV-III Infection*. Publication no. DHHS(ADM)85-1432. Rockville MD: Alcohol, Drug Abuse and Mental Health Administration, 1986.

58. Makadon HJ. Assessing HIV infection in primary care practice. *J Gen Int Med* 6 (suppl):S2–S7, 1991.
59. Makadon HJ, Silin J. Prevention of HIV in primary care: Current practices, future possibilities. *Ann Intern Med* In press.

Infection Control and Risk Reduction for Health Care Workers

36

Robert A. Burke, Gail M. Garvin, Carol A. Sulis

The potential for occupational transmission of HIV is a serious concern among health care workers (HCW) [1–5]. In 1988, the Centers for Disease Control (CDC) estimated a 0.42 percent risk of infection following occupational exposure to HIV-infected blood or bloody body fluids [6]. As of December 1994, 133 cases of occupationally acquired HIV infection in HCW had been reported in the United States (Table 36-1). In 42 instances, HCW had a negative baseline HIV test at the time of exposure [7]. Most were the result of needlestick or other sharps injuries. The timing and source of acquisition of HIV infection for the other 91 HCW are not well documented. In addition to percutaneous injuries, a small number of HIV seroconversions following mucous membrane or nonintact skin occupational exposure have also been reported. Factors that are believed to influence the risk of occupational HIV transmission include the type and extent of exposure and the immunologic characteristics of both the source ("donor") and recipient [6, 8–39] (Table 36-2).

Universal Precautions/Body Substance Isolation

Health care workers can reduce their risk of exposure to blood and body fluids through the use of basic safety measures, barrier precautions, and technologically safer instruments [8, 13–28, 33, 38–59]. In 1987, the CDC issued a set of infection control guidelines designed to prevent or minimize the risk of occupational exposure to blood-borne pathogens [13]. These guidelines, known as "universal precautions," are reflected

Table 36-1 *Occupationally acquired HIV infection in US health care workers*

Clinical status	No.	Type of exposure	No.	Occupation	No.
Documented seroconversion[a]					
AIDS	17	Percutaneous	36	Laboratory worker	17
HIV infection	25	Mucocutaneous	4	Nurse	13
		Both	1	Physician	6
		Unknown	1	Other	6
Presumed seroconversion[b]					
HIV infection	91	Not available		Not available	

[a]Requires a baseline negative HIV antibody test.
[b]Includes HCW with HIV infection who have not reported other risk factors and who describe a history of occupational exposure to blood, body fluids, or HIV-infected laboratory material but for whom seroconversion after exposure was not documented.
Data reported to the Centers for Disease Control as of December 1994.

in a series of regulations enacted by the Occupational Safety and Health Administration (OSHA) [25, 44] (Table 36-3).

Universal precautions are based on the premise that all patients are potentially infectious. Recommendations include the use of protective clothing and equipment, and special techniques to prevent contamina-

Table 36-2 *Assessing significance of occupational exposure to HIV*

Risk factor	Commentary
Number of exposures	Single vs. multiple
Type of exposure	Percutaneous
	Mucosal
	Cutaneous
Type of fluid	Concentrated virus (e.g., tissue culture)
	Blood
	Other body fluid
	Age of fluid (e.g., fresh sample)
Severity of injury or exposure	Depth of wound (superficial vs. deep)
	Size of wound
	Duration of contact (brief vs. prolonged)
	Evident infectious material introduced? How much?
Source (donor) characteristics	Stage of HIV disease
	Presence of viremia
	Presence of antigenemia
	Use of antiretroviral therapy
HCW characteristics	Hygiene
	First aid procedure following exposure
	Skin integrity
	Use of barriers at the time of exposure
	Immunologic status

Table 36-3 *Methods to reduce the risk of occupational exposure to infection*

Procedure*	Precautionary measure
Any direct patient contact	10-sec hand wash before and after patient contact
Handling blood or body fluid, or equipment contaminated with blood or body fluid	Wear gloves; remove immediately after task, and wash hands
If soiling of clothes or arms is likely	Wear a fluid-resistant gown or apron; discard or launder after use
If splash to the face is likely	Wear a mask and protective eyewear
Direct contact with a lesion, rash, or mucous membrane	Wear gloves; remove immediately after, and wash hands
Phlebotomy, insertion of intravenous catheter	Wear gloves; do not recap, bend or cut needle; discard all needles and sharps in a puncture-resistant container located at the point of use
Arterial puncture or cannulation	Wear gloves, mask, and protective eyewear
Aerosol drug treatment in an immunosuppressed patient	Treat patient in a booth or room with negative pressure and external exhaust; HCW entering room or providing direct care during or immediately after treatment should wear snugly fitting 1–5 μ filtration mask or particulate respirator
Reusable equipment and devices Device enters the bloodstream or normally sterile body cavity	Wash thoroughly and sterilize
Device touches intact mucosa but does not penetrate the body	Wash thoroughly and perform high-level disinfection
Device touches only intact skin	Clean with a hospital-grade disinfectant

*In all cases, sterile equipment should be used with aseptic technique.

tion of mucous membranes and skin with potentially infectious body fluids or laboratory preparations. HIV has been isolated from blood; semen; vaginal secretions; amniotic fluid; cerebrospinal, synovial, pleural, peritoneal, and pericardial fluids; and organs for transplant [25, 27, 60]. The risk of transmission of HIV from feces, nasal secretions, sputum, saliva, sweat, tears, urine, or vomitus is very low unless they contain visible blood [25]. However, some institutions have expanded the CDC recommendation of universal precautions into a policy called "body substance isolation," which requires that protective clothing or barrier devices be used whenever skin or mucous membrane exposure to *any* body fluid, tissue, or culture is anticipated [53].

A comprehensive program of universal precautions is burdensome, difficult to implement, and expensive, and not all of the procedures are equally effective [43, 45–47, 52, 61–72]. Compliance with universal precautions may reduce the incidence of skin and mucous membrane exposures, but may also promote a false sense of security [38, 39, 45–47, 59, 62, 65–68, 70–72]. Most sharp devices, including disposable needle/syringe combinations, winged steel needle intravenous sets, intravenous catheter stylets, scalpels, and suture needles, can cause injuries, which often occur during recapping or disposal [45, 52, 54, 61]. Despite implementation of aggressive infection control education programs and protective sharps disposal systems, some investigators have reported a significant increase in occupational injuries [45, 70].

Because percutaneous exposures account for 80 percent of occupationally acquired HIV infection, more emphasis needs to be placed on measures to reduce sharps injuries [50, 56, 62]. OSHA requires that health care institutions purchase devices with incorporated safety features if available; design changes could eliminate 85 to 95 percent of injuries [44, 52]. Safety design modifications should be automatic and not depend on the interest or cooperation of the user. Examples include needleless systems and needles that recess or resheathe spontaneously [42]. Institutions should attempt to prevent sharps-related injuries in all work areas, including the operating room [45, 46, 52, 65].

The approach listed below is recommended when performing invasive procedures or when handling blood, body fluids, or contaminated equipment [13, 25, 50, 57]. OSHA requires that employers document HCW compliance with these measures [44].

1.   Hand washing (10-second scrub with hand soap) should be performed before and after patient contact. If intact skin is contaminated with blood or body fluid, the area should be washed immediately. Health care workers with exudative lesions or weeping dermatitis should not perform direct patient care or invasive procedures [28].

2.   Gloves should be worn whenever blood or body fluid is handled. No differences have been reported in permeability between *intact* latex and vinyl gloves [25]. Gloves should be worn for a single procedure and removed carefully to avoid skin contamination. Hands should be thoroughly washed after removing gloves. Some institutions require several pairs of gloves or cotton liners for extra protection during certain procedures. If maximum tactile sensation is not essential, steel mesh gloves that can be sterilized are available for procedures associated with a high risk of cuts or punctures.

3.   Needles, scalpels, and other sharp instruments should be handled carefully to prevent injuries. Whenever possible, open needles should be replaced with devices that include a safety feature to prevent accidental puncture of the user. Although injuries that occur during recapping or disposal have been recognized for years, HCW compliance with safety measures is

difficult to achieve [58, 61, 62, 70, 71]. *Needles should never be recapped, bent, broken, or removed from syringes by hand.* Needles and sharps should be disposed of immediately after use in a puncture-resistant container, located at the point of use. Availability of containers may significantly decrease injuries related to disposal, but they must be designed to avoid jamming and be emptied or replaced by properly trained personnel on a regular basis [42, 45].

4. Surgical procedures that require blind manipulations and hand-held sharps should be modified whenever possible [28].

5. A fluid-resistant gown or protective apron should be worn if soiling is anticipated, and it should be discarded after a single use.

6. Protective eyewear and a mask should be worn if a blood or body fluid splash to the mouth, nose, or eyes is likely.

7. To avoid mouth-to-mouth resuscitation, barrier devices or resuscitation bags should be strategically located in areas where the need for resuscitation is predictable.

8. Surgical procedures should include appropriate barrier precautions. For some subspecialties, universal precautions require additional or enhanced precautions. For example, the US Public Health Service recommends the use of protective wear and barrier devices to prevent transmission of blood-borne organisms during dental and oral surgical procedures [22, 57]. Other examples include the use of face shields during orthopedic surgery with electric saws and vacuum devices to recover flume during cautery [46, 49, 65, 68].

9. Postmortem procedures for all patients should include complete protective wear for any HCW at risk for fluid or tissue contamination. All cadavers should be considered potentially infectious, as should all surfaces and equipment that were used during autopsy.

10. All HCW should receive annual education about infection control and safe work practices [2, 42, 44, 70].

The HIV-Infected Health Care Worker

Following an investigation of a cluster of HIV infections among patients of a Florida dentist, there has been great public concern about HIV-infected HCW performing invasive procedures [73–75]. In response, the CDC has recommended that HCW who perform exposure-prone procedures know their HIV status and voluntarily refrain from performing them unless they have sought counsel from an expert review panel [28]. As of December 1994, 14,591 of the persons reported with AIDS in the United States had been employed in health care services (CDC Information Service). However, several "look back" investigations have failed to identify additional cases of HIV transmission from HCW to patients [76–81]. Extensive debate has yet to produce either a list of "exposure-prone" procedures or a consensus on the means to enforce the CDC recommendation [8, 28, 82–89]. Each institution should develop its own policies and resources regarding HIV-infected personnel.

Cleaning and Disinfection

Reusable instruments and equipment used in patient care should be appropriately cleaned, and then disinfected or sterilized. All practices related to cleaning and reprocessing of equipment should be rigorously monitored [44]. Equipment and devices that enter the bloodstream or body cavities should be sterilized [90]. Equipment and devices that touch intact mucous membranes but do not penetrate the body should at least undergo high-level disinfection or be sterilized if possible. Equipment and devices that only touch intact skin should be cleaned with a detergent or as indicated by the manufacturer [13].

Once outside the human body, HIV is sensitive to heat and light, and is easily killed by many hospital-grade and some "household" disinfectants [13, 50, 91–94]. Germicides that are effective against HIV on precleaned, environmental surfaces usually have Environmental Protection Agency labels that include directions for use [91]. Hospital-grade chemical disinfectants that have been shown to deactivate HIV include quaternary ammonium chloride, 0.3% hydrogen peroxide, 50% ethanol, 35% isopropanol, paraformaldehyde, phenolic sodium hypochlorite, and 50 ppm sodium hypochlorite, which is equivalent to household bleach diluted 1:100 with water [24, 92–94]. Spills of blood or body fluids should be cleaned immediately. The HCW should wear heavy-duty rubber gloves, wipe up the spill with absorbent material, and wash the area with a hospital-grade disinfectant. Disposable cleaning material that is grossly soiled with blood should be discarded as hazardous infectious waste [13, 25, 44, 51]. Operators of machines such as a centrifuge used in specimen preparation must be trained to clean the equipment thoroughly and safely should breakage or accidental contamination with blood or body fluids occur.

Detergent and hot-water washing (160 °F) of dishes and laundry is adequate decontamination for HIV [20, 40]. Laundry that is soiled with blood or body fluids should be transported in leak-proof bags and handled as little as possible. It should be washed for 25 minutes with detergent and hot water (160°F). If a low-temperature water cycle is used, detergents that are suitable for this type of washing should be employed [13].

Protection of Ancillary Staff

Specimen Preparation

All fluid and tissue specimens should be considered potentially infectious. Specimens should be placed in a tightly closed container, which in turn is sealed within a leak-proof transport bag labeled with an easily recognizable biohazard warning [21, 44]. Requisition forms attached to the outside of the bag need not contain any reference to the patient's HIV status, since universal precautions or body substance isolation procedures should be used by all laboratory personnel.

Hazardous/Infectious Waste Disposal

All needles and sharps should be placed in a puncture-resistant container immediately after use, and containers handled in accordance with federal, state, and local regulations. Material that is grossly contaminated with blood must be discarded in bags or containers colored or marked according to applicable health authority regulations. Some local regulators allow the disposal of bulk blood and blood products directly into the municipal sewerage system [20]. However, in most laboratory areas, any fluid that could contain HIV or hepatitis B virus (HBV) may be poured into the sanitary sewer system only after a disinfectant is added [51]. Gloves should be worn, as well as protective eyewear and a mask, if splashing is anticipated.

While there has been a great deal of public concern over the environmental impact of medical waste, there is no evidence to suggest that it is any more infectious than community waste. Viruses such as HIV require living cells for survival and are not likely to endure long enough to become a significant environmental health problem [50, 95].

Management of Accidental Exposures

Occupational exposure to HIV through accidental needlesticks is common and often unreported by HCW [96]. Every institution should have a protocol that clearly defines the procedure to be followed in the event that HCW are exposed to blood or bloody body fluid [44]. The protocol should be easily accessible to HCW and consistent in application. Routine care, including thorough washing and clinical evaluation of injury, should be performed immediately after a percutaneous or mucous membrane exposure. The HCW supervisor and employee health service should be informed, and the institution's protocol for potential HIV/HBV exposure followed [25, 29, 44, 97, 98]. The source patient should be assessed to determine the likelihood of HIV/HBV infections. If there is no record of recent negative serologies, the patient should be tested for HBV and asked to consent to HIV antibody testing. If the source patient is HIV negative, follow-up evaluation may be unnecessary [98–101]. If the source patient cannot be identified, refuses testing, or is HIV infected, further evaluation of the exposed health care worker should begin immediately. A baseline HIV antibody test should be performed as soon as possible, with follow-up at 6 weeks, 3 months, and 6 months if negative [6, 8, 13, 27]. While the risk of seroconversion for exposed HCW is very low, the CDC suggests that Public Health Service recommendations for reducing HIV transmission, such as practicing safe sex and refraining from blood or organ donation, be followed during this period [27, 102, 103].

Reporting of potentially significant exposures should be encouraged [70]. Information must be confidential and not used in a punitive manner. Epidemiologic data about such injuries are few [8, 45, 46, 98]. Within an individual institution, such information could be used to assure that the "blood and body fluid exposure" protocol is being implemented consistently, while providing an opportunity to change unsafe practices. On a national level, better information might permit more rational design and implementation of prevention programs.

Many health care institutions now offer antiretroviral chemoprophylaxis with zidovudine (ZDV) to HCW who have potentially been exposed to HIV. There are no compelling data to support or discourage the use of ZDV for preventive purposes [27, 98]. In a CDC surveillance study of occupational exposure to HIV infection, the use of postexposure ZDV increased from 5 percent in 1988 to 43 percent in 1992 [99]. During this period, one health care worker who received ZDV prophylaxis seroconverted, making eight such cases reported to date. Seventy-five percent of HCW taking ZDV described adverse drug reactions, including nausea, myalgias, and headache. In general, the ZDV dose administered is 200 mg orally every 4 hours for 6 weeks; recipients must be monitored for hematologic toxicity. Health care workers who have suffered a significant parenteral or mucous membrane exposure should carefully weigh the potential risks and benefits of postexposure chemoprophylaxis [27, 33, 98, 99, 104–107].

Opportunistic Infections that Require Additional Precautionary Measures

Varicella-Zoster Virus

Persons who are susceptible to varicella-zoster virus may contract chickenpox by direct, unprotected contact with a zoster patient. Health care workers who provide direct care to patients with zoster should wear gloves. Because zoster may disseminate more readily in the immunocompromised host, HIV-infected patients should be isolated in a private negative-pressure room with external venting for the duration of their illness. Nonimmune HCW should avoid entering the room.

Mycobacterium tuberculosis

Although the annual incidence of *M. tuberculosis* infection in the United States is 9 in 100,000, the rate among HIV-infected patients is much higher. Tuberculosis (TB) may occur in early HIV disease and differ in clinical presentation from TB in an immunocompetent host [108–113]. Clinicians must maintain a high index of suspicion for TB in all HIV-infected patients with pulmonary symptoms. Strict respiratory isolation precautions should be used for patients with suspected or confirmed pulmonary TB. Because of the increased prevalence of multidrug-resistant TB among AIDS patients, isolation precautions should be used until clinical and bacteriologic response to therapy is documented or until three successive sputum smears are negative for acid-fast organisms (AFB) [112–116]. Infectious patients should not be discharged to residential facilities, such as a nursing home, hospice, or correctional institution, unless appropriate AFB precautions can be implemented [113, 114, 117].

Techniques that reduce the number of air-borne droplet nuclei should be used. Examples include requesting that patients cover the nose and mouth when coughing or sneezing, and placing patients in a private room with the door closed. The room should have negative pressure and external venting with five to six air exchanges per hour. Some authorities recommend ultraviolet irradiation of the air in the upper part of the room. Persons entering the room should wear 1- to 5-µ filtration particulate respirators or filtered masks [44, 112, 114].

Sputum induction and aerosol pentamidine treatments that induce cough may facilitate transmission of TB [114, 118]. These procedures should be performed in a negative-pressure room or booth with external venting. Health care workers who provide direct care during or immediately after such treatments should wear filtration particulate respirators or filtered masks and use appropriate barrier precautions [109, 112–114, 118].

All HCW who have potential exposure to TB should participate in an organized screening program and have at least one purified protein derivative (PPD) skin test every year. Each institution should rigorously monitor compliance, and data should be analyzed to evaluate the effectiveness of infection control practices [112–114].

Other Diseases

AIDS-indicative diseases that do not require special infection control precautions include extrapulmonary TB, atypical mycobacterial infection, candidiasis, coccidioidomycosis, cryptosporidiosis, cryptococcosis, histoplasmosis, toxoplasmosis, Kaposi's sarcoma and other malignancies, and progressive multifocal leukoencephalopathy [119].

References

1. Brennan TA. Transmission of the human immunodeficiency virus in the health care setting: Time for action. *N Engl J Med* 324:1504–1509, 1991.
2. Hayward RA, Shapiro MF. A national study of AIDS and residency training: Experiences, concerns, and consequences. *Ann Intern Med* 114:23–32, 1991.
3. Granich R. Students' attitudes about AIDS (letter). *Ann Intern Med* 114:1066, 1991.
4. Singh V, Hamadeh R. AIDS and residency training (letter). *Ann Intern Med* 114:605–606, 1991.
5. Hoffman-Terry M, Rhodes LV, Reed JF. Impact of human immunodeficiency virus on medical and surgical residents. *Arch Intern Med* 152:1788–1796, 1992.
6. Marcus R, CDC Cooperative Needlestick Surveillance Group. Surveillance of health care workers exposed to blood from patients infected with human immunodeficiency virus. *N Engl J Med* 319:1118–1123, 1988.
7. Centers for Disease Control. *HIV/AIDS Surveillance Report* 5:19, 1994.
8. Bell DM. Human immunodeficiency virus transmission in health care settings: Risk and risk reduction. *Am J Med* 91 (suppl 3B):294S–300S, 1991.
9. Weiss SH, Saxinger WC, Rechtman D, et al. HTLV-III infection among health care workers: Association with needlestick injuries. *JAMA* 254:2089–2093, 1985.
10. McCray E, CDC Cooperative Needlestick Surveillance Group. Special report: Occupational risk of the acquired immunodeficiency syndrome among health care workers. *N Engl J Med* 314:1127–1132, 1986.
11. Gerberding JL, Bryant-LeBlanc CE, Nelson K, et al. Risk of transmitting the human immunodeficiency virus, cytomegalovirus, and hepatitis B virus to health care workers exposed to patients with AIDS and AIDS-related conditions. *J Infect Dis* 156:1–8, 1987.
12. Centers for Disease Control. Update: Human immunodeficiency virus infections in health care workers exposed to blood of infected patients. *MMWR* 36:285–289, 1987.
13. Centers for Disease Control. Recommendations for prevention of HIV transmission in health-care settings. *MMWR* 36 (suppl 2):3–18, 1987.
14. Centers for Disease Control. Update: Acquired immunodeficiency syndrome and human immunodeficiency virus infection among health care workers. *MMWR* 37:229–239, 1988.
15. Klein RS, Phelan JA, Freeman K, et al. Low occupational risk of human immunodeficiency virus infection among dental professionals. *N Engl J Med* 318:86–90, 1988.
16. Gerberding JL. Occupational health issues for providers of care to patients with HIV infection. *Infect Dis Clin North Am* 2:321–328, 1988.
17. Henderson DK, Fahey BJ, Willy M, et al. Risk for occupational transmis-

sion of human immunodeficiency virus type 1 (HIV-1) associated with clinical exposures: A prospective evaluation. *Ann Intern Med* 133:740–746, 1990.

18. Beekmann SE, Fahey BJ, Gerberding JL, Henderson DK. Risky business: Using necessarily imprecise casualty counts to estimate occupational risks for HIV-1 infection. *Infect Control Hosp Epidemiol* 11:371–379, 1990.

19. Ippolito G, Puro V, De Carli G, and the Italian Study Group on Occupational Risk of HIV Infection. The risk of occupational human immunodeficiency virus infection in health care workers. *Arch Intern Med* 153:1451–1458, 1993.

20. Centers for Disease Control. Recommendations for preventing transmission of infection with T-lymphotropic virus type III/lymphadenopathy-associated virus in the workplace. *MMWR* 34:682–686, 691–695, 1985.

21. Conte JE. Infection with human immunodeficiency virus in the hospital. *Ann Intern Med* 105:730–736, 1986.

22. Centers for Disease Control. Recommended infection-control practices for dentistry. *MMWR* 35:237–242, 1986.

23. Kuhls TL, Viker S, Parris NB, et al. Occupational risk of HIV, HBV, and HSV-2 infections in health care personnel caring for AIDS patients. *Am J Public Health* 77:1306–1309, 1987.

24. McCray E, Martone W. Infection Control Considerations in HIV Infection. In G Wormser, R Stahl, E Bottone (eds), *AIDS and Other Manifestations of HIV Infection*. Park Ridge, NJ: Noyes Publications, 1987. Pp 950–974.

25. Centers for Disease Control. Update: Universal precautions for prevention of transmission of human immunodeficiency virus, hepatitis B virus, and other bloodborne pathogens in health-care settings. *MMWR* 37:377–388, 1988.

26. Centers for Disease Control. Guidelines for prevention of transmission of human immunodeficiency virus and hepatitis B virus to health-care workers and public safety workers. *MMWR* 38 (suppl 6):1–37, 1989.

27. Centers for Disease Control. US Public Health Service statement on management of occupational exposure to human immunodeficiency virus (HIV), including considerations regarding zidovudine post-exposure use. *MMWR* 39(RR-1):1–14, 1990.

28. Centers for Disease Control. Recommendations for preventing transmission of human immunodeficiency virus and hepatitis B virus to patients during exposure-prone invasive procedures. *MMWR* 40(RR8):1–9, 1991.

29. Sullivan MT, Williams AE, Fang CT, et al. Transmission of human T-lymphotropic virus types I and II by blood transfusion: A retrospective study of recipients of blood components (1983 through 1988). *Arch Intern Med* 151:2043–2048, 1991.

30. Gaughwin MD, Gowans E, Ali R, Burrell C. Bloody needles: The volumes of blood transferred in simulations of needlestick injuries and shared use of syringes for injection of intravenous drugs. *AIDS* 5:1025–1027, 1991.

31. Colebunders R, Ryder R, Francis H, et al. Seroconversion rate, mortality, and clinical manifestations associated with the receipt of a human immunodeficiency virus-infected blood transfusion in Kinshasa, Zaire. *J Infect Dis* 164:450–456, 1991.

32. Hagan MD, Meyer KB, Kopelman RI, Pauker SG. Human immunodeficiency virus infection in health care workers: A method for estimating individual occupational risk. *Arch Intern Med* 149:1541–1544, 1989.

33. Henderson DK, Gerberding JL. Prophylactic zidovudine after occupational exposure to the human immunodeficiency virus: An interim analysis. *J Infect Dis* 160:321–327, 1989.

34. Clark SJ, Kelen GD, Henrard DR, et al. Unsuspected primary human immunodeficiency virus type 1 infection in seronegative emergency department patients. *J Infect Dis* 170:194–197, 1994.

35. Nelsing S, Nielsen TL, Nielsen JO. Occupational exposure to human immunodeficiency virus among health care workers in a Danish hospital (letter). *J Infect Dis* 169:478, 1994.

36. Chamberland ME, Petersen LR, Munn VP, et al. Human immunodeficiency virus infection among health care workers who donate blood. *Ann Intern Med* 121:269–273, 1994.

37. Palmer DL, Hjelle BL, Wiley CA, et al. HIV-1 infection despite immediate combination antiviral therapy after infusion of contaminated white cells. *Am J Med* 97:289–295, 1994.

38. Adegboye AA, Moss GB, Soyinka F, Kreiss JK. The epidemiology of needlestick and sharp instrument accidents in a Nigerian hospital. *Infect Control Hosp Epidemiol* 15:27–31, 1994.

39. Marcus R, Culver DH, Bell DM, et al. Risk of human immunodeficiency virus infection among emergency department workers. *Am J Med* 94:363–370, 1993.

40. *Guidelines for Handwashing and Hospital Environmental Control, 1985.* Hospital Infections Program, Centers for Disease Control, US Government Printing Office.

41. Infection control measures for all patients. *AIDS Policy and the Law.* July 15, 1987:3.

42. Special report and product review: Needlestick prevention devices. *Health Devices* 20:154–167, 1991.

43. Klein RS. Universal precautions for preventing occupational exposures to human immunodeficiency virus type 1 (editorial). *Am J Med* 80:141–144, 1991.

44. Department of Labor. Occupational Safety and Health Administration. 29 CFR Part 1910.1030. Occupational exposure to bloodborne pathogens. *Federal Register* 56:64004–64182, December 6, 1991.

45. McCormick RD, Meisch MG, Ircink FG, Maki DG. Epidemiology of hospital sharps injuries: A 14-year prospective study in the pre-AIDS and AIDS eras. *Am J Med* 91 (suppl 3B):301S–307S, 1991.

46. Panlilio AL, Foy DR, Edwards JR, et al. Blood contacts during surgical procedures. *JAMA* 265:1533–1537, 1991.

47. Wong ES, Stotka JL, Chinchilli VM, et al. Are universal precautions effective in reducing the number of occupational exposures among health care workers? A prospective study of physicians on a medical service. *JAMA* 265:1123–1128, 1991.

48. US Department of Labor. OSHA Instruction CPL 2-2.44B, February 1990.

49. AAOS Task Force on AIDS and Orthopedic Surgery. *Recommendations for the Prevention of Human Immunodeficiency Virus (HIV) Transmission in the*

Practice of Orthopedic Surgery. Park Ridge, IL: American Academy of Orthopedic Surgeons, 1989.

50. Becker CE, Cone JE, Gerberding J. Occupational infection with human immunodeficiency virus (HIV): Risks and risk reduction. *Ann Intern Med* 110:653–656, 1989.

51. Agent summary statement for human immunodeficiency viruses (HIVs) including HTLV-III, LAV, HIV-1, and HIV-2. *MMWR* 37 (suppl 4):1–17, 1988.

52. Jagger J, Hunt EH, Brand-Elnaggar J, Pearson RD. Rates of needle-stick injury caused by various devices in a university hospital. *N Engl J Med* 319:284–288, 1988.

53. Lynch P, Jackson MM, Cummings MJ, Stamm WE. Rethinking the role of isolation practices in the prevention of nosocomial infections. *Ann Intern Med* 107:243–246, 1987.

54. Makofsky D, Cone JE. Installing needle disposal boxes closer to the bedside reduces needle-recapping rates in hospital units. *Infect Control Hosp Epidemiol* 14:140–144, 1993.

55. Mast ST, Woolwine JD, Gerberding JL. Efficacy of gloves in reducing blood volumes transferred during simulated needlestick injury. *J Infect Dis* 168:1589–1592, 1993.

56. Owens-Schwab E, Fraser VJ. Needleless and needle protection devices: A second look at efficacy and selection. *Infect Control Hosp Epidemiol* 14:657–660, 1993.

57. Centers for Disease Control. Recommended infection-control practices for dentistry, 1993. *MMWR* 42 (RR-8):1–12, 1993.

58. Hersey JC, Martin LS. Use of infection control guidelines by workers in healthcare facilities to prevent occupational transmission of HBV and HIV: Results from a national survey. *Infect Control Hosp Epidemiol* 15:243–252, 1994.

59. Beekmann SE, Vlahov D, Koziol DE, et al. Temporal association between implementation of universal precautions and a sustained, progressive decrease in percutaneous exposure to blood. *Clin Infect Dis* 18:562–569, 1994.

60. Erice A, Rhame FS, Heussner RC, et al. Human immunodeficiency virus infection in patients with solid-organ transplants: Report of five cases and review. *Rev Infect Dis* 13:537–547, 1991.

61. Willy ME, Dhillon GL, Loewen NL, et al. Adverse exposures and universal precautions practices among a group of highly exposed health professionals. *Infect Control Hosp Epidemiol* 11:351–356, 1990.

62. Becker MH, Janz NK, Band J, et al. Noncompliance with universal precautions policy: Why do physicians and nurses recap needles? *Am J Infect Control* 18:232–239, 1990.

63. Kelen GD, DiGiovanna TA, Celentano DD, et al. Adherence to universal (barrier) precautions during interventions on critically ill and injured emergency department patients. *J Acquir Immune Defic Syndr* 3:987–994, 1990.

64. Doebbeling BN, Wentzel RP. The direct costs of universal precautions in a teaching hospital. *JAMA* 264:2083–2087, 1990.

65. Gerberding JL, Littell C, Tarkington A, et al. Risk of exposure of surgical

personnel to patients' blood during surgery at San Francisco General Hospital. *N Engl J Med* 322:1788–1793, 1990.

66. Kelen GD, Green GB, Hexter DA, et al. Substantial improvement in compliance with universal precautions in an emergency department following institution of policy. *Arch Intern Med* 151:2051–2056, 1991.
67. Popejoy SL, Fry DE. Blood contact and exposure in the operating room. *Surg Gynecol Obstet* 172:480–483, 1991.
68. Gerberding JL, Schecter WP. Surgery and AIDS: Reducing the risk (editorial). *JAMA* 265:1572–1573, 1991.
69. Samuels ME, Koop CE. Hartsock PI. Single use syringes (letter). *N Engl J Med* 324:996–997, 1991.
70. Mangione CM, Gerberding JL, Cummings SR. Occupational exposure to HIV: Frequency and rates of underreporting of percutaneous and mucocutaneous exposures by medical housestaff. *Am J Med* 90:85–90, 1991.
71. Gerberding JL. Does knowledge of human immunodeficiency virus infection decrease the frequency of occupational exposure to blood? *Am J Med* 91 (suppl 3B):308S–311S, 1991.
72. Fahey BJ, Koziol DE, Banks SM, Henderson DK. Frequency of nonparenteral occupational exposures to blood and body fluids before and after universal precautions training. *Am J Med* 90:145–153, 1991.
73. Centers for Disease Control. Possible transmission of human immunodeficiency virus to a patient during an invasive dental procedure. *MMWR* 39:489–493, 1990.
74. Centers for Disease Control. Update: Transmission of HIV infection during an invasive dental procedure—Florida. *MMWR* 40:21–33, 1991.
75. Ciesielski C, et al. Transmission of human immunodeficiency virus in a dental practice. *Ann Intern Med* 116:798–805, 1992.
76. Rogers AS, et al. Investigation of potential HIV transmission to the patients of an HIV-infected surgeon. *JAMA* 269:1795–1801, 1993.
77. Dickinson CM, et al. Absence of HIV transmission from an infected dentist to his patients. *JAMA* 269:1802–1806, 1993.
78. von Reyn CF, et al. Absence of HIV transmission from an infected orthopedic surgeon. *JAMA* 269:1807–1811, 1993.
79. Mishu B, Schaffner W. HIV transmission from surgeons and dentists to patients: Can models predict the risk? *Infect Control Hosp Epidemiol* 15:144–146, 1994.
80. Schulman KA, McDonald RC, Lynn LA, et al. Screening surgeons for HIV infection: Assessment of a potential public health program. *Infect Control Hosp Epidemiol* 15:147–155, 1994.
81. Longfield JN, Brundage J, Badger G, et al. Look-back investigation after human immunodeficiency virus seroconversion in a pediatric dentist. *J Infect Dis* 169:1–8, 1994.
82. New York Academy of Medicine. The risk of contracting HIV infection in the course of health care. *JAMA* 265:1872–1873, 1991.
83. Danila RN, MacDonald KL, Rhame FS, et al. A look-back investigation of patients of an HIV-infected physician. *N Engl J Med* 325:1406–1411, 1991.
84. Gostin L. The HIV-infected health care professional. Public policy, discrimination, and patient safety. *Arch Intern Med* 151:663–665, 1991.

85. Lowenfels AB, Wormser G. Risk of transmission of HIV from surgeon to patient (letter). *N Engl J Med* 325:888–889, 1991.
86. Cowen DN, Brundage JF, Pomerantz RS, et al. HIV infection among members of the US Army Reserve components with medical and health occupations. *JAMA* 265:2826–2830, 1991.
87. Henderson DK. HIV screening for healthcare providers: Can we provide sense and sensibility without pride or prejudice? *Infect Control Hosp Epidemiol* 15:631–634, 1994.
88. Sell RL, Jovell AJ, Siegel JE. HIV screening of surgeons and dentists: A cost-effectiveness analysis. *Infect Control Hosp Epidemiol* 15:635–645, 1994.
89. Phillips KA, Lowe RA, Kahn JG, et al. The cost-effectiveness of HIV testing of physicians and dentists in the United States. *JAMA* 271:851–858, 1994.
90. Marcus R, Favero MS, Banerjee S, et al. Prevalence and incidence of human immunodeficiency virus among patients undergoing long-term hemodialysis. *Am J Med* 90:614–619, 1991.
91. Environmental Protection Agency. Clarification of HIV (AIDS virus) labeling policy for antimicrobial pesticide products. *Federal Register* 54:6288–6290, 1989.
92. Resnick L, Veren K, Salahuddin SZ, et al. Stability and inactivation of HTLV-III/LAV under clinical and laboratory environments. *JAMA* 255:1887–1891, 1986.
93. Sattar SA, Springthorpe VS. Survival and disinfectant inactivation of the human immunodeficiency virus: A critical review. *Rev Infect Dis* 13:430–447, 1991.
94. Rutala WA. APIC guideline for selection and use of disinfectants. *Am J Infect Control* 18:99–117, 1990.
95. Keene JH. Medical waste: A minimum hazard. *Infect Control Hosp Epidemiol* 12:682–685, 1991.
96. O'Neill TM, et al. Risk of needlesticks and occupational exposures among residents and medical students. *Arch Intern Med* 152:1451–1456, 1992.
97. Centers for Disease Control. Hepatitis B virus: A comprehensive strategy for eliminating transmission through universal childhood vaccination: Recommendations of the Immunization Practices Advisory Committee (ACIP). *MMWR* 40(RR-13):1–25, 1991.
98. Fahey BJ, Beekmann SE, Schmitt JM, et al. Managing occupational exposures to HIV-1 in the healthcare workplace. *Infect Control Hosp Epidemiol* 14:405–412, 1993.
99. Tokars JI, et al. Surveillance of HIV infection and zidovudine use among health care workers after occupational exposure to HIV-infected blood. *Ann Intern Med* 118:913–919, 1993.
100. Imagawa DT, Lee MH, Wolonsky SM, et al. Human immunodeficiency virus type 1 infection in homosexual men who remain seronegative for prolonged periods. *N Engl J Med* 320:1458–1462, 1989.
101. Manian FA, Meyer L, Jenne J. Puncture injuries due to needles removed from intravenous lines: Should the source patient routinely be tested for bloodborne infections? *Infect Control Hosp Epidemiol* 14:325–330, 1993.
102. Centers for Disease Control. Additional recommendations to reduce sexual

and drug abuse-related transmission of human T-lymphotropic virus type III/lymphadenopathy-associated virus. *MMWR* 35:152–155, 1986.

103. Centers for Disease Control. Provisional public health service interagency recommendations for screening donated blood and plasma for antibody to the virus causing acquired immunodeficiency syndrome. *MMWR* 34:1–5, 1985.

104. Allen UD, Guerriere M, Read SE, Detsky AS. Percutaneous injuries among health care workers: The real value of human immunodeficiency virus testing of "donor" blood. *Arch Intern Med* 151:2033–2040, 1991.

105. White AC, Miller SM. HIV infection after needlesticks (letter). *Ann Intern Med* 114:253, 1991.

106. Durand E, LeJeunne C, Hugues FC. Failure of prophylactic zidovudine after suicidal self-inoculation of HIV-infected blood (letter). *N Engl J Med* 324:1062, 1991.

107. Henderson DK. Postexposure chemoprophylaxis for occupational exposure to human immunodeficiency virus type 1: Current status and prospects for the future. *Am J Med* 91 (suppl 3B):312S–319S, 1991.

108. DesPrez RM, Heim CR. *Mycobacterium tuberculosis.* In GL Mandell, RG Douglas, JE Bennett (eds), *Principles and Practice of Infectious Diseases* (3rd ed). New York: Churchill Livingstone, 1990. Pp 1879–1880.

109. Centers for Disease Control. Tuberculosis and human immunodeficiency virus infection: Recommendations of the Advisory Committee for the Elimination of Tuberculosis (ACET). *MMWR* 38:236–238, 243–250, 1989.

110. Centers for Disease Control. Tuberculosis and acquired immunodeficiency syndrome—New York City. *MMWR* 36:785–790, 795, 1987.

111. US Dept. of Health and Human Services. *Core Curriculum on Tuberculosis* (2nd ed). Document 00-t 5763, April 1991. P 11.

112. Centers for Disease Control. Guidelines for preventing the transmission of tuberculosis in health-care settings, with special focus on HIV-related issues. *MMWR* 39(RR-17):1–29, 1990.

113. Centers for Disease Control. Nosocomial transmission of multidrug-resistant tuberculosis to health-care workers and HIV-infected patients in an urban hospital—Florida. *MMWR* 39:718–722, 1990.

114. Department of Health and Human Services, Centers for Disease Control. Draft guidelines for preventing the transmission of tuberculosis in health care facilities (2nd ed); notice of comment period. *Federal Register* 58:52810–52854, 1993.

115. Coronado VG, Beck-Sague CM, Hutton MD, et al. Transmission of multidrug-resistant *Mycobacterium tuberculosis* among persons with human immunodeficiency virus infection in an urban hospital: Epidemiologic and restriction fragment length polymorphism analysis. *J Infect Dis* 168:1052–1055, 1993.

116. Weltman AC, Rose DN. Tuberculosis susceptibility patterns, predictors of multidrug resistance, and implications for initial therapeutic regimens at a New York City hospital. *Arch Intern Med* 154:2161–2167, 1994.

117. Valway SE, Greifinger RB, Papania M, et al. Multidrug-resistant tuberculosis in the New York state prison system, 1990–1991. *J Infect Dis* 170:151–156, 1994.

118. Centers for Disease Control. *Mycobacterium tuberculosis* transmission in a health clinic—Florida, 1988. *MMWR* 38:256–264, 1989.
119. Centers for Disease Control. *CDC Guidelines for Isolation Precautions in Hospitals.* US Dept of Health and Human Services, 1986.

The Homosexual or Bisexual Patient

37

Jon D. Fuller

Background

Since 1973, when the American Psychiatric Association removed homosexuality as a disorder from its *Diagnostic and Statistical Manual*, attention has focused on better understanding long-term, stable relationships among gay men and women, and clinicians have become more familiar with promoting healthy lifestyles for homosexuals [1–5]. Before the AIDS epidemic, the training of health care workers in the treatment of gay and bisexual patients frequently emphasized those medical conditions to which these persons, especially gay men, were more prone than the general public.

When the gay community was first affected by AIDS in the early 1980s, other issues became prominent as well, including the observation that certain clinical manifestations, such as Kaposi's sarcoma (KS), salmonellosis, and anal squamous cell carcinoma, occurred more frequently in gay men. The AIDS epidemic has also had an impact on gay and bisexual women, with HIV infection transmitted through injection drug use, sexual contact with men, and, rarely, sexual contact between women. Some of the unique challenges in providing health care to these persons include incorporating a homosexual patient's partner into the medical decision-making process; recognizing the psychological effect of persistent, heavy losses on the gay community; and anticipating the need for a substitute decision maker by identifying a health care proxy.

HIV/AIDS and the Gay and Bisexual Male Population

Epidemiology

The majority of AIDS cases in the United States has been reported in men who have sex with men. Through June 1994, cumulative AIDS cases included 211,779 gay and bisexual men and 25,447 gay and bisexual male injection drug users (IDUs). These represent, respectively, 53 and 6 percent of the total cases reported in adults and adolescents [6]. However, if one analyzes annual epidemiologic trends, the proportion contributed by men who have sex with men has been gradually declining over time. For example, from May 1984 through April 1985, gay and bisexual men represented 74 percent of all adult cases; during a similar period 9 years later, they accounted for only 45 percent [6, 7].

This decreased proportion of AIDS cases attributed to gay/bisexual men has been interpreted by some authorities as indicating that educational efforts emphasizing safer sexual practices have been effective. Behavioral changes documented in this population include a decreased number of sexual partners, decreased frequency of sexual intercourse involving the exchange of body fluids, decreased frequency of anal intercourse, and increased condom usage [8–15].

The decline in percentage of cases attributable to gay and bisexual men is also, in part, secondary to an increased number of cases in other behavioral categories. For example, the number of annual reported AIDS cases in men who have sex with men increased by 900 percent between 1984–85 and 1993–94, from 4,199 to 37,991 [6, 7]. Thus, while gay and bisexual men constitute a decreasing proportion of the total HIV-infected population in the United States, they continue to represent a large total number of cases, estimated in 1990 to be 630,000 [16].

Prevention

Despite the adoption of safer sex practices by many members of the gay male community, recent studies also indicate that a significant percentage are still engaging in high-risk sexual activity [17]. Among men aged 25 years or older, maintenance of safer sexual behaviors may be more difficult than initiation, and relapse to high-risk activities, such as unprotected anal intercourse, has been observed in 16 to 50 percent of sampled populations [13, 18–21]. Relapse has been associated with less consistency in maintaining safer sex practices, a perceived sense of invulnerability, and survivor guilt. In the San Francisco gay community, persons participating in focus groups have also described failure to maintain safer sex practices being related to the difficulty in imagining a future devoid of their closest friends [22]. In addition, some individuals may feel a certain attraction to becoming part of the HIV-infected community, which is perceived by some as receiving preferential social treatment.

Young Gay Men

In contrast to the changes in sexual behavior demonstrated among members of the gay population who are 25 years and older, younger men, especially members of minority communities, appear to be especially vulnerable to acquisition of HIV through unsafe sexual practices and have higher rates of sexually transmitted diseases (STDs) in general [10, 13, 23–26]. Studies of gay men aged 13 to 25 conducted between 1989 and 1991 demonstrated that 34 to 43 percent had engaged in unprotected anal intercourse during the previous year, a practice associated with the highest risk of HIV transmission for both insertive and receptive partners [27–31]. A blinded survey of more than 2,500 blood specimens collected over a 2-year period from an adolescent crisis center in New York City revealed an HIV seroprevalence rate of 5.3 percent, ranging from 1.3 percent for 15-year-olds to 8.6 percent for 20-year-olds [32]. Of the men who were HIV-infected, 27 of 59 (45%) were gay or bisexual and had no history of drug use. A summary of blinded serologic surveys from 38 metropolitan areas in 1988 and 1989 showed that, among 20- to 24-year-old gay or bisexual male STD clinic patients, HIV seroprevalence rates ranged from 9.7 to 55.6 percent, compared to 0.48 percent for heterosexual men of the same age group [33].

A number of factors have been identified that appear to contribute to the susceptibility of young gay men to HIV infection [34, 35]:

1. This population, like most youth, lives with a sense of invulnerability. Despite the recognition that they engage in high-risk activity and know individuals who are suffering the effects of HIV infection, the notion that "it can't happen to me" may contribute to unsafe behavior.
2. Most gay men diagnosed with AIDS are in their thirties or older. Unfortunately, this has led some persons to believe that sex with other young men is unlikely to expose them to HIV.
3. Gay and bisexual adolescents discovering their sexual identity are at increased risk for a variety of problems. These include social isolation and internalized homophobia, strong negative attitudes by family and friends, sexual abuse, verbal and physical abuse, school and institutional harassment, employment discrimination, homelessness, prostitution, STDs, substance abuse, compromised mental health, and difficulties with the law [4, 5, 35–37]. Gay and lesbian adolescents are two to three times more likely to attempt suicide than their peers and have been estimated to account for up to 30 percent of all successful suicides in this age group [38]. Some young gays may resort to high-risk, anonymous sexual encounters in their search for affirmation and affection [28].

In order for young homosexual men to benefit from directed educational efforts, they must consciously perceive themselves as members of the gay community. However, this identification is frequently discouraged by family, church, and society, and individuals may not become fully conscious of their homosexual orientation until after a period of high-risk experimentation. For these reasons, clinicians who work with adolescents should sensitively inquire about their developing sexual identity and provide a safe context in which they can ask questions and receive information in a nonjudgmental manner [39, 40]. In addition, patients should be assisted in developing the self-confidence, communication, and negotiation skills necessary to decline unwanted sexual advances. They should also be reminded of the increased frequency of high-risk sexual activity associated with alcohol or drug use [27, 41, 42].

HIV-Seronegative Persons
Clinicians who work with seronegative gay and bisexual patients should concentrate their prevention efforts on safer sexual practices and on the prevention of relapse in those who have already modified their behavior. In addition, since 2 to 52 percent of HIV-infected persons engage in unprotected intercourse without informing sexual partners of their serostatus, all persons should be reminded of the need to be personally responsible for protecting themselves when engaging in any sexual activity [43, 44].

HIV-Seropositive Persons
Health care providers should discuss safer sex practices with their HIV-seropositive patients on a regular basis in order to decrease the likelihood of HIV transmission to seronegative sexual partners. HIV-infected patients should also be encouraged to use barrier methods during sex with other seropositive persons. This approach is intended to prevent acquisition of other sexually transmitted agents that could affect HIV disease progression and to guard against being coinfected with other HIV strains [45–48].

Clinical Care

General Considerations
Knowing that a male patient is homosexual or bisexual is important in considering certain clinical issues. This has been particularly well appreciated for STDs. For example, since approximately 20 percent of pharyngeal or rectal gonococcal infections among homosexual men may be asymptomatic, regular cultures of the throat, urethra, and rectum have been suggested as part of the health care maintenance of sexually active gay and bisexual men [49, 50].

In order to take an adequate medical history and evaluate a patient's risk for specific medical conditions, clinicians need to be comfortable with inquiring in a nonjudgmental manner about sexual orientation and activities, including the use of toys or instruments and exposure to urine or feces. Oral-anal intercourse may lead to infection with bacterial pathogens, parasites, chlamydia, hepatitis A virus, or herpes simplex virus. Oral-penile exposure may result in gonococcal pharyngitis, and rectal intercourse predisposes to gonococcal, chlamydial, and herpetic proctitis, as well as condyloma acuminatum (human papillomavirus infection). Exposure to blood or semen may result in hepatitis B, cytomegalovirus (CMV), human T-lymphotropic virus, type 1 (HTLV-1), hepatitis C virus [51–53], or HIV infections [54–56]. Noninfectious complications of anal intercourse include prolapsed hemorrhoids, nonspecific proctitis, anorectal fissures and fistulas, and foreign bodies [57].

Identifying the means by which a patient has become infected with HIV can help focus educational efforts to reduce the risk of viral transmission to others. In addition, because some HIV-related conditions occur with increased frequency among homosexual and bisexual men, knowledge of an individual's sexual orientation should prompt the clinician to be especially alert for KS, salmonellosis, and anal carcinoma.

Kaposi's Sarcoma

In the early years of the HIV epidemic, KS was reported as the initial AIDS-defining diagnosis in 30 to 40 percent of homosexual and bisexual men, in only 3 to 4 percent of heterosexual men, and very rarely in hemophiliacs; greater than 90 percent of all epidemic KS occurs among gay men [58–61]. Although the reason for this epidemiologic disparity is not known, at least three explanations have been offered. First, CMV may serve as a cofactor in the development of KS following HIV infection. Supporting this hypothesis is the finding of CMV DNA in some KS tumor specimens and the observation of a high incidence of CMV infection (> 90%) among homosexual men [62–65]. Secondly, amyl nitrate inhalants ("poppers"), which are used by some homosexual men to produce a "rush" and relaxation of the anal sphincter, may also predispose to the development of KS [66–69]. Since education in the gay community has stressed avoidance of the exchange of body fluids and counseled against the use of poppers, the incidence of KS as a presenting AIDS diagnosis has decreased to approximately 10 percent [70–72]. The third suggestion, that a sexually transmitted agent may be a cofactor in the development of KS, derives from the observation that KS has occasionally been reported from HIV-seronegative homosexual men, but virtually never from seropositive recipients of infected blood products. Additionally, most women and children who have been diagnosed with AIDS-related KS come from well-delineated geographic areas or, in the case of women with KS, have had sexual contact with bisexual men [73]. Taken together, these data imply that a virus that is sexually transmitted but not spread through blood products may be necessary or even sufficient in itself to lead to the development of KS [74]. Recent identification of herpesvirus-like DNA from KS tissue in people with and without AIDS further supports this hypothesis [74a].

Salmonella Infection

Individuals who have had oral-anal contact with a *Salmonella* carrier are at risk for acquiring salmonellosis [75–77]. Salmonellosis may cause bacteremia with or without gastrointestinal symptoms.

Anal Carcinoma

Aggressive squamous cell carcinoma of the anus has been reported among HIV-infected individuals who have had prior exposure to human papillomavirus [78–81]. Persons at risk for this tumor include men and women with a history of receptive anal intercourse, as well as those diagnosed with condyloma acuminatum.

HIV/AIDS and the Female Gay and Bisexual Population

Increased attention has been focused on lesbians and bisexual women in recent years regarding their risk of HIV infection.

Epidemiology

It is difficult to ascertain precisely how many gay and bisexual women have been diagnosed with AIDS, since the Centers for Disease Control (CDC) does not routinely provide data about women who have sex with women. In the largest published subset study of AIDS cases in lesbians, the CDC analyzed surveillance data for all women diagnosed with AIDS between 1980 and 1989. Of 9,717 persons interviewed, 8,475 responded to two questions inquiring whether they had ever had sexual relations with a male partner or with a female partner after the year 1977 and before being diagnosed with AIDS. The percentage of women with AIDS who had sexual relations exclusively with female partners was reported to be quite low (79 cases, or 0.8%), as was the proportion of bisexual women (103 cases, or 1%) [73]. Among those with exclusively female partners, 95 percent were IDUs and 5 percent had received HIV-infected blood products; among bisexuals, 79 percent were IDUs, 16 percent had male sex partners at risk for HIV or known to be HIV-infected, and 4 percent had received infected blood products.

HIV seroprevalence estimates for gay and bisexual women have been presented in a number of different series. In one review of 960,000 female blood donors, 144 were found to be HIV-positive [82]. Of 106 seropositive individuals who could be interviewed, none reported sex exclusively with women, whereas three (2.8%) reported sexual contact with women, as well as with men who were bisexual or IDUs. The CDC has published data collected during HIV antibody testing of women at 47 sentinel STD clinics and women's health centers in 24 US metropolitan areas between 1989 and 1991 [83]. Among 15,685 sexually active women who were interviewed and tested, 511 (3.3%) reported having had sex with women since 1978; 41 of the 511 (8%) described relationships exclusively with women. There were no cases of HIV infection in gay women, whereas 13 of 470 (2.8%) of bisexual women were HIV-seropositive.

The San Francisco Department of Public Health found that among 498 lesbians and bisexual women 17 years of age and older who were randomly surveyed during 1993, 0.9 percent of lesbians and 2.8 percent of bisexual women were infected with HIV [84]. These rates were three to eight times higher than the prevalence estimated at 0.35 percent for all adult or adolescent women in San Francisco. In New Jersey, among 115 women interviewed and tested for HIV infection in two high-prevalence cities, 57.4 percent were seropositive [85]. The seroprevalence rate was considerably higher among the lesbian/bisexual group (17 of 19, or 89%) than in the exclusively heterosexual group (49 of 96, or 51%), with injection drugs having been used by 84 percent of the former as compared with 35.4 percent of the latter.

These data suggest that a relatively small number of AIDS cases reported in women have occurred among lesbians and bisexuals. However, HIV seroprevalence rates in lesbian and bisexual women, at least in some areas, appear higher than expected for heterosexual women. The increased incidence of injection drug use in this population may account for a large proportion of these cases, but, even in women who self-identify as lesbians, sexual contact with men is not infrequent [86–89]. Through June 1990, among women diagnosed with AIDS who had heterosexually acquired HIV infection, 11 percent reported that sex with a bisexual man was their only risk behavior [90, 91].

Woman-to-Woman Sexual Transmission of HIV

Although the epidemiologic studies described above suggest that HIV infection among women who have sex with women can largely be attributed to injection drug use or heterosexual contact, this has been interpreted as implying that there is no risk of HIV transmission during woman-to-woman sexual contact [82, 83]. A prospective evaluation of the seronegative partners of 18 HIV-discordant female couples, among whom no seroconversions were demonstrated over a 6-month observation period, supports such a position [92]. However, HIV has been isolated from cervical secretions and endocervical swabs, and HIV transmission during woman-to-woman sexual activity has been implicated in several anecdotal reports [93–100]. In all cases, oral-genital contact had occurred between partners, and one case also included the sharing of insertive instruments.

Prevention

Women who have sex with women should be informed of the possibility of HIV transmission during sex, and methods should be encouraged to decrease the risk of viral acquisition. These include avoiding contact with blood and cervical secretions by using barrier methods such as dental dams, condoms, or gloves during oral or digital genital contact [101]. In addition, educational efforts should also be directed to minimizing the risk of HIV transmission through injection drug use, and women who have sex with both women and men should be reminded of the higher risks of HIV infection that they may face with bisexual male partners.

Clinical Care

There are no gynecologic manifestations unique to lesbians, but a number of STDs, including candidal and *Trichomonas* vaginitis, are common in this population [101]. In addition, women who have sex with multiple partners may be vulnerable to the full spectrum of STDs. As discussed in Chap. 39, certain gynecologic manifestations may be more frequent in the context of HIV infection, including vaginal candidiasis, pelvic inflammatory disease, and cervical dysplasia and neoplasia [102–106].

Health Care Providers and the Gay or Bisexual Patient

Many studies before the AIDS era reported that gay and bisexual persons were reluctant to share their sexual identity with health care providers and that clinicians frequently presumed a heterosexual identity of their patients. However, there is also evidence that gay/bisexual persons believe that their quality of care is enhanced when their sexual identity is known [107–109]. While simply knowing that a patient is gay or bisexual may be helpful, it is critical that clinicians move beyond the "gay" identifier in order to understand the individual's development as a person. Just as there is no "typical" heterosexual person or lifestyle, it is important to recognize that a gay patient's lifestyle, sexual activity, or psychological development may not fit one's preconceived notions of homosexuality. Gay and bisexual male and female members of minority communities may tread an especially difficult path in adjusting to a homosexual life compared to their white counterparts. Some homosexual persons of color may feel that they have been forced to choose between identifying with their minority community or the largely white, "high-profile" gay community [110].

The goal for the clinician should be to understand the patient's sexuality as it is experienced by that individual. For the health care provider, relevant aspects of a gay or bisexual man or woman's personal life include some sense of how comfortable the individual is with his/her sexual identity and, if the person has "come out," for how long a period? To what degree is the person known to be gay or bisexual in his or her family of birth, and what has been their response? Does the family know the individual's HIV status? What is the impact of their knowledge level and response? If the person is employed, to what extent are others in the workplace aware that the person is gay or bisexual, HIV-infected, or both, and what has been their response? Is the individual in a relationship at present, and, if so, for how long? What is the HIV serostatus of the partner, and what effect has the AIDS epidemic had on their relationship? Is the individual sexually active, and, if so, are risk reduction techniques understood and employed? What is the person's level of support and connection with the larger gay and bisexual community? What has been the individual's experience with the HIV/AIDS epidemic to date? Has the person lost friends or partners to the disease? How does this personal experience affect the individual's anticipation of the future [111–114]?

Substitute Decision Making

An especially important issue for health care providers to discuss with their gay and bisexual patients is substitute decision making in the event of incompetence resulting from deterioration of their medical condition. If no prior arrangements have been made, a gay or bisexual person's birth family is often given authority as next of kin and may countermand the wishes of the patient's life partner, even to the extent of forbidding visiting privileges. In many states, a durable power of attorney for health care may be executed to allow for transfer of decision making to an individual of the patient's choosing. Clinicians should make a special effort to anticipate such eventualities and to discuss the patient's wishes for resuscitation and substitute decision making early in the course of HIV disease.

References

1. McWhirter DP, Mattison AM. *The Male Couple.* Englewood Cliffs, NJ: Prentice-Hall, 1984.
2. Council on Scientific Affairs, American Medical Association. Health care needs of a homosexual population. *JAMA* 248:726–739, 1982.

3. Owen WF. The clinical approach to the homosexual patient. *Ann Intern Med* 93:90–92, 1980.
4. Committee on Adolescence, American Academy of Pediatrics. Homosexuality and adolescence. *Pediatrics* 72:249–250, 1983.
5. Gonsiorek JC. Mental health issues of gay and lesbian adolescents. *J Adolesc Health Care* 9:114–122, 1988.
6. Centers for Disease Control. *HIV AIDS Surveillance Report.* 6 (mid-year edition), 1994.
7. Centers for Disease Control. Update: Acquired immunodeficiency syndrome—United States. *MMWR* 34:245–248, 1985.
8. Martin JL. The impact of AIDS on gay male sexual behavior patterns in New York City. *Am J Public Health* 77:578–581, 1987.
9. Schechter MT, Craib KJP, Willoughby B, et al. Patterns of sexual behavior and condom use in a cohort of homosexual men. *Am J Public Health* 78:1535–1538, 1988.
10. McKusick L, Coates TJ, Morin SF, et al. Longitudinal predictors of reductions in unprotected anal intercourse among gay men in San Francisco: The AIDS Behavioral Research Project. *Am J Public Health* 80:978–983, 1990.
11. Winkelstein W, Samuel M, Padian S, et al. The San Francisco Men's Health Study: Reduction in human immunodeficiency virus transmission among homosexual/bisexual men, 1982–1986. *Am J Public Health* 76:685–689, 1987.
12. Becker MH, Joseph JG. AIDS and behavioral change to reduce risk: A review. *Am J Public Health* 78:394–410, 1988.
13. Ekstrand ML, Coates TJ. Maintenance of safer sexual behaviors and predictors of risky sex: The San Francisco Men's Health Study. *Am J Public Health* 80:973–977, 1990.
14. Centers for Disease Control. Self-reported behavioral change among gay and bisexual men—San Francisco. *MMWR* 34:613–615, 1985.
15. Stall RD, Coates TJ, Hoff C. Behavioral risk reduction for HIV infection among gay and bisexual men. *American Psychol* 43:878–885, 1988.
16. Brookmeyer R. Reconstruction and future trends of the AIDS epidemic in the United States. *Science* 253:37–42, 1991.
17. Silvestre AJ, Kingsley LA, Wehman P, et al. Changes in HIV rates and sexual behavior among homosexual men, 1984 to 1988/92. *Am J Public Health* 83:578–580, 1992.
18. Peterson JL, Coates TJ, Catania JA. High-risk sexual behavior and condom use among gay and bisexual African-American men. *Am J Public Health* 82:1490–1494, 1992.
19. Adib SM, Joseph JG, Ostrow DG, et al. Relapse in sexual behavior among homosexual men: A 2-year follow-up from the Chicago MACS/CCS. *AIDS* 5:757–760, 1991.
20. Stall R, Ekstrand M, Pollack L, et al. Relapse from safer sex: The next challenge for AIDS prevention efforts. *J Acquir Immune Defic Syndr* 3:1181–1187, 1990.
21. Goldman EL. HIV upsurge tied to "psychological epidemic" in gay men. *Fam Pract News* 24:5, 1994.
22. Van Gorder D, Cloutier M, Bellinger G, et al. A call for a new generation

of AIDS prevention for gay and bisexual men in San Francisco. City of San Francisco.

23. Rompalo AM, Price CB, Roberts PL, Stamm WE. Potential value of rectal-screening cultures for *Chlamydia trachomatis* in homosexual men. *Br J Med Psychol* 153:888–892, 1986.

24. Koblin BA, Taylor PE, Stevens CE. The effect of age on high-risk sexual behavior and HIV-1 infection among gay men. Ninth International Conference on AIDS, Berlin, Germany, June 6–11, 1993.

25. Steiner S, Lemke AL, Roffman RA, et al. Risk behavior for HIV transmission among gay men surveyed in Seattle bars. *Public Health Rep* 109:563–566, 1994.

26. Steiner S, Lemke AL, Roffman RA, et al. Risk behavior for HIV transmission among gay men surveyed in Seattle bars. *Public Health Rep* 109:563–566, 1994.

27. Remafedi G. Predictors of unprotected intercourse among gay and bisexual youth: Knowledge, beliefs, and behavior. *Pediatrics* 94:163–168, 1994.

28. Hays RB, Kegeles SM, Coates TJ. High HIV risk-taking among young gay men. *AIDS* 4:901–907, 1990.

29. Winkelstein W, Lyman DM, Padian N, et al. Sexual practices and risk of infection by the human immunodeficiency virus: The San Francisco Men's Health Study. *JAMA* 257:321–325, 1987.

30. Kingsley LA, Detels R, Kaslow R, et al. Risk factors for seroconversion to human immunodeficiency virus among male homosexuals. *Lancet* 1:345–348, 1987.

31. Coates RA, Calzavara LM, Read SE, et al. Risk factors for HIV infection in male sexual contacts of men with AIDS or an AIDS-related condition. *Am J Epidemiol* 128:729–739, 1988.

32. Stricof RL, Kennedy JT, Nattell TC, et al. HIV seroprevalence in a facility for runaway and homeless adolescents. *Am J Public Health* 81:50–53, 1991.

33. Wendell DA, Onorato IM, McCray E, et al. Youth at risk: Sex, drugs, and human immunodeficiency virus. *Am J Dis Child* 146:76–81, 1992.

34. Remafedi G, Farrow JA, Deisher RW. Risk factors for attempted suicide in gay and bisexual youth. *Pediatrics* 87:869–875, 1991.

35. Remafedi G. Adolescent homosexuality: Psychosocial and medical implications. *Pediatrics* 79:331–337, 1987.

36. Prenzlauer S, Drescher J, Winchel R. Suicide among homosexual youth. *Amer J Psychiatr* 149:1416, 1992.

37. Remafedi G. Male homosexuality: The adolescent's perspective. *Pediatrics* 79:326–330, 1987.

38. Feinleib MR. Report of the Secretary's Task Force on Youth Suicide. US Department of Health and Human Services, 1989.

39. Cwayna K, Remafedi G, Treadway L. Caring for gay and lesbian youth. *Medical Aspects of Human Sexuality* July 1991; 50–57.

40. Tartagni D. Counseling gays in a school setting. *School Counselor* 26:26–32, 1978.

41. Remafedi GJ. Preventing the sexual transmission of AIDS during adolescence. *J Adolesc Health Care* 9:139–143, 1988.

42. Zenilman J. Sexually transmitted diseases in homosexual adolescents. *J Adolesc Health Care* 9:129–138, 1988.
43. Marks G, Ruiz MS, Richardson JL, et al. Anal intercourse and disclosure of HIV infection among seropositive gay and bisexual men. *Soc Sci Med* 7:866–869, 1994.
44. Marks G, Richardson JL, Naldonada N. Self-disclosure of HIV infection to sexual partners. *Am J Public Health* 81:1321–1322, 1991.
45. Cleghorn FR, Blattner WA. Does human T-lymphotropic virus type 1 and human immunodeficiency virus type 1 coinfection accelerate acquired immunodeficiency syndrome? *Arch Intern Med* 152:1372–1373, 1992.
46. Page JB, Lai S, Chitwood DD, et al. HTLV-I/II seropositivity and death from AIDS among HIV-1 seropositive intravenous drug users. *Lancet* 335:1439–1441, 1990.
47. Gotuzzo E, Escamilla J, Phillips IA, et al. The impact of human T-lymphotropic virus type I/II infection on the prognosis of sexually acquired cases of acquired immunodeficiency syndrome. *Am J Epidemiol* 152:1429–1432, 1992.
48. Richman DD, Bozzette SA. The impact of the syncytium-inducing phenotype of human immunodeficiency virus on disease progression. *J Infect Dis* 169:968–974, 1994.
49. Dritz S. Medical aspects of homosexuality. *N Engl J Med* 302:463–464, 1980.
50. Sohn N, Robilotti JG. The gay bowel syndrome: A review of colonic and rectal conditions in 200 male homosexuals. *Am J Gastroenterol* 67:478–484, 1977.
51. Centers for Disease Control. Human T-lymphotropic virus type 1 screening in volunteer blood donors—United States, 1989. *MMWR* 39:915–924, 1990.
52. Eyster ME, Alter HJ, Aledort LM, et al. Heterosexual co-transmission of hepatitis C virus (HCV) and human immunodeficiency virus (HIV). *Ann Intern Med* 115:764–768, 1991.
53. Murphy EL, Figueroa JP, Gibbs WN, et al. Sexual transmission of human T-lymphotropic virus type 1 (HTLV-1). *Ann Intern Med* 111:555–560, 1989.
54. Corey L, Holmes KK. Sexual transmission of hepatitis A in homosexual men: Incidence and mechanism. *N Engl J Med* 302:435–438, 1980.
55. Owen WF. Sexually transmitted diseases and traumatic problems in homosexual men. *Ann Intern Med* 92:805–808, 1980.
56. Weller IVD. The gay bowel. *Gut* 26:869–875, 1985.
57. Rompalo AM, Stamm WE. Anorectal and enteric infections in homosexual men. *West J Med* 142:647–652, 1985.
58. Centers for Disease Control. Kaposi's sarcoma and *Pneumocystis carinii* pneumonia among homosexual men—New York City and California. *MMWR* 30:305–308, 1981.
59. Centers for Disease Control. Epidemiologic aspects of the current outbreak of Kaposi's sarcoma and opportunistic infections. *N Engl J Med* 306:248–252, 1982.
60. Haverkos HW, Pinsky PF, Drotman DP, Bregman J. Prevalence of Kaposi's sarcoma among patients with AIDS. *N Engl J Med* 312:1518, 1985.
61. Des Jarlais DC, Marmor M, Thomas P, et al. Kaposi's sarcoma among four different AIDS risk groups. *N Engl J Med* 310:1119, 1984.

62. Brodie HR, et al. Prevalence of Kaposi's sarcoma in AIDS patients reflects differences in rates of cytomegalovirus infection in high risk groups. *AIDS Memorandum* 1:12, 1984.

63. Collier AC, Meyers JD, Corey L, et al. Cytomegalovirus infection in homosexual men: Relationship to sexual practices, antibody to human immunodeficiency virus, and cell-mediated immunity. *Am J Med* 82:593–601, 1987.

64. Giraldo G, Beth E. The involvement of cytomegalovirus in acquired immune deficiency syndrome and Kaposi's sarcoma. *Prog Allergy* 37:319–331, 1986.

65. Mintz L, Drew WL, Miner RC, Braff EH. Cytomegalovirus infections in homosexual men: An epidemiologic study. *Ann Intern Med* 99:326–329, 1983.

66. Marmor M, Laubenstein L, William DC, et al. Risk factors for Kaposi's sarcoma in homosexual men. *Lancet* 1:1083–1086, 1982.

67. Haverkos HW, Pinsky PF, Drotman P, Bregman DJ. Disease manifestations among homosexual men with acquired immunodeficiency syndrome: A possible role of nitrites in Kaposi's sarcoma. *Sex Transm Dis* 12:203–208, 1985.

68. Durack DT. Opportunistic infections and Kaposi's sarcoma in homosexual men. *N Engl J Med* 305:1465–1467, 1981.

69. Jorgensen KA, Lawesson SO. Amyl nitrite and Kaposi's sarcoma in homosexual men. *N Engl J Med* 307:893–894, 1982.

70. Rutherford GW, Schwarcz SK, Lemp GF, et al. The epidemiology of AIDS-related Kaposi's sarcoma in San Francisco. *J Infect Dis* 159:569–572, 1989.

71. Des Jarlais DC, Stoneburner R, Thomas P. Declines in proportion of Kaposi's sarcoma among cases of AIDS in multiple risk groups in New York City. *Lancet* 2:1024–1025, 1987.

72. Drew WL, Mills J, Hauer LB, et al. Declining prevalence of Kaposi's sarcoma in homosexual AIDS patients paralleled by fall in cytomegalovirus transmission. *Lancet* 1:66, 1988.

73. Chu SY, Buehler JW, Fleming PL, Berkelman RL. Epidemiology of reported cases of AIDS in lesbians, United States 1980–1989. *Am J Public Health* 80:1380–1381, 1990.

74. Beral V, Peterman TA, Berkelman RI, Jaffe HW. Kaposi's sarcoma among persons with AIDS: A sexually transmitted infection? *Lancet* 335:123–128, 1990.

74a. Moore PS, Chang Y. Detection of herpesvirus-like DNA sequences in Kaposi's sarcoma in patients with and those without HIV infection. *N Engl J Med* 332:1181–1185, 1995.

75. Sperber SJ, Schleupner CJ. Salmonellosis during infection with human immunodeficiency virus. *Rev Infect Dis* 9:925–934, 1987.

76. Nadelman RB, Mathur-Wagh U, Yancovitz SR, Mildvan D. *Salmonella* bacteremia associated with the acquired immunodeficiency syndrome (AIDS). *Arch Intern Med* 145:1968–1971, 1985.

77. Levine WC, Buehler JW, Bean NH, Tauxe RV. Epidemiology of nontyphoidal *Salmonella* bacteremia during the human immunodeficiency virus epidemic. *Ann Intern Med* 164:81–87, 1991.

78. Daling JR, Weiss MS, Hislop G, et al. Sexual practices, sexually transmit-

ted diseases, and the incidence of anal cancer. *N Engl J Med* 317:973–977, 1987.

79. Leichman L, Nigro N, Vaitkevicius VK, et al. Cancer of the anal canal. *Am J Med* 78:211–215, 1985.
80. Melbye M, Cote TR, Kessler L, et al. High incidence of anal cancer among AIDS patients. *Lancet* 343:636–639, 1994.
81. Palefsky JM, Gonzales J, Greenblatt RM, et al. Anal intraepithelial neoplasia and anal papillomavirus infection among homosexual males with group IV disease. *JAMA* 263:2911–2916, 1990.
82. Petersen LR, Doll L, White C, et al. No evidence for female-to-female HIV transmission among 960,000 female blood donors. *J Acquir Immune Defic Syndr* 5:853–855, 1992.
83. McCombs SB, McCray E, Wendell DA, et al. Epidemiology of HIV-1 infection in bisexual women. *J Acquir Immune Defic Syndr* 5:850–852, 1992.
84. Lemp G, Jones M, Kellogg T, et al. HIV seroprevalence and risk behaviors among lesbians and bisexual women: The 1993 San Francisco/Berkeley Women's Survey. San Francisco: San Francisco Department of Public Health, 1993.
85. Weiss SH, Vaughn A, Reyelt C, et al. Risk of HIV and other sexually transmitted diseases among lesbian and heterosexual women. Ninth International Conference on AIDS, Berlin, June 1993.
86. Cochran SD, Mays VM. Disclosure of sexual preference to physicians by black lesbian and bisexual women. *West J Med* 149:616–619, 1988.
87. Johnson SR, Guenther SM, Laube DW, Keettel WC. Factors influencing lesbian gynecologic care: A preliminary study. *Am J Obstet Gynecol* 140:20–28, 1981.
88. Chu SY, Diaz T, Schable B, and the SHAS Project Group. Risk behaviors among women with HIV/AIDS who report sex with women. Tenth International Conference on AIDS, Yokohama, August 1994.
89. Hunter J, Rosano M, Rotheram-Borus MJ. Sexual and substance abuse acts that place adolescent lesbians at risk for HIV. Ninth International Conference on AIDS, Berlin, June 1993.
90. Chu SY, Peterman TA, Doll LS, et al. AIDS in bisexual men in the United States: Epidemiology and transmission to women. *Am J Public Health* 82:220–224, 1992.
91. Wood RW, Krueger LE, Pearlman TC. HIV transmission: Women's risk from bisexual men. *Am J Public Health* 83:1757–1759, 1993.
92. Raiteri R, Fora R, Sinicco A. No HIV-1 transmission through lesbian sex. *Lancet* 344:270, 1994.
93. Blaser MJ. Isolation of human immunodeficiency virus from cervical secretions during menses. *Ann Intern Med* 106:912, 1987.
94. Marmor M, Laubenstein L, William DC, et al. Possible female-to-female transmission of human immunodeficiency virus. *Ann Intern Med* 105:969, 1986.
95. Monzon OT, Capellan JMB. Female-to-female transmission of HIV. *Lancet* 2:40–41, 1987.
96. Vogt MW, Witt DJ, Craven DE, et al. Isolation of HTLV-III/LAV from cervical secretions of women at risk for AIDS. *Lancet* 1:525–527, 1986.
97. Wofsy CB, Cohen JB, Hauer LB, et al. Isolation of AIDS-associated

retrovirus from genital secretions of women with antibodies to the virus. *Lancet* 1:527–529, 1986.

98. Clemetson DBA, Moss GB, Willerford DM, et al. Detection of HIV DNA in cervical and vaginal secretions: Prevalence and correlates among women in Nairobi, Kenya. *JAMA* 269:2860–2864, 1993.

99. Zorr B, Schafer APA, Habermehl KO, Kosh M. HIV-1 detection in endocervical swabs and mode of HIV-1 infection. *Lancet* 343:852, 1994.

100. Rich JD, Buck A, Tuomala RE, Kazanjian PH. Transmission of human immunodeficiency virus infection presumed to have occurred via female homosexual contact. *Clin Infect Dis* 17:1003–1005, 1993.

101. White J, Levinson W. Primary care of lesbian patients. *J Gen Intern Med* 8:41–47, 1993.

102. Hankins CA. Issues involving women, children, and AIDS primarily in the developed world. *J Acquir Immune Defic Syndr* 3:443–448, 1990.

103. Imam N, Carpenter CCJ, Mayer KH, et al. Hierarchical pattern of mucosal candida infections in HIV-seropositive women. *Am J Med* 89:142–146, 1990.

104. Rhoads JL, Wright DC, Redfield RR, Burke DS. Chronic vaginal candidiasis in women with human immunodeficiency virus infection. *JAMA* 257:3105–3107, 1987.

105. Minkoff HL, DeHovitz JA. Care of women infected with the human immunodeficiency virus. *JAMA* 266:2253–2258, 1991.

106. Centers for Disease Control. Risk for cervical disease in HIV-infected women—New York City. *MMWR* 39:846–849, 1990.

107. Smith EM, Johnson SR, Guenther SM. Health care attitudes and experiences during gynecologic care among lesbians and bisexuals. *Am J Public Health* 75:1085–1087, 1985.

108. Dardick L, Gradey KE. Openness between gay persons and health professionals. *Ann Intern Med* 93:115–119, 1980.

109. McGhee RD, Owen WF. Medical aspects of homosexuality. *N Engl J Med* 303:50–51, 1980.

110. Mays VM, Cochran SD. Black gay and bisexual men coping with more than just a disease. *Focus* 4:1–3, 1988.

111. Nichols SE. Psychosocial reactions of persons with the acquired immunodeficiency syndrome. *Ann Intern Med* 103:765–767, 1985.

112. Cassens BJ. Social consequences of the acquired immunodeficiency syndrome. *Ann Intern Med* 103:768–771, 1985.

113. Forstein M. The psychosocial impact of the acquired immunodeficiency syndrome. *Semin Oncol* 11:77–82, 1984.

114. Schwartzberg SS. AIDS-related bereavement among gay men: The inadequacy of current theories of grief. *Psychotherapy* 29:422–429, 1992.

The Drug-Using Patient *38*

Alan A. Wartenberg, Jeffrey H. Samet

In the past, interaction between the health care system and injection drug users (IDUs) was relatively limited, and acute medical issues, such as cellulitis, pneumonia, endocarditis, and drug overdose, predominated. Once treatment was initiated, the IDU would often leave the hospital or emergency room as soon as he or she was physically able, and little thought was given to the management of chronic medical problems. The HIV epidemic has dramatically changed this situation [1].

Many individuals have either switched to or started using cocaine in the form of freebase or "crack" in recent years. Use of alcohol, benzodiazepines, barbiturates, and oral opiates is also very prevalent. Disinhibited sexual behavior associated with these agents may result in increased HIV transmission [2]. However, since sharing of injection equipment remains the predominant drug-related risk behavior for acquiring HIV infection, the IDU serves as the paradigm for the drug-using patient in this chapter.

Injection drug users with HIV disease are presenting for care in increasing numbers and, to the surprise of many physicians, are often highly compliant [3–4, 5]. Health care professionals must learn to deal with the patient who has drug problems in a way that builds mutual respect and reduces animosity. Five basic concepts are involved in this effort:

1. Understanding addiction as a process and the addict as someone with a disease.
2. Understanding how to deal with difficult behaviors and set limits for the patient.
3. Developing a knowledge base to recognize and manage the common medical complications of drug use.
4. Understanding treatment options and how they can be accessed.

5.   Recognizing the special health care issues of the drug user with HIV disease.

Addiction as a Process and the Addict as a Patient

Chemical dependency is not universally accepted as a disease [6, 7]. The repetition of self-destructive behaviors, whether involving the ingestion of substances or pathologic gambling, is understood by some as poor decision making that is socially conditioned rather than a disease manifestation. However, intoxication, withdrawal, and medical complications of drug addiction clearly fit a disease model; the addiction process has a natural history with a characteristic pattern of behavior and response to intervention. The "moral" or criminalization model that prevailed earlier resulted in preventable deaths in "drunk tanks" and the development of abysmal prison drug treatment programs. This perspective may be the basis of therapeutic nihilism regarding the addict [8].

The attitude of the health professional toward the IDU has an impact on the quality of care provided. Development of a nonjudgmental posture and the use of positive interpersonal skills, such as empathy, legitimization, respect, support, and partnership, are important [9]. The clinician should attempt to understand the language and culture of the addict. Physicians or nurses who do not comprehend this jargon should ask what is meant; a dictionary of street drug use is available [10]. If the health care provider maintains a professional and nonjudgmental attitude toward the IDU, treats him or her with the same respect accorded other patients, and creates an atmosphere of caring and concern for the individual's well-being, a positive outcome is more likely.

Limit Setting and Dealing with Difficult Behaviors

The responsibilities of the clinician and IDU should be delineated early in the relationship. The tone of conversation should be professional, calm, and reassuring; anger and hostility are counterproductive. The rules of the clinic or inpatient unit should be clearly stated and include absolute intolerance of drug use in the health care setting. Violence, threats of violence, and abusive or threatening language are not acceptable and should lead to sanctions, including discharge from care, if warranted. The health care team, including the physician, nurse, and social worker, must collaborate in determining appropriate regulations and responses, and be unified in their approach to the patient.

Guidelines should be considered in advance for psychoactive drugs, including analgesics, anxiolytics, hypnotics, and antidepressants. When possible, drugs that do not produce significant mood alteration and are less addictive are preferred. Examples include the use of nonsteroidal antiinflamatory drugs for pain, buspirone for long-term anxiety, and low-dose sedating antidepressants for sleep. When possible, nonpharmacologic treatments, such as relaxation tapes, physiotherapy, acupuncture, local heat, and biofeedback, should be used to control symptoms. Patients should be informed in advance if urine toxicology screens are to be performed, and care should be taken to ensure that a legitimate specimen is provided [11]. Limitations of toxicology studies include failure to detect drugs with short half-lives; specimen substitution or adulteration; and false-positive test results [12].

The health care team must decide in advance how it will respond to negative behaviors. If the patient refuses to cooperate after limits have been set and understood, or repeatedly violates the treatment contract, consideration should be given to discharging him or her from care as soon as medically feasible. If a patient uses drugs in the hospital setting or is involved in behavior that is dangerous to self or others, discharge may be necessary even if he or she has a serious continuing medical condition. Every effort should be made to prevent this outcome, but if necessary, such an action must be taken without anger and recrimination. The patient should be informed that it is the consequence of his or her violation of the contract [13].

Understanding the motivation of the patient with difficult behaviors can result in a more professional response by the clinician [14]. A positive finding on urine toxicology screen or other evidence of recent drug use should lead to a discussion with the patient about factors that precipitated the incident. In some cases, drug use or other negative behaviors may indicate that detoxification is not proceeding properly and that the patient is being either overtreated, which may produce disinhibition, or undertreated, with resultant craving, anxiety, and agitation.

Medical Evaluation and Treatment

In addition to the general medical history, obtaining a complete history of drug use is necessary. Specific questions regarding opiates, cocaine, alcohol, sedative-hypnotics, and inhalants should be asked, with particular attention to quantity, duration, and last use; social and medical consequences; and previous attempts at abstinence.

When assessing the quantity of drug use, the clinician should be aware of the packaging and concentration of street drugs. Heroin is sold in "bags," with 10 bags to a "bundle." A bag may cost $10 to $20 and contains from 2 to 15 mg of heroin, but cost and purity are highly variable. An average bag in New England presently contains 7 to 10 mg of heroin. Cocaine is sold in fractions of an ounce, with "eighths," "sixteenths," and "quarters" being common sizes. An eighth contains approximately 3.5 gm of 50 to 80 percent cocaine but may vary considerably in purity; currently, cocaine costs approximately $50 to $75 per gram. A patient on a cocaine binge or "run" may use more than $500 of cocaine in 1 to 3 days.

General care of all patients with a history of drug or alcohol abuse should include adequate nutrition, as well as the provision of thiamine and multivitamins. The ability of the health care professional to spend time with the patient and to project reasonable optimism regarding the future is important for a successful outcome. However, while a caring clinician may facilitate behavioral change in the addict, the drug user must take primary responsibility for these efforts.

Opiate Use

Determining the patient's prior experience with drug withdrawal is extremely important [15–17]. Opiate withdrawal, while not life threatening, may be very uncomfortable and lead to drug-seeking behavior. Methadone is the treatment of choice, although clonidine and high-dose benzodiazepines have been advocated as alternative therapies [18–21]. In the inpatient setting, the initial oral dose of methadone is 20 mg; intramuscular methadone is almost twice as potent as the oral preparation, and its dose should be adjusted accordingly [22]. The patient should be examined for objective signs of withdrawal, such as piloerection, mydriasis, rhinorrhea, and lacrimation. Additional methadone may be administered if clinical symptoms and signs of opiate withdrawal are evident 1 hour after the initial oral dose. Rarely is a starting dose of more than 40 mg per day required. Methadone overtreatment may lead to respiratory depression and aspiration. Nonsteroidal antiinflammatory agents, antispasmodics, and sedatives can be used on a short-term basis to control the pain, abdominal cramps, diarrhea, and insomnia of opiate withdrawal.

If the patient receives outpatient methadone treatment, the program should be notified of his or her hospitalization, and the dose level should be confirmed. If this is not possible, 40 mg of methadone per day in two to three divided doses is generally sufficient to cover the first few days of hospitalization, even for individuals receiving higher doses in an outpatient treatment program. If the patient is unable to take anything by mouth, the total daily dose of methadone should be reduced approximately 40 to 50 percent and given intramuscularly in three to four divided doses per day. Patients who need narcotic analgesics for pain should receive an appropriate agent; drug tolerance may require a 50 to 100 percent increase over the usual dosage. The maintenance dose of methadone will not provide analgesia for patients with significant pain. Mixed agonist-antagonists, such as pentazocine, butorphanol, and nalbuphine, may precipitate a withdrawal syndrome and should be avoided. If the patient is being discharged from an inpatient setting, the staff of the methadone program should be notified in advance, so that they can plan readmission to their facility.

A regimen utilizing clonidine and naltrexone in an outpatient setting has been described for the management of opiate withdrawal [23]. Buprenorphine is also being studied as an alternative to methadone [24, 25]. While investigators have evaluated the sublingual form, an intramuscular preparation is currently available. It is given at the dose of 0.15–0.30 mg initially and can be titrated upward to 2.4 to 4.8 mg in three or four divided doses, then tapered 15 to 25 percent per day. In addition to treating heroin withdrawal, buprenorphine may reduce cocaine craving, but this indication is controversial [24].

If naloxone is used to treat respiratory depression resulting from narcotic overdose, it may produce an abrupt withdrawal syndrome. Following acute treatment with bolus naloxone, a continuous infusion with 4 mg of naloxone in 1,000 ml of 5% dextrose in water (D5W) at 100 ml per hour can be titrated to maintain adequate ventilation without precipitating significant withdrawal [26]. In severe overdose, large doses of naloxone (2 mg) may be necessary, with repeated administration every 20 to 40 minutes. If the patient is taking methadone or propoxyphene, up to a 4-mg bolus of naloxone may be required to reverse respiratory depression.

Cocaine Use

Cocaine craving and postcocaine depression may be severe. Anticraving agents such as bromocriptine, amantadine, and tricyclic antidepressants, particularly desipramine, have been used with some success in the treatment of postcocaine symptoms [27, 28]. An initial dose of bromocriptine, 1.25 mg, can be given orally, and if tolerated, 2.5 to 5.0 mg every 8 to 12 hours may be effective. Alternatively, amantadine, 100 to 200 mg, can be given orally two to three times daily. Desipramine is given orally at 25 to 50 mg initially, increasing the dose by 25 to 50 mg every 2 or 3 days until a dose of 100 to 150 mg per day is attained. Other antidepressants can be used in equivalent doses if desipramine is not tolerated. Some of these agents, such as desipramine and fluoxetine, are stimulating and should be given early in the day, whereas others, such as amitriptyline, nortriptyline, and doxepin, are sedating and should be given in the evening or at bedtime. Bromocriptine or amantadine should be continued until the antidepressant begins to work or cocaine craving has spontaneously subsided.

The optimal duration of antidepressant therapy in this setting is unknown, but 3 months appears adequate. Tricyclic antidepressants may have serious toxicity in some patients, including cardiac dysrhythmias and seizures, and their efficacy in the treatment of postcocaine symptoms has not been definitively established. The judicious use of short-term anxiolytic agents is warranted in the presence of severe anxiety. Psychotic symptoms can be managed with neuroleptics, but these agents sometimes worsen postcocaine craving and depression. It should be emphasized that all pharmacotherapy of cocaine craving is optimally used in conjunction with psychosocial counseling.

Referral to Drug Treatment

Understanding addiction treatment options and how to access them is an important skill for primary care providers. If the patient has a supportive social structure and no serious medical or psychiatric disabilities, outpatient treatment may be appropriate. For an individual with extensive opiate use, methadone detoxification with evaluation for maintenance should be considered [18, 29]. If the patient is placed on methadone in the hospital, it should be with a rapid detoxification over 5 to 10 days, unless there has been consultation with the staff of an approved methadone program who agree to "maintain" drug treatment after discharge.

If hospital detoxification is warranted, methadone should be given orally in a single daily dose, preferably in liquid form, and the patient should swallow the entire dose while under observation. In general, the dose can be decreased by 2.5 to 5.0 mg per day. Clonidine may be useful in patients being detoxified from short-acting opiates or for those receiving lower-dose methadone ($\leq$ 40 mg) [19, 20]. In general, an initial dose of 0.1 mg of clonidine can be given if the systolic blood pressure is 100 mm Hg or higher, followed by 0.1 to 0.2 mg every 2 to 4 hours, titrating the dose based on clinical response and blood pressure. The optimal daily dose should be maintained for 24 to 48 hours and then tapered over the next 7 to 10 days. Clonidine transdermal patches may be better tolerated in some patients. Initially a 0.1-mg patch is placed, and the dose doubled every 2 days until symptomatic improvement occurs; 0.4 to 0.6 mg may be required. Patients may need oral clonidine supplementation for the first 24 to 48 hours. Use of nonsteroidal antiinflammatory agents, antispasmodics, antidiarrheal agents, and hypnotics is usually necessary as part of clonidine detoxification.

For patients with less extensive opiate histories or with primary cocaine or other drug problems, referral to a drug-free program is appropriate. If the patient does not live in a supportive setting or if outpatient therapy has failed, residential treatment is preferred. Such programs are readily available to those with health insurance, but may be harder to find for those receiving medical assistance or those without the capacity to pay. The hospital social work staff or addiction service should be familiar with local programs.

Self-help programs, such as Narcotics Anonymous, Cocaine Anonymous, and Alcoholics Anonymous, are almost universally available, and patients should be encouraged to attend meetings, join a group, and obtain a sponsor [30, 31]. Programs for family members and significant others, including Nar-Anon and Al-Anon, are often invaluable. Involvement of family and significant others in treatment programs may increase the chance of success [32]. For patients who have difficulty with the "spiritual" nature of these programs, others, such as Rational Recovery, Secular Organizations for Sobriety, and Women for Sobriety, may be useful.

In patients in whom less restrictive treatment has failed, therapeutic communities (long-term residential programs that offer highly structured programs) may be the best option [33]. Communities that are members of Therapeutic Communities of America adhere to accepted standards of care and are preferred. Abstinence rates in highly structured residential programs are better than 90 percent at 1 year and 70 percent 3 years after treatment [33].

If immediate placement in a treatment program is not available referral to self-help groups, family referral, outpatient detoxification using clonidine, and/or other symptomatic measures should be offered. Temporizing measures may be successful until more appropriate treatment options become available.

In well-motivated patients, treatment with naltrexone may be effective in reducing or eliminating illicit opiate use [34]. This drug blocks the opioid receptor, preventing its physiologic effects. Naltrexone should be prescribed only for patients who have been detoxified from opiates, preferably with clonidine. If naltrexone is given to a patient who is still dependent on opiates, it may precipitate a severe and long-lasting withdrawal syndrome. The dose is 50 mg given orally once a day; in supervised programs, patients may receive 100 mg on Mondays and Wednesdays and 150 mg on Fridays. Gastrointestinal distress may limit dosing, and liver function should be monitored periodically.

If treatment is refused, the primary care provider should continue to educate, persuade, and support the patient, while promoting appropriate options at each visit. Improvement in behavior may be gradual, and the clinician may need to accept relatively modest changes over time [35]. Treatment should be viewed as an ongoing process rather than as an isolated event. It may be possible to refer family members into counseling and self-help groups; the reduction in "enabling behaviors" may prompt a previously resistant patient to seek treatment. Cultural and ethnic sensitivity is important; patients may be more likely to accept treatment in self-help groups if they are composed of people of similar backgrounds or have a counselor who is linguistically and culturally sensitive.

For patients still injecting drugs, careful instruction in the use of dilute bleach to clean paraphernalia is important. Referral to needle exchange programs may be appropriate and result in reduced transmission of HIV and increased acceptance of drug treatment [36]. There is no evidence that such programs promote increased injection drug use [37, 38].

The Drug User with HIV Infection

Clinicians who deal with drug-using patients should be familiar with the medical complications that may ensue (Table 38-1); several excellent reviews are available [39–43]. In addition to injection drug use, crack cocaine dependence and alcoholism appear to be independent risk behaviors for the transmission of HIV infection and have their own sequelae [44, 45].

Medical Issues

The manifestations of HIV disease in drug users are similar to those described in other affected populations. In a study that compared HIV-infected IDUs with CD4 cell counts less than 200/mm^3 to seropositive

Table 38-1 *Medical complications in the drug-using patient*

Bacterial infections
    Pneumonia
    Endocarditis
    Skin and soft tissue infections
    Osteomyelitis/septic arthritis
Tuberculosis
Sexually transmitted diseases
    Syphilis
    Gonorrhea
    Chlamydia
    Herpes simplex virus
    Human papillomavirus
Hepatitis
    Viral hepatitis (A, B, C, delta)
    Alcoholic
Central and peripheral nervous system diseases
Retroviral infections
    HIV infection and its medical complications
    HTLV-I
    HTLV-II
Malignancies
    Lymphoma
    Solid tumors (oropharynx, larynx, lungs)
Miscellaneous
    Constitutional symptoms
    Lymphadenopathy
    Renal disease
    Thrombocytopenia

Source: Adapted from PA Selwyn, PG O'Connor. Diagnosis and treatment of substance users with HIV infection. *Primary Care* 19:119–156, 1992.

homosexual control subjects, the only more common clinical finding in IDUs was oral candidiasis [46].

The frequency of bacterial pneumonias in HIV-infected drug users appears to be increased and contributes significant morbidity and mortality [47]. Smoking illicit drugs, including marijuana, cocaine, and crack, may be a contributing factor [48]. More than 80 percent of the bacterial pneumonias in a New York City IDU cohort were caused by *Streptococcus pneumoniae* or *Haemophilus influenzae* [47]. Bacterial endocarditis, skin and soft tissue infections, and osteomyelitis and septic arthritis also occur more often in IDUs.

Tuberculosis (TB) exposure is common among HIV-infected drug users, and this observation has both personal and public health implications. Evidence supporting the use of isoniazid prophylaxis in HIV-infected persons with a positive purified protein derivative (PPD) initially came from a group of patients in a New York City methadone maintenance treatment program [49]. The empiric finding of a high risk for active TB among anergic HIV-infected IDUs in the same program led to the recommendation to provide prophylaxis for this group as well [50]. Compliance with 12-month treatment regimens for TB may be problematic in drug users, but success has been reported in specialized clinical settings [51–53].

Sexually transmitted diseases, including syphilis, gonorrhea, chlamydia infection, herpes simplex virus infection, and human papillomavirus infection, are common in drug users. False-positive findings on syphilis screening tests, such as the rapid plasma reagin (RPR), occur in approximately 10 percent of IDUs. Serologic evidence of past or current hepatitis B and C infection is present in the vast majority of IDUs with HIV infection, and the risk of progressing to chronic hepatitis is increased in this population [54].

Kaposi's sarcoma is an infrequent finding in drug users without a history of homosexual or bisexual activity. Oropharyngeal, laryngeal, and lung cancers occur more commonly in drug users than in the general population, probably reflecting the high prevalence of concomitant alcohol and tobacco use.

Constitutional symptoms may be the result of drug use or withdrawal, opportunistic disease, or HIV infection itself. Miscellaneous conditions, including lymphadenopathy, renal disease, and thrombocytopenia, may be related to drug use or HIV infection. Preliminary evidence suggests that the rate of decline of CD4 cell counts among HIV-infected drug users appears to be no more rapid than in other seropositive populations [55]. Independent predictors of progression to AIDS in drug users based on the pre-1993 case definition include CD4 cell count, lack of zidovudine use, oral candidiasis, bacterial infections, and TB [47].

Potential drug interactions of concern in HIV-infected drug users relate to methadone. Rifampin enhances methadone metabolism and reduces plasma levels in patients by the induction of hepatic microsomal enzymes [56]. The clinician should anticipate precipitation of withdrawal syndrome in a methadone patient begun on rifampin; daily methadone dosing may need to be increased by 50 percent or another antituberculous drug substituted. While it is not known whether rifabutin significantly affects methadone metabolism, we are familiar with several cases of apparent opioid withdrawal related to rifabutin therapy. Phenytoin and phenobarbital may have similar but less dramatic effects [57]. There is no evidence of a clinically significant interaction between methadone and zidovudine.

Perspective must be maintained when assuming primary care responsibility for the HIV-infected drug user, as the priorities of the patient may be quite different from those of the clinician. Psychosocial issues, including housing, family and financial problems, social isolation, victimization, and legal difficulties, may be dominant concerns on presentation. The IDU spends much, if not most, of his or her time securing drugs, making it difficult for the actively using patient to devote sufficient time or energy to health promotion. Similarly, the IDU who is trying to recover will be expending most of his or her energy on staying clean and in treatment. Thus it is not surprising that drug-using patients with HIV disease often present for primary medical care years after becoming infected [43].

Every effort should be made to keep the IDU with known HIV infection in drug treatment, since continued drug use threatens both the individual's health and medical compliance. Because a patient has declined treatment on one occasion does not mean that treatment should not be offered again at every opportunity; involvement of the patient's family or significant other or the enlistment of counselors may improve the likelihood of acceptance. However, the clinician should be cognizant of confidentiality requirements of federal and state laws regarding substance abuse [58].

Chronic Pain and Psychiatric Issues

The treatment of pain, anxiety, and depression in a population with a history of abusing mood-altering drugs presents special problems for the clinician. In general, pain should be managed in accordance with recognized principles [59, 60]. Initially, salicylates or acetaminophen can be given; if the patient has chronic pain, these agents should be prescribed on a continuing basis. Nonsteroidal antiinflammatory agents are an acceptable alternative and may be better tolerated by some patients. If acute pain is severe, short-acting opiates, such as codeine, hydrocodone, or oxycodone, can be added to the nonnarcotic analgesics already given. Oral opiates are equally effective in equipotent doses, but codeine tends to cause more nausea and pruritus than other agents. In general, it is better to avoid fixed combinations of salicylates or acetaminophen with an opiate, since the patient may end up taking toxic doses of the nonnarcotic agent to provide adequate doses of the opiate.

The treatment of chronic, moderate to severe pain in the HIV-infected drug user is a particular challenge. No single approach has been broadly adopted. The appropriateness of opiate analgesia depends on the stage of the patient's HIV disease, availability of alternative regimens, and history of prescription drug misuse. In general, narcotic analgesia should be administered with caution for the treatment of chronic pain in patients with recent or active drug use. If short-acting opiates are given and pain cannot be controlled with four or five daily doses, consideration should be given to switching to a longer-acting agent, such as methadone or sustained-action morphine sulfate. If methadone is used, patients should be dosed every 6 to 8 hours for analgesic effect; once-daily dosing is usually not effective. Doses of 5 to 10 mg of methadone are generally sufficient for pain control, as is 30 to 60 mg of sustained-action morphine sulfate every 8 to 12 hours. Patients should be started at a lower dose, and the dose titrated upward.

Anxiety may be situational or part of a phobic, panic, or generalized disorder [61]. Situational anxiety is best treated with reassurance and counseling. Phobic disorder may respond to desensitization therapy, and panic disorder to antidepressants. Generalized anxiety can be treated with buspirone, which is nonaddicting, but takes 2 to 3 weeks to be effective. Depression, whether unipolar or bipolar, is treated in standard fashion, although patients with advanced HIV disease may have difficulty with tricyclic agent side effects, such as dry mouth and orthostatic hypotension [62, 63]. Many psychiatric disorders, including bipolar and personality disorders, are overrepresented in this population, and posttraumatic stress disorder may occur in combat veterans or patients with a history of childhood sexual trauma.

Patients whose conditions have been stable with mood-altering drugs, even those that produce dependency, need not be switched to other agents. If there is evidence of dose escalation, concomitant abuse of alcohol, or frequent abuse or intoxication, the clinician should proceed with gradual detoxification and substitution of a safer agent or therapy. Patients should be informed in advance that prescriptions for analgesics and mood-altering drugs will not be refilled before the appropriate time interval; prescriptions that are "lost," "stolen," "fell in the toilet," or "were eaten by the dog" are the patient's responsibility. The clinician should, however, provide medications in doses and quantities sufficient to last until the next appointment. It may be preferable to give prescriptions that are to be refilled several times, rather than a 2- or 3-month supply. An agreement to use only one pharmacy is often a helpful part of the therapeutic contract.

Conclusion

HIV-infected patients who have a history of drug use can be success-fully managed by primary care physicians. Enhancement of one's knowledge base, use of interpersonal skills, and appreciation of ap-proaches to drug treatment are all important. Interested health care providers may find it useful to do a rotation on a specialized drug treatment unit, particularly one where medical and psychiatric prob-lems are comanaged [64]. Improved attitudes, skills, and behaviors of health professionals who provide care for drug-using patients are es-sential.

References

1. Schoenbaum EE, et al. Risk factors for human immunodeficiency virus infection in intravenous drug users. *N Engl J Med* 321:874–879, 1989.
2. Chaisson RE, Bachetti P, Osmond D, et al. Cocaine use and HIV infection in intravenous drug users in San Francisco. *JAMA* 261:561–565, 1989.
3. Selwyn PA, et al. Primary care for patients with human immunodeficiency virus (HIV) infection in a methadone maintenance treatment program. *Ann Intern Med* 111:761–763, 1989.
4. Broers B, Morabia A, Hirschel B. A cohort study of drug users' compli-ance with zidovudine treatment. *Arch Intern Med* 154:1121–1127, 1994.
5. Samet JH, Libman H, Steger KA, et al. Compliance with zidovudine therapy in patients infected with HIV type 1: A cross-sectional study in a municipal hospital clinic. *Am J Med* 92:495–502, 1992.
6. Fingarette H. *Heavy Drinking: The Myth of Alcoholism as a Disease.* Berke-ley: University of California Press, 1988.
7. Peele S. *Diseasing of America: Addiction Treatment out of Control.* Lexington, MA: Lexington Books, 1989.
8. Senay EC. The Treatment of Drug Abuse. In S Aneti (ed), *American Hand-book of Psychiatry.* New York: Basic Books, 1976.
9. Novack DH. Therapeutic aspects of the clinical encounter. *J Gen Intern Med* 2:346–355, 1987.
10. Johnson NP, Davis CW, Michels PJ. *Dictionary of Street Alcohol and Drug Terms.* Columbia, SC: University of South Carolina Press, 1989.
11. Mackenzie RG, Cheng M, Haftel AJ. The clinical utility and evaluation of drug screening techniques. *Pediatr Clin North Am* 34:423–437, 1987.
12. Verebey K, Martin DM, Gold MS. Interpretation of drug abuse testing: Strengths and limitations of current methodology. *Psychiatr Med* 3:287–297, 1987.
13. Quill TE. Partnerships in patient care: A contractual approach. *Ann Intern Med* 98:228–234, 1983.
14. Groves JE. Taking care of the hateful patient. *N Engl J Med* 298:883–887, 1978.

15. Wartenberg AA. Detoxification of the chemically dependent patient. *RI Med J* 42:451–456, 1989.
16. Sullivan JT, Sellers EM. Treating alcohol, barbiturate and benzodiazepine withdrawal. *Rational Drug Ther* 20:1–9, 1986.
17. Wartenberg AA, Nirenberg TD, Liepman MR, et al. Detoxification of alcoholics: Improving care by symptom-triggered sedation. *Alcohol Clin Exp Res* 14:71–75, 1990.
18. Cooper JR. Methadone treatment and acquired immunodeficiency syndrome. *JAMA* 262:1664–1668, 1989.
19. Washton AM, Resnick RB. Clonidine for opiate detoxification: Outpatient clinical trials. *Am J Psychiatry* 137:1121–1122, 1980.
20. Kleber HD, et al. Clonidine in outpatient detoxification from methadone maintenance. *Arch Gen Psychiatry* 42:391–394, 1985.
21. Drummond DC, Turkington D, Rahman MZ, et al. Chlordiazepoxide versus methadone in opiate withdrawal: A preliminary double-blind trial. *Drug Alcohol Depend* 23:63–71, 1989.
22. O'Connor PG, Samet JH, Stein MD. Management of hospitalized intravenous drug users: Role of the internist. *Am J Med* 96:551–558, 1994.
23. O'Connor PG, Waugh ME, Schottenfeld RS, et al. Ambulatory opiate detoxification and primary care: A role for the primary care physician. *J Gen Intern Med* 7:532–534, 1992.
24. Gastfriend DR, Mendelson NK, Teoh SK, Reif S. Buprenorphine pharmacotherapy for concurrent heroin and cocaine dependence. *Am J Addict* 2:269–278, 1993.
25. Banys P, Clark HW, Tusel DJ, et al. An open trial of low dose buprenorphine in treating methadone withdrawal. *J Subst Abuse Treat* 11:9–15, 1994.
26. Goldfrank LR, Bresnitz EA. Opioids. In LR Goldfrank, et al (eds), *Toxicologic Emergencies: A Comprehensive Handbook in Problem Solving*. New York: Appleton-Century-Crofts, 1986. Pp 126–127.
27. Tennant FS Jr, Saherian AA. Double-blind comparison of amantadine and bromocriptine for ambulatory withdrawal from cocaine maintenance. *Arch Intern Med* 147:109–112, 1987.
28. Gawin FH, et al. Desipramine facilitation of initial cocaine abstinence. *Arch Gen Psychiatry* 46:117–121, 1989.
29. Novick DM, et al. Absence of antibody for human immunodeficiency virus in long-term socially rehabilitated methadone maintenance patients. *Arch Intern Med* 150:97–99, 1990.
30. Bean MH. Alcoholics anonymous. *Psychiatr Ann* 5:7–61, 1975.
31. Zweben JE. Recovery orientated psychotherapy: Facilitating the use of 12-step programs. *J Psychoactive Drugs* 19:243, 1987.
32. Usher ML, Jay J, Glass DR. Family therapy as a treatment modality for alcoholism. *J Stud Alcohol* 43:927–938, 1982.
33. Rosenthal MS. Therapeutic communities: A treatment alternative for many but not all. *J Subst Abuse Treat* 1:55–58, 1984.
34. O'Brien CP. A new approach to the management of opioid dependence: Naltrexone. *J Clin Psychiatry* 45:57–58, 1984.
35. Goldstein MG, Guise BJ, Ruggiero L, et al. Behavioral Medicine Strategies for Medical Patients. In A Stoudemire (ed), *Clinical Psychiatry for Medical Students*. Philadelphia: Lippincott, 1990. Pp 609–629.

36. DesJarlais DC, Friedman SR, Sotheran JL, et al. Continuity and change within an HIV epidemic: Injecting drug users in New York City, 1984 through 1992. *JAMA* 271:121–127, 1994.
37. Watters JK, Estilo MJ, Clark GL, Lorvick J. Syringe and needle exchange as HIV/AIDS prevention for injection drug users. *JAMA* 271:115–120, 1994.
38. Wartenberg AA. "Into Whatever Houses I Enter": HIV and injecting drug use (editorial). JAMA 271:151–152, 1994.
39. O'Connor PG, Selwyn PA, Schottenfield RS. Medical care for injection drug users with human immunodeficiency virus infection. *N Engl J Med* 331:450–459, 1994.
40. Cushman P. The major medical consequences of opioid addiction. *Drug Alcohol Depend* 5:239–254, 1980.
41. Wartenberg AA, Liepman MR. Medical Complications of Substance Abuse. In WD Lerner, MA Barr (eds), *Handbook of Hospital Based Substance Abuse Treatment.* New York: Pergamon Press, 1990. Pp 45–65.
42. Stein MD. Clinical review: Medical complications of intravenous drug use. *J Gen Intern Med* 5:249–257, 1990.
43. Selwyn PA, O'Connor PG. Diagnosis and treatment of substance users with HIV infection. *Primary Care* 19:119–156, 1992.
44. Edlin BR, et al. Intersecting epidemics: crack cocaine use and HIV infection among inner-city young adults. *N Engl J Med* 331:1422–1427, 1994.
45. Avins AL, et al. HIV infection and risk behaviors among heterosexuals in alcohol treatment programs. *JAMA* 271:515–518, 1994.
46. Palenicek J, Nelson KE, Vlahov D, et al. Comparison of clinical symptoms of human immunodeficiency virus disease between intravenous drug users and homosexual men. *Arch Intern Med* 153:1806–1812, 1993.
47. Selwyn PA, Alcabes P, Hartel D, et al. Clinical manifestations and predictors of disease progression in drug users with human immunodeficiency virus infection. *N Engl J Med* 327:1697–1703, 1992.
48. Caiaffa WT, et al. Drug smoking, *Pneumocystis carinii* pneumonia, and immunosuppression increase risk of bacterial pneumonia in HIV-seropositive injection drug users. *Am J Respir Crit Care Med* 150:1493–1498, 1994.
49. Selwyn PA, Hartel D, Lewis VA, et al. A prospective study of the risk of tuberculosis among intravenous drug users with HIV infection. *N Engl J Med* 320:545–550, 1989.
50. Centers for Disease Control. The use of preventive therapy for tuberculosis infection in the United States: Recommendations of the Advisory Committee for the Elimination of Tuberculosis (ACET). *MMWR* 39:6–8, 1990.
51. Brudney K, Dobkin J. Resurgent tuberculosis in New York City: Human immunodeficiency virus, homelessness, and the decline of tuberculosis control programs. *Am Rev Respir Dis* 144:745–749, 1991.
52. O'Connor PG, Molde S, Henry SP, et al. Human immunodeficiency virus infection in intravenous drug users: A model for primary care. *Am J Med* 93:382–386, 1992.
53. Selwyn PA, Feingold AR, Iezza A, et al. Primary care for patients with

human immunodeficiency virus (HIV) in a methadone maintenance program. *Ann Intern Med* 110:761–763, 1989.

54. Hadler SC, et al. Outcome of hepatitis B virus infection in homosexual men and its relation to prior human immunodeficiency virus infection. *J Infect Dis* 163:454–459, 1991.

55. Margolick JB, Munoz A, Vlahov D, et al. Changes in T-lymphocyte subsets in intravenous drug users with HIV-1 infection. *JAMA* 267:1631–1636, 1992.

56. Baciewicz AM, Self TH, Bekemeyer WR. Update on rifampin drug interactions. *Arch Intern Med* 147:565–568, 1987.

57. Liu SS, Wang RI. Case report of barbituate-induced enhancement of methadone metabolism and withdrawal syndrome. *Am J Psychiatry* 141:1287–1288, 1984.

58. Blume SB, American Medical Society on Alcoholism and Other Drug Dependencies and the National Council on Alcoholism. *Confidentiality of Patients Records in Alcoholism and Drug Treatment Programs*. New York: 1987.

59. Portnoy RK. Drug treatment of pain syndromes. *Semin Neurol* 7:139–149, 1987.

60. Amadio P Jr, Cummings DM, Amadio P. A framework for the management of chronic pain. *Am Fam Physician* 38:155–160, 1988.

61. Roth M, Argyle N. Anxiety, panic and phobic disorders: An overview. *J Psychiatr Res* 22(suppl 1):333–354, 1988.

62. Dilsaver SC, Votolato N, Coffman S. Depression in medical practice. *Am Fam Physician* 38:117–124, 1988.

63. Liepman MR, Nirenberg TD, Porges R, Wartenberg A. Depression Associated with Substance Abuse. In OG Cameron (ed), *Presentations of Depression*. New York: Wiley, 1987, Pp 131–167.

64. Dans PE, Matricciani RM, Otter SE, Reuland DS. Intravenous drug abuse and one academic health center. *JAMA* 263:3173–3176, 1990.

HIV Infection in Women   *39*

Beth Zeeman, Lisa R. Hirschhorn

In recent years, the greatest increase in reported AIDS cases in the United States has been among women. The threat that HIV poses to women's health is formidable, and perinatal transmission of the virus is an increasing problem worldwide. Despite these trends, the impact of HIV infection on the female population is perhaps the most inadequately studied aspect of the epidemic. While more is known now about HIV infection in women than in the past, large gaps remain in our knowledge about its medical, psychological, and social consequences.

Epidemiology

It is estimated that 4 million women are infected with HIV worldwide. In the United States, more than 46,000 women have been diagnosed with AIDS, representing 13 percent of all cases reported to date [1]. In women of childbearing age, AIDS has become the fourth leading cause of death, and it is the second leading cause for black women in this group [2]. Among women with AIDS in the United States, 35 percent are from large urban areas, and 85 percent are between 15 and 44 years old; 72 percent of cases are in blacks and Latinas [3, 4].

Seroprevalence surveys have contributed important information about the HIV epidemic. Among hospitalized women in the United States from 1989 through 1991, HIV seroprevalence rates ranged from 0.1 to 10.7 per 1,000, with the highest rates in the Northeast region [5, 6]. In 1989, seroprevalence studies of neonatal cord blood revealed that 1.5 per 1,000 women who gave birth in the United States were infected with HIV. In 1987, Donegan and colleagues [7] found that 1.8 percent of cord blood samples at Boston City Hospital were positive for HIV antibody; more recent data indicate that the seroprevalence rate at the institution is now higher than 3 percent. Of note, the ratio of HIV-infected women to men in adolescents is 1:1, the same pattern described in countries where heterosexual contact is the most common route for HIV transmission [8].

The epidemiology of HIV infection and AIDS in US women is changing. Earlier in the epidemic, injection drug use was the most frequent mode of transmission. More recently, increasing numbers of women diagnosed with AIDS have reported heterosexual contact as their only risk behavior. There is also evidence of increasing numbers of cases in smaller cities and rural areas [9, 10]. In 1993, the Centers for Disease Control (CDC) expanded the case definition for AIDS to include for the first time all persons with CD4 cell counts less than 200/mm³ and women with invasive cervical cancer [10]. This new definition incorporates many women who were previously excluded, resulting in a proportional increase in the number of AIDS cases reported in women [1, 11].

Sexual Transmission of HIV

Several studies suggested that transmission of HIV from men to women occurs more easily than from women to men, with ratios ranging from 1.9 to 18.7 [12–14]. The probability that an HIV-infected man will transmit the virus to an uninfected woman during a single episode of vaginal intercourse is estimated to be 0.2 percent [15]. Factors that appear to increase the rate of sexual transmission of HIV include failure to use a condom regularly, the presence or a history of genital ulcers, the practice of anal intercourse, increased number of sexual exposures, and intercourse with an infected partner with more advanced disease [16–19]. The estimated risk of becoming infected with HIV after several years of unprotected sex with the same seropositive partner ranges from 10 to 45 percent [20]. Although infrequent, transmission of HIV from a woman to another woman, possibly through oral sex, has been documented [21].

Natural History of HIV Infection in Women

Knowledge of the natural history, prognosis, and treatment of HIV infection is based primarily on studies of men, and the applicability of this information to women is unknown.

Initial studies found decreased survival in women following the diagnosis of AIDS. Rothenberg and colleagues [22] reported that survival time after a diagnosis of AIDS was significantly shorter for women than for men (298 vs. 374 days). Female gender remained an independent risk factor for mortality even after controlling for race, age, and risk behavior. In Massachusetts, Seage and coworkers [23] also found that the median survival time following an AIDS diagnosis was shorter for women than for men (347 vs. 411 days), although this difference did not reach statistical significance. More recent studies suggested that survival in women is equivalent to that of men, with any observed differences the result of poorer access to health care [24–27]. HIV-infected women had decreased rates of private insurance, increased emergency room utilization, increased treatment in hospitals with less AIDS experience, and in some studies, delayed presentation for care [26–28].

In general, there do not appear to be significant gender differences in HIV disease progression as measured by CD4 cell count decline or in the frequency of complications. Whereas *Pneumocystis carinii* pneumonia (PCP) is the most common opportunistic infection in women, several studies showed increased rates of candidal esophagitis and HIV wasting syndrome and decreased rates of Kaposi's sarcoma [29–31]. In addition, a higher percentage of HIV-infected women have a history of injection drug use or come from populations at increased risk for exposure to tuberculosis (TB). Therefore, higher rates of certain infections, including TB and bacterial pneumonia, might be anticipated [32]. Finally, several female-specific complications of HIV infection have been described, including chronic or recurrent vaginal candidiasis, pelvic inflammatory disease, and cervical neoplasia.

Barriers to Care

With the advent of zidovudine (ZDV) and prophylaxis for PCP, progression to AIDS has slowed, and survival has been prolonged [33, 34]. However, many HIV-infected women do not engage in primary care or, once in care, utilize fewer resources [35]. It is unclear whether this problem represents a lack of awareness or an inability or reluctance to access care. Common impediments to health care for HIV-infected women include ongoing drug use, lack of available drug treatment programs, child care responsibilities, and psychological barriers such as guilt over HIV transmission to children. Strategies that have been utilized to deal with these issues include use of neighborhood outreach workers; establishment of clinic day care and food pantry facilities; coordination of HIV, obstetrics-gynecology, and pediatric care; and improved social services.

Selected Gynecologic Diseases

Chronic Vaginal Candidiasis

Candida albicans is a normal colonizer of the female genital tract. While recurrent candidal vaginitis is common in healthy women, it may also be a presenting symptom in women who are HIV infected, occurring at all stages [36, 37]. Either topical antifungal therapy with clotrimazole or terconazole or an oral imidazole, such as ketoconazole or fluconazole, is generally effective for vulvovaginal candidiasis. However, relapse is common after cessation of treatment, and intermittent or continuous maintenance therapy is sometimes necessary [38]. Resistance to oral imidazoles has been reported, especially in patients on long-term fluconazole therapy [39].

Pelvic Inflammatory Disease

Two studies showed that a significant percentage of women (6.7–17.0%) who require hospitalization for pelvic inflammatory disease (PID) are HIV positive [40, 41]. HIV-infected women with PID may present with less abdominal tenderness, lower white blood cell counts, and decreased rates of isolation of *Neisseria gonorrhoeae*, and have higher rates of surgical intervention compared to seronegative patients [42, 43]. In addition, increased frequencies of endometritis and endocervical human papillomavirus (HPV) infection have been reported among HIV-infected women with PID [44].

Herpes Simplex Virus

Herpes simplex virus (HSV) has been shown to be an independent risk factor for the acquisition of HIV infection [45, 46]. HIV-infected women with HSV may have frequent and severe outbreaks. Treatment with higher than conventional doses of acyclovir is sometimes necessary, and chronic maintenance therapy may reduce the frequency of recurrences [47, 48]. Acyclovir-resistant strains of HSV have been isolated from HIV-infected women receiving long-term treatment [49].

Syphilis

Genital ulcers caused by *Treponema pallidum* have also been shown to be an independent risk factor for HIV infection [45, 50]. The clinical manifestations, natural history, serologic response, and treatment of syphilis may be altered in the context of HIV disease (see Chap. 23).

Gonorrhea, Chlamydia, and Trichomoniasis

Nonulcerative sexually transmitted diseases also increase the risk of acquisition and transmission of HIV [51, 52]. There are limited data on the effect of HIV infection on the clinical course of these conditions [53].

Human Papillomavirus and Cervical Dysplasia

Infection with HPV, the etiologic agent of genital warts, is a risk factor for cervical squamous intraepithelial lesion (SIL; also known as cervical intraepithelial neoplasia [CIN]), a precursor to cervical cancer. Early information about the course of HPV in immunocompromised renal transplant recipients suggested an increased risk of SIL, complicated by more aggressive disease and decreased response to standard treatment [54]. More recent studies have shown that this increased risk exists in HIV-infected women coinfected with HPV. Vermund and colleagues [55] compared 51 HIV-infected women with 45 HIV-negative women from similar demographic and risk groups. While HIV or HPV infection alone was associated with an increased risk of SIL, coinfection resulted in a 12-fold increased risk compared with that in control subjects without HIV and HPV infections. Other studies confirmed this synergistic effect and also demonstrated an increasing prevalence of SIL and cervical carcinoma associated with decreasing CD4 cell counts [56, 57]. This increased risk for cervical cancer was reflected in the addition of invasive cervical carcinoma to the 1993 CDC case definition for AIDS [11].

Appropriate screening protocols for cervical disease in HIV-infected women remain controversial. Maiman and colleagues [58] performed concurrent Papanicolaou's (Pap) smears and colposcopic biopsies in 32 HIV-infected women. In this population, only 3 (9%) had abnormalities on Pap smears, while on colposcopic biopsy, 13 (41%) had SIL and 15 (47%) had chronic cervicitis. These researchers recommended routine colposcopy for HIV-infected women, given the low sensitivity of Pap smear in detecting SIL in their population. However, other studies suggest that the sensitivity of Pap smears is not significantly different from that in HIV-negative women [59]. An expert panel convened by the Agency for Health Care Policy and Research (AHCPR) recommended semiannual Pap smears with aggressive follow-up for abnormal cytology in HIV-infected women, but did not advocate the use of colposcopy as an initial screening tool [59].

Similar uncertainty exists regarding the appropriate treatment for women with SIL or cervical carcinoma. Maiman and associates [60] studied 84 women under the age of 50 with documented invasive cervical cancer, of whom 16 (19%) were HIV infected. They found that HIV-positive women presented with a more advanced stage of disease and had a poor response to treatment, with higher rates of recurrence and death. These risks were higher in patients with CD4 cell counts below $500/mm^3$. More frequent recurrences have also been described in HIV-positive women with SIL receiving standard therapy, with rates of 18 percent in women with CD4 counts higher than $500/mm^3$ and 45 percent in women with counts lower than $500/mm^3$ [61]. The role of intravaginal 5-fluorouracil to prevent recurrent disease after standard ablative treatment is currently being evaluated in clinical trials.

Other Gynecologic Problems

A number of other gynecologic abnormalities have been found to be more frequent or severe in HIV-infected women. In a case-control study, 41 percent of HIV-positive women compared to 24 percent of control subjects had menstrual abnormalities, including amenorrhea or bleeding between periods [62]. Stein and colleagues [63] noted that, even in HIV-infected women without specific complaints, abnormal gynecologic findings were common. Severe and persistent sexual dysfunction has also been described [64]. In addition, rates of spontaneous abortion in HIV-positive injection drug users (IDUs) have been found to be higher than those for HIV-negative control subjects [65].

Family Planning

The CDC and American College of Obstetricians and Gynecologists (ACOG) recommend HIV antibody testing for women of reproductive age who are at high risk and for all pregnant women regardless of risk. Knowledge of HIV serostatus may not have a significant impact on the decision to terminate a pregnancy. Selwyn and associates [66] reported that among patients in a methadone clinic, HIV-positive patients were no more likely to have an elective abortion than seronegative ones; Johnstone and colleagues [67] found similar results.

For couples with discordant HIV serostatus, attempts to achieve pregnancy mean exposing the uninfected partner to the virus. HIV transmission through artificial insemination with washed semen from an HIV-positive man to his HIV-negative spouse has been documented, although preliminary results using processed semen have been encouraging [68, 69].

The condom is the only method that has been proved to decrease transmission of HIV and other sexually transmitted diseases. Impediments to condom use include lack of perceived risk; partner rejection; the perception that condoms are unpleasant, unreliable, and expensive, and offer incomplete protection; and religious objections [70, 71]. Therefore, other methods may need to be considered in some patients.

Certain contraceptives may pose specific health hazards for the HIV-infected woman. Estrogen in oral contraceptive pills (OCPs) increases cervical ectropion and may predispose to acquisition of HIV. Simonsen and associates [72], in a study of 418 prostitutes in Nairobi, found OCP use to be an independent risk factor for HIV infection, and Clemetson and coworkers [73] reported increased shedding of HIV in vaginal and cervical secretions in Kenyan women who used OCPs.

The intrauterine contraceptive device (IUD) is probably a poor family planning choice for HIV-infected women, as the IUD string may serve as a nidus for ascending infection or cause penile abrasions, which increase the risk of HIV transmission. Concern has also been raised that nonoxynol-9 and contraceptive sponges may enhance HIV transmission through irritation of the vaginal mucosa [74–76], although there is also evidence that spermicides may have anti-HIV activity [77]. The Food and Drug Administration recently approved the female condom as a barrier contraceptive for the prevention of HIV infection and other sexually transmitted diseases, and its effectiveness in preventing pregnancy is comparable to that of other barrier methods. In addition, the female condom has the distinct advantage of being the first barrier method that can be controlled by the woman [78].

HIV Infection in Pregnancy

The issue of HIV infection in women is complicated by the fact that more than 80 percent of women with AIDS are in their childbearing years [79]. Providing medical care to the HIV-infected pregnant woman is a challenging endeavor. Practitioners are limited by a paucity of clinical trials involving pregnant women and by a general reluctance to use drugs for which safety during pregnancy has not been established. As the incidence of HIV infection in women rises, so does the number of HIV-infected infants. Up to 1 in 57 US women delivering babies in inner-city hospitals are infected with HIV [80]. In sub-Saharan African cities, as many as 10 percent of infants born are seropositive [81].

Normal pregnancy alters immune status, causing a change in lymphocyte response to infection and a decrease in CD4 cell counts [82]. While these effects could potentially result in a more rapid progression of HIV infection during pregnancy, this has not been demonstrated, at least in the women studied to date [83, 84].

Vertical transmission of HIV from mother to fetus is well established, and can occur transplacentally throughout gestation, during birth, or through breast feeding after delivery [85–88]. Recent data suggest that transmission predominantly occurs during the intrapartum period [89, 90]. A working definition of early (in utero) infection versus late (intrapartum) infection has been developed based on the presence or absence of HIV in the infant's blood within the first 2 days following birth [91]. The overall transmission rate from an HIV-infected mother to her fetus is 15 to 40 percent [89–92]. There is evidence that transmission rates are higher among symptomatic HIV-infected women and those with more advanced disease [89, 92]. In addition, early infant gestational age (< 34 weeks) appears to correlate independently with an increased risk of HIV transmission [92].

Initial studies assessing the effect of HIV infection on pregnancy outcome revealed higher rates of preterm labor and low-birth-weight infants, and more frequent prematurely ruptured membranes [93, 94]. However, more recent reports from both the United States and sub-Saharan Africa showed no difference in rates of prematurely ruptured membranes, gestational age, Apgar scores, congenital abnormalities, or stillbirths after controlling for substance abuse [95, 96].

The treatment of pregnant HIV-infected women is often complicated by psychosocial problems, such as poverty, homelessness, drug use, domestic violence, and isolation. Realistic goals in treating HIV-infected pregnant women include

1. Provision of up-to-date statistics about the risks of maternal-fetal transmission and possible effects of pregnancy on maternal health.
2. Education in methods to prevent adult transmission.
3. Clinical staging and assessment of the risks and benefits of antiretroviral treatment and prophylaxis for opportunistic infections.
4. Provision of prenatal services with an emphasis on nutrition, as well as monitoring for and treatment of opportunistic diseases.
5. Provision of psychological and social support.
6. Access to drug treatment if necessary.

The following sections focus on the medical issues related to HIV infection in pregnancy, including the role of antiretroviral therapy and the prophylaxis and management of selected opportunistic infections. Complete clinical guidelines for the care of pregnant HIV-infected women are described elsewhere [97–99].

Antepartum Care

Many of the "normal" complaints of pregnancy, such as fatigue, may mimic symptoms of HIV infection, and careful history and physical examination are essential. In HIV-infected women, screening for TB, syphilis, chlamydia, gonorrhea, and viral hepatitis should be done routinely, and antibody titers to cytomegalovirus and *Toxoplasma gondii* should be considered. CD4 lymphocyte counts should be performed at least once each trimester and more frequently in patients with counts near $500/mm^3$ and $200/mm^3$. Serum alpha-fetoprotein testing should be offered to all patients at the appropriate gestational age. However, both amniocentesis and chorionic villus sampling are associated, in theory, with a risk of HIV transmission to the fetus. Antepartum testing to ensure fetal well-being should be performed for the usual obstetric indications recognizing that many of the risk factors for HIV infection may independently affect pregnancy.

Antiretroviral Therapy

Antiretroviral therapy that is clinically indicated should not be withheld from a woman on the basis of pregnancy. Fertility in rabbits and rats is diminished with very high doses of ZDV, but teratogenic effects have not been demonstrated [100]. Zidovudine has been shown to cross the placenta [101], and data concerning its effect on maternal and fetal health are beginning to emerge. In a multicenter survey of ZDV use in 43 HIV-infected pregnant women, no teratogenic abnormalities were noted in any of the 12 infants with first-trimester exposure, and only 2 (4.6%) of 43 mothers experienced dose-limiting drug toxicity [102].

Results from a recent AIDS Clinical Trial Group (ACTG) protocol indicate that ZDV is effective in reducing perinatal HIV transmission [103]. This study compared ZDV with placebo in a selected group of HIV-positive pregnant women with CD4 cell counts higher than 200/ mm^3. It was designed to determine whether ZDV could prevent HIV transmission when administered to pregnant women between 14 and 34 weeks' gestation, continued intrapartum, and given to their infants during the first 6 weeks of life.

ACTG 076 showed a highly significant reduction in risk of HIV transmission from mother to infant in the ZDV treatment group compared with the placebo group (25.5 vs. 8.3%), representing a 67.5 percent decrease in the risk of transmission in this select population. The study reported similar side effects in both the ZDV and placebo groups, with the exception of somewhat decreased hemoglobin levels in infants treated with ZDV. Zidovudine did not appear to have any significant effect on HIV disease progression in women at 6 months postpartum, and its long-term consequences in the newborn are unknown.

This information, as well as current recommendations for antiretroviral use [104], should be discussed with pregnant HIV-infected women, with ZDV offered after the first trimester. Patients who elect to take ZDV should be monitored closely with complete blood cell counts. The optimal management of ZDV-intolerant women or women already receiving ZDV at the time of pregnancy is presently uncertain, and there are no data on the use of other antiretroviral agents during pregnancy.

Prophylactic Antimicrobial Therapy

Attention to prophylaxis against opportunistic infections is important in all HIV-infected patients, and in pregnant women treatment choices should be made based on their benefits and risks [105]. Because of its superior efficacy, trimethoprim-sulfamethoxazole (TMP-SMX) is the drug of choice for primary and secondary PCP prophylaxis [106]. Whereas TMP-SMX has been reported to cause fetal malformations in rats and kernicterus in the newborn when administered during the third trimester, one study in humans found no increase in fetal abnormalities [107].

Other options for PCP prophylaxis include aerosol pentamidine and dapsone. Very little pentamidine is systemically absorbed when given as an aerosol treatment, making its potential risk for the fetus small, although its efficacy may be diminished given the decreased lung volumes in pregnant women. The safety of dapsone during pregnancy is unknown, although it has been used to treat leprosy without reports of fetal harm. Until more data are available, established guidelines for PCP prophylaxis should be applied to pregnant women with HIV infection [34, 106].

HIV-infected patients with *Mycobacterium tuberculosis* are at an increased risk for both primary and reactivation disease. Active TB poses a serious health danger to the mother, the fetus, and the general public. For all HIV-infected pregnant women with a positive purified protein derivative (PPD) or who are anergic and at high risk for having been exposed to TB, a chest x-ray, with abdominal shielding should be performed to exclude active pulmonary disease [108]. The decision whether to delay preventive treatment with isoniazid in a pregnant HIV-infected woman with a positive PPD or anergy should be individualized.

HIV-infected patients have a greater likelihood of developing a number of conventional bacterial infections, including pneumonia, salmonellosis, and cutaneous disease with *Staphylococcus aureus*. Pregnant women should receive pneumococcal and *Haemophilus influenzae* vaccines. In addition, they should be counseled regarding safe dietary practices, including avoiding undercooked meat, raw eggs, and unpasteurized dairy products.

HIV-infected patients may be prone to recurrent genital HSV infection requiring chronic suppressive therapy with oral acyclovir. While not approved for use in pregnancy, acyclovir has been given to many pregnant women without any evidence of teratogenicity [109].

In 1993 an expert panel recommended that HIV-infected persons with CD4 cell counts lower than $100/mm^3$ should be offered prophylaxis for *Mycobacterium avium* complex (MAC) infection with rifabutin [110]. However, this recommendation has not been uniformly accepted by clinicians, and the safety of this agent during pregnancy is unknown.

Intrapartum and Postpartum Care

In light of the potential for intrapartum transmission of HIV, sampling of fetal scalp blood and the use of scalp electrodes should be avoided, if possible. One study concluded that the rate of perinatal transmission is higher with vaginal delivery than cesarean section [111]. The authors suggested less invasive alternatives to cesarean section, such as cleansing of the birth canal, as a means of reducing HIV transmission.

Women who receive ZDV during pregnancy should continue the drug intrapartum. The recommended regimen is a loading dose of 2 mg/kg initiated during labor, followed by an infusion of 1 mg/kg/hr until delivery. This should be followed by administration of oral ZDV (2 mg/kg every 6 hours) to the infant [100]. While there are no data on the efficacy of ZDV during delivery in patients who have not received it during pregnancy, in light of ACTG 076 results, this option should be considered. Antiretroviral therapy postpartum should be managed based on the patient's clinical status and published guidelines, as discussed in Chapter 31.

Both the CDC and ACOG recommend bottle feeding for children of HIV-infected women in areas where safe alternatives to breast feeding exist [112, 113]. During the first postpartum visit with the patient, a barrier contraceptive method should be recommended and health maintenance issues for the mother and newborn addressed.

Infectious Complications

HIV-infected women who are pregnant are at similar risk of opportunistic infections as nonpregnant HIV-infected women at a similar stage of disease. The prevention, diagnosis, and treatment of these infections may be compromised by a number of factors, including the decreased use of prophylactic agents because of concern for the fetus, delay in diagnosis because of nonspecific symptoms attributed to pregnancy or deferred procedures because of perceived risk to the fetus, and withholding of certain medicines not approved for use in pregnancy. The risks and benefits of each treatment and procedure should be carefully weighed, remembering that fetal well-being is almost always best served by optimal medical management of the mother [102].

Pneumocystis carinii pneumonia should be treated with TMP-SMX or intravenous pentamidine. The theoretic risks of teratogenicity and kernicterus associated with TMP-SMX are small compared with the potential for hypoxemia and death from untreated PCP. Patients should initially receive parenteral TMP-SMX since absorption of oral medications is unpredictable in pregnancy.

Candidiasis of the pharynx or vagina should be treated initially with topical therapy. Oral ketoconazole or fluconazole should be considered for resistant mucosal infection or esophagitis, but the safety of these agents in pregnancy is unknown. Amphotericin B is the drug of choice for life-threatening fungal infections such as cryptococcus, and it has not been shown to cause fetal damage in studies of a small number of pregnant women [114].

Central nervous system infection with toxoplasmosis is usually caused by reactivation of latent infection and should be managed with pyrimethamine and sulfadiazine with folinic acid. Whereas the risks of these drugs during pregnancy are uncertain, one large study failed to demonstrate teratogenic effects [115]. Sulfadiazine should be replaced by clindamycin in patients intolerant to sulfonamides.

Acyclovir is indicated for the treatment of mucocutaneous HSV and varicella-zoster virus infections and appears to be safe in pregnancy [109]. Ganciclovir or foscarnet is indicated for the treatment of invasive cytomegalovirus infection, including retinitis and gastrointestinal disease. No data are available regarding the safety of either of these agents in pregnant women.

The natural history of syphilis may be altered in HIV-infected individuals; there are case reports of treatment failure with standard drug regimens [116]. In light of the risk to both the mother and fetus, women with untreated syphilis, or in whom serologic titers have not responded to therapy, should receive the appropriate penicillin regimen. Management should be individualized, based on the stage of syphilis, serology results, treatment history, and trimester of pregnancy [18, 59].

Treatment of active TB should not be delayed because of pregnancy. In general, a four-drug regimen is recommended for initial management. Isoniazid, ethambutol, and rifampin are probably safe; there is less experience with pyrazinamide in pregnancy, although it has been used when drug resistance is suspected [108, 117].

There is little information on the course and treatment of MAC infection in pregnant women with HIV disease. Similarly, there are few data regarding the safety of the newer macrolides, clarithromycin and azithromycin, when used as part of a multidrug regimen in this setting. If possible, quinolone antibiotics should be avoided during pregnancy because of their potential for fetal harm.

Clinical Trials

Relatively few HIV-infected women have been involved in clinical studies to date. Cotton and Finkelstein [118] reported that from 1987 through 1990, only 6.7 percent of participants in ACTG-sponsored trials were women. As a result, study results have had to be extrapolated to women, and there is limited information regarding gender-specific differences in drug efficacy or toxicity, or the effect of hormonal changes on pharmacokinetics. Barriers to access and enrollment that have contributed to this underrepresentation include transportation problems, child care responsibilities, the exclusion of women of childbearing age from earlier studies, and a general distrust of clinical trials. It is important that strategies be developed to address these issues in the future.

References

1. Massachusetts Department of Health. AIDS surveillance summary. *AIDS Newslett* 1994;10.
2. Centers for Disease Control. Update: Mortality attributable to HIV infection among persons aged 24–55 years—United States, 1991 and 1992. *MMWR* 42:869–872, 1993.

3. Ellerbrock TV, Bush TJ, Chamberland ME, Oxtoby MJ. Epidemiology of women with AIDS in the United States, 1981 through 1990: A comparison with heterosexual men with AIDS. *JAMA* 265:2971–2972, 1991.
4. Centers for Disease Control. Update: Acquired immunodeficiency syndrome—United States, 1992. *MMWR* 42:547–551, 1993.
5. Janssen RS, St. Louis ME, Satten GA et al. HIV infection among patients in US acute care hospitals. *N Engl J Med* 327:445–452, 1992.
6. Gwinn M, Pappaioanou M, George JR, et al. Prevalence of HIV infection in childbearing women in the United States: Surveillance using newborn blood samples. *JAMA* 265:1704–1708, 1991.
7. Donegan SP, Edelin KC, Craven DE. HIV seroprevalence rate at the Boston City Hospital (letter). *N Engl J Med* 319:653, 1988.
8. Burke DS, Brundage JF, Goldenbaum M, et al. HIV infections in teenagers: Seroprevalence among applicants for the US military service. *JAMA* 263:2074–2077, 1990.
9. Ellerbrock TV, Lieb S, Harrington PE, et al. Heterosexually transmitted human immunodeficiency virus infection among pregnant women in a rural Florida community. *N Engl J Med* 327:1704–1709, 1992.
10. Centers for Disease Control. 1993 Revised classification system for HIV infection and expanded surveillance case definition for AIDS among adolescents and adults. *MMWR* 41 (RR-17) :1–19, 1993.
11. Centers for Disease Control. Update: Impact of the expanded AIDS surveillance case definition for adolescents and adults on case reporting—United States, 1993. *MMWR* 43 (9) :160–170,1994.
12. European Study Group on Heterosexual Transmission of HIV. Comparison of female to male and male to female transmission in 563 stable couples. *Br Med J* 304:809–813, 1992.
13. Padian NS, et al. Female-to-male transmission of human immunodeficiency virus. *JAMA* 266:1664–1667, 1991.
14. Wenstrom KD, Gall SA. HIV infection in women. *Obstet Gynecol Clin North Am* 16:627–643, 1989.
15. Hearst W, Halley SB. Preventing the heterosexual spread of AIDS: Are we giving our patients the best advice? *JAMA* 259:2428–2432, 1988.
16. Saracco A, Musicco M, Nicolosi A. Man-to-woman sexual transmission of HIV: Longitudinal study of 343 steady partners of infected men. *J Acquir Immune Defic Syndr* 6:497–502, 1993.
17. Kreiss JK, et al. AIDS virus infection in Nairobi prostitutes: Spread of the epidemic in East Africa. *N Engl J Med* 314:414–418, 1986.
18. Centers for Disease Control. 1993 Sexually transmitted diseases treatment guidelines. *MMWR* 42 (RR-14) :1–102, 1993.
19. Padian NS, Shiboski SC, Jewell NP. The effect of number of exposures on the risk of HIV transmission. *J Infect Dis* 161:883–887, 1990.
20. Wofsy CB. Human immunodeficiency virus in women. *JAMA* 257:2074–2076, 1987.
21. Chu S, Hammett T, Buehler J. Update: Epidemiology of reported cases of AIDS in women who report sex only with other women, United States, 1980–1991. *AIDS* 6:518–519, 1992.
22. Rothenberg R, et al. Survival with the acquired immunodeficiency syndrome. *N Engl J Med* 317:1297–1302, 1987.

23. Seage GR, Oddleifson S, Carr E, et al. Survival with AIDS in Massachusetts, 1979–1989. *Am J Public Health* 83:72–78, 1993.
24. Melnick SL, et al. Survival and disease progression according to gender of patients with HIV infection. *JAMA* 272:1915–1921, 1994.
25. Lepri AC, et al. HIV disease progression in 854 women and men infected through injecting drug use and heterosexual sex and followed for up to nine years from seroconversion. *Brit Med J* 309:1537–1542, 1994.
26. Lemma GF, et al. Survival for women and men with AIDS. *J Infect Dis* 166:74–79, 1992.
27. Bastian L, Bennett CL, Adams J, et al. Difference between men and women with HIV-related *Pneumocystis carinii* pneumonia: Experience from 3, 070 cases in New York City in 1987. *J Acquir Immune Defic Syndr* 6:617–623, 1993.
28. Stone VE, Seage GR, Hertz T, Epstein AM. The relation between hospital experience and mortality for patients with AIDS. *JAMA* 268:2655–2661, 1992.
29. Chu SY, Buchler JW, Berkelman RL. Impact of the human immunodeficiency virus epidemic on mortality in women of reproductive age, United States. *JAMA* 264:225–229, 1990.
30. Carpenter CCJ, et al. Natural history of acquired immunodeficiency syndrome in women in Rhode Island. *Am J Med* 86:771–775, 1989.
31. Fleming PL, Ciesielski CA, Byers RH, et al. Gender differences in reported AIDS indicator diagnoses. *J Infect Dis* 168:61–67, 1993.
32. Selwyn PA, Alcabes P, Hartel D, et al. Clinical manifestations and predictors of disease progression in drug users with human immunodeficiency virus infection. *N Engl J Med* 327:1697–1703, 1992.
33. Fischl M, Ricjman DD, Greico MH, et al. The efficacy of AZT in the treatment of patients with AIDS and ARC. *N Engl J Med* 317:185–198, 1987.
34. Centers for Disease Control. Recommendations for prophylaxis against *Pneumocystis carinii* pneumonia for adults and adolescents infected with human immunodeficiency virus. *MMWR* 41 (RR-4) :1–11, 1992.
35. Hellinger FJ. The use of health services by women with HIV infection. *Health Serv Res* 28:543–561, 1993.
36. Rhoads JL, Wright CW, Redfield RR, Burke DS. Chronic vaginal candidiasis in women with human immunodeficiency virus infection. *JAMA* 257:3105–3107, 1987.
37. Imam N, Carpenter CC, Mayer KH, et al. Hierarchical pattern of mucosal candida infections in HIV-seropositive women. *Am J Med* 89:142–146, 1990.
38. Sobel D. Recurrent vulvovaginal candidiasis: A prospective study of the efficiency of maintenance ketoconazole therapy. *N Engl J Med* 315:1455–1458, 1986.
39. Newman S, Fisher A, Rinaldi M, et al. Clinically significant candida mucositis resistant to high dose fluconazole in patients with AIDS (abstract). Ninth International Conference on AIDS, Berlin, June 1993.
40. Allen MH. Primary care of women infected with the human immunodeficiency virus. *Obstet Gynecol Clin North Am* 117:557–569, 1990.
41. Safrin S, Dattel BJ, Hauer L, Sweet RL. Seroprevalence and epidemiologic correlates of human immunodeficiency virus infection in women with pelvic inflammatory disease. *Obstet Gynecol* 75:666–670, 1990.

42. Korn AP, Lander DV, Green JR, Sweet RL. Pelvic inflammatory disease in human immunodeficiency virus infected women. *Obstet Gynecol* 82:765–768, 1993.

43. Hoegsberg B, Abulafia O, Sedlis A, et al. Sexually transmitted diseases and human immunodeficiency virus infection among women with pelvic inflammatory disease. *Am J Obset Gynecol* 163:1135–1139, 1990.

44. Moorman A, Rui R, Irwin K, et al. The microbiologic etiology of pelvic inflammatory disease in HIV-positive and HIV-negative women: Preliminary findings of a multicenter study (abstract). Ninth International Conference on AIDS, Berlin, June 1993.

45. Quinn TC, Glasser D, Cannon RO, et al. Human immunodeficiency virus infection among patients attending clinics for sexually transmitted diseases. *N Engl J Med* 318:197–203, 1988.

46. Hook EW, Cannon RU, Nahmias AJ, et al. Herpes simplex virus infection as a risk factor for human immunodeficiency virus infection. *J Infect Dis* 165:251–255, 1992.

47. Thin RN. Management of genital herpes simplex infections. *Am J Med* 85(suppl 2A) :3–6, 1988.

48. Bartlett JG. *The Johns Hopkins Hospital Guide to Medical Care of Patients with HIV Infection* (4th ed). Baltimore: Williams & Wilkins, 1994.

49. Erlich KS, Mills J, Chatis P, et al. Acyclovir-resistant herpes simplex virus infections in patients with the acquired immunodeficiency syndrome. *N Engl J Med* 320:293–296, 1989.

50. Kreiss JK, Coombs R, Plummer F, et al. Isolation of human immunodeficiency virus from genital ulcers in Nairobi prostitutes. *J Infect Dis* 160:380–384, 1989.

51. Laga M, Nzila N, Manoka AT, et al. Non ulcerative sexually transmitted diseases (STD) as risk factors for HIV infection (abstract). Seventh International Conference on AIDS, Florence, June 1991.

52. Dolei A, Serra C, Mattana A, et al. *In vitro* interactions between HIV and *Trichomonas vaginalis* (abstract). Seventh International Conference on AIDS, Florence, June 1991.

53. Wald A, Corey L, Handsfield HH, Holmes KK. Influence of HIV infection on manifestations and natural history of other sexually transmitted diseases. *Annu Rev Public Health* 14:19–42, 1993.

54. Silman FH, Sedlis A. Anogenital papilloma virus infection and neoplasia in immunodeficient women. *Obstet Gynecol Clin North Am* 14:537–558, 1987.

55. Vermund S, Kelly K, Klein R, et al. High risk of human papillomavirus infection and cervical squamous intraepithelial lesions among women with symptomatic human immunodeficiency virus infection. *Am J Obstet Gynecol* 165:392–400, 1991.

56. Mandleblatt JS, Fahs M, Garibaldi K, et al. Association between HIV infection and cervical neoplasia: Implications for clinical care of women at risk for both conditions. *AIDS* 6:173–178, 1993.

57. Marte C, Kelly P, Cohen M, et al. Papanicolaou smear positive abnormalities in ambulatory care sites for women infected with the human immunodeficiency virus. *Am J Obstet Gynecol* 166:1232–1237, 1992.

58. Maiman M, Tarricone N, Viera J, et al. Colposcopic evaluation of human

immunodeficiency virus-seropositive women. *Obstet Gynecol* 78:84–88, 1991.

59. El-sadr W, Oleske JM, Agins BD, et al. *Evaluation and Management of Early HIV Infection.* US Department of Health and Human Services, Public Health Service, Agency for Health Policy and Research, 1994 (US Department of Health and Human Services PHS Agency for Health Policy and Research [ed]. *Clinical Practice Guideline* [Vol 7]. Washington, DC: AHCPR publication no. 94-0572.

60. Maiman M, Fruchter RG, Guy L, et al. Human immunodeficiency virus infection and invasive cervical carcinoma. *Cancer* 71:402–406, 1993.

61. Maiman M, Fruchter R, et al. Recurrent cervical intraepithelial neoplasia in human immunodeficiency virus-seropositive women. *Obstet Gynecol* 82:1170–1174, 1993.

62. Warne PA, Ehrhardt A, Schechter D, et al. Menstrual abnormalities in HIV+ and HIV– women with a history of intravenous drug use (abstract). Seventh International Conference on AIDS, Florence, June 1991.

63. Stein J, Roche N, Mathur-Wagh U, et al. Gynecologic findings in an HIV-positive outpatient population (abstract). Seventh International Conference on AIDS, Florence, June 1991.

64. Brown GR, Rundell JR. A prospective study of the aspects of early HIV disease in women. *Gen Hosp Psychiatry* 15:139–147, 1993.

65. Casolati E, Agarossi A, Muggiasca L, et al. Sexual behavior in HIV-positive intravenous drug abuser women (abstract). Seventh International Conference on AIDS, Florence, June 1991.

66. Selwyn PA, Schoenbaum EE, Davenny K, et al. Prospective study of human immunodeficiency virus infections and pregnancy outcomes in intravenous drug users. *JAMA* 261:1289–1294, 1989.

67. Johnstone FD, et al. Women's knowledge of their HIV antibody state: Its effect on their decision whether to continue the pregnancy. *Br Med J* 300:23–24, 1990.

68. Semprini AE, et al. Insemination of HIV-negative women with processed semen of HIV-positive partners. *Lancet* 340:1317–1319, 1992.

69. Centers for Disease Control. HIV-1 infection and artificial insemination with processed semen. *MMWR* 39:249–252, 1990.

70. Ehrhardt A, Yingling S, Zawadzki R, et al. Barriers to safer heterosexual sex for women from high HIV prevalence communities (abstract). Seventh International Conference on AIDS, Florence, June 1991.

71. Mehryar AH, Carballo M, Carael M, Ferry B. Acceptability and use of condoms in sub-Saharan Africa: A review (abstract). Seventh International Conference on AIDS, Florence, June 1991.

72. Simonsen JN, et al. HIV infection among lower socioeconomic strata prostitutes in Nairobi. *AIDS* 4:139–144, 1990.

73. Clemetson D, et al. Detection of HIV DNA in cervical and vaginal secretions. *JAMA* 269:2860–2864, 1993.

74. Niruthisard S, Roddy RE, Fortney JA, Chutivongse S. A randomized comparative trial of mucosal irritation of N-9 and placebo (abstract). Seventh International Conference on AIDS, Florence, June 1991.

75. Brown RC, Brown JE. The use of intra-vaginal irritants as a risk factor for

the transmission of HIV infection in Zairian prostitutes (abstract). Seventh International Conference on AIDS, Florence, June 1991.

76. Kreiss J, et al. Efficiency of nonoxynol-9 contraceptive sponge use in preventing heterosexual acquisition of HIV in Nairobi prostitutes. *JAMA* 268:477–482, 1992.

77. Zekeng L, et al. Barrier contraceptive use and HIV infection among high-risk women in Cameroon. *AIDS* 7:725–731, 1993.

78. Gollub PH, Stein ZA. Commentary: The new female condom—item 1 on a women's AIDS prevention agenda. *Am J Public Health* 84:498–500, 1993.

79. Centers for Disease Control. AIDS in women. *MMWR* 39:845–846, 1990.

80. Hoff R, et al. Seroprevalence of human immunodeficiency virus among childbearing women: Estimation by testing samples of blood from newborns. *N Engl J Med* 318:525–530, 1988.

81. Ryder RW, et al. Perinatal transmission of the human immunodeficiency virus type I to infants of seropositive women in Zaire. *N Engl J Med* 320:1637–1642, 1989.

82. Strelkankas AJ, et al. Longitudinal studies showing alterations in the levels and functional response of T and B lymphocytes in human pregnancy. *Clin Exp Immunol* 32:531–539, 1978.

83. Berrebi A, Chraibi J, Kobuch WE, et al. Influence of pregnancy on HIV disease (abstract). Seventh International Conference on AIDS, Florence, June 1991.

84. Hocke C, Morlat P, et al. Influence of pregnancy on the progression of HIV infection: A retrospective cohort study (abstract). Ninth International Conference on AIDS, Berlin, June 1993.

85. Hill WC, et al. Isolation of acquired immunodeficiency syndrome virus from the placenta. *Am J Obstet Gynecol* 157:10–11, 1987.

86. Lapointe W, et al. Transplacental transmission of HTLV-III virus. *N Engl J Med* 312:1325–1326, 1985.

87. Van de Perre P, Simonson A, et al. Post-natal transmission of human immunodeficiency virus type-1 from mother to infant. *N Engl J Med* 325:593–598, 1991.

88. Dunn DT, Newell ML, Ades AE, Peekham CS. Risk of human immunodeficiency virus type-1 transmission through breast feeding. *Lancet* 340:585–588, 1992.

89. European Collaborative Study. Risk factors for mother-to-child transmission of HIV-1. *Lancet* 339:1007–1012, 1992.

90. Ehrnet A, Lindgren S, Pictor M, et al. HIV in pregnant women and their offspring: Evidence for late transmission. *Lancet* 338:203–207, 1991.

91. Bryson YL, Luzuraga K, Sullivan J, Wara DW. Proposed definitions for in utero versus intrapartum transmission of HIV. *N Engl J Med* 327:1247–1249, 1992.

92. Blanche S, et al. A prospective study of infants born to women seropositive for human immunodeficiency virus type I. *N Engl J Med* 32:1643–1648, 1989.

93. Gloeb J, et al. Human immunodeficiency virus infection in women. *Am J Obstet Gynecol* 159:756–761, 1988.

94. Minkoff H, Nanda D, Menez R, et al. Pregnancies resulting in infants with

acquired immunodeficiency syndrome or AIDS-related complex. *Obstet Gynecol* 69:285–287, 1987.

95. Minkoff HL, Henderson C, Mendez H, et al. Pregnancy outcomes among mothers infected with human immunodeficiency virus and uninfected control subjects. *Am J Obstet Gynecol* 163:1598–1604, 1990.

96. Braddock MR, et al. Impact of maternal HIV infection on obstetrical and early neonatal outcome. *AIDS* 4:1001–1005, 1990.

97. Nanda D. Human immunodeficiency virus infection in pregnancy. *Obstet Gynecol Clin North Am* 3:617–626, 1990.

98. Minkoff H. Care of pregnant women infected with human immunodeficiency virus. *JAMA* 258:2714–2717, 1987.

99. Boyer PVJ. HIV infection in pregnancy. *Pediatr Ann* 22:406–412, 1993.

100. Maha M. Conference presentation on pregnancy and treatment. National Conference of Women and HIV Infection, Washington, DC, 1990.

101. Bawdon RE, Sobhi S, Dax J. The transfer of anti-human immunodeficiency virus nucleoside compounds by the term human placenta. *Am J Obstet Gynecol* 167:1570–1574, 1992.

102. Sperling RS, et al. A survey of zidovudine use in pregnant women with human immunodeficiency virus infection. *N Engl J Med* 326:857–861, 1992.

103. Connor EM, et al. Reduction of maternal-infant transmission of human immunodeficiency virus type 1 with zidovudine treatment: Pediatric AIDS Clinical Trials Protocol 076 Study Group. *N Engl J Med* 331:1173–1180, 1994.

104. Sande MA, Carpenter CJ, Cobbs CG, et al. Antiretrovirual therapy for adult HIV-infected patients: Recommendations from a state-of-the-art conference. *JAMA* 270:2583–2589, 1993.

105. Minkoff HL, Moreno JD. Drug prophylaxis for human immunodeficiency virus-infected pregnant women: Ethical considerations. *Am J Obstet Gynecol* 163:1111–1114, 1990.

106. Gallant JE, Moore R, Chaisson RE. Prophylaxis for opportunistic infections in patients with HIV infection. *Ann Intern Med* 120:932–944, 1994.

107. Ocho P. Trimethoprim and sulfamethoxazole in pregnancy. *JAMA* 217:1244, 1971.

108. Centers for Disease Control. Tuberculosis among pregnant women—New York City, 1985–1992. *MMWR* 42(31):605–612, 1993.

109. Centers for Disease Control. Pregnancy outcome following systemic prenatal acyclovir exposure. *MMWR* 42:806–809, 1993.

110. Centers for Disease Control. Recommendations on prophylaxis and therapy for disseminated *Mycobacterium avium* complex for adults and adolescents infected with human immunodeficiency virus. *MMWR* 42 (RR-9) :3–20, 1993.

111. The European Collaborative Study. Caesarean section and the risk of vertical transmission of HIV-1 infection. *Lancet* 343:1464–1467, 1994.

112. American College of Obstetricians and Gynecologists (ACOG). Prevention of HIV infection and AIDS. ACOG Committee Statement, 1987.

113. Centers for Disease Control. Recommendations for assisting in the prevention of perinatal transmission of human lymphotrophic virus type III/ lymphadenopathy associated virus and acquired immune deficiency syndrome. *MMWR* 34:681–699, 1985.

114. Amphotericin B. In *Physicians' Desk Reference*. Oradell, NJ: Medical Economics, 1995.
115. Daffos F, et al. Prenatal management of 746 pregnancies at risk for congenital toxoplasmosis. *N Engl J Med* 318:271–275, 1988.
116. Musher DM, Hamill RJ, Baughn RE. Effect of human immunodeficiency virus (HIV) infection on the course of syphilis and on the response to treatment. *Ann Intern Med* 113:872–881, 1990.
117. Hamadeh MA, Glassroth J. Tuberculosis and pregnancy. *Chest* 4:1114–11120, 1992.
118. Cotton DJ, Finkelstein DM. Determinants of accrual of women to a large multicenter clinical trials program of HIV infection. *J Acquir Immune Defic Syndr* 6:1322–1328, 1993.

Overview of Pediatric HIV Infection

40

Ellen R. Cooper, Stephen I. Pelton

The medical and psychosocial implications of HIV disease frequently involve the entire family. Most HIV-infected women are of childbearing age, and the number of affected children continues to grow. Reduction in the frequency of vertical transmission by administration of zidovudine (ZDV) to the mother and neonate has been demonstrated, and programs to identify pregnant women with HIV disease are in the process of development. The purpose of this chapter is to present an overview of pediatric HIV infection for the adult health care practitioner.

Epidemiology

Widespread recognition of pediatric AIDS was delayed until 1982 because of difficulty in differentiating it from other congenital immunodeficiencies. As of December 1994, 6,209 children and adolescents in the United States had been diagnosed with AIDS, but the number of children infected with HIV who do not meet the case definition of AIDS may be 10 times greater [1]. Approximately 50 percent of children with AIDS have died. Although children represent less than 2 percent of all cases of AIDS reported to the Centers for Disease Control (CDC), this disease is expected to be among the five leading causes of death in 1- to 4-year-olds in the United States in 1995 [1].

Human immunodeficiency virus can be transmitted to children perinatally, through transfusion of contaminated blood products, through the use of shared needles, and sexually. Approximately 80 percent of children under the age of 13 with AIDS were infected perinatally, and 15 percent through blood products. In Massachusetts, anonymous cord blood screening indicates that 2.5 of 1,000 newborns have HIV-infected mothers. However, this rate varies considerably with patient population [2]. For example, at Boston City Hospital, 2.5 to 3.0 of 100 newborns are born to HIV-seropositive mothers. Transfusion-related transmission has become rare since the advent of routine HIV screening of blood products in 1985, but children infected before that time are still being identified. Needle sharing and sexual transmission, principally of concern in adolescents, have also been described in younger children [3–5].

Current estimates of the rate of maternal-fetal transmission are between 13 and 43 percent; most prospective studies show it to be 25 to 30 percent [6, 7]. Women who have previously given birth to an HIV-infected child may be at greater risk of the same outcome with subsequent pregnancies. Vertical transmission may also be increased in mothers who deliver vaginally, have more advanced disease, have a higher plasma HIV titer, or develop primary HIV infection during or just before pregnancy [8, 9].

Preliminary results from a randomized, multicenter, double-blind trial of ZDV to prevent HIV transmission from mother to infant were released in February 1994 [10]. Eligibility was limited to women with a CD4 lymphocyte count greater than $200/mm^3$. The rate of HIV transmission was 25.5 percent among children receiving placebo compared with 8.3 percent in children in the ZDV group, constituting a 67 percent relative risk reduction. Based on these interim findings, the trial was terminated early.

The ZDV regimen included

1. Antepartum ZDV (100 mg given orally five times daily) initiated at 14 to 34 weeks' gestation and continued for the remainder of the pregnancy.
2. Intravenous ZDV during labor (administered as a loading dose of 2 mg/kg of body weight given over 1 hour, followed by continuous infusion of 1 mg/kg of body weight until delivery).
3. Oral administration of ZDV to the newborn (ZDV syrup at 2 mg/kg of body weight given every 6 hours) for the first 6 weeks of life, beginning 8 to 12 hours after birth.

Uncertainties remain regarding the relative importance of the three components of the regimen, its efficacy in women with a CD4 count less than $200/mm^3$ or who have been previously treated with ZDV, and its potential long-term toxicity in the newborn.

The precise timing of HIV transmission from mother to infant is not well established. The virus has been demonstrated in fetal tissue from first- and second-trimester aborted fetuses [11]. Some investigators believe that a significant proportion of children are infected during the intrapartum period. Data supporting transmission during the birth process include the disparity in infection rate between first and second twins (twin A being infected 50% more frequently than twin B) and the detection of HIV-specific immunoglobulin M (IgM) between 6 and 12 weeks after birth [7, 12]. Postnatal transmission by breast feeding has been documented in a small number of cases, leading to the recommendation that HIV-infected women abstain from this practice if a suitable alternative exists [13].

Natural History and Prognosis

Maternal HIV disease stage and viral burden appear to have a significant effect on the course of infection in the newborn [14]. Data suggest that the latency period following transfusion-acquired infection is significantly shorter in children than in adults (24 vs. 54 months) [15]. The duration of the latency period appears to be inversely related to the age at seroconversion [16]. Studies showed that the latency period for perinatally acquired HIV infection can be from 3 to perhaps as long as 8 years [17, 18].

In the United States, there seems to be a subpopulation of children in whom HIV infection presents early in life and progresses quickly. Opportunistic infections are the cause of death in more than 60 percent of HIV-infected children, and 75 percent of those in whom an opportunistic infection develops do not survive longer than 1 year [19, 20]. Of 172 children diagnosed with symptomatic HIV infection in Miami, Florida, 18 percent died before the age of 1 year [21]. The median survival time for children in whom symptoms of clinical disease appeared before their first birthday was 24.8 months, while the median survival time for children who were asymptomatic was 6 years. A more recent study including asymptomatic HIV-infected children found the median survival time to be 8 years [22]. The factors responsible for long-term survival with perinatally acquired HIV infection have yet to be elucidated [23].

Diagnosis of HIV Infection in Children

The diagnosis of HIV infection is complicated by the passive transfer of HIV antibody from infected mothers to their newborn infants. The presence of antibody to HIV detected by enzyme-linked immunosorbent assay (ELISA) and Western blot techniques may not be diagnostic of HIV infection in children under the age of 24 months, in contrast to adults and older children. The CDC has used the classification "PO" to designate an asymptomatic infant less than 15 months born to an HIV-infected mother [24]. The CDC case definition for AIDS in children differs from that in adults by its inclusion of recurrent serious bacterial infections and lymphoid interstitial pneumonitis (LIP) [25].

Figure 40-1 illustrates the decay in ELISA and Western blot activity in children of HIV-infected women who are eventually found to serorevert [6]. Ten months represents the age at which 50 percent of uninfected children revert to seronegativity, and 24 months is the maximum age at which seroreversion generally occurs. Children who remain ELISA and Western blot seropositive after the age of 15 months meet the CDC criteria for HIV infection.

Culture of peripheral white blood cells for HIV, polymerase chain reaction (PCR) testing, IgA-specific HIV antibody assays, and p24 antigen testing have been evaluated for their ability to distinguish asymptomatic HIV-infected from uninfected infants. In studies performed by Comeau and colleagues [26] in conjunction with Boston City Hospital and the Massachusetts State Laboratory, viral culture and PCR testing during the first 6 months of life successfully identified the majority of children subsequently proved to be HIV infected. Immunoglobulin A–specific antibody to HIV was of limited usefulness during the first 12 weeks of life. However, after this time, IgA antibody testing was very sensitive, with 26 of 27 HIV-infected children showing positive results. All of these techniques were quite specific, and there were no false-positive tests. Other reports confirmed the usefulness of PCR testing and IgA antibody assays in the early diagnosis of HIV infection in children [27–30]. Immune complex-dissociated p24 antigen testing may also provide early and accurate diagnosis of neonatal HIV infection [31].

A child less than 18 months old who is born to an HIV-infected mother is considered to be infected if there are positive results on two separate

Figure 40-1. Decay of antibody to HIV in uninfected children born to HIV-infected mothers. (Adapted from European Collaborative Study. Children born to women with HIV-1 infection: Natural history and risk of transmission. *Lancet* 337:253–260, 1991.)

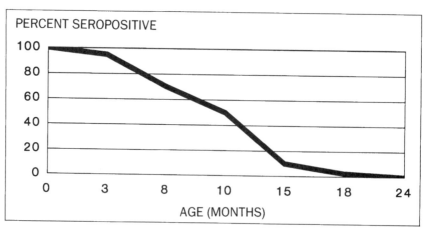

determinations (excluding cord blood) using one or more of the following HIV detection tests: viral culture, PCR, and p24 antigen. With increasing sensitivity and specificity of laboratory detection techniques, diagnosis of HIV infection in even the asymptomatic infant can often be made by the age of 2 to 4 months.

Clinical Manifestations

The onset of clinical manifestations of perinatally acquired HIV infection is extremely variable. Over 80 percent of such children have symptoms and signs of disease before the age of 24 to 36 months; approximately 10 percent remain asymptomatic for as long as 4 to 10 years [6, 32] (Fig. 40-2). Clinical manifestations of HIV disease in children are often nonspecific (Fig. 40-3). Oral candidiasis, generalized lymphadenopathy, organomegaly, poor weight gain, and developmental delay occur in approximately 40 percent [21]. As many as 10 percent of children have recurrent episodes of invasive bacterial disease, including sepsis, pneumonia, meningitis, and sinusitis. Opportunistic infections, including *Pneumocystis carinii* pneumonia (PCP) and candidal esophagitis, may also be early disease manifestations [21].

Lymphoid interstitial pneumonitis, a chronic, progressive inflammatory disease, is sometimes the initial disorder [33]. It is characterized by tachypnea, absence of fever and cough, interstitial densities on chest x-ray, increased serum immunoglobulin levels, and occasionally, digital clubbing, adenopathy, and parotid swelling. Lung pathology shows

Figure 40-2. Age at diagnosis of pediatric HIV infection. (Reprinted with permission of MJ Oxtoby, Perinatally Acquired HIV Infection. In PA Pizzo, CM Wilfert [eds], *Pediatric AIDS*. Copyright 1991, the Williams & Wilkins Co., Baltimore.)

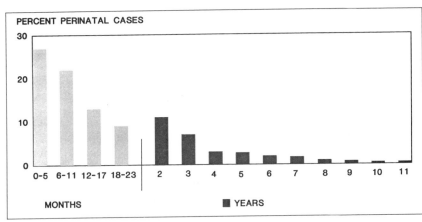

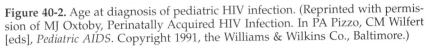

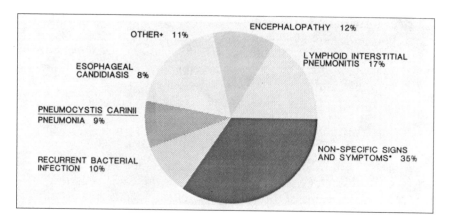

Figure 40-3. Clinical presentations in children with HIV infection.* = Oral candidiasis, poor weight gain, hepatomegaly, splenomegaly, lymphadenopathy, developmental delay; + = other AIDS-defining conditions, such as disseminated herpes simplex, cytomegalovirus disease. (Adapted from GB Scott et al. Survival in children with perinatally acquired HIV-1. *N Engl J Med* 321:1791–1796, 1989.)

diffuse alveolar infiltration with lymphocytes, plasma cells, plasmacytoid lymphocytes, and immunoblasts.

Encephalopathy may also be an early manifestation of HIV disease [34]. Acquired microcephaly with or without cerebral calcification detected by computed tomography, delayed development or loss of already achieved milestones, and/or signs of pyramidal tract disease, such as increased toxicity and hyperreflexia, have all been described.

Heart disease related to HIV infection may manifest as myocarditis, cardiomyopathy with or without congestive failure, pericardial effusion, or sudden death [35]. Renal disease may present as nephrotic syndrome, acute nephritis, acute renal failure, renal tubular dysfunction, or recurrent urinary tract infection [36]. Electrolyte and acid-base abnormalities are common, frequently precipitated by rapid fluid shifts associated with vomiting or diarrhea. Pancreatitis, hepatitis, unusual skin conditions (especially chronic fungal infections), and hematologic abnormalities have also been described.

Organ System Approach to Care

Human immunodeficiency virus infection in children is a multisystem disease that requires comprehensive care by a multidisciplinary team. The management plan should address the medical needs of the child, coordination of care for family members with HIV infection, and attention to psychosocial needs. An organ system approach to selected medical issues is presented in the following sections.

Gastrointestinal/Nutrition

Nutritional assessment is of special importance in the management of pediatric HIV infection. It should include a detailed nutritional history, evaluation of growth parameters and anthropometric measurements, and selected laboratory studies, including measurements of serum albumin, iron, and ferritin. Failure to maintain growth along the child's standard curve requires prompt intervention. HIV-infected children often need some type of nutritional support. This may range from multivitamin supplements to a high-calorie, high-protein, nutrient-dense formula or food regimen. Enteral feeding via gastrostomy tube has proved to be a successful technique when caloric supplements and nutritional counseling have not resulted in adequate weight gain. Total parenteral nutrition may be necessary during acute illness when oral or enteral feedings are not tolerated.

Central Nervous System/Neurodevelopment

Children with HIV infection require frequent monitoring for central nervous system disease and neurodevelopmental abnormalities. A neurologic examination and neurodevelopmental assessment should be obtained as part of the initial evaluation. Computed tomography or magnetic resonance imaging of the head is performed in children with neurologic or developmental abnormalities. Reevaluation of neurodevelopment at regular intervals is important for monitoring disease progression. Individualized treatment strategies should be developed for each child. Ongoing assessment for supportive services, including home-based occupational therapy, physical therapy, and speech therapy, is an important aspect of care.

Pulmonary

Careful respiratory assessment is an important part of the clinical evaluation. Because of an increased risk of tuberculosis, a skin test (purified protein derivative [PPD]) with control panel should be performed every 6 months in HIV-infected children who previously tested negative; anergy may develop over time as a result of waning immune function. Early identification of lung disease is facilitated by monitoring chest radiographs, pulse oximetry, and pulmonary function.

Cardiovascular

Myocardial dysfunction is sometimes first identified during periods of acute illness, when anemia, hypoxemia, or sepsis produces cardiac decompensation. HIV-infected children with acute illness or chronic pulmonary disease require close monitoring of cardiac function. Electrocardiographic screening should be performed in these settings; children with dysrhythmias may require Holter monitoring. Echocardiography is useful to detect ventricular or valvular dysfunction, hypertrophy or dilation of heart chambers, and pericardial effusion.

Renal

Because of the increased risk of renal disease and urinary tract infection in HIV-infected children, blood pressure measurements, urinalysis, and renal function and electrolyte tests should be monitored.

Hematologic

Initial and follow-up measurements of the complete blood cell count to identify hematologic abnormalities are an important component of care. Anemia, neutropenia, and lymphopenia may be caused by progression of HIV disease or drug-induced bone marrow suppression.

Other Organ Systems

Screening ophthalmologic examinations are necessary for early identification and treatment of cytomegalovirus (CMV) retinitis. Nonspecific HIV-associated retinal lesions have also been described, and uveitis has been reported as a toxicity of rifabutin therapy. Hearing evaluation should be performed in the child who has a history of recurrent otitis media. Routine dental care is important for the early diagnosis of oral lesions and dental decay, as is close inspection of skin for infectious, neoplastic, or drug-induced eruptions.

Common Diagnostic Issues

Fever

An acute febrile illness in an HIV-infected child may represent a serious bacterial infection, a life-threatening opportunistic disease, or a self-limited condition. HIV infection is associated with both cellular and humoral immune defects, and vaccines may fail to induce protective levels of antibody. HIV-infected children may suffer serious bacterial infections, including sepsis, meningitis, pneumonia, visceral abscess, urinary tract infection, and cellulitis. As in other children, encapsulated bacteria, such as *Haemophilus influenzae* type b and *Streptococcus pneumoniae*, are frequent pathogens; gram-negative enteric bacilli may also cause invasive disease [37]. Common opportunistic diseases to which they are prone include mucocutaneous candidiasis, tuberculosis, PCP, and CMV infection. HIV-infected children are also at risk for recurrent typical childhood infections, including otitis media, sinusitis, and purulent nasopharyngitis [38].

The initial evaluation of the HIV-infected child with fever should have three goals: to assess the severity of illness, to identify a likely focus of infection, and to determine its microbiologic etiology. The majority of bacteremic episodes are not associated with localized infection and are manifested by nonspecific findings, such as decreased feeding, lethargy, or irritability [20].

Special attention is given to the head and neck, skin, respiratory, and gastrointestinal examinations. Identification of thrush generally indicates poor cellular immune function and increases suspicion of esophageal candidiasis if vomiting, anorexia, or painful swallowing is present. Tachypnea and abnormal auscultatory findings suggest a respiratory focus, such as bacterial pneumonia, PCP, or LIP. Vomiting and abdominal pain may be associated with hepatitis or pancreatitis related to HIV infection or drug therapy. Urinary tract infection is frequently manifested by nonspecific symptoms such as abdominal pain and diarrhea.

Initial laboratory evaluation consists of complete blood cell count, blood cultures, urinalysis, and urine culture. Oximetry and chest x-ray studies are indicated when respiratory symptoms or signs are present. Additional diagnostic tests, such as lumbar puncture, esophagoscopy, or needle aspiration, are individualized based on history and physical examination.

If the child is clinically stable, has a normal white blood cell count and baseline oxygenation, and the family can reliably observe him or her, initial outpatient management is appropriate. In the absence of specific focal findings, following appropriate cultures, a single dose of ceftriaxone or other age-appropriate antibiotic can be administered, and a return visit arranged within 48 hours.

When unusual pathogens are suggested by history or physical examination, meningitis is suspected because of irritability or lethargy, or fever occurs in the presence of a permanent intravascular catheter, hospitalization is necessary. Empiric therapy consists of a parenteral antistaphylococcal penicillin in combination with a third-generation cephalosporin. In children on chronic antibiotics or in regions where pneumococcal resistance is a problem, consideration should be given to adding vancomycin to the regimen. Despite earlier concerns, acetaminophen is now considered safe for the treatment of febrile episodes in patients receiving ZDV [39]. Response of bacterial diseases to antimicrobial therapy in HIV-infected children should be carefully monitored. One report described the failure of amoxicillin in more than 50 percent of children with otitis media, despite in vitro sensitivity of pathogens to the drug [40].

Respiratory Symptoms

Children with HIV infection are at risk for common respiratory pathogens, including respiratory syncytial virus, adenovirus, parainfluenza virus, *Bordetella pertussis, S. pneumoniae,* and *H. influenzae.* They are also susceptible to PCP, CMV, tuberculosis, *Mycobacterium avium* complex infection, candidiasis, and LIP. When an HIV-infected child has respiratory symptoms, initial laboratory evaluation should include a chest x-ray, oximetry, and blood cultures. An interstitial pattern on chest x-ray in the presence of hypoxemia, tachypnea, and increased serum lactate dehydrogenase level suggests PCP but does not exclude other diagnoses. A nasal wash or deep tracheal aspirate should be obtained for viral and bacterial cultures, as well as silver stain or fluorescent antibody stain for PCP.

Age-appropriate antimicrobial therapy, such as ceftriaxone, should be empirically started. In addition, trimethoprim-sulfamethoxazole (TMP-SMX) should be administered if clinical or radiologic findings suggest PCP. If the etiology remains unclear after 24 to 48 hours and the child's condition does not improve significantly, plans should be made to perform bronchoscopy or open lung biopsy. Clinically active LIP, marked by tachypnea and hypoxia, is an indication for corticosteroid therapy. The dose of oral prednisone is gradually tapered to alternate-day therapy after clinical improvement.

Common Therapeutic Issues

Mucocutaneous Candidiasis

Mucocutaneous candidiasis is one of the most common manifestations of pediatric HIV infection. Initial treatment of oropharyngeal candidiasis includes the use of nystatin suspension or clotrimazole troches. Systemic therapy with ketoconazole or fluconazole is necessary for relapsing disease or esophageal involvement documented by endoscopy. Many children will require maintenance therapy to avoid recurrences. Cutaneous candidiasis may present as diaper dermatitis or inflammation in skinfold areas. Treatment requires meticulous hygiene and frequent diaper changes in addition to a topical antifungal agent.

Pneumocystis Prophylaxis

Pneumocystic carinii pneumonia occurs most often in infants aged 3 to 6 months with perinatally acquired HIV infection. Initial guidelines for PCP prophylaxis in children were published by the CDC in 1991 [41]. However, the continued occurrence of PCP in this age group and in children less than 5 months old who had CD4 lymphocyte counts greater than $1,500/mm^3$ prompted a reassessment of the guidelines, and in April 1995 revised recommendations were published [42]. These guidelines cite failure to identify the at-risk status of children in 59 percent of PCP episodes as the major reason no decrease in the number of new cases was achieved. In young infants, almost 25 percent of the cases had CD4 cell counts higher than 1500/mm³, the previously recommended level for starting prophylaxis.

The revised guidelines stress the need for early identification of infants born to HIV-infected mothers, prompt evaluation and monitoring of HIV-infection status with viral culture or PCR, and initiation of PCP prophylaxis in all at-risk infants beginning at age 4 to 6 weeks (Table 40-1). If HIV infection is considered unlikely (negative PCR or viral culture on at least two occasions, with both tests performed when the infant is > 1 month old and with at least one test performed at > 4 months), and the CD4 cell count is normal for age, then PCP prophylaxis is discontinued. If HIV infection is confirmed, PCP prophylaxis is maintained through the age of 12 months. In children older than 12 months, only those with significant immunodeficiency are continued

Table 40-1 *Recommendations for PCP prophylaxis and CD4 monitoring for HIV-exposed infants and HIV-infected children, by age and HIV-infection status*

Age/HIV-infection status	PCP prophylaxis	CD4 monitoring
Birth to 4–6 wk, HIV exposed	No prophylaxis	1 mo
4–6 wk to 4 mo, HIV exposed	Prophylaxis	3 mo
4–12 mo		
HIV infected or indeterminate	Prophylaxis	6, 9, and 12 mo
HIV infection reasonably excluded[a]	No prophylaxis	None

1–5 yr, HIV infected	Prophylaxis if:
	  CD4 count < 500/mm³
	  or
	  CD4 percentage < 15%[c,d]
		q3–4 mo[b]

6–12 yr, HIV infected	Prophylaxis if:
	  CD4 count < 200/mm³
	  or
	  CD4 percentage < 15%[d]
		q3–4 mo[b]

[a]HIV infection can be reasonably excluded among children who have had two or more negative HIV diagnostic tests (HIV culture or PCR), both of which are performed at ≥ 1 month of age and one of which is performed at ≥ 4 months, or two or more negative HIV IgG antibody tests performed at > 6 months of age among children who have no clinical evidence of HIV disease.
[b]More frequent monitoring (e.g., monthly) is recommended for children whose CD4 counts or percentages are approaching the threshold at which prophylaxis is recommended.
[c]Children 1–2 years of age who were receiving PCP prophylaxis and had a CD4 count of < 750/mm³ or percentage of < 15% at < 12 months of age should continue prophylaxis.
[d]Prophylaxis should be considered on a case-by-case basis for children who might otherwise be at risk for PCP, such as those with rapidly declining CD4 counts or percentages or those with category C conditions. Children who have had PCP should receive lifelong PCP prophylaxis.
Source: Centers for Disease Control. 1995 Revised guidelines for prophylaxis against *Pneumocystis carinii* pneumonia for children infected with or perinatally exposed to human immunodeficiency virus. *MMWR* 44(RR-4):6, 1995.

on preventive therapy. All HIV-infected children with a prior episode of PCP should receive lifelong prophylaxis.

Because of its safety profile, efficacy, and ease of administration, TMP-SMX is the drug of choice. If rash or neutropenia occurs, the drug should be discontinued for 2 weeks and the patient rechallenged. Complete blood cell and differential counts should be performed monthly to monitor for hematologic toxicity. Neutropenia has been a frequent observation in children taking TMP-SMX for PCP prophylaxis, especially when it is prescribed concurrently with ZDV. Aerosol pentamidine in children over the age of 5 years and oral dapsone are alternative regimens for those who are intolerant to TMP-SMX.

Intravenous Immunoglobulin

Children with HIV infection often have recurrent serious bacterial infections caused by encapsulated organisms. Although the majority of HIV-infected children have hypergammaglobulinemia, their response to immunizations is usually impaired [43]. Intravenous immunoglobulin (IVIG) has been advocated by some authorities for use in children with AIDS or symptomatic HIV disease to prevent recurrent bacterial infections [44, 45].

In January 1991, the National Institute of Child Health and Development terminated a randomized, double-blind, controlled trial of IVIG in 372 children with symptomatic HIV disease after demonstrating that those receiving IVIG who had CD4 counts of $200/mm^3$ or higher had a significantly prolonged period of time free from serious bacterial infection [46]. IVIG was found to be most effective against invasive pneumococcal disease and acute pneumonia, but no improvement in survival could be demonstrated. Viral and minor bacterial infections affecting the ears, skin, soft tissue, and upper respiratory tract were also found to be reduced in IVIG recipients [47]. However, a recently concluded National Institutes of Health study suggested IVIG offered no additional protection against serious bacterial infection beyond that achieved with thrice-weekly TMP-SMX [48].

The American Academy of Pediatrics task force on pediatric AIDS recommends IVIG treatment for children with symptomatic HIV infection and a CD4 cell count of $200/mm^3$ or higher [49]. Other groups suggest that HIV-infected infants and children with evidence of humoral immune dysfunction or significant recurrent bacterial infections may be appropriate candidates for IVIG [43–45]. Adverse reactions are generally mild. Patients who experience toxicity from IVIG infusions may benefit from pretreatment with antihistamines or antipyretics.

Antiretroviral Therapy

Zidovudine, didanosine (ddI), zalcitabine (formerly dideoxycytidine [ddC]), and stavudine (d4T) have all been approved by the Food and

Drug Administration (FDA) for treatment of HIV disease [49a]. In addition, lamivudine (3TC) and two protease inhibitors are available as investigational new drugs. Except for ZDV, the experience with these agents in children has been limited. Surrogate markers of disease activity, including p24 antigenemia and CD4 cell count, are followed in conjunction with clinical parameters to determine therapeutic response. Evidence of a favorable therapeutic response includes weight gain, increase in neurodevelopmental scores, and a decrease in the size of lymph nodes and organomegaly [50]. Antiretroviral drug levels, which are affected by patient age and drug interactions, can be monitored [51].

Zidovudine

Studies of ZDV in pediatric patients were initiated in 1986 after preliminary results from adult protocols demonstrated efficacy in delaying the onset of opportunistic infections [52, 53]. The first study in children involved intravenous administration of ZDV, with the majority showing increased appetite and weight, reduction in immunoglobulin levels, and increased CD4 cell counts [52]. Neurodevelopmental abnormalities also improved with ZDV therapy. The largest study of ZDV in children evaluated the efficacy of oral ZDV in patients with AIDS or symptomatic HIV disease. The majority increased or maintained their weight, demonstrated a reduction in p24 antigen levels, and had a rise in mean CD4 cell counts [54].

Antiretroviral therapy is currently indicated for children for whom a definitive diagnosis of HIV infection has been made and who have evidence of either significant immunodeficiency or HIV-related symptoms. The use of CD4 lymphocyte parameters in children is complicated because they are normally higher in infants than in adults and they decline through the first 6 years of life [55] (Table 40-2). The most commonly prescribed dose of ZDV is 180 mg/m^2 four times a day. However, there is considerable disagreement regarding the optimal regimen, and an ongoing AIDS Clinical Trials Group (ACTG) study is comparing high-dose (180 mg/m^2) and low-dose (90 mg/m^2) therapy. Dosing of infants aged 3 months or younger should be adjusted for age-related renal function. In children under the age of 1 month, a 2 mg/kg/dose, and in infants 1 to 3 months old, a 3 mg/kg/dose give blood levels of ZDV that are comparable to a 180 mg/m^2/dose in chil-

Table 40-2 *Suggested CD4 lymphocyte values for the initiation of antiretroviral therapy*

Age (yr)	CD4 (%)	CD4 (cells/mm^3)
< 1	< 30	< 1,750
1–2	< 25	< 1,000
2–6	< 20	< 750
> 6	< 20	< 500

dren over 3 months old [56]. Children receiving ZDV therapy in whom viral resistance develops are at increased risk for poor clinical outcome [57].

The major toxicity associated with ZDV administration in children has been myelosuppression. At the dose of 180 mg/m^2, as many as 26 percent of children have significant anemia or neutropenia that requires dosage adjustment or temporary discontinuation of the drug [54]. Children should have a complete blood cell count every 2 weeks during the initial 2 months of ZDV therapy and monthly thereafter. Dose reduction to 120 mg/m^2 is necessary if there is evidence of significant hematologic toxicity.

Didanosine
Experience with ddI in HIV-infected children has been limited. Investigators at the National Cancer Institute (NCI) published results of a study involving the use of ddI in 43 children with symptomatic HIV infection [58]. Antiretroviral activity was demonstrated after 20 to 24 weeks of therapy by significant improvement in CD4 cell counts and p24 antigenemia. While the number of children enrolled in the NCI study was small, the drug was well tolerated. Peripheral neuropathy was not observed, but pancreatitis, which resolved following discontinuation of ddI, developed in two children. The ACTG is currently conducting a trial of two doses of ddI in symptomatic HIV-infected children who are intolerant of or unresponsive to ZDV. In a preliminary study, combination therapy with ZDV and ddI had a good antiviral effect and limited toxicity [59].

Didanosine has been approved by the FDA for use in HIV-infected children more than 6 months old who demonstrate ZDV intolerance or disease progression after 6 months of treatment with ZDV. The current recommended dose is 200 mg/m^2/day in divided doses every 12 hours. Didanosine is unstable in gastric acid. Oral formulations contain buffering agents to provide maximal absorption. The drug should be taken on an empty stomach, and food should not be eaten 1 hour before or until 2 hours after its administration.

Zalcitabine
Zalcitabine was first studied at the NCI in 15 children with symptomatic HIV infection [60]. During this 8-week trial, antiretroviral activity was demonstrated by increased CD4 cell counts in 8 of 15 children and by a decrease in p24 antigenemia in 6 of 9. In addition, 2 of 3 children with neurodevelopmental delay improved with ddC. At this time, the ACTG is conducting a trial of two doses of ddC in children with symptomatic HIV infection who are intolerant of ZDV or who demonstrate disease progression while receiving ZDV. In the NCI study, no children developed peripheral neuropathy; mouth sores and rashes occurred when higher doses were used.

Possible indications for the use of ddC in children with HIV infection include ZDV intolerance or disease progression evidenced by lack of clinical or laboratory improvement after 6 months of ZDV therapy. The current dose of ddC under investigation by the ACTG is 0.005 mg/kg or 0.01 mg/kg orally every 8 hours. Zalcitabine is supplied as a raspberry-flavored syrup in a concentration of 0.1 mg/ml. It is recommended that ddC be administered directly into the child's mouth without dilution. If mixture with food is necessary, ddC can be combined with applesauce, in which it is known to be stable.

Immunizations

The safety of immunizations in HIV-infected children have been questioned because live-virus vaccination of immunosuppressed persons is associated with the potential risk of viral replication. To evaluate the frequency of serious adverse effects, a retrospective review of vaccination histories in 200 HIV-infected children was performed by the New York City Department of Health [61]. No serious sequelae were identified following administration of oral polio (OPV) and measles-mumps-rubella (MMR) vaccines. Many unanswered questions persist regarding the ability of HIV-infected children to mount a protective antibody response. While inactivated vaccines are generally not considered to be harmful for immunosuppressed persons, concern has been expressed by some authorities that their stimulatory effect may accelerate deterioration in immune function [62]. At this time, there are insufficient data to support this hypothesis.

Based on currently available information, the Advisory Committee on Immunization Practice (ACIP) recommends routine immunization of HIV-infected children [63] (see Table 32-8). Previous ACIP guidelines did not include MMR vaccine in symptomatic children because of the potential risk of live vaccines. However, several reports of severe measles in unimmunized HIV-infected children resulted in modification of these recommendations. In general, MMR should be administered to HIV-infected children at the age of 15 months. In areas where the likelihood of measles exposure is high, children 6 to 11 months old should be immunized with monovalent measles vaccine, followed by MMR vaccine at 15 months.

The enhanced inactivated poliovirus (e-IPV) vaccine is recommended by the ACIP for all HIV-infected children. In addition, any child who lives in a household with an HIV-infected individual should receive e-IPV. Live poliovirus may be excreted in the stool of the OPV recipient for 6 weeks, thereby placing an immunocompromised household contact at risk for vaccine-related polio.

In addition to the routine childhood immunizations for all HIV-infected children, pneumococcal vaccine is recommended at the age of 2 years. Influenza vaccine is suggested annually for children older than 6 months and should also be considered for other members of the household. The need for hepatitis B vaccine in HIV-infected children is individualized based on serologic results, although immunization of all newborns is becoming standard practice in the United States.

Despite strict adherence to immunization schedules, the possibility exists that HIV-infected children will remain unprotected against many infectious diseases. Once it has been determined that a child with HIV infection has had a significant exposure to varicella, measles, hepatitis B, or tetanus, appropriate postexposure prophylaxis should be initiated [49].

Psychosocial Care

The diagnosis of a child with HIV infection often identifies an entire family at risk. Parents are immediately faced with not only their child's diagnosis of a chronic progressive illness but also the likelihood of infection in themselves and other family members. Additionally, they are burdened by concerns for the future care of their family. Parents may experience shock, denial, fear, anger, and guilt. They may be physically and emotionally stressed by their own illness and experience significant guilt for their role in transmitting the virus to their child. The social stigma associated with HIV disease promotes feelings of isolation and fear of family and community abandonment.

In addition to dealing with the stress of medical illness, families often must cope with the lack of basic social support. Social service assessment is essential. Home-based services, including a visiting nurse and homemaker, are helpful to reduce the stress and demands of everyday care. Families may need advocacy related to school and legal issues. Crises frequently occur with disease progression or death of a parent and may require that extended family or the welfare system assume custody of the child.

A psychosocial assessment of the strengths, stressors, losses, coping abilities, and concrete service needs of the family is important. Many children and families require supportive psychotherapy, bereavement counseling, and crisis intervention. Children with HIV infection often endure frequent blood drawing, intravenous therapies, and invasive diagnostic tests and need honest preparation, explanation, and support. Play therapy has been useful in helping them work through fears related to their medical care.

References

1. Centers for Disease Control. HIV/AIDS Surveillance Report, December 1994.
2. Massachusetts Newborn Screening Program, Massachusetts Department of Public Health. Theobald Smith Research Institute, Boston, MA.
3. Gutman LT, St. Claire KK, Weedy C, et al. The epidemiologic intersection in children of sexual abuse and AIDS. In the American Pediatric Society and the Society for Pediatric Research Abstracts. Anaheim, CA: 1990. P 172A.
4. St. Louis ME, et al. Human immunodeficiency virus infection in disadvantaged adolescents. *JAMA* 266:2387–2391, 1991.
5. Centers for Disease Control. Selected behaviors that increase risk for HIV infection among high school students—United States, 1990. *MMWR* 41:231–240, 1992.
6. European Collaborative Study Group. Children born to women with HIV-1 infection: Natural history and risk of transmission. *Lancet* 337:253–260, 1991.
7. Johnson JP, Nair P, Hines SE, et al. Natural history and serologic diagnosis of infants born to human immunodeficiency virus–infected women. *Am J Dis Child* 143:1147–1153, 1989.
8. The European Collaborative Study. Caesarean section and the risk of vertical transmission of HIV-1 infection. *Lancet* 343:1464–1467, 1994.
9. Boyer P, et al. Factors predictive of maternal-fetal transmission of HIV-1. *JAMA* 271:1925–1930, 1994.
10. Centers for Disease Control. Zidovudine for the prevention of HIV transmission from mother to infant. *MMWR* 43(16):285–287, 1994.
11. Sprecher S, Soumenkoff G, Puissant F, et al. Vertical transmission of HIV in 15-week fetus. *Lancet* 2:288–289, 1986.
12. Goedert JJ, Duliege AM, Amos CI, et al. High risk of HIV-1 infection for first-born twins. *Lancet* 338:1471–1475, 1991.
13. Zregler JB, Stewart GJ, Penny R, et al. Breastfeeding and transmission of HIV from mother to infant. Fourth International Conference on AIDS, Stockholm, June 1988.
14. Blanche S, et al. Relation of the course of HIV infection in children to the severity of the disease in their mothers at delivery. *N Engl J Med* 330:308–312, 1994.
15. Rogers MF, Thomas PA, Starcher ET, et al. AIDS in children: Report of the CDC national surveillance 1982–1985. *Pediatrics* 79:1008–1014, 1987.
16. Medley GF, Anderson RM, Cox DR, et al. Incubation period of AIDS in patients infected via blood transfusions. *Nature* 328:719–721, 1987.
17. Centers for Disease Control. Revision of the CDC surveillance case definition for AIDS. *MMWR* 36 (suppl 15):3–15, 1987.
18. MaWhinney S, Pagano M. Incubation time for vertically infected AIDS. Seventh International Conference on AIDS, Florence, June 1991.
19. Lampert R, Milben J, O'Donnell R, et al. Life table analysis of children with AIDS. *Pediatr Infect Dis J* 5:374–375, 1986.

20. Krasinski K, Borkowsky W, Bork S, et al. Bacterial infection in HIV-infected children. *Pediatr Infect Dis J* 7:323, 1988.
21. Scott GB, Hutto C, Makuch RW, et al. Survival in children with perinatally acquired HIV-1. *N Engl J Med* 321:1791–1796, 1989.
22. Tovo PA, et al. Prognostic factors and survival in children with perinatal HIV-1 infection. *Lancet* 339:1249–1253, 1992.
23. The Italian Register for HIV Infection in Children. Features in children perinatally infected with HIV-1 surviving longer than 5 years. *Lancet* 343:191–194, 1994.
24. Centers for Disease Control. Classification system for HIV infection in children under 13 years of age. *MMWR* 36:225–236, 1987.
25. Centers for Disease Control. Revision of CDC surveillance case definition for acquired immunodeficiency syndrome. *MMWR* 36:3S–15S, 1987.
26. Comeau AM, Harris JS, McIntosh K, et al. Polymerase chain reaction in detecting HIV infection among seropositive infants: Relation to clinical status and age and to results of other assays. *J Acquir Immune Defic Syndr* 5:271–278, 1992.
27. Cassol SA, et al. Diagnosis of vertical HIV-1 transmission using the polymerase chain reaction and dried blood spot specimens. *J Acquir Immune Defic Syndr* 5:113–119, 1992.
28. Comeau AM, et al. Polymerase chain reaction in detecting HIV infection among seropositive infants: Relation to clinical status and age and to results of other assays. *J Acquir Immune Defic Syndr* 5:271–278, 1992.
29. Quinn TC, et al. Early diagnosis of perinatal HIV infection by detection of viral specific IgA antibodies. *JAMA* 266:3439–3442, 1991.
30. Landesman S, et al. Clinical utility of HIV-IgA immunoblot assay in the early diagnosis of perinatal HIV infection. *JAMA* 266:3443–3446, 1991.
31. Miles SA, et al. Rapid serologic testing with immune-complex-dissociated HIV p24 antigen for early detection of HIV in neonates. *N Engl J Med* 328:297–302, 1993.
32. Oxtoby MJ. Perinatally Acquired HIV Infection. In PA Pizzo, CM Wilfert (eds), *Pediatric AIDS: The Challenge of HIV Infection in Infants, Children and Adolescents*. Baltimore: Williams & Wilkins, 1991.
33. Connor EM, Marquis I, Oleske JM. Lymphoid Interstitial Pneumonitis. In PA Pizzo, CM Wilfert (eds), *Pediatric AIDS: The Challenge of HIV Infection in Infants, Children and Adolescents*. Baltimore: Williams & Wilkins, 1991.
34. Brouwers P, Belman AL, Epstein LG. Central Nervous System Involvement: Manifestations and Evaluation. In PA Pizzo, CM Wilfert (eds), *Pediatric AIDS: The Challenge of HIV Infection in Infants, Children and Adolescents*. Baltimore: Williams & Wilkins, 1991.
35. Kavanaugh-McHugh A, Ruff AJ, Rowe SA, et al. Cardiovascular Manifestations. In PA Pizzo, CM Wilfert (eds), *Pediatric AIDS: The Challenge of HIV Infection in Infants, Children and Adolescents*. Baltimore: Williams & Wilkins, 1991.
36. Salcedo JR, Conner EM, Oleske JM. Renal Complications. In PA Pizzo, CM Wilfert (eds), *Pediatric AIDS: The Challenge of HIV Infection in Infants, Children and Adolescents*. Baltimore: Williams & Wilkins, 1991.
37. Bernstein LT, Krieger BZ, Novick B, et al. Bacterial infection in the ac-

quired immunodeficiency syndrome of children. *Pediatr Infect Dis J* 4:472–475, 1985.

38. Barnett ED, Klein JO, Pelton SI, Luginbuhl LM. Otitis media in children born to HIV infected mothers. *Pediatr Infect Dis J* 11:360–364, 1992.

39. Steffe EM, King JH, Inciardo JK, et al. The effect of acetaminophen on zidovudine metabolism in HIV-infected patients. *J Acquir Immune Defic Syndr* 3:691–694, 1990.

40. Principi N, Marchisio P, Tornaghi R, et al. Acute otitis media in human immunodeficiency virus–infected children. *Pediatrics* 88:566–571, 1991.

41. Centers for Disease Control. Guidelines for prophylaxis against *Pneumocystis carinii* pneumonia for children infected with human immunodeficiency virus. *MMWR* 40 (RR-2):1–13, 1991.

42. Centers for Disease Control. 1995 Revised guidelines for prophylaxis against *Pneumocystis carinii* pneumonia for children infected with or perinatally exposed to human immunodeficiency virus. *MMWR* 44(RR-4):1–11, 1995.

43. Berkman SA, Lee ML, Gale RP. Clinical uses of intravenous immunoglobulins. *Ann Intern Med* 112:278–292, 1990.

44. Calvell TA, Rubinstein A. Intravenous gamma-globulin in infant acquired immunodeficiency syndrome. *Pediatr Infect Dis J* 5 (suppl):S207–S210, 1986.

45. Gupta A, Novick BE, Rubinstein A. Restoration of suppressor T-cell functions in children with AIDS following intravenous gamma globulin treatment. *Am J Dis Child* 140:143–146, 1986.

46. The National Institute of Child Health and Human Development Intravenous Immunoglobulin Study Group. Intravenous immune globulin for the prevention of bacterial infections in children with symptomatic human immunodeficiency virus infection. *N Engl J Med* 325:73–80, 1991.

47. Mofenson LM. Prophylactic intravenous immunoglobulin in HIV-infected children with CD4 counts of 0.20 X 10^9/L or more. *JAMA* 268:483–488, 1992.

48. Spector SA, et al. A controlled trial of intravenous immune globulin for the prevention of serious bacterial infections in children receiving zidovudine for advanced HIV infection. *N Engl J Med* 331:1181–1187, 1994.

49. American Academy of Pediatrics. *Report of the Committee on Infectious Diseases* (22nd ed), 1991.

49a. Pizzo PA, Wilfert C. Antiretroviral therapy for infection due to HIV in children. *Clin Infect Dis* 19:177–196, 1994.

50. Pizzo PA, Wilfert C. Treatment Considerations for Children with HIV Infection. In PA Pizzo, CM Wilfert (eds), *Pediatric AIDS: The Challenge of HIV Infection in Infants, Children and Adolescents*. Baltimore: Williams & Wilkins, 1991.

51. Balis FM, Blaney SM, Poplack DG. Antiretroviral drug development and clinical pharmacology. *Pediatr Infect Dis J* 10:849–857, 1991.

52. Pizzo PA, Eddy J, Falloon J, et al. Effect of continuous intravenous infusion of zidovudine in children with symptomatic HIV infection. *N Engl J Med* 319:889–896, 1988.

53. McKinney PE, Pizzo PA, Scott GB, et al. Safety and tolerance of intermittent intravenous and oral zidovudine therapy in human immunodeficiency

virus infected pediatric patients: A phase I study. *J Pediatr* 116:641–647, 1990.

54. McKinney RE Jr, Maha MA, Connor EM, et al. A multicenter trial of oral zidovudine in children with advanced human immunodeficiency virus disease. *N Engl J Med* 324:1018–1025, 1991.

55. Working Group on Antiretroviral Therapy, National Pediatric HIV Resource Center. Antiretroviral therapy and medical management of the human immunodeficiency virus-infected child. *Pediatr AIDS HIV Infect Fetus Adolesc* 5(1):20–32, 1994.

56. Boucher FD, Mudlin JA, Ruff A, et al. A phase one evaluation of zidovudine administered to infants exposed at birth to the human immunodeficiency virus. *J Pediatr* 122:137–144, 1993.

57. Tudor-Williams G, et al. HIV-1 sensitivity to zidovudine and clinical outcome in children. *Lancet* 339:15–19, 1992.

58. Butler KM, Husson RN, Balis FM, et al. Dideoxyinosine in children with symptomatic human immunodeficiency virus infection. *N Engl J Med* 323:137–144, 1991.

59. Hussein RN, et al. Zidovudine and didanosine combination therapy in children with human immuno-deficiency virus infection. *Pediatrics* 93:316–322, 1994.

60. Pizzo PA, Butler K, Balis F, et al. Dideoxycytidine alone and in an alternating schedule with zidovudine in children with symptomatic HIV infection. *J Pediatr* 117:799–808, 1990.

61. McLaughlin M, Thomas P, Onorato I, et al. Live virus vaccines in human immunodeficiency virus–infected children: A retrospective survey. *Pediatrics* 82:229–233, 1988.

62. Advisory Committee on Immunization Practice. Immunization of children infected with human T-lymphotropic virus type III/lymphadenopathy-associated virus. *MMWR* 35:595–606, 1986.

63. Advisory Committee on Immunization Practice. General recommendations on immunization. *MMWR* 38:205–228, 1989.

HIV Infection in Communities of Color 41

John A. Rich

This chapter addresses the problem of HIV infection in communities of color.* Persons of color, including African-Americans, Haitian-Americans, and Latinos account for a disproportionate share of AIDS cases in the United States, and their numbers continue to grow. Many from these groups are also burdened by poverty, discrimination, and limited access to medical care. Though the diversity among people of color makes it difficult to make valid broad generalizations, this chapter examines possible reasons for the high prevalence of AIDS in communities of color and highlights issues that may be important in the prevention and primary care of HIV infection in these groups.

Epidemiology

Black and Latino persons make up 13 and 7 percent, respectively, of the US population. However, among newly diagnosed AIDS patients, 39 percent are black and 19 percent are Latino [1] (Fig. 41-1). This translates into a risk of AIDS that is three times greater for black men than for white men, and risks for Latino and black women that are, respectively, 8 times and 13 times greater than those of their white counterparts [2]. Though early studies showed that black and Latino persons

---

*The term *communities of color* refers to persons of African, Caribbean, Haitian, and Latin American origin and is used here in preference to the term *minority*. Many of the data presented in the following sections, however, were gathered using the terms *black, Hispanic*, and *white. Black* is understood to include not only African-Americans but also Caribbean-Americans and Haitian-Americans. The terms *Hispanic* and *Latino* include individuals from Puerto Rico, Dominican Republic, and other islands with Spanish-speaking populations, as well as persons from Central and South America.

651

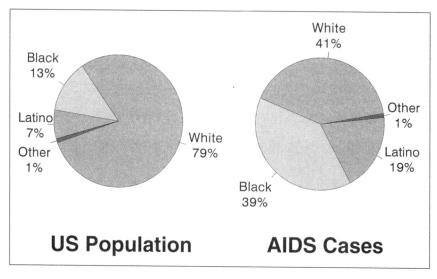

Figure 41-1. Comparison of ethnic composition of the US population and reported AIDS cases. (Data from Centers for Disease Control. HIV/AIDS Surveillance Report, December 1994.)

also had shorter survival times following an AIDS-defining diagnosis, more recent data fail to confirm this difference [3]. Rather, apparent differences in survival for blacks probably reflected more limited access to health care because of lower socioeconomic status [4]. Studies of US military recruits have documented a rate of HIV seroprevalence that is 3.9 in 1,000 for black persons, compared to 0.9 in 1,000 for white persons [5]. However, since enlistment in the military may be influenced by a number of social factors, such studies may be subject to bias and not be generalizable to the population at large.

As of 1994, 78 percent of white men with AIDS acquired HIV infection through sex with another man and only 8 percent via injection drug use, whereas 37 percent of black and 38 percent of Latino men acquired the disease through drug use, and 40 percent and 45 percent respectively, through sex with another man [1] (Fig. 41-2). Also of note is the fact that a relatively greater proportion of men of color with AIDS identify themselves as bisexual (30% for blacks, 20% for Latinos, and 14% for whites), as opposed to exclusively homosexual. This factor may contribute to the higher reported rate of heterosexual HIV transmission in communities of color.

Women of color are strikingly overrepresented among the population with AIDS [1]. Blacks constitute 54 percent of AIDS cases in women, and Latinas comprise 21 percent. For all women with AIDS, regardless of ethnicity, the most common risk factor is injection drug use, and heterosexual contact with an injection drug user (IDU) ranks second. Children of color predominate among AIDS patents less than 13 years

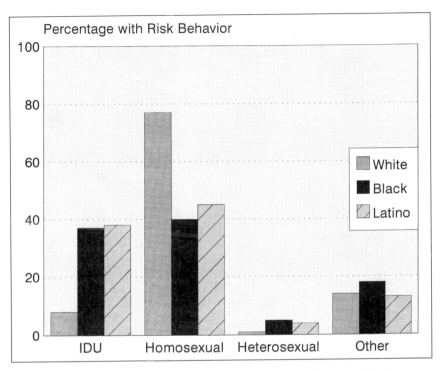

Figure 41-2. Comparison of HIV risk behaviors for white, black, and Latino men. IDU = injection drug user. (Data from Centers for Disease Control. HIV/AIDS Surveillance Report, December 1994.)

old, with black and Latino children comprising 55 and 25 percent of cases, respectively. Almost all of these children were born to HIV-infected mothers [1].

A number of reasons have been cited for the disproportionate prevalence of HIV disease in persons of color. While drug abuse is a problem in white communities as well as communities of color, injection drug use appears to be more common in urban areas plagued by despair and economic uncertainty. Data gathered by the Drug Abuse Warning Network of the National Institute on Drug Abuse showed that more than 80 percent of persons presenting to selected emergency rooms throughout the nation with cocaine- or heroin-related complaints are black or Latino [6]. Since these drugs are frequently injected and, by their very nature, may alter judgment with regard to sexual behavior, they are important contributors to the acquisition of HIV infection. This risk may be further enhanced by the practice of using "shooting galleries," proprietary inner-city locations where IDUs gather and may rent syringes and other apparatus ("works") from the gallery's operator. Needle sharing and the use of contaminated syringes are common in this setting.

Other drugs such as crack cocaine and alcohol may also enhance HIV transmission. Crack has been directly linked to an increased risk of HIV infection through its well-known ability to enhance sexual arousal and inhibit climax [7]. High levels of sexual activity have been reported in "crack houses" (locations where crack users gather for the sale and use of the drug), and the direct exchange of sex for drugs is common.

Other factors may also play a role in the increased prevalence of HIV infection in specific ethnic groups. It is possible that since a significant number of African-American and Latino men have been involved with the penal system, some may have had homosexual experiences while incarcerated. In 1991, 2.2 percent of federal and state inmates were estimated to be infected with HIV [8]. It is also well known that the presence of ulcerative genital lesions may facilitate the transmission of HIV infection, and diseases, such as herpes simplex virus and syphilis are endemic in inner-city, low-income communities.

Despite these possible explanations for the higher prevalence of HIV in persons of color, it is important to note that they do not seem to account for all of the increased risk observed. Several studies have noted that even among IDUs, HIV infection is more prevalent among blacks and Latinos than among whites, even when controlled for needle sharing [7, 9]. Similarly, black homosexual and bisexual men have a higher prevalence of HIV infection than their white counterparts [10]. Far from suggesting any biologic or genetic predisposition to HIV infection, Selik and associates [2] concluded that

> the wide range of relative risks of AIDS in Blacks and Hispanics for different exposure categories, and the variation in these relative risks by geographic area of residence, support the view that the higher risks of AIDS in Blacks and Hispanics are due primarily to behavioral and perhaps environmental differences between racial/ethnic groups, rather than genetic differences.

Etiology: Cultural Versus Sociopolitical

It has long been assumed that disparities between rates of disease for persons in different ethnic groups reflect differences in culture. More recently, however, emphasis has been placed on sociopolitical issues that may have an important impact on behaviors and attitudes. Framing differences in behavior as manifestations of cultural differences is problematic since, as De La Cancela [11] points out, cultural explanation "creates the image of minorities as having certain static, exotic, racial or ethnic features that serve as barriers to their accepting an AIDS prevention message." This problem extends also to the care of patients with AIDS. Such cultural characterizations have led to stereotyped notions about taboos concerning discussions of sexuality among Latino families or the reluctance to use condoms among African-Americans.

Notions of "machismo" and fatalism have been applied to Latinos regardless of their country or origin [11].

It is perhaps more useful to view the problem of AIDS in communities of color in the context of the complex economic, social, and political realities of the inner city. For example, as Mays and Cochran [12] point out, an economically oppressed woman of color in the inner city may determine that insisting that her partner use a condom could endanger the relationship itself. Given the low ratio of "available" men to women (75 men to 100 women for African-Americans) and the fact that women may depend on their partners for both emotional and financial support, the wisdom of potentially endangering this relationship is questionable at best. Important interpersonal decisions appear related to economic and political realities rather than to cultural issues [11]. Such circumstances need to be considered in the education of persons with or at risk for HIV infection.

Similarly, Dalton [13] notes that homophobia in the African-American community may stem more from the unequal ratio of men to women and less from a strict cultural bias. He argues that men who are perceived as having "chosen" homosexuality in the midst of a paucity of available heterosexual African-American men due to incarceration and homicide may be resented for their sexual orientation. Certainly, the strong presence of the church in African-American and Latino communities and its general opposition to homosexuality also adds to the perceived intolerance of gay or bisexual men.

Attitudes about HIV/AIDS in Communities of Color

Much has been written about the difficulties of addressing HIV in communities of color and their seeming reluctance to "own the issue of AIDS" [13]. Clearly, one of the strongest influences is racism. With regard to AIDS, this was exemplified in the minds of many African-Americans and Latinos by the delayed response to the epidemic on the part of federal officials at a time when it was clearly growing among inner-city drug users. Skepticism and mistrust grew further when some scientists insisted that HIV had originated in Africa and when Haitians were labeled as a distinct risk group [14]. These incidents were interpreted by many as an attempt to hold people of color responsible for AIDS. To make matters worse, HIV-infected IDUs and homosexual/bisexual men were often portrayed by the media as being less "innocent" than afflicted infants and recipients of tainted blood products.

Seemingly more extreme are the persistent feelings in some communities of color that HIV infection represented a conspiracy of biologic engineering designed to eliminate those who are less valued by society. Such a view was based on the precedent of the Tuskegee syphilis experiment, wherein African-American men were observed without treatment for syphilis, despite the availability of penicillin, in order to define the natural history of the disease [15]. Theories of a conspiracy to infect Africans with HIV have been advanced by a number of authors and are prevalent in the United States and abroad [16]. These speculations undoubtedly play a role in distrust for the health care system.

The inner city is awash with other issues that compete with AIDS as prime concerns. Economic instability has spawned what sociologist William Julius Wilson [17] termed the "underclass," a group of persons in the inner city who are increasingly set apart from the surrounding community by lack of training and skills, unemployment, involvement in street crime, prolonged periods of poverty, and welfare dependence. Contact with the criminal justice system is common as evidenced by a study that found that 24 percent of black men aged 20 to 29 are in jail, on probation, or on parole [18]. In addition, 300,000 blacks are incarcerated in the United States, representing 47 percent of the total prison population [19]. Violence in the inner city is widespread; 1 of 30 black men now living will die as a victim of homicide. Access to medical care is limited, exacerbating problems of sexually transmitted diseases and infant mortality. High dropout rates from school and lack of economic opportunity may lead to involvement with the illicit economies of drug trafficking and prostitution, despite their attendant dangers. All of these factors contribute to a general sense of powerlessness and hopelessness in the inner city. HIV infection, in contrast, may seem to some an abstract and distant risk given its long latency. Effective strategies are needed that foster empowerment around a broad spectrum of health and socioeconomic issues in these communities [20].

Issues for Health Care Providers

Family and Community Support

Health care providers must be sensitive to the previously mentioned issues in managing HIV disease in patients of color. Many of these patients, regardless of route of infection, depend heavily on family and friends for support. However, given the ongoing stigma that accompanies homosexuality and drug use within communities, patients may fear acknowledgment of such behaviors, and HIV infection may alienate families at a critical time. The situation in communities of color is thus different from that in the white gay community, where there are often better-established means of group support. The lack of an advocacy system for HIV-infected persons of color makes it all the more important that clinicians attempt to identify and foster available social supports [21].

Substance Abuse Treatment

Substance abuse should always be regarded as an important and separate diagnosis. Active use will undoubtedly compromise medical compliance and likely increase morbidity and mortality. However, the choice of drug treatment should be individualized depending on the patient's needs and preferences, which may be influenced by community attitudes. Methadone, although effective for many patients, has been viewed by some communities as simply substituting one addiction for another. This preference for "drug-free" programs is reflected in the difficulties that city and state public health officials have faced in finding sites for methadone treatment. Such an attitude was apparent in the resistance of New York City residents to a needle exchange program in the late 1980s [13]. While the effectiveness of needle exchange programs remains unproved, there is evidence that they may be useful in reaching IDUs who are most out of touch with the health care system. Such programs do not appear to increase the frequency of drug use, but community resistance to them, reflecting AIDS knowledge deficits and attitudinal barriers, is common [22]. These impediments are often amenable to change through education and community involvement in the developmental process [23].

Opposition to needle exchange programs exemplifies the complex relationship that inner-city communities have with drug use and abuse. As Harlan Dalton [13] so aptly points out:

> We as a community have a complex relationship with drug abuse. On the one hand, we are scared to even admit the dimensions of the problem for fear that we will all be treated as junkies and our culture viewed as pathological. On the other, we desperately want to find solutions. For us, drug abuse is a curse far worse than you can imagine. Addicts prey on our neighborhoods, sell drugs to our children, steal our possessions, and rob us of hope. We despise them. We despise them because they hurt us and because they are us. They are a constant reminder of how close we all are to the edge. And "they" are "us" literally as well as figuratively; they are our sons and daughters, our sisters and brothers. . . . Can we possibly cast out the demons without casting out our own kin? (From "AIDS in Blackface." Reprinted by permission of *Daedalus*, Journal of the American Academy of Arts and Sciences, from the issue entitled, "Living with AIDS: Part II," Summer 1989, Vol. 118, No. 3.)

Other important considerations in the choice of a drug treatment program include residential versus outpatient and behavioral versus insight oriented. Individuals who live in settings where there is ongoing drug use and trafficking are probably best served by a program that removes them from such an environment. Residential programs are more costly and tend to be more difficult to find. Programs with a strong behavior modification component may be particularly helpful for crack/cocaine users, for whom the presence of any drug-associated images may evoke strong cravings. Such stimuli may include the site where drugs were purchased, money itself, and even drug prevention commercials that feature drug use symbols or paraphernalia. Usually, these programs exist in conjunction with programs such as Cocaine Anonymous and Narcotics Anonymous, which are crucial supports to recovering drug users.

The Role of the Church

The church, both Catholic and Protestant denominations, is a strong institution in African-American and Latino communities. Much has been written about the opposition of the church to education about sexual issues, condom distribution, and acceptance of members of the gay community. Nevertheless, some congregations have been active and successful in counseling and supporting HIV-infected persons, and these resources should not be overlooked. Furthermore, a number of church-affiliated drug treatment programs rely heavily on religious principles in rehabilitation. Many of these programs have been particularly receptive to HIV-infected clients. Drug rehabilitation programs are most successful when they are culturally specific and linguistically appropriate.

Other Issues

Maintaining access to medical care for economically disadvantaged, inner-city, HIV-infected patients is essential. This requires that primary care providers, nurses, and social workers be well versed in financial assistance programs, such as general relief, Social Security Disability Insurance, and Medicaid, as well as sources of support and assistance from local community and charitable agencies. For patients who are still able to work, job referrals can be an important source of income and a way to maintain independence and self-esteem.

Many individuals from inner-city communities of color have had unpleasant interactions with the health care system and may be very apprehensive and distrustful of providers in an AIDS clinic [21]. The nature of the disease itself and fears about breaches in confidentiality may deepen this distrust. Development of a safe and trusting environment is therefore crucial to providing good medical care. This may require repeated explanations to patient, family, and partner(s) about the side effects of medications, prognosis of the disease, and methods of risk reduction. However, skepticism on the part of patients should not lead providers to abandon efforts to institute effective therapy or fail to consider enrollment in clinical trials. The building of a trusting patient-doctor relationship, even for IDUs, can lead to improved medical compliance and broad acceptance of diagnostic and treatment modalities.

Discussion of preventing the spread of HIV infection is also an important part of the encounter. Language that suggests the patient to be a "vector" of disease is counterproductive and alienating. Many HIV-infected patients have stable sexual partners and are concerned about spreading the virus to others. For those not in monogamous relationships, emphasis on protection from potentially morbid infections such as hepatitis B, in addition to protecting others, may be useful in encouraging condom use and limiting unprotected sexual encounters.

Clinicians should be aware of the potent stigma associated with HIV infection in communities of color [24]. Some men of color, because of their denial about homosexuality, may not identify with words such as "gay," "bisexual," or "homosexual," or may attribute their infection to another risk behavior. Use of more neutral phrases, such as "sex with another man," may be more acceptable. Many AIDS patients, already affected by racial discrimination, find themselves further alienated by health care workers who may treat them differently because of their diagnosis. Hospital and clinic staff should be educated about the transmission of HIV infection in order to allay fears. Non–English-speaking persons may be further estranged by their language. The use of appropriate interpreters or, ideally, polylingual clinicians, is essential in this setting.

Finally, any maneuver that can enhance medical compliance should be explored. Data suggest that a history of injection drug use does not predict poor compliance with zidovudine, and the option of antiretroviral and other therapies should not be withheld from appropriate patients [25]. Such simple devices as a pillbox with an alarm can be very effective in improving compliance.

HIV Prevention Efforts

Attempts to prevent HIV infection must focus on reducing high-risk behaviors. Within communities of color, such efforts should target the modes of transmission that are the most prevalent, including injection drug use with needle sharing, unprotected sex between men, and heterosexual sex with IDUs. To date, the major strategies for prevention have concentrated on HIV education and protective measures such as condoms. However, studies demonstrated that among African-Americans and Latinos, levels of knowledge are already quite high [26]. Unfortunately, rates of condom use remain discouragingly low, even among those who know about the specifics of viral transmission. One study suggested that levels of knowledge about HIV are significantly lower among Asians and other recent immigrants [27].

It is clear that knowledge alone is insufficient to alter complex behaviors, particularly in the face of alcohol or other drug use. It is also evident that behavior modification programs must be multifaceted and intensive to attain desired results. A study of a New York program for adolescent runaways showed that behavioral change in this population was related to the number of intensive counseling sessions and that increases in consistent condom use required 15 or more sessions [28]. While this population of largely minority youths has special issues and problems, the study indicated that inducing behavioral change is a difficult challenge and requires a powerful, sustained effort.

Future prevention programs will need to employ strategies that empower individuals to act on the knowledge they possess. This may be as simple as teaching a person both how to use a condom and how to discuss using a condom with an indifferent partner. Other programs have used peer educators in an attempt to break through social norms regarding multiple sexual partners or condoms. The courageous revelation by former Los Angeles Laker guard Earvin "Magic" Johnson that he is HIV positive and is devoting his life to increasing awareness about AIDS may have a profound impact on the acceptability of safe sex and condoms, especially among young men of color who view him as a hero and role model. In his own words,

> I didn't know that **half** of the Americans currently suffering with this disease are either black or Hispanic. Like most other blacks, I was denying that AIDS was spreading through our community like wildfire while we ignored the flames. . . . My doctors have told me that there are more than 1 million people in the U.S.—many of them black—who are infected with the AIDS virus but don't know because they refuse to get tested. Maybe that will change soon. . . . [29].

Magic Johnson's story reinforces the notion that anybody can get HIV disease and HIV-infected individuals may appear healthy. Such realizations are important to adolescents and adults who continue to believe that they can choose "clean" partners and thus avoid exposure to HIV infection.

Conclusion

Communities of color are disproportionately affected by HIV disease. Persons of color, particularly those from the inner city, are confronted with a number of difficult economic and political issues. Such factors may account for the high prevalence of HIV infection and necessitate innovative strategies for prevention and treatment. An understanding of community perceptions about disease, drug abuse, and the health care system is critical to the provision of primary care. HIV-infected persons with limited previous experience with the health care system can be managed successfully in clinics and community health centers.

References

1. Centers for Disease Control. HIV/AIDS Surveillance Report, December 1994.
2. Selik RM, Castro KG, Pappaiouanou M. Racial/ethnic differences in the risk of AIDS in the United States. *Am J Public Health* 78:1539–1545, 1988.
3. Rothenberg R, et al. Survival with the acquired immunodeficiency syndrome: Experience with 5833 cases in New York City. *N Engl J Med* 317:1297–1302, 1987.
4. Curtis JR, Patrick DL. Race and survival time with AIDS: A synthesis of the literature (review). *Am J Public Health* 83:1425–1428, 1993.
5. Leads from the *MMWR*. Human T-lymphotrophic virus type III/lymphadenopathy-associated virus antibody prevalence in U.S. military recruit applicants. *JAMA* 356:975–977, 1986.
6. National Institute on Drug Abuse Statistical Series: Data from Drug Abuse Warning Network Series 1, No. 7. DHHS Publication No. ADM 88-1584, 1987.
7. Chaisson RE, Bacchetti P, Osmond D, et al. Cocaine use and HIV infection in intravenous drug users in San Francisco. *JAMA* 261:561–565, 1989.
8. Bureau of Justice Statistics, Department of Justice. HIV in U.S. Prisons and Jails, September 1993.
9. Brown LS, Murphy DL, Primm BJ. Needle sharing and AIDS in minorities (letter). *JAMA* 258:1474–1475, 1987.
10. Samuel M, Winkelstein W. Prevalence of human immunodeficiency virus infection in ethnic minority homosexual and bisexual men (letter). *JAMA* 257:1901–1902, 1987.
11. De La Cancela V. Minority AIDS prevention: Moving beyond cultural perspectives toward sociopolitical empowerment. *AIDS Educ Prev* 1:141–153, 1989.
12. Mays VM, Cochran SD. Issues in the perception of AIDS risk reduction activities by black and Hispanic/Latino women. *Am Psychol* 43:949–957, 1988.
13. Dalton H. AIDS in blackface. *Daedalus* 118:205–227, 1989.
14. Chirimuita R. *AIDS, Africa and Racism*. London: Free Association Books, 1989.
15. Jones J. *Bad Blood: The Tuskegee Syphilis Experiment*. New York: New York Free Press, 1981.
16. Madhubuhti HR. *Black Men: Obsolete, Single, Dangerous?* Chicago: Third World Press, 1990.
17. Wilson WJ. *The Truly Disadvantaged*. Chicago: The University of Chicago Press, 1987. P 8.
18. *Young Black Men and the Criminal Justice System: A Growing National Problem*. Washington, DC: The Sentencing Project, 1990.
19. Bureau of Justice Statistics, Department of Justice. Correctional Populations in the United States, 1986.
20. Braithwaite RL, Lythcott N. Community empowerment as a strategy for health promotion for black and other minority populations. *JAMA* 261:282–283, 1989.

21. Mays VM, Cochran SD. Acquired immunodeficiency syndrome and black Americans: Special psychosocial issues. *Public Health Rep* 102:224–231, 1987.

22. Schwartz RH. Syringe and needle exchange programs: Part 1 (review). *South Med J* 86:318–322, 1993.

23. Thomas SB, Quinn SC. The burdens of race and history on black Americans' attitudes toward needle exchange policy to prevent HIV disease. *J Public Health Policy* 14:320–347, 1993.

24. Peterson JL, Marin G. Issues in the prevention of AIDS among black and Hispanic men. *Am Psychol* 43:871–877, 1988.

25. Samet JH, Libman H, Steger KA, et al. Compliance with zidovudine therapy in patients infected with human immunodeficiency virus, type 1: A cross-sectional study in a municipal hospital clinic. *Am J Med* 92:495–502, 1992.

26. Hardy A. AIDS knowledge and attitudes for April–June 1989. Advance Data from the Vital and Health Statistics of the National Center for Health Statistics. 179:1–7, 1989.

27. Hingson RW, Strunin L, Grady M, et al. Knowledge beliefs and behavioral risks for human immunodeficiency virus 1 infection of Boston public school students born outside the United States mainland. Presented at the American Public Health Association 118th Annual Meeting: School Health Education and Services Section, October 1, 1990.

28. Rotheram-Borus MJ, Koopman C, Haignere C, Davies M. Reducing HIV sexual risk behaviors among runaway adolescents. *JAMA* 226:1237–1241, 1991.

29. *Sports Illustrated*, November 18, 1991. Pp 19, 25–26.

Legal Issues Regarding HIV Infection

42

Leonard H. Glantz

Unlike any other disease, HIV infection has resulted in a large amount of legal commentary and action. This has occurred for a variety of reasons. First, AIDS has primarily afflicted homosexual men and injection drug users, groups that have historically been the victims of discrimination. Second, AIDS is communicable and fatal. Finally, the AIDS epidemic evolved after the concepts of individual and civil rights had been firmly rooted in the social values and law of the United States. All of these factors have contributed to the development of laws designed to avoid or alleviate the stigmatization associated with HIV infection.

For the most part AIDS has produced few new legal issues. Concerns about confidentiality of medical information, informed consent for medical procedures, and discrimination against people with disabilities predated the AIDS epidemic. However, AIDS has compelled us to reexamine our approach to these issues and has raised questions as to whether existing laws have been vigorously enforced.

AIDS has led to the development of many specific state statutes and regulations, which are in a constant process of revision. Because of this, it is not possible to write a complete or definitive chapter on the legal aspects of HIV infection. Should questions arise in practice regarding the rights or obligations of a particular patient or practitioner, it is essential to obtain the advice of an attorney who is knowledgeable about applicable state laws and policies regarding HIV infection. This chapter discusses many of the general legal issues presented by AIDS and describes how a variety of state and federal laws have attempted to address them.

Testing for HIV

One of the earliest controversies to come out of the AIDS epidemic was the testing of persons to determine their serologic status. Health care practitioners, prisons, mental health facilities, employers, insurance companies, and others presented arguments supporting the need to know the HIV status of individuals with whom they dealt. On the other hand, advocates for patients, employees, and insurance policy holders argued that no individual should undergo HIV antibody testing without informed consent because (1) testing could have adverse emotional effects in those identified as HIV positive, in that they would be learning of a potentially life-threatening condition, and (2) testing could result in a discrimination against them, with devastating social and financial consequences. As a result of these strong arguments, a number of states, including New York, Massachusetts, California, Illinois, and Maine, have required that persons may not be tested for HIV without their fully informed consent [1–3].

The potential impact on the life of a person being tested for HIV is so great that general rules regarding informed consent probably require that it be provided before testing, even in the absence of a specific state statute. The potential risks and benefits of HIV testing and alternatives should be communicated, as should information that testing is voluntary and confidential. Public health authorities have stated that HIV antibody testing should never be done in the absence of appropriate pretest and post-test counseling, and several states have made counseling a prerequisite to testing [1].

Some states have legislated exceptions to the above rules and permit mandatory testing in certain defined circumstances [1]. Testing may be mandated for persons arrested for prostitution and persons who are indicted or convicted of sexual assault or rape. Additionally, some states permit involuntary testing when a health care worker can document "significant exposure" to blood or infectious bodily fluids during the performance of his or her occupation. However, these statutes have significant procedural requirements. For example, in Rhode Island, the health care worker who is concerned about a "significant exposure" to a patient must do the following:

1. Complete an incident report within 48 hours of the exposure, describing the events in question.
2. Submit to a baseline HIV test within 72 hours, with the results being negative.
3. Demonstrate that there has been a "significant puncture or mucous membrane exposure" of a type and in sufficient concentration to result in transmission of the AIDS virus.
4. Have an exposure evaluation group made up of three impartial health care providers determine that a "significant exposure"

has occurred and that the patient has refused to grant informed consent.

Once these steps are taken, if a sample of the patient's blood is available, it may be tested for the presence of HIV antibody. If no sample of blood is available, the health care worker may petition the superior court for an order mandating the test [4]. This complex procedure, which is indicative of the importance placed on voluntary testing, is an attempt to balance the rights of patients with the need for information by exposed workers.

Confidentiality

All modern courts that have dealt with this issue have held that the information a physician possesses about a patient is confidential and may not be divulged without consent [5–7]. This legal rule is derived from a long history of medical ethics and practice, licensing statutes, and the contractual obligations that are implied in the doctor-patient relationship. The purpose of the rule assuring patients that information they share with their physicians will remain confidential is to make them secure in disclosing very sensitive facts about themselves that may be needed to make diagnostic and treatment decisions. Information related to the diagnosis of HIV infection would certainly be considered in this realm of protection.

However, confidentiality of medical information is not absolute, and courts and legislatures have made exceptions to the general rule. For example, all states have statutes that require physicians to report suspected cases of child abuse [8]. Similarly, all states require reporting an AIDS diagnosis to public health authorities, similar to the regulations pertaining to other communicable diseases [9]. Such requirements have never been legally challenged and if they were would no doubt be upheld as originating from the public health powers of the state, so long as the information was protected from general disclosure [10].

A number of states have statutes that specifically ensure HIV antibody test results are confidential [3]. New York includes in its definition of confidential HIV-related information not just the fact that a person "has HIV infection" or an "HIV-related illness," but also the fact that a person has been the subject of an HIV test [11]. States with such confidentiality protections usually require that HIV-related information not be released without written authorization of the patient. These authorizations generally need to specifically identify to whom the disclosure is being made, the purpose for the disclosure, and the time period during which such disclosure can be made [3, 12]. General forms used to authorize the release of other types of medical information are usually insufficient to meet the demands of these specific statutes.

The purpose of these statutes is to limit the disclosure of HIV-related information outside the hospital, not to impede its transfer among clinicians involved in the care of a specific patient. However, health care workers and institutions must be very careful to limit this highly sensitive information to only those who have "a need to know." As an example, in one case, a physician was diagnosed as having AIDS when he was a patient in the hospital in which he practiced. This information was widely disseminated in the health care community, causing his patients and staff to desert him. A court held that this was sufficient grounds to demonstrate that the hospital did not act appropriately to protect his confidentiality [13]. Similarly, when police officers disclosed to neighbors that a person they were arresting had AIDS, the court held that the officers violated that individual's rights and also found the town that employed the officers liable for failing to adequately train them about AIDS [14].

As important as confidentiality is for people with HIV infection, their right to keep this information secret is not absolute. For example, a number of state statutes permit disclosure to health care workers who have been exposed to a risk of infection [9]. Similarly, there are statutes that give emergency care providers or "first responders," such as emergency medical technicians, paramedics, fire fighters, lifeguards, and police officers, access to a patient's HIV status if they have been significantly exposed to blood or other bodily fluids.

Individual states have different procedures regarding how the first responder gains access to this confidential information. In some cases, a committee or physician must certify the seriousness of the exposure. In Massachusetts, an exposed first responder must file an exposure report form with the facility to which the patient was delivered. If the facility knows the patient's HIV status, it may be disclosed to the exposed first responder without the patient's name [15]. It is the obligation of the first responder who learns of the HIV status of a particular patient not to disclose this information to another person. Given the complexity and specificity of state laws, health care practitioners who are in the position of making decisions regarding the release of HIV-related information need to be knowledgeable about the regulations of their individual state.

Partner Notification

There has been a good deal of professional and scholarly speculation about the duty to warn sexual or needle-sharing partners of patients who are HIV infected [16, 17]. Many practitioners who deal with HIV disease believe that it is their ethical or professional obligation to ensure that others are not placed at risk unknowingly. Before determining if there is a duty to warn, a physician clearly has other obligations to reduce the risk of HIV transmission. The patient should be informed about the ways in which HIV infection is acquired and means to reduce the risk of transmission, including safer sexual practices and avoidance of needle sharing. Also part of the discussion should be the *patient's* obligation to disclose his or her status to partners. Failure to provide such information would constitute a breach of good medical practice, similar to a failure to caution an epileptic about the dangers of driving [18].

Having taken these steps, the question still remains of whether there is a duty to warn known sexual or needle-sharing partners of the patient's HIV serostatus and the potential danger to them. The traditional route to partners at risk of contracting sexually transmitted diseases has been public officers who engage in contact tracing. It has not been the individual physician's responsibility to serve this role.

The argument that physicians have a "duty to warn," which means that failure to do so could result in liability, is usually based on the California case, *Tarasoff v. The Regents of the University of California* [19]. In this case, a student told a psychologist working for the student health clinic that he intended to kill his girlfriend. The psychologist and the psychiatrist colleagues with whom he had consulted believed that the threat was real, but did little to protect the intended victim. After the murder of the girlfriend, her parents brought suit, arguing that the psychologist should have committed his dangerous patient to a mental hospital. This argument was rejected by the court because of a California law that forbids lawsuits on this basis. The parents then argued that the psychologist should have warned the potential victim of the danger so that she could have taken steps to protect herself. While ultimately decided as a duty-to-warn case, the court's decision did not focus on warning alone. Rather, it held that once a therapist in fact determines that

> . . . a patient poses a serious danger of violence to others, he bears *a duty to exercise reasonable care to protect the foreseeable victim* of that danger [emphasis added]. While the discharge of this duty will necessarily vary with the facts of each case, in each instance the adequacy of the therapist's conflict must be measured against the traditional negligence standard of the rendition of reasonable care under the circumstances.

The duty, then, according to *Tarasoff*, is the exercise of reasonable care to protect potential victims. In most cases, providing the HIV-infected person with the information described above will be all the "reasonable care" necessary to protect sexual partners. In contrast to *Tarasoff*, which is about a mentally deranged, homicidal man, there is no reason to believe that a typical HIV-infected person desires to harm his or her partners. *Tarasoff* was meant to deal with the unusual case, not to obliterate confidentiality for all psychiatric patients, and applies to a victim who could in no way know she was in any danger. Such a description would not pertain to injection drug users who share needles with others. In summary, *Tarasoff* should not be interpreted as a mandate to transform every physician into a public health officer.

It is notable that there are no cases charging that a physician has failed to warn an HIV-infected patient's sex or needle-sharing partner. Furthermore, no state statute *requires* physicians to warn partners that they are at risk. Several states have adopted statutes that permit, but do not require, physicians to make certain disclosures to a known partner. Once again, it is essential to know the specifics of these statutes and what they permit. For example, in Connecticut, a physician may disclose HIV-related information to a partner if both the partner and the HIV-infected person are patients. Before informing the partner, the physician must believe that there is a significant risk of transmission and must have counseled the HIV-infected person to notify the partner. The physician must reasonably believe that no such notification will occur and must tell the infected person of his or her plans to inform the partner. Alternatively, the physician may request a public health officer to contact the partner. However, neither the physician nor the public health officer is permitted to disclose the identity of the original patient [20].

In states with strong confidentiality laws that contain no exceptions to the requirement of patient consent for release of HIV-related information, such disclosures may not be made if they would expose the nature of the patient's condition to others. Furthermore, it should be remembered that when a statute permits or requires obtaining information for a particular purpose, it may not be used for another aim. For example, under New York law, AIDS cases are reported to the state Department of Health for epidemiologic and statistical purposes. Disclosure by the Department of Health of a child's HIV serostatus to a school board was deemed to constitute a violation of that law [21].

Discrimination

Confidentiality of a person's HIV test result is considered important because knowledge of it could lead to discriminatory practices by employers, landlords, schools, and even health care practitioners. Whether or not discrimination is prohibited depends on the specific scope of the antidiscrimination law in question. For example, while the federal Rehabilitation Act of 1973 has been instrumental in protecting the jobs of handicapped people, it only applies to federal employees, federal contractors, and programs receiving federal financial assistance [22, 23]. In addition to their presence in federal laws, antidiscrimination regulations may also be part of state statutes and city ordinances.

The complexity of antidiscrimination law can be demonstrated by posing the question of whether physicians have an obligation to treat patients with HIV infection. Strong ethical and policy arguments have been made arguing that physicians have such an obligation [24]. In 1988, the American Medical Association (AMA) took the position that a physician may not ethically refuse to treat a patient solely because he or she is HIV infected [25]. This position is notable because Principle VI of the 1980 AMA Principles of Medical Ethics states that, except in emergencies, a physician is "free to choose whom to serve . . . ." However, the 1988 position argues that this principle does not permit "categorical discrimination." While the AMA's position does not set a legal requirement, it does establish a professional standard of care for the medical community. Some medical licensing boards, including those in New Jersey and Massachusetts, have taken the position that physicians may not categorically refuse to treat AIDS patients [26].

As a general matter of law, physicians do have the right to choose whom they wish to treat with some exceptions. For example, patients who come to an emergency room have a legal right to care, and, because of this, health care providers who work there have an obligation to provide it. Furthermore, once a physician has established a relationship with a patient, the physician must continue to provide necessary care or be liable for abandonment. A practitioner may terminate a relationship with a patient, but only if the patient has been given adequate notice so that alternative care can be arranged.

A number of antidiscrimination laws prohibit discrimination by "public accommodations." There has been controversy as to whether a physician's office is a public accommodation for purpose of these laws. However, a sweeping federal law enacted in July 1990, the Americans with Disabilities Act (ADA), prohibits discrimination based on disability "in the full and equal enjoyment of the . . . services, facilities, privileges, advantages, or accommodations of any place of public accommodation . . . " [27]. The term *public accommodation* includes both hospitals and the "professional office of a health care worker" [28]. While these provisions of the ADA have not yet been interpreted by a court, it is likely that this section would be found to prohibit discrimination by health care providers.

The laws prohibiting discrimination against people with handicaps or disabilities tend to define these terms expansively, so that the maximum number of individuals can benefit from them. Thus, the ADA, like the earlier federal Rehabilitation Act of 1973, defines the term *disability* to mean (1) a physical or mental impairment that substantially limits one or more major life activities and (2) a situation in which the person has a *record* of such an impairment or is *regarded* as having such an impairment [29]. Therefore, one need not be impaired at all to be "disabled" but need only be treated as a disabled person to be protected by the law. Thus, there is no question that a person with AIDS is disabled, and even an asymptomatic HIV-positive person might be considered "disabled" for purposes of this and other antidiscrimination laws.

The fact that a person is protected by antidiscrimination laws does not mean that he or she is entitled to a job. The individual must still be able to perform the essential functions that the position requires. Thus, in a landmark Supreme Court case, in which a teacher with tuberculosis was fired from her job, the court found that she was a "handicapped individual" under the federal Rehabilitation Act and, therefore, protected against discrimination [30]. However, to maintain her position she would also need to be "otherwise qualified" to perform the functions of her job. The court found that if a person poses a "significant risk" of communicating an infectious disease to others in the workplace and, if "reasonable accommodations" would not eliminate the risk, that person is not "otherwise qualified." As the court said, "The Act would not require a school board to place a teacher with active, contagious tuberculosis in a classroom with elementary school children" [30]. The court ruled that a finding regarding the presence of a significant risk should be "based on reasonable medical judgment" about (1) how the disease is transmitted, (2) the duration of the risk, (3) the severity of the potential harm if the disease is transmitted, and (4) the probability of transmission.

The ADA takes a similar approach. Otherwise protected individuals can be excluded from the workplace if they pose a "direct threat" to the health or safety of others. To be a direct threat, a person must present a high probability of substantial harm. Mere fear of harm is not enough to exclude people from their jobs. As a result of these types of policies and laws, schoolchildren who are HIV positive can continue to attend school, teachers who are HIV positive can continue to teach, and employees in schools for the mentally retarded cannot be forced to take an HIV antibody test as a condition of employment because they do not present a significant risk of harm to anyone [20, 30, 32].

Ironically, it appears that when health care practitioners are HIV infected, the courts seem to give their employers the most flexibility in excluding them from the workplace. In one case, a person was diagnosed as having AIDS, and the hospital in which this occurred knew that one of its nurses, Kevin Leckelt, was a homosexual and had been this patient's roommate for 8 years [33]. The hospital demanded that Leckelt be tested for HIV or disclose the results of a test he had previously obtained himself, both of which he refused to do. The hospital fired him for insubordination, which was upheld by the US Court of Appeals. The court acknowledged that the risk of transmission of HIV from a nurse to a patient is "extremely low and can be minimized by the use of universal precautions," which Leckelt regularly employed. However, the court apparently believed that, since the potential harm— death—was so serious, the extremely low risk was irrelevant. This court's analysis is generally viewed as incorrect in that failure to assess the probability of harm violates antidiscrimination laws.

Similarly, a hospital in New Jersey suspended the privileges of a surgeon who was diagnosed with AIDS in June 1987. The physicians on various hospital committees concluded that the risk of transmission of HIV from the surgeon to a patient was so low that he should be able to continue his work and did not need to disclose this very minimal risk as part of informed consent. The hospital's president and lawyer disagreed with this finding because of "legal and social conditions." Ultimately, the hospital trustees concurred with the president, and the physician never practiced again. Once again, a court upheld this hospital's action, failing to evaluate adequately the low probability of harm to patients [13].

There are several explanations for these outcomes. First, the disclosure that a dentist in Florida appears to have infected five of his patients with HIV has shaken many people's ability to assess the low probability of this risk [34]. Second, reactions from both the Centers for Disease Control and AMA have made it appear that even the most minimal risks of transmission need to be avoided [35, 36]. Finally, no legal cases have yet been decided solely on the basis of the antidiscrimination laws discussed earlier. For example, Nurse Leckelt was not fired for having AIDS but for being insubordinate. How courts will ultimately decide cases of HIV-infected health care workers based on antidiscrimination laws is unknown. However, it is likely that they will rely to a great extent on how medical and public health authorities define and present the risks of HIV transmission.

Death and Dying

The high mortality of AIDS requires a discussion of the rights of dying patients. Unlike many areas of the law that apply to HIV-infected patients, there is a good deal of uniformity among the states regarding the rights of patients to refuse treatment.

Since the Karen Quinlan case was decided in 1976, a large and consistent body that recognizes the rights of individuals to decline life-prolonging treatment has developed [37]. Courts are unanimous that competent people can reject any type of medical intervention, including amputation, resuscitation, assisted ventilation, dialysis, and artificial means of nutrition. A patient's refusal of such interventions does not constitute suicide but is rather the decision to let a disease take its natural course.

Whether or not to accept medical treatment is seen by the courts as an option a patient is free to exercise, rather than an obligation. If a patient is able to understand the nature and consequences of a decision to refuse treatment, then he or she is competent; that is, a patient must be capable of understanding that he or she has an illness or condition, that treatment is available, and the consequences if a treatment is accepted or declined [38]. Competence is a factual issue in each case that does not necessarily require consultation with a mental health expert. If a patient has a relationship with a physician or nurse, that person may be well suited to determine the ability of the patient to understand the issues relevant to competence.

The most difficult and controversial treatment decisions arise when a patient is incompetent. This is because it may be difficult to identify an appropriate surrogate to make life-and-death decisions on behalf of another person. In the case of AIDS, decisions on behalf of incompetent patients may be even more difficult than in other situations because traditional family members who are called on to make proxy decisions may be unavailable or inappropriate.

However, the crisis situation of having to make a treatment decision on behalf of an incompetent AIDS patient is virtually always avoidable. It is crucial for physicians to talk to HIV-infected patients about end-of-life treatment decisions when they are competent. By doing so, the patient will be more comfortable knowing that the physician understands and supports his or her decisions, and the physician will not be left guessing what the patient would have wanted done.

Every state has a law authorizing the use of living wills, in which persons can state their treatment directives, and/or durable power of attorney or health care proxy laws, in which one person designates another to make health care decisions for him/her if he/she is incompetent. If a person decides to write a living will, it should be as detailed as possible and deal explicitly with matters such as resuscitation, ventilation, use of antibiotics, and artificial nutrition. It is in the area of withholding or withdrawing artificial nutrition that the courts have been most insistent on knowing the patient's actual desires.

It is also advisable for AIDS patients to identify a health care proxy. For example, if a homosexual patient has a long-term companion, that person may well have no legal standing to make health care decisions, particularly in the face of family opposition. Designating the companion as health care proxy grants him or her sole legal authority to make such decisions. It is the joint obligation of health care practitioners and patients to ensure that these matters are addressed appropriately. Legal difficulties that arise at the end of life are generally predictable and preventable.

Conclusion

Just as the AIDS epidemic has necessitated changes in the practice of medicine, it has also required legal innovations. In some instances, it has meant new applications of old laws and in others, the development of entirely new legislation. For the most part, these rules have been designed to protect the dignity and social well-being of those afflicted with HIV infection. Physicians owe it to themselves and their patients to be aware of the relevant laws and policies in this area.

References

1. Field M. Testing for AIDS: Uses and abuses. *Am J Law Med* 16:34–106, 1990.
2. Mass. Rev. St. Title 5, Section 19230-A.1.
3. Mass. Gen. Laws, Chap. 111, Section 70F.
4. RI Gen. Laws 23-6-14.
5. *Horne v. Patton*, 287 So 2d 824 (Ala., 1974).
6. *Alberts v. Devine*, 395 Mass. 59, 1985.
7. Annas GJ. *The Rights of Patients*. Carbondale: Southern Illinois University Press, 1989.
8. Mnookin R, Weisberg D. *Child, Family and State*. Boston: Little, Brown, 1988. P 299.
9. Edgar H, Sandomire H. Medical privacy issues in the age of AIDS: Legislative options. *Am J Law Med* 16:155–222, 1990.
10. *Whalen V. Roe*, 429 US 589, 1977.
11. NY Pub. Health Law Section 2780(7).
12. NY Pub. Health Law Section 2780(9).
13. *Estate of Behringer v. The Medical Center at Princeton*, 592 A 2d 1251, (Superior Ct. NJ 1991).
14. *Doe v. Borough of Barrington*, 729 F Suppl 377, (D, NJ, 1990).
15. Mass. Gen. Laws, Chap. 111, Section 111c.
16. Dickins B. Legal limits of AIDS confidentiality. *JAMA* 259:3449–3451, 1988.
17. Gostin L, Curren W. AIDS screening, confidentiality, and the duty to warn. *Am J Public Health* 77:361–365, 1987.
18. *Freese v. Lemmon*, 210 NW 2d 576 (Iowa, 1973).
19. *Tarasoff v. The Regents of the University of California*, 551 P 2d 334, 1976.
20. Conn. Gen. Stat. Sec. 19a—584(a)(b).
21. *District 27 Comm. School v. Board of Educ*, 502 NYS 2d 325 (Sup., 1986).
22. 29 USC Section 701, et seq.
23. Leonard A. AIDS in the Workplace. In HL Dalton, S Burris (eds), *AIDS and the Law*. New Haven: Yale University Press, 1987. Pp 109–125.
24. Emanuel E. Do physicians have an obligation to treat patients with AIDS? *N Engl J Med* 318:1686–1690, 1988.
25. Council on Ethical and Judicial Affairs. Ethical issues involved in the growing AIDS crisis. *JAMA* 259:1360–1361, 1988.
26. Annas GJ. Not saints, but healers: The legal duties of health care professionals in the AIDS epidemic. *Am J Public Health* 78:844–849, 1988.
27. 42 USC 12182(a).
28. 42 USC 12181(7).
29. 42 USC 12102(2).

30. *School Board of Nassau County v. Arline*, 107 S Ct 1123, 1987.
31. *Chaulk v. US District Court*, 840 F 2d 701, (9th Cir., 1988).
32. *Glover v. Eastern Nebraska Community Office of Mental Retardation*, 686 F Suppl 243 (D, Neb., 1988).
33. *Leckelt v. Board of Commissioners of Hospital District* 1, 909 F 2d 820 (5th Cir., 1990).
34. Ciesielski C, et al. Transmission of human immunodeficiency virus in a dental practice. *Ann Intern Med* 116:798–805, 1992.
35. Centers for Disease Control. Recommendations for preventing transmission of human immunodeficiency virus and hepatitis B virus to patients during exposure-prone invasive procedures. *MMWR* 40:1–9, 1991.
36. Glantz L, Mariner W, Annas G. Risky business: Setting public health policy for HIV-infected health care professionals. *Milbank Q* 70:43–79, 1992.
37. In the matter of *Quinlan*, 355 A 2d 647 (NJ, 1976).
38. *Lane v. Candura*, 376 NE 2d 1232 (Mass. App., 1978).

Appendixes

Beth Israel Hospital HIV Drug Information Guide

A

Note: See text and package inserts for drug interactions and for dosage modifications in patients with hepatic or renal disease.

Drug	Indications	Dosage	Toxicities	Contraindications	Pregnancy category[a]
Antiviral therapy					
Acyclovir (Zovirax)	Treatment of primary and recurrent episodes of genital HSV infection Treatment of VZV infection	Induction: 200 mg PO q4h while awake × 7–10 days; maintenance: 400 mg PO bid Induction: 800 mg PO q4h while awake × 7–10 days IV administration should be considered for severe or disseminated HSV or VZV infection (10 mg/kg q8h)	GI intolerance, renal dysfunction with high-dose therapy; irritation at infusion site	Known hypersensitivity	C
Didanosine, ddI (Videx)	Treatment of HIV infection in patients who are intolerant to or have shown evidence of disease progression on ZDV; ddI may also be of benefit in patients who have received prolonged ZDV therapy Evaluation of ddI in combination with other antiretroviral agents is currently in progress	Based on weight: ≥ 60 kg → 200 mg PO bid; < 60 kg → 125 mg PO bid of buffered wafers that must be chewed or dissolved in water and taken on an empty stomach Also available as a buffered powder to be dissolved in water for oral solution Recommended dose of buffered powder based on weight: ≥ 60 kg → 250 mg PO bid; < 60 kg → 167 mg PO bid	Pancreatitis, peripheral neuropathy, hepatic dysfunction, GI intolerance	Known hypersensitivity; history of pancreatitis or significant peripheral neuropathy	B

Drug	Indication	Dose	Toxicity	Contraindications	
Foscarnet (Foscavir)	Treatment of CMV infection	Induction: 60 mg/kg q8h or 90 mg/kg q12h IV × 2 wk; maintenance: 90–120 mg/kg IV qd	Renal insufficiency, hypocalcemia, hypophosphatemia, hypomagnesemia, hypokalemia; seizure activity; penile ulcers	Known hypersensitivity; history of active seizure disorder or renal failure; concurrent use of IV pentamidine	C
	Treatment of acyclovir-resistant HSV or VZV infection	60 mg/kg IV q12h × 3 wk Foscarnet should be administered over number of min = mg/kg To minimize risk of renal toxicity, IV hydration should be given before and during each infusion			
Ganciclovir, DHPG (Cytovene)	Treatment of CMV infection	Induction: 5 mg/kg IV bid × 2–3 wk; maintenance: 5 mg/kg IV qd or 6 mg/kg IV qd 5 days/wk	Neutropenia, thrombocytopenia, CNS dysfunction, hepatic dysfunction	Hypersensitivity to ganciclovir or acyclovir; severe neutropenia	C
	Oral ganciclovir is currently being evaluated for CMV prophylaxis	Oral dose[b] for maintenance therapy: 1 gm PO tid			
Interferon-alpha	Treatment of AIDS-related KS in patients with CD4 count > 200/mm^3	30–36 million units IM or SC 3–7 times/wk until lesions resolve	Flulike syndrome, GI intolerance, CNS dysfunction, bone marrow suppression, hepatic dysfunction	Known hypersensitivity	C
	Treatment of chronic hepatitis B infection	5 million units IM or SC qd or 10 million units 3 times/wk × 4 mo			
	Treatment of chronic hepatitis C infection	3 million units IM or SC 3 times/wk × 6 mo			

Drug	Indications	Dosage	Toxicities	Contraindications	Pregnancy category[a]
Lamivudine, 3TC	Currently available in the US for treatment of HIV infection through clinical trial protocols. Several studies using 3TC in combination with ZDV show increased CD4 counts and decreased plasma HIV RNA levels sustained at 24 wk	150 mg PO bid or 300 mg PO bid. Studies comparing doses suggest equal efficacy with possibly less toxicity at lower dose	Headache, fatigue, nausea, diarrhea, rash, restlessness, abdominal pain; there are also reports of peripheral neuropathy	Unknown	—
Stavudine, d4T (Zerit)	Treatment of advanced HIV infection in patients who are intolerant to or who have shown evidence of disease progression on other antiretroviral agents. At present, there are no data from controlled trials regarding the effect of d4T on clinical progression of HIV disease or survival	Based on weight: ≥ 60 kg→ 40 mg PO bid; < 60 kg→ 30 mg PO bid	Peripheral neuropathy, pancreatitis, hepatic dysfunction	Known hypersensitivity; concurrent ZDV use	C
Trifluridine (Viroptic)	Treatment of acyclovir-resistant HSV infection	Apply 2–3 times/day to lesions and cover with occlusive dressing	Local irritation	Known hypersensitivity	C

Drug	Indications	Dose	Adverse effects	Contraindications	Pregnancy category
Zalcitabine, ddC (Hivid)	Treatment of HIV infection (with or without ZDV) in patients who are intolerant to or have shown evidence of disease progression on ZDV; Evaluation of ddC in combination with other antiretroviral agents is currently in progress	0.75 mg PO tid	Peripheral neuropathy, aphthous ulcerations, pancreatitis, hepatic dysfunction	Known hypersensitivity; significant peripheral neuropathy	B
Zidovudine, ZDV, AZT, (Retrovir)	Treatment of HIV infection in patients with CD4 counts < 500/mm^3; In some studies, ZDV has been shown to delay progression to AIDS in asymptomatic patients with CD4 count < 500/mm^3; for patients with AIDS-related complex, ZDV has been demonstrated to delay the progression to AIDS; for patients with AIDS, ZDV has been shown to prolong survival	Adults: 200 mg PO tid	GI intolerance, headache, anemia, leukopenia, myopathy, hepatic dysfunction, macrocytosis, fingernail discoloration, insomnia	Known hypersensitivity	C

Drug	Indications	Dosage	Toxicities	Contraindications	Pregnancy category[a]
Zidovudine, ZDV, AZT (Retrovir) *(continued)*	ZDV may benefit patients with HIV-related thrombocytopenia or encephalopathy Prophylaxis of perinatal transmission when given during pregnancy and delivery to HIV-infected mother and after birth to infant	Pregnancy wk 14-34: 100 mg PO q4h while awake During labor: 2 mg/kg IV loading dose, then 1 mg/kg/hr IV through delivery Infant: 2 mg/kg syrup PO q6h × 6 wk			

Pneumocystis pneumonia: Treatment and prophylaxis

Drug	Indications	Dosage	Toxicities	Contraindications	Pregnancy category[a]
Atovaquone (Mepron)	Treatment of mild to moderate PCP in patients who cannot tolerate TMP-SMX Atovaquone is currently being evaluated for PCP prophylaxis in TMP-SMX intolerant patients	750 mg tabs PO tid taken with food; dose of suspension is 750 mg PO bid	GI intolerance, rash, headache, fever	Known hypersensitivity	C
Dapsone	Treatment of mild to moderate PCP in combination with TMP Prophylaxis of PCP Prophylaxis of toxoplasmosis in combination with pyrimethamine	100 mg PO qd in combination with TMP 15–20 mg/kg/day 50–100 mg PO qd or 100 mg 2 times/wk 50 mg PO qd *plus* pyrimethamine 50 mg PO/wk with folinic acid 25 mg PO/wk	Rash, fever, GI intolerance, neutropenia, methemoglobinemia	Known hypersensitivity; G6PD deficiency	C

Drug	Use	Dosage	Toxicity	Contraindications	Category
Pentamidine, aerosol; AP (Nebupent)	Prophylaxis of PCP; AP has been shown to be inferior to TMP-SMX for this indication	300 mg via Respirgard II nebulizer once monthly	Because the drug is poorly absorbed through the pulmonary alveoli; the most frequent side effects are local, including bronchospasm, particularly in patients with history of asthma or COPD; pharyngeal irritation; metallic taste	Severe asthma or bronchospasm, active pulmonary TB; patients should be screened for TB prior to initiating AP	C
Pentamidine, intravenous (Pentam)	Treatment of PCP	3–4 mg/kg/day IV × 3 wk; dilute in 100–250 ml D5W and administer over a period of at least 60 min	Renal dysfunction, hypotension with rapid infusion, hypoglycemia/hyperglycemia, GI intolerance, bone marrow suppression, pancreatitis	Known hypersensitivity; concurrent use of foscarnet	C
Prednisone	Adjunctive treatment of moderate to severe PCP as defined by $PaO_2 < 70$ mm Hg or $A-aO_2$ gradient > 35 mm Hg at time of presentation	Days 1–5: 40 mg PO bid; days 6–10: 40 mg PO qd; days 11–21: 20 mg PO qd If necessary, IV methylprednisolone can be used in substitution at 75% of the above doses	Exacerbation of mucocutaneous HSV infection and candidiasis; increased frequency of other opportunistic diseases has not been reported; usual toxicities of steroid preparations may occur	None	—
Primaquine	Treatment of PCP in combination with clindamycin in patients intolerant to TMP-SMX and pentamidine	30 mg (base) PO qd × 3 wk in combination with clindamycin 900 mg IV q8h or 450–600 mg PO tid	Hemolytic anemia, GI dysfunction	Known hypersensitivity; G6PD deficiency	—

Drug	Indications	Dosage	Toxicities	Contraindications	Pregnancy category[a]
Trimethoprim	Treatment of mild to moderate PCP in combination with dapsone	15–20 mg/kg/day PO in 4 divided doses × 3 wk	Rash, GI intolerance, bone marrow suppression	Known hypersensitivity; megaloblastic anemia	C
Trimethoprim-sulfamethoxazole, TMP-SMX (Bactrim, Septra)	Treatment of PCP	15–20 mg/kg/day (based on TMP component) IV in 4 divided doses × 3 wk; oral regimen: 2 DS tabs tid-qid (dose determined by above regimen)	Side effects are increased in frequency in patients with HIV disease	Hypersensitivity to TMP or sulfonamides; megaloblastic anemia	C; avoid use at term because of risk of kernicterus in newborn
	Prophylaxis of PCP	1 DS tab PO qd; 1 SS tab or 1 DS tab 3 times/wk may also be effective	GI intolerance; rash, urticaria, photosensitivity, toxic epidermal necrolysis; fever; leukopenia, thrombocytopenia, hemolytic anemia; hepatic dysfunction; renal dysfunction, interstitial nephritis; aseptic meningitis		
	Treatment of *Isospora belli* enteritis (isosporiasis)	2 DS tab PO qid × 2–4 wk; may require maintenance therapy following			
	Treatment of respiratory tract infections due to pneumococcus or *Haemophilus influenzae*	1 DS tab PO bid	Some patients with history of mild to moderate toxicity may be successfully desensitized to TMP-SMX (see Table 19-4)		
Trimetrexate (Neutrexin)	Treatment of moderate to severe PCP in combination with high-dose leucovorin (folinic acid) in patients intolerant or refractory to TMP-SMX	45 mg/m²/IV qd in combination with leucovorin 20 mg/m² IV/PO q6h × 3 wk Leucovorin should be continued for 72 hr after completing trimetrexate	Bone marrow suppression, GI ulceration, renal dysfunction, hepatic dysfunction	Known hypersensitivity; severe bone marrow suppression; concurrent use of other myelosuppressive drugs	D

Drug	Indication/Dosage	Comments	Toxicity/Adverse effects	Contraindications	
Trimetrexate (Neutrexin) (*continued*)		In a study comparing trimetrexate/leucovorin to TMP-SMX, trimetrexate had more treatment failures but fewer treatment-terminating adverse events than TMP-SMX (*J Infect Dis*, 170:165–172, 1994)	Dosage of trimetrexate needs to be modified for hematologic toxicity (see package insert)		

Antifungal therapy

Drug	Indication	Dosage	Comments	Toxicity/Adverse effects	Contraindications	Category
Amphotericin B (Fungizone)	Treatment of cryptococcosis, histoplasmosis, coccidioidomycosis	0.7–1.0 mg/kg IV qd	Dosage and mode of administration vary depending on type of infection treated; a test dose of 1 mg amphotericin in 100–250 ml D5 should be given prior to administration of full-dose therapy	Fever, chills, GI intolerance, hypotension with infusion; thrombophlebitis at infusion site; renal dysfunction, hypocalcemia, hypomagnesemia, hypokalemia, anemia; nephrotoxicity may be reduced by prehydration with normal saline	Known hypersensitivity	B
	Treatment of severe of refractory candidal infection (esophagitis and fungemia)	0.3–0.5 mg/kg IV qd				
	Treatment of aspergillosis	0.7–1.5 mg/kg IV qd				

Drug	Indications	Dosage	Toxicities	Contraindications	Pregnancy category[a]
Clotrimazole (Mycelex, Lotrimin)	Treatment of oropharyngeal candidiasis (thrush)	1 troche dissolved in mouth 3–5 times/day	Local irritation	Known hypersensitivity	C (oral troche) B (vaginal suppository or cream)
	Treatment of vaginal candidiasis	100 mg suppository intravaginally qd × 3–7 days or cream 5 gm intravaginally at bedtime × 7–14 days			
Flucytosine (Ancobon)	Treatment of severe cryptococcal meningitis in combination with amphotericin	25.0–37.5 mg/kg PO q6h (monitor serum levels)	Bone marrow suppression, GI intolerance, rash, hepatic dysfunction	Known hypersensitivity; renal failure, bone marrow suppression	C
Fluconazole (Diflucan)	Induction treatment of cryptococcal meningitis not associated with mental status changes or focal neurologic abnormalities; maintenance treatment of cryptococcal meningitis	Induction: 400 mg PO qd; maintenance: 200 mg PO qd	GI intolerance, hepatic dysfunction	Hypersensitivity to imidazoles; concurrent use of terfenadine or astemizole	C
	Treatment of mucocutaneous candidal infection refractory to topical therapy	50–200 mg PO qd			
	Fluconazole may also be effective in the prophylaxis of systemic fungal infections in patients with advanced HIV disease				

Drug	Indication	Dose	Toxicity	Contraindications	
Itraconazole (Sporanox)	Treatment of histoplasmosis; Under investigation for treatment of other mycoses	Optimal dose for treatment of fungal infections in HIV-infected patients has not been established; Treatment in non–HIV-infected patients: 200 mg PO bid	Hepatic dysfunction, GI intolerance	Hypersensitivity to imidazoles; concurrent use of terfenadine or astemizole	C
Ketoconazole (Nizoral)	Treatment of mucocutaneous candidiasis not responsive to topical agents	200–400 mg PO bid; Poorly absorbed in achlorhydric states	GI intolerance; dose-dependent depression of serum testosterone and ACTH levels; hepatic dysfunction	Hypersensitivity to imidazoles; concurrent use of terfenadine or astemizole	C
Nystatin (Mycostatin)	Treatment of oral candidiasis	2 ml (100,000 units/ml) PO qid; dose should be retained in the mouth as long as possible prior to swallowing; Alternatively, 2 pastilles can be used 4 times/day	GI intolerance	Known hypersensitivity	—
	Treatment of vaginal candidiasis	100,000 unit suppositories intravaginally 1–2 times/day × 7–14 days			

Toxoplasmosis treatment

Drug	Indication	Dose	Toxicity	Contraindications	
Clindamycin (Cleocin)	Treatment of cerebral toxoplasmosis in combination with pyrimethamine in patients with history of sulfa drug intolerance	First 2–4 wk: 600–1200 mg IV q6–8h with pyrimethamine (see below); thereafter, 300–450 mg PO q6–8h with pyrimethamine	GI intolerance, including pseudomembranous colitis; rash; hepatic dysfunction	Known hypersensitivity	—

Drug	Indications	Dosage	Toxicities	Contraindications	Pregnancy category[a]
Clindamycin (Cleocin) (*continued*)	Treatment of PCP in combination with primaquine in patients with history of TMP-SMX and pentamidine intolerance	900 mg IV q8h in combination with primaquine 30 mg PO qd × 3 wk; dose may be decreased to 450–600 mg PO tid as PCP improves			
Pyrimethamine (Daraprim)	Treatment of toxoplasmosis in combination with sulfadiazine or clindamycin Prophylaxis of toxoplasmosis in combination with dapsone (see Dapsone)	Induction: sulfadiazine 6–8 gm/day PO or IV in 4 divided doses and pyrimethamine 75–100 mg PO qd; maintenance: pyrimethamine 50 mg PO qd and sulfadiazine 2 gm/day in 2–4 divided doses Pyrimethamine should always be given with leucovorin (folinic acid) 5–10 mg PO qd to prevent bone marrow suppression	GI intolerance, bone marrow suppression, neurocognitive dysfunction	Known hypersensitivity	C
Sulfadiazine	Treatment of toxoplasmosis in combination with pyrimethamine	See pyrimethamine	Side effects are increased in frequency in patients with HIV disease GI intolerance; rash, urticaria, toxic epidermal necrolysis; leukopenia, thrombocytopenia, hemolytic anemia; fever; hepatic and renal dysfunction	Hypersensitivity to sulfa drugs; if necessary, patient can be desensitized	C; avoid use at term because of risk of kernicterus in newborn

TB and MAC infection: Treatment and prophylaxis

Drug	Indication	Dose	Adverse effects	Contraindications	Category
Amikacin (Amikin)	Treatment of MAC infection in combination with other antimycobacterial agents	7.5–10.0 mg/kg/day IV × first 4 wk of therapy	Ototoxicity especially with larger total dose (> 10 gm) and longer duration; nephrotoxicity	Hypersensitivity to aminoglycosides	D
Azithromycin (Zithromax)	Treatment of MAC infection in combination with other antimycobacterial agents	500–1000 mg PO qd	GI intolerance, hepatic dysfunction	Hypersensitivity to azithromycin or other macrolide antibiotics; concurrent use of terfenadine or astemizole	B
	Treatment of bacterial respiratory tract infections	250–500 mg PO qd			
	Experimental for treatment of cerebral toxoplasmosis and cryptosporidiosis	1000–1500 mg PO qd			
Ciprofloxacin (Cipro)	Treatment of MAC infection in combination with other antimycobacterial agents	500–750 mg PO bid in combination with other agents	GI intolerance, CNS dysfunction	Known hypersensitivity	C
Clarithromycin (Biaxin)	Treatment of MAC infection in combination with other antimycobacterial agents	500–1000 mg PO bid in combination with other agents	GI intolerance; hepatic dysfunction	Hypersensitivity to clarithromycin or other macrolide antibiotics; concurrent use of terfenadine	C
	Treatment of bacterial respiratory tract infections	250–500 mg PO bid			
	Experimental for prophylaxis of MAC infection in patients with CD4 count <75/mm³	500 mg PO bid			

Drug	Indications	Dosage	Toxicities	Contraindications	Pregnancy category[a]
Clarithromycin (Biaxin) (*continued*)	Experimental for treatment of cerebral toxoplasmosis	1000 mg PO bid in combination with pyrimethamine			
Clofazimine (Lamprene)	Treatment of MAC infection in combination with other antimycobacterial agents	100 mg PO qd in combination with other agents	Skin pigmentation; GI intolerance; rash, pruritus, photosensitivity	Known hypersensitivity	C
Ethambutol (Myambutol)	Treatment of TB in combination with other antimycobacterial agents	25 mg/kg/day PO × first 2 mo followed by 15 mg/kg/day × rest of course	Optic neuritis, rash	Known hypersensitivity; history of optic neuritis	—; teratogenic in animals
	Treatment of MAC infection in combination with other agents	15–25 mg/kg/day PO			
Isoniazid, INH	Treatment of TB in combination with other antimycobacterial agents	5–10 mg/kg/day, usually 300 mg PO qd in combination with other agents	Hepatotoxicity, especially in alcoholics and persons older than 50; peripheral neuropathy; fever, skin rash, positive ANA	Known hypersensitivity; significant hepatic disease	C
	Prophylaxis of TB in patients with positive PPD or anergy associated with high risk of TB exposure	300 mg PO qd × 12 mo Pyridoxine 10–50 mg PO qd should be given concurrently for prevention of peripheral neuropathy if patient is malnourished or alcoholic			
Pyrazinamide, PZA	Treatment of TB in combination with other antimycobacterial agents	20–35 mg/kg PO qd in combination with other agents	Hepatic dysfunction, hyperuricemia, rash	Known hypersensitivity; significant hepatic disease	C

Drug	Indications	Dose	Toxicity	Contraindications	Category
Rifabutin (Mycobutin)	Treatment of MAC infection in combination with other antimycobacterial agents Prophylaxis of MAC infection in patients with CD4 count $<75/mm^3$	300–600 mg PO qd in combination with other agents 300 mg PO qd	Orange discoloration of body secretions, hepatic dysfunction, GI intolerance; uveitis which presents with red, painful eye, blurring vision, or photophobia, appears to be dose-related and may be more common when used in association with clarithromycin	Known hypersensitivity	B
Rifampin (Rimactane)	Treatment of TB in combination with other antimycobacterial agents	600 mg PO qd in combination with other agents	Orange discoloration of body secretions, hepatic dysfunction, GI intolerance, rash	Known hypersensitivity	C
Streptomycin	Treatment of MAC infection in combination with other agents Treatment of TB in combination with other antimycobacterial agents	15 mg/kg IM qd in combination with other agents	Ototoxicity, vestibular toxicity	Hypersensitivity to aminoglycoside antibiotics	D
Management of GI disorders					
Albendazole	Experimental for treatment of microsporidiosis Albendazole is only available by expanded access from SmithKline Beecham (Philadelphia) at 1-610-832-3909	400–800 mg PO bid × 4 wk minimum duration	GI intolerance, CNS dysfunction, reversible alopecia	Known hypersensitivity; contraindicated in pregnancy	—
Dronabinol (Marinol)	Management of anorexia and weight loss	2.5–5.0 mg PO bid	CNS dysfunction	Hypersensitivity to sesame oil	C

Drug	Indications	Dosage	Toxicities	Contraindications	Pregnancy category[a]
Megestrol acetate (Megace)	Management of anorexia and weight loss	120–800 mg/day PO in 3 divided doses	Rare thromboembolic phenomena, GI intolerance, edema, hyperglycemia, alopecia, rash	Known hypersensitivity	D
Octreotide (Sandostatin)	Experimental for treatment of cryptosporidiosis and HIV-associated diarrhea of unknown etiology	50 μg SC bid–tid; dose may be doubled every 48 hr up to max of 1500 μg/day until control of diarrhea	GI intolerance, injection site pain, dysglycemia, cholelithiasis	Known hypersensitivity	B
Paromomycin (Humatin)	Experimental for treatment of cryptosporidiosis	250 mg–1 gm PO qid	GI intolerance, rash	Known hypersensitivity	—
Thalidomide	Treatment of aphthous ulcerations not responsive to topical steroid therapy	100–200 mg PO qd × 7–14 days	GI intolerance, peripheral neuropathy, rash, fever, eosinophilia	Absolutely contraindicated in pregnancy	X
Bone marrow stimulants					
Erythropoietin (Epogen, Procrit)	Treatment of ZDV-associated anemia Effective only in patients with endogenous erythropoietin level < 500 mU/ml	50–100 U/kg SC 3 times/wk; adjust regimen monthly based on response	Flulike syndrome, rash	Known hypersensitivity	C

Drug	Indication/Comments	Dose	Toxicity	Contraindications	Pregnancy category
Erythropoietin (Epogen, Procrit) (*continued*)	Expanded access data reveal that the anemia of HIV disease also responds to erythropoietin, although somewhat more slowly and at a higher dose than ZDV-associated anemia				
G-CSF (Filgrastim, Neupogen)	Treatment of ganciclovir-associated neutropenia Treatment of KS and lymphoma chemotherapy-induced neutropenia	5 µg/kg/day SC; dose may be increased to 10 µg/kg/day over 2 wk based on response	Bone pain, although side effects are generally fewer than with GM-CSF	Known hypersensitivity	C

ACTH = adrenocorticotropic hormone; ANA = antinuclear antibodies; CMV = cytomegalovirus; COPD = chronic obstructive pulmonary disease; D5 = 5% dextrose; D5W = 5% dextrose in water; DS = double strength; G6PD = glucose 6-phosphate dehydrogenase; G-CSF = granulocyte colony stimulating factor; GM-CSF = granulocyte-macrophage colony stimulating factor; HSV = herpes simplex virus; KS = Kaposi's sarcoma; MAC = *Mycobacterium avium* complex; PCP = *Pneumocystis carinii* pneumonia; PPD = purified protein derivative; RNA = ribonucleic acid; SS = single strength; TB = tuberculosis; TMP-SMX = trimethoprim-sulfamethoxazole; VZV = varicella-zoster virus; ZDV = zidovudine.

[a]Pregnancy categories: A = controlled studies show no risk; B = no evidence of risk in humans; C = risk cannot be excluded; D = positive evidence of risk; X = contraindicated in pregnancy.

[b]Oral ganciclovir is now FDA-approved for maintenance therapy for CMV retinitis in HIV-infected patients. Preliminary data indicate that time to disease progression is comparable on oral and IV therapies. However, there may be a trend toward higher rates of progression from unilateral to bilateral involvement on oral regimen.

Source: Adapted from HIV Information Option, Center for Clinical Computing, Beth Israel Hospital, Boston, 1995. Developed with support from the Agency for Health Care Policy and Research (grant RO1 HS 06288). Data compiled by Drs. Judith Currier, David Ives, Helen Jacoby, Howard Libman, Peter Piliero, and Sharon Weissman.

Rationale, Safety, and Efficacy of Alternative Medical Therapies

B

Immunologic claims

Remedies	Descriptions	Claimed rationale	Safety	Efficacy
Vitamins A, C, B, E, B12	Megadoses	Restores cell-mediated immunity by increasing T-cell number and activity	Toxicity associated with chronic vitamin A intakes over 50,000 IU/day	Undemonstrated
Selenium	Megadoses		Toxicity associated with chronic elevated selenium intakes; toxic amounts unknown	
Zinc	Megadoses		Toxicity associated with chronic zinc intakes over 2 g/day	
Dr. Berger's Immune Power Diet	21-day elimination diet for food purporting to cause allergies, followed by a reintroduction phase then a maintenance diet with a 4-day cycle	Prevents food sensitivity and "revitalizes" the immune system	? Undernutrition Consumption of moldy foods to test for allergy to mold may be hazardous to immunocompromised persons	Undemonstrated
Maximum immunity diet	Vitamin C megadoses	Strengthens the immune system	? Rebound scurvy on cessation of megadoses	Undemonstrated
Herbal remedies	Supplied as pills or teas; commonly used with acupuncture	Regenerates immune system; contains vitamins, minerals, and enzymes that enrich blood	May contain traces of lead, cadium, and beryllium that could lead to toxicity	Undemonstrated
Miscellaneous	Dietary supplements	Strengthens the immune system	? Purity	Undemonstrated

Inhibitors of cancer growth

Laetrile (Vitamin B17)	Strict vegan diet with vitamin supplements	Supposedly destroys a tumor enzyme (ß-glucuronidase)	Possible deficiencies of calcium, iron, vitamins B2, B12, D, energy; toxicities of zinc, vitamins B1, C, and A; contains naturally occurring poisons (cyanide), which may cause nausea, vomiting, headache, or dizziness	None
Gerson method	Restricts all foods other than uncanned fresh fruits, vegetables, and oatmeal; uses enemas, especially coffee enemas	Detoxifies and creates internal milieu hostile to malignant cells	Questionable	Undemonstrated
Kelly regimen	Nutrition supplements including vitamins, minerals, almonds to replace meat and pancreatic enzymes; diet is devoid of meat, milk in all forms (except yogurt), and peanuts	Overcomes putative pancreatic deficiency	Possible deficiencies of protein, calcium; fluid and electrolyte losses; megadoses of vitamin A and possible toxicity; no toxicities to date	Undemonstrated
ß-Carotene	Megadoses	Chemopreventive in animals; clinical trials in progress	No toxicities to date	Some inhibition of cancer promotion in experimental animals; none yet in humans

Remedies	Descriptions	Claimed rationale	Safety	Efficacy
Inhibitors of cancer growth (*continued*)				
Colonic irrigation	Enema performed by passing a rubber tube into rectum (up to 20–30 in) and pumping approximately 20+ gallons of warm water through tube (sometimes coffee or herbs are used)	Detoxifies the body, cleansing it of impurities	Infection of pathogenic microorganisms transferred from contaminated equipment; perforation or rupture of colon; colitis from additives; fluid and electrolyte abnormalities	No toxins ever specified or scientifically demonstrated
Dr. Emanuel Revici therapy	"Biologically guided chemotherapy"; adjustment of the acid-alkaline level in patients through administration of lipids	Controls certain types of cancer, reflecting an acid or an alkaline imbalance	Questionable	No objective benefit in the treatment of cancer in human beings
Antiviral, antiinfective, and homeostatic claims				
Homemade AL 721	Made from soy or egg yolk lecithin	Reduces or inhibits HIV replication	AZ 721 is approved by FDA for clinical trials; homemade AL 721 is of unknown purity	
BHT (butylated hydroxytoluene)	Oral supplements	Kills HIV by attacking the "coating" on virus	Has promoted cancer in some animals	Undemonstrated
Lecithin	Oral supplements	Kills HIV by "membrane fluidization"	Anorexia, vomiting, bloating, diarrhea, fatty stools from large doses	Undemonstrated
Yeast-free diet	Eliminates "high carbohydrate and yeast-containing foods in diet	Prevents opportunistic yeast infections, such as candidiasis	? Undernutrition ? Weight loss	Undemonstrated

Therapy	Description	Rationale	Safety	Efficacy
Macrobiotic diet	Diet includes: 50% by volume whole grain cereals; 20–30% vegetables; 10–15% cooked beans or seaweed; 5% miso (fermented soy paste) or tamari broth soup Note: This diet is very low in fat and high in bulk	Restores balance and harmony between yin and yang forces and therefore ameliorates disease	Possible protein calorie malnutrition; inadequate intake of riboflavin, niacin, calcium in adults; inadequate intake of above, as well as pyridoxine, vitamins B12 and D in children	None for cancer; undemonstrated in HIV-infected patients
Iscador (mistletoe extract)	Natural fermentation product of the leaves of the *viscum album L.* (Loranthaceae) by *Lactobacillus* culture	Enhances immune system and may decrease or block the reproduction of the HIV virus within the cell	Initially may cause strong skin reaction; lack of specific information on the raw materials used in the preparation, their fermentation, and pharmaceutical treatment, and the chemical contents and standardization of the remedy; proteins in plant are toxic	Some inhibition of cancer promotion in humans; undemonstrated in HIV-infected patients
Hypericin	Chemical found in *Hypericum perforatum* (a plant traditionally used as a medicinal herb)	Found strongly to inhibit retroviral infections in animal and laboratory tests; may be effective AIDS therapy	Large doses have poisoned grazing animals feeding on it; safe and effective doses for humans not established; elevated hepatic transaminases	Shown antiretroviral properties in vivo in mice and anti-HIV activity in vitro; undemonstrated in humans

Source: JT Dwyer, AM Salvato-Schille, A Coulston, et al. The use of unconventional remedies among HIV-positive men living in California. *J Assoc Nurses AIDS Care* 6:25–26, 1995.

Index

Note: Page numbers followed by f indicate figures; page numbers followed by t indicate tables.